T0228175

Hematopoietic Stem Cell Transplantation

Hematopoietic Stem Cell Transplantation

edited by

Anthony D. Ho
University of Heidelberg
Heidelberg, Germany

Rainer Haas
Heinrich Heine University
Düsseldorf, Germany

Richard E. Champlin
University of Texas M.D. Anderson Cancer Center
Houston, Texas

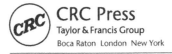

CRC Press
Taylor & Francis Group
Boca Raton London New York

CRC Press is an imprint of the
Taylor & Francis Group, an **informa** business

CRC Press
Taylor & Francis Group
6000 Broken Sound Parkway NW, Suite 300
Boca Raton, FL 33487-2742

First issued in paperback 2019

© 2000 by Taylor & Francis Group, LLC
CRC Press is an imprint of Taylor & Francis Group, an Informa business

No claim to original U.S. Government works

ISBN-13: 978-0-8247-0273-1 (hbk)
ISBN-13: 978-0-367-39831-6 (pbk)

Visit the Taylor & Francis Web site at
http://www.taylorandfrancis.com

and the CRC Press Web site at
http://www.crcpress.com

Preface

The existence of hematopoietic stem cells (HSCs) was demonstrated 40 years ago. In a seminal article published in 1961, Till and McCulloch described the presence of clonogenic bone marrow (BM) precursors that were able to reconstitute the marrow function of lethally irradiated mice. Such BM precursors possess the dual capacity of self-renewal as well as multilineage differentiation. This has remained the definition of stem cells to this day. The observation of these authors has also led to the idea of bone marrow transplantation in humans: If patients with leukemia were given a lethal dose of total body irradiation, which would eliminate the malignant cells as well as normal marrow precursors, an infusion of healthy BM cells would be expected to protect the patients from death.

Since then, a vast amount of knowledge has been gained through basic laboratory research and clinical trials. A gradual understanding of transplantation immunology, of human leukocyte antigen (HLA) system, of controlling opportunistic infections, and of transfusion medicine evolved in the late 1960s and early 1970s. Interest in bone marrow transplant as a treatment option for leukemia grew in the late 1970s. In the 1980s the discovery of novel cytokines as well as novel blood cell populations, and recognition of their roles in proliferation, differentiation, and regulation of hematopoietic stem cells and lineage-committed progenitors spawned another wave of interest in stem cell technology. This was accompanied in the early 1980s by advances in identification, enrichment, and amplification of hematopoietic stem and progenitor cells. Translation of such knowledge into clinical practice has been occurring at a breathtaking pace.

In the last ten years, we have witnessed an exponential growth in the numbers of transplants performed worldwide, both allogeneic and autologous, as well as in the number of transplant centers. Ten years ago, blood-derived stem cells for transplantation, CD34$^+$ separation, tumor cell purging, and progenitor cell expansion, among others, were novel ideas and their clinical applicability and relevance had yet to be proven. Some of these technologies have become clinical routine, while others have been discarded. Meanwhile, the immunological sequelae of allogeneic transplantation have been recognized as the major contributing factor for its therapeutic efficacy, whereas the long-term benefits of high-dose chemotherapy and autologous transplants for solid tumors have been questioned. The present trend is moving toward selective exploitation of the immunomodulatory effect of allogeneic stem cell transplantation. The goal is to establish chimerism and conditioning regimens that induce immunoablation only without myeloablation. Donor-derived lymphocytes or subpopulations will be used for ultimate cure. Although early attempts have generated encouraging data, this strategy needs thorough evaluation in a larger number of patients and in randomized studies.

Finally, advances in molecular biology have made it feasible to correct human diseases by gene transfer. The hematopoietic system is a prime target of somatic gene therapy, because the developmental biology of hematopoiesis is well understood, HSC transplantation is a well-established procedure, and the stem cells are readily accessible.

We hope that this volume will serve as an introduction to all these fascinating aspects of hematopoietic stem cell transplantation and will be a resource for scientists and physicians alike who are searching for an overview of the scientific background, clinical advances in allogeneic and autologous transplantation, and future prospects of hematopoietic stem and progenitor cell technology.

Anthony D. Ho
Rainer Haas
Richard E. Champlin

Contents

Preface   *iii*

Contributors   *ix*

Novel Cytokines and Cellular Components

1. Thrombopoietin: Basic Biology and Clinical Effects   1
    Kenneth Kaushansky and C. Glenn Begley

2. Preclinical Biology and Potential Clinical Utility of flt3 Ligand   23
    Douglas E. Williams

3. Stem Cell Factor   31
    Leo Lacerna, Jr., Russell Basser, C. Glenn Begley, Jeffrey Crawford,
    George Demetri, Craig H. Moskowitz, Guido Tricot, Andrew Weaver,
    William P. Sheridan, and John A. Glaspy

4. Cytokine Modulation of Hematopoietic Stem Cell Phenotype   47
    Ahmad-Samer Al-Homsi and Peter J. Quesenberry

5. Homing and Self-Renewal of Hematopoietic Stem Cells   69
    Anthony D. Ho, Michael Punzel, Stefan Fruehauf, Shiang Huang, and
    Bernhard Palsson

6. Requirements for Hematopoietic Stem Cell Engraftment and Graft
    Engineering: Role of Facilitating Cells   87
    Michael Neipp, Christina L. Kaufman, Marianne Bergheim, Beate G.
    Exner, and Suzanne T. Ildstad

7. Ins and Outs of Hematopoietic Stem Cells: Regulation by Genes and
    Stromal Cells   111
    Christa E. Müller-Sieburg and Rajeev Soni

8. Cell-Signaling by Adhesion Receptors in Normal and Leukemic
    Hematopoiesis   125
    Catherine M. Verfaillie, Yuehua Jiang, Robert C. H. Zhao, Felipe
    Prosper, and Ravi Bhatia

9. Detection of Infrequent Cells in Blood and Bone Marrow by Flow
    Cytometry   137
    Leon W. M. M. Terstappen

Animal Models

10. Human/Sheep Hematopoietic Chimeras   153
    Graça Almeida-Porada, Christopher D. Porada, Nam D. Tran, João
    L. Ascensao, and Esmail D. Zanjani

11. Canine Models for Transplantation and Gene Therapy   171
    Hans-Peter Kiem and Rainer Storb

12. Murine Model of In Utero Transplantation   195
    Ewa Carrier

CD34+ Selection

13. CD34 Selection Using Immunomagnetic Beads   223
    Robert A. Preti, Andrew L. Pecora, Tauseef Ahmed, and Timothy
    J. Farley

14. Autologous and Allogeneic Transplantation with Blood CD34+
    Cells: A Pediatric Experience   239
    Yoshifumi Kawano, Yoichi Takaue, Tsutomu Watanabe, Yasuhiro
    Okamoto, Takanori Abe, Yasuhiro Kuroda, and Arata Watanabe

15. Using Allogeneic Graft Engineering to Improve Long-Term
    Survival   251
    Stephen J. Noga

Purging

16. Detection and Significance of Minimal Residual Disease from Solid
    Tumor Malignancies in Stem Cell Autografts 275
    Amy A. Ross

17. Stem Cell Isolation with Immunomagnetic Beads and Tumor Cell
    Contamination 291
    *Gunnar Kvalheim, Anne Pharo, Harald Holte, Elisabeth Lenschow,
    Mengyu Wang, Bjorn Erikstein, Stein Kvaloy, John Magne Nesland, and
    Erlend Smeland*

Ex Vivo Expansion

18. CD34 Cell Culture: Clinical Needs and Applications 303
    Dennis E. Van Epps

19. Critical Parameters Influencing the Expansion and Differentiation of
    Cultured Human CD34+ Cells 321
    Jane S. Lebkowski and Lisa R. Schain

Advances in Allogeneic Transplantation

20. Mobilization of Peripheral Blood Stem Cells from Normal Donors 333
    Thomas A. Lane and Ping Law

21. Innovative Approaches for Allogeneic Blood and Marrow
    Transplantation for Treatment of Hematological Malignancies: Graft
    Engineering and Nonmyeloablative Preparative Regimens 361
    Richard E. Champlin

22. Peripheral Blood Stem Cells for Allogeneic Transplantation 383
    *Lutz Uharek, Peter Dreger, Bertram Glass, Matthias Zeis, and
    Norbert Schmitz*

23. Mechanisms of Cure of Acute Myeloid Leukemia with Allogeneic
    Transplantation 403
    Frederick R. Appelbaum

24. Late Complications of Hematopoietic Stem Cell Transplantation 413
    Emin Kansu and Keith M. Sullivan

GVHD, GVL

25. Prevention of Acute Graft-Versus-Host Disease by Delayed or
    Selected Lymphocyte Add Back   435
    John Barrett and Dimitrios Mavroudis

Advances in Autologous Transplantation

26. Blood Stem Cell Versus Bone Marrow Transplantation: A Critical
    Appraisal   447
    Anne Kessinger

27. Autologous Peripheral Blood Stem Cell Collection and Engraftment   457
    Stefan Hohaus, Maria Teresa Voso, Simona Martin, and Rainer Haas

28. Stem Cell Transplantation for Hodgkin's Disease   479
    Ram Kancherla and Tauseef Ahmed

29. Stem Cell Transplantation for Multiple Myeloma—10 Years Later   499
    *David S. Siegel, Seah H. Lim, Guido Tricot, K. R. Desikan, A. Fassas,
    Jayesh Mehta, Seema Singhal, Elias Anaissie, Sundar Jagannath, and
    Barthel Barlogie*

30. High-Dose Therapy for Primary and Metastatic Breast Cancer   517
    Gary Spitzer, Kenneth Meehan, and Douglas Adkins

Genetic and Immune Therapy

31. Gene Therapy Using Hematopoietic Stem Cells   537
    Donald B. Kohn, Gay M. Crooks, and Jan A. Nolta

32. Gene Therapy for Human Immunodeficiency Virus Infection Using
    Stem Cell Transplantation   553
    Alain Gervaix and Flossie Wong-Staal

33. Autografting Followed by Low-Intensity Conditioning Regimen for
    Allografting   569
    Angelo M. Carella

34. Development of Retroviral Vectors that Target Hematopoietic Stem
    Cells   575
    *Chris A. Benedict, Yi Zhao, Nori Kasahara, Paula M. Cannon, and
    W. French Anderson*

Index   595

Contributors

Takanori Abe, M.D. Clinical Fellow, Department of Pediatrics, University of Tokushima, Tokushima, Japan

Douglas Adkins Division of BMT and Stem Cell Biology, Washington University
School of Medicine, St. Louis, Missouri

Tauseef Ahmed, M.D. Professor of Medicine, Division of Hematology/Oncology, New
York Medical College, Valhalla, New York

Ahmad-Samer Al-Homsi, M.D. Assistant Professor of Medicine, University of Massachusetts Medical Center, Worcester, and Milford-Whitinsville Regional Hospital, Milford,
Massachusetts

Graça Almeida-Porada, M.D., Ph.D. Assistant Professor of Medicine, Department of
Veterans Affairs Medical Center and University of Nevada School of Medicine, Reno,
Nevada

Elias Anaissie, M.D. Myeloma and Transplantation Research Center, University of Arkansas for Medical Sciences, Little Rock, Arkansas

W. French Anderson, M.D. Professor of Biochemistry and Pediatrics, Gene Therapy
Laboratories, Norris Cancer Center, University of Southern California School of Medicine,
Los Angeles, California

Frederick R. Appelbaum, M.D.   Director, Clinical Research Division, Fred Hutchinson Cancer Research Center, Seattle, Washington

João L. Ascensao, M.D., Ph.D., F.A.C.P.   Professor of Medicine, Pathology, Microbiology, and Immunology, Department of Internal Medicine, Department of Veterans Affairs Medical Center and University of Nevada School of Medicine, Reno, Nevada

Barthel Barlogie, M.D., Ph.D.   Myeloma and Transplantation Research Center, University of Arkansas for Medical Sciences, Little Rock, Arkansas

John Barrett, M.D., F.R.C.P., F.R.C.Path.   Chief, Blood and Marrow Transplantation Unit, Hematology Branch, National Heart, Lung and Blood Institute, National Institutes of Health, Bethesda, Maryland

Russell Basser, M.D.   Centre for Developmental Cancer Therapy, Royal Melbourne Hospital, Melbourne, Australia

C. Glenn Begley, M.D., P.L.D.   Western Australia Institute for Medical Research, Perth, Australia

Chris A. Benedict, Ph.D.   Postdoctoral Fellow, Department of Biochemistry and Molecular Biology, University of Southern California School of Medicine, Los Angeles, California

Marianne Bergheim   Department of Surgery and Institute for Cellular Therapeutics, University of Louisville, Louisville, Kentucky

Ravi Bhatia, M.D., M.B.B.S.   Division of Hematology and Bone Marrow Transplantation, City of Hope National Medical Center, Duarte, California

Paula M. Cannon   Norris Cancer Center, University of Southern California School of Medicine, Los Angeles, California

Angelo M. Carella, M.D.   Department of Hematology, N.O.A. Hematology/ABMT Unit, Ospedale San Martino, Genoa, Italy

Ewa Carrier, M.D.   Assistant Professor of Medicine and Pediatrics, Department of Medicine, University of California, San Diego, La Jolla, California

Richard E. Champlin, M.D.   Chairman, Department of Blood Marrow and Transplantation, University of Texas M.D. Anderson Cancer Center, Houston, Texas

Gay M. Crooks   Children's Hospital Los Angeles and University of Southern California, Los Angeles, California

Jeffrey Crawford, M.D.   Duke Comprehensive Cancer Center, Duke University Medical Center, Durham, North Carolina

George Demetri, M.D.   Sarcoma Center, Dana-Farber Cancer Institute, Boston, Massachusetts

K. R. Desikan, M.D.   Myeloma and Transplantation Research Center, University of Arkansas for Medical Sciences, Little Rock, Arkansas

Peter Dreger, M.D.   Department of Internal Medicine II, Christian Albrechts University of Kiel, Kiel, Germany

Bjorn Erikstein, M.D., Ph.D.   Department of Radiotherapy and Oncology, The Norwegian Radium Hospital, Oslo, Norway

Beate G. Exner, M.D.   Department of Surgery and Institute for Cellular Therapeutics, University of Louisville, Louisville, Kentucky

Timothy J. Farley, Ph.D.   Clinical Services Division, New York Blood Center, Valhalla, New York

A. Fassas, M.D.   Myeloma and Transplatation Research Center, University of Arkansas for Medical Sciences, Little Rock, Arkansas

Stefan Fruehauf, M.D.   Department of Internal Medicine, University of Heidelberg, Heidelberg, Germany

Alain Gervaix, M.D.   Department of Pediatrics, University Hospital of Geneva, Geneva, Switzerland

John A. Glaspy, M.D., M.P.H.   University of California School of Medicine, Los Angeles, California

Bertram Glass, M.D.   Department of Internal Medicine II, Christian Albrechts University of Kiel, Kiel, Germany

Rainer Haas, Ph.D., M.D.   Professor and Head, Department of Hematology, Oncology, and Clinical Immunology, Heinrich Heine University, Düsseldorf, Germany

Anthony D. Ho, M.D.   Professor of Medicine and Chair, Department of Internal Medicine V, University of Heidelberg, Heidelberg, Germany

Stefan Hohaus, M.D.   Department of Hematology, Catholic University "S. Cuore," Rome, Italy

Harald Holte, M.D., Ph.D.   Department of Radiotherapy and Oncology, The Norwegian Radium Hospital, Oslo, Norway

Shiang Huang, M.D.   Department of Medicine, University of California, San Diego, La Jolla, California

Suzanne T. Ildstad, M.D. Department of Surgery and Director, Institute for Cellular Therapeutics, University of Louisville, Louisville, Kentucky

Sundar Jagannath, M.D. Myeloma and Transplantation Research Center, University of Arkansas for Medical Sciences, Little Rock, Arkansas

Yuehua Jiang, M.D. Postdoctoral Fellow, Department of Medicine, University of Minnesota, Minneapolis, Minnesota

Ram Kancherla, M.D. Assistant Professor, Department of Medicine, New York Medical College, Valhalla, New York

Emin Kansu, M.D., F.A.C.P. Professor of Hematology, Department of Medicine, and Chairman, Department of Basic Oncology, Hacettepe University, Hacettepe, Ankara, Turkey

Nori Kasahara Norris Cancer Center, University of Southern California School of Medicine, Los Angeles, California

Christina L. Kaufman, Ph.D. Assistant Professor, Department of Surgery, and Institute for Cellular Therapeutics, University of Louisville, Louisville, Kentucky

Kenneth Kaushansky, M.D. Professor of Medicine, Department of Hematology, University of Washington, Seattle, Washington

Yoshifumi Kawano, M.D. Department of Pediatrics, University of Tokushima, Tokushima, Japan

Anne Kessinger, M.D. Professor, Department of Oncology/Hematology, University of Nebraska Medical Center, Omaha, Nebraska

Hans-Peter Kiem, M.D. Assistant Member, Fred Hutchinson Cancer Research Center, and Assistant Professor, University of Washington, Seattle, Washington

Donald B. Kohn, M.D. Professor of Pediatrics and Molecular Microbiology/Immunology, Children's Hospital Los Angeles and University of Southern California School of Medicine, Los Angeles, California

Yasuhiro Kuroda, M.D. Professor, Department of Pediatrics, University of Tokushima, Tokushima, Japan

Gunnar Kvalheim, M.D., Ph.D. Director, Clinical Stem Cell Laboratory, Department of Radiotherapy and Oncology, The Norwegian Radium Hospital, Oslo, Norway

Stein Kvaløy, M.D., Ph.D. Department of Radiotherapy and Oncology, The Norwegian Radium Hospital, Oslo, Norway

Leo Lacerna, Jr., M.D. Amgen Inc., Thousand Oaks, California

Thomas A. Lane, M.D.   Professor, Department of Pathology, University of California, San Diego, La Jolla, California

Ping Law, Ph.D.   Director, Stem Cell Processing Laboratory, Department of Medicine, University of California, San Diego, La Jolla, California

Jane S. Lebkowski, Ph.D.   Vice President, Cell and Gene Therapy, Geron Corporation, Menlo Park, California

Elisabeth Lenschow   Clinical Stem Cell Laboratory, Department of Radiotherapy and Oncology, The Norwegian Radium Hospital, Oslo, Norway

Seah H. Lim, M.R.C.P. (U.K.), F.R.C.Path, M.D., Ph.D.   Associate Professor, Myeloma and Transplantation Research Center, University of Arkansas for Medical Sciences, Little Rock, Arkansas

Simona Martin, M.D.   Department of Hematology, Oncology, and Clinical Immunology, Heinrich Heine University, Düsseldorf, Germany

Dmitrios Mavroudis, M.D., Ph.D.   Attending Physician in Medical Oncology, University General Hospital of Heraklion, Crete, Greece

Kenneth Meehan   Bone Marrow Transplantation Program, Georgetown University Medical Center, Washington, D.C.

Jayesh Mehta, M.D.   Myeloma and Transplantation Research Center, University of Arkansas for Medical Sciences, Little Rock, Arkansas

Craig H. Moskowitz, M.D.   Memorial Sloan-Kettering Cancer Center, New York, New York

Christa E. Müller-Sieburg, Dr. rer.nat.*   Medical Biology Institute, La Jolla, California

Michael Neipp, M.D.   Department of Surgery and Institute for Cellular Therapeutics, University of Louisville, Louisville, Kentucky

John Magne Nesland, M.D., Ph.D.   Professor, Department of Pathology, The Norwegian Radium Hospital, Oslo, Norway

Stephen J. Noga, M.D., Ph.D.   Associate Professor, Oncology and Pathology, Oncology Director, Hematopoietic and Therapeutic Support Service, Department of Oncology, The Johns Hopkins University, Baltimore, Maryland

---

* *Current affiliation*: Sidney Kimmel Cancer Center, San Diego, California.

Jan A. Nolta, Ph.D.   Children's Hospital Los Angeles and University of Southern California School of Medicine, Los Angeles, California

Yasuhiro Okamoto, M.D.   Clinical Fellow, Department of Pediatrics, University of Tokushima, Tokushima, Japan

Bernhard Palsson, Ph.D.   Department of Bioengineering, University of California, San Diego, La Jolla, California

Andrew L. Pecora, M.D.   Hackensack University Medical Center, Hackensack, New Jersey

Anne Pharo   Clinical Stem Cell Laboratory, Department of Radiotherapy and Oncology, The Norwegian Radium Hospital, Oslo, Norway

Christopher D. Porada, Ph.D.   Assistant Scientist, Research Department, Department of Veterans Affairs Medical Center and University of Nevada School of Medicine, Reno, Nevada

Robert A. Preti, Ph.D.   President and Chief Scientific Officer, Progenitor Cell Therapy, L.L.C., Hackensack, New Jersey

Felipe Prosper, M.D.   Assistant Professor, Department of Hematology and Medical Oncology, Hospital Clinico Universitario, Valencia, Spain

Michael Punzel, M.D.   Department of Internal Medicine V, University of Heidelberg, Heidelberg, Germany

Peter J. Quesenberry, M.D.   Professor of Medicine and Head, University of Massachusetts Medical Center, Worcester, Massachusetts

Amy A. Ross, Ph.D.   Vice President, Department of Diagnostics, Nexell Therapeutics Inc., Irvine, California

Lisa R. Schain   Supervisor, Stem Cell Laboratory, Research Department, RPR Gencell, Hayward, California

Norbert Schmitz, M.D.   Professor, Department of Internal Medicine II, Christian Albrechts University of Kiel, Kiel, Germany

William P. Sheridan, M.B., B.S., F.R.A.C.P.   Senior Director Product Development, Amgen Inc., Thousand Oaks, California

David S. Siegel, M.D., Ph.D.   Myeloma and Transplantation Research Center, University of Arkansas for Medical Sciences, Little Rock, Arkansas

Seema Singhal, M.D.   Myeloma and Transplantation Research Center, University of Arkansas for Medical Sciences, Little Rock, Arkansas

Erlend Smeland, M.D., Ph.D. Director, Department of Immunology, The Norwegian Radium Hospital, Oslo, Norway

Rajeev Soni Medical Biology Institute and LIDAK Pharmaceuticals, La Jolla, California

Gary Spitzer, M.D. Director of Transplantation, Cancer Centers of the Carolinas, Greenville, South Carolina

Rainer Storb, M.D. Member and Head, Transplantation Biology Program, Fred Hutchinson Cancer Research Center, and Professor of Medicine, University of Washington, Seattle, Washington

Keith M. Sullivan, M.D. Clinical Professor of Medicine, and Chief, Division of Medical Oncology and Transplantation, Duke University Medical Center, Durham, North Carolina

Yoichi Takaue, M.D. Division Chief, Hematopoietic Stem Cell Transplant/Immunotherapy Unit, Department of Medical Oncology, National Cancer Center Hospital, Tokyo, Japan

Leon W. M. M. Terstappen, M.D., Ph.D. Senior Vice President, Department of Research & Development, Immunicon Corporation, Huntingdon Valley, Pennsylvania

Nam D. Tran, Ph.D. Assistant Scientist, Research Department, Department of Veterans Affairs Medical Center and University of Nevada School of Medicine, Reno, Nevada

Guido Tricot, M.D., Ph.D. Myeloma and Transplantation Research Center, University of Arkansas for Medical Sciences, Little Rock, Arkansas

Lutz Uharek, M.D. Department of Internal Medicine II, University of Leipzig, Leipzig, Germany

Dennis E. Van Epps, Ph.D. Vice President, Research, Nexell Therapeutics Inc., Irvine, California

Catherine M. Verfaillie, M.D. Professor, Department of Medicine, University of Minnesota, Minneapolis, Minnesota

Maria Teresa Voso, M.D. Department of Hematology, Catholic University "S. Cuore," Rome, Italy

Mengyu Wang, M.D. Department of Tumor Biology, The Norwegian Radium Hospital, Oslo, Norway

Arata Watanabe, M.D. Director, Department of Pediatrics, University of Akita and Naka-dori Hospital, Akita, Japan

Tsutomu Watanabe, M.D.   Assistant Pediatrician, Department of Pediatrics, University of Tokushima, Tokushima, Japan

Andrew Weaver, M.D.   Christie Hospital, Manchester, England

Douglas E. Williams, Ph.D.   Executive Vice President, Chief Technology Officer, Immunex Corporation, Seattle, Washington

Flossie Wong-Staal, Ph.D.   Professor of Medicine and Biology, Department of Medicine, University of California, San Diego, La Jolla, California

Esmail D. Zanjani, Ph.D.   Professor of Medicine and Physiology, Department of Veterans Affairs Medical Center and University of Nevada School of Medicine, Reno, Nevada

Matthias Zeis, M.D.   Department of Internal Medicine II, University of Leipzig, Leipzig, Germany

Robert C. H. Zhao, M.D., Ph.D.   Assistant Professor, Department of Medicine, University of Minnesota, Minneapolis, Minnesota

Yi Zhao   Norris Cancer Center, University of Southern California School of Medicine, Los Angeles, California

1

Thrombopoietin
Basic Biology and Clinical Effects

KENNETH KAUSHANSKY

University of Washington, Seattle, Washington

C. GLENN BEGLEY

Western Australia Institute for Medical Research, Perth, Australia

I. PHYSIOLOGY OF MEGAKARYOCYTE DEVELOPMENT

The generation of platelets from their marrow progenitors is an enormously important and complex process. Each day the adult human produces 2×10^{11} platelets, a number which can increase 10-fold in times of heightened demand. Megakaryocyte (MK) and platelet formation is dependent on the productive interaction of hematopoietic stem and progenitor cells, marrow stromal elements, and multiple endocrine and paracrine hormones. Our evolving understanding of the humoral regulation of megakaryocyte development and how we might manipulate this process for therapeutic benefit will form the focus of this chapter.

Current models of blood cell development stress the stochastic nature of hematopoietic stem cell commitment to individual blood cell lineages (1). Although this progressive loss of pluripotency is believed to be driven by mechanisms independent of the cellular environment, it is clear that the survival and proliferation of developing stem and progenitor cells of each hematopoietic lineage are dependent on the action of at least two members of several groups of related growth factors. One group of cytokines, for the most part restricted to hematopoiesis and including interleukin-3 (IL-3), stem cell factor (SCF; also known as mast cell growth factor, steel factor, and kit ligand), granulocyte-macrophage colony-stimulating factor (GM-CSF), flt3 ligand (FL), and IL-4 act directly on immature multipotent progenitors to support their survival, proliferation, and differentiation into cells restricted to a single lineage. More recently, several pleiotropic cytokines, which act not only on hematopoiesis but also on metabolism, the liver and on the inflammatory system, including IL-6, IL-11, and leukemia inhibitory factor (LIF), have been shown to act in synergy with IL-3, FL, or SCF to enhance the proliferation of primitive and mature cells. And a group of true hormones, including granulocyte colony-stimulating factor (G-CSF), erythropoietin, IL-5, and macrophage colony-stimulating factor (M-CSF), support the final stages of cellular development, with each protein being primarily committed to a single hematopoietic lineage. Although correct in principle, this schema is marked by exceptions; for example, G-CSF, a lineage-specific late-acting hormone for the neutrophilic lineage also acts in synergy with IL-3 to accelerate the entry of primitive hematopoietic cells into the cell cycle (2).

Several cytokines and hormones have been reported to influence the development of the megakaryocytic lineage. Classically, these had been divided into MK-CSFs and MK potentiators. IL-3, GM-CSF, and SCF have been shown by several investigators to display MK colony-stimulating activity (3–7). MK potentiators, defined by the capacity to augment MK colony numbers when added to cultures containing MK-CSFs, include IL-6, IL-11, LIF, and SDF-1 (8–10a). However, none of these agents were felt to fulfill the role of thrombopoietin, posited some 42 years ago to be the primary regulator of MK and platelet formation (11,12).

II. CLONING OF THROMBOPOIETIN

Thrombopoietin was initially defined as the substance in blood responsible for platelet recovery following thrombocytopenic stress. Assays based on the incorporation of ^{75}Se or ^{35}S methionine into new platelets were devised to measure its presence in physiological samples. Based on this rather cumbersome assay, several groups attempted to purify the substance from physiological sources. Although none of the attempts using this assay was ultimately successful, they did provide partially purified thrombopoietin sufficient to identify some of its biological properties (11,12). Thrombopoietin was thought to promote the differentiation of marrow cells into large highly polyploid MKs, with each being capable of producing thousands of platelets (Fig. 1). However, thrombopoietin was not originally believed to be a MK-CSF; it was not thought to stimulate the proliferation of MK progenitors, only their differentiation. The sine qua non of thrombopoietin is its capacity to stimulate platelet production in vivo. As the physiological regulator of this process, its levels should be inversely related to platelet count, or mass, or some measure of hemostatic adequacy. And like the other hematopoietic differentiation factors, such as erythropoietin, thrombopoietin was predicted to be lineage specific.

As noted, owing to the difficult nature of the assay, and to its scarcity in even the richest physiological sources, purification of thrombopoietin to homogeneity proved to be quite difficult; leading some in the field to doubt its existence. Nevertheless, occasionally in science, a finding from one area of research, important in itself, provides the catalytic spark in a seemingly unrelated field of investigation. Study of the myeloproliferative leukemia virus (MPLV) by Wendling and her colleagues in the late 1980s (13) provided the critical catalyst for the discovery of thrombopoietin and our first understanding of its biology. Cloning of the cellular homologue (c-*mpl*) of the transforming gene (v-*mpl*) of MPLV yielded an orphan cytokine receptor in 1992 (14). The expression of c-*mpl* in MKs, their precursors, and progeny, and its antisense elimination leading to reductions in MK colony formation (15) led investigators working in the field to predict that the product of the c-*mpl* gene might correspond to the thrombopoietin receptor. Within 2 years of publication of the mpl structure, its ligand was cloned or purified by five separate groups and

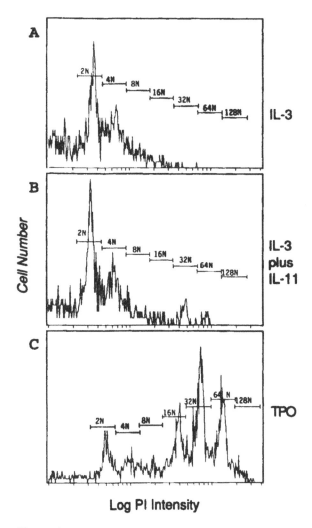

Figure 1 Ploidy analysis of marrow MKs grown in the presence and absence of multiple cytokines. Murine marrow cells were obtained and cultured in the presence of IL-3 (A), IL-3 plus IL-11 (B), or thrombopoietin (C). Suspension cultures of marrow contain accessory cells capable of cytokine production. Preliminary experiments indicated that thrombopoietin and gp130-related cytokines were present in such cultures. To eliminate the contribution of these cytokines, a monoclonal antibody (Ab) that neutralizes the signaling component of the IL-6, IL-11, and LIF receptors (RX187; provided by Dr. Tetsuya Taga) was added to cultures (A) and (C), and a soluble form of the Mpl receptor (MPLsol; provided by Dr. Catherine Lofton-Day) that neutralizes thrombopoietin activity was added to cultures (A) and (B). Following 4 days of culture, cells were stained with a murine platelet-specific antibody (1C2; provided by Dr. Junichiro Fujimoto) and with propidium iodide to assess DNA content per cell. The individual ploidy classes are indicated.

shown to be identical to thrombopoietin (16–18). With the availability of this hormone, investigators could test the relative effects of multiple cytokines in supporting the proliferation and differentiation of MK in vitro.

III.   MEGAKARYOPOIETIC ACTIVITIES OF THROMBOPOIETIN

Two types of hematopoietic assays have been commonly used to characterize megakaryocytic cytokines, an agar or plasma clot–based colony-forming assay, and a serum-free suspension culture system in which rodent MKs are quantitated by acetylcholinesterase content and human cells identified by specific immunofluorescence. Cultures containing IL-3 and thrombopoietin were found to maximize murine MK colony formation in our hands (19). Subsequent studies have shown that at optimal levels thrombopoietin supports proliferation of about 75% of the maximal number of assayable colony-forming unit (CFU)–MKs; IL-3 alone induces approximately 40% of this number of progenitors to form colonies. Thus, the two cytokines were additive; suggesting that each could support a subpopulation of progenitors not responsive to the other. Other investigators obtained similar results, although occasionally quantitatively different (20). To further investigate whether the MK progenitor cell targets of IL-3 and thrombopoietin are distinct, we evaluated individual MK colonies derived from cultures of murine marrow cells containing either of these proteins. Colonies supported by thrombopoietin alone were invariably small to medium in size, with 3–20 large MKs per colony. In contrast, colonies which developed in the presence of IL-3, either alone or together with thrombopoietin, often contained up to 200 MKs. This result suggests that IL-3 acts on developmentally more immature CFU-MKs than does thrombopoietin, a premise confirmed by examination of the responsiveness of separated populations of early and late CFU-MKs (21). Substitution of purified IL-6 or IL-11 for thrombopoietin also augmented the number of MK colonies in IL-3–containing cultures, but not to the level seen with thrombopoietin alone. These results were echoed by studies using suspension culture assays. Purified stem cell factor (SCF) was also used alone and together with thrombopoietin, IL-6, and IL-11 in both colony-forming and suspension culture systems. Alone, SCF was found to be a poor stimulus of MK colony formation. However, in the presence of IL-6, IL-11, and especially thrombopoietin, MK colony formation was greatly augmented over that seen with any of these proteins used alone (22). Finally, although not capable of supporting the formation of MKs in either colony-forming or suspension culture systems alone, both IL-11 and erythropoietin were found to act in synergy with thrombopoietin to augment MK production (22).

IV.   IS THROMBOPOIETIN ESSENTIAL FOR MK FORMATION?

In order to investigate the relative contributions of these cytokines to MK formation, we utilized a serum-free murine marrow culture system composed of purified cytokines and agents which neutralize each of the proteins known to affect megakaryopoiesis in vitro (18,23). The use of neutralizing antibodies to murine SCF and IL-3, and an antibody which neutralizes the effect of the gp130 receptor (the signaling subunit of the IL-6, IL-11, and LIF receptors) revealed that recombinant thrombopoietin alone is sufficient for the formation of large highly polyploid MKs. Because whole marrow culture systems contain stromal elements which contribute thrombopoietin to developing hematopoietic cells, we employed a soluble form of the Mpl receptor to neutralize thrombopoietin activity in order to assess the capacity of several other cytokines to induce MK formation in the absence of any source of thrombopoietin. Without the effect of endogenous thrombopoietin, combinations of cytokines, including SCF, IL-6, or IL-11, failed to support the development of MKs in either semisolid colony-forming or suspension culture assays.

In contrast to the results obtained using SCF, cultures containing IL-3 maintained a basal level of MK formation despite neutralization of thrombopoietin. This was especially true if the cultures also contained IL-6 or IL-11. Together with the findings that IL-3 increases the number of MK colonies over that seen with thrombopoietin alone, these results indicate that IL-3 induces MK formation independent of thrombopoietin. However, this conclusion ignores the state of MK differentiation in the IL-3–containing cultures. To assess the level of MK differentiation in the absence of thrombopoietin, ploidy analysis and electron microscopic studies of cultures containing IL-3 were performed, and to eliminate the effects of endogenous cytokines, the soluble Mpl receptor and the gp130 neutralizing antibody were added. Although multiple cells binding the murine platelet-specific 4A5 monoclonal antibody were identified in such cultures, their ploidy values were restricted to the 2N and 4N classes (Fig. 1A). The removal of the anti-gp130 antibody (not shown) or the addition of IL-11 to the cultures (Fig. 1B) improved ploidy values somewhat, but the mean geometrical ploidy was consistently several classes less than that seen in thrombopoietin/anti-gp130–containing cultures (Fig. 1C). On an ultrastructural level, thrombopoietin appeared to be essential for the full development of platelet-specific granules, demarcation membranes, and platelet fields. Despite their display of the 4A5 antigen, IL-3–induced MKs failed to display any ultrastructural features of specific maturation; the addition of IL-11 led to modest demarcation membrane formation, but only poorly formed platelet-specific granules were detected, and few if any platelet fields were found (24). Taken together, these data suggest that thrombopoietin is both necessary and sufficient for full MK maturation from a primitive hematopoietic stem or progenitor cell. Of the cytokines classically defined as MK-CSFs, IL-3 appears to be most important, at least in vitro. By itself the cytokine can induce hematopoietic stem cell development into immature MK; however, in the absence of thrombopoietin, these cells fail to develop the ultrastructural characteristics of platelet-producing MKs. And although they can act synergistically to influence primitive hematopoietic cell development, the gp130-related cytokines fail to promote MK growth or differentiation in the absence of other cytokines or thrombopoietin.

Although these studies were underway, scientists at Genentech and at the Walter and Eliza Hall Institute of Medical Research in Melbourne were able genetically to eliminate the *tpo* and/or c-*mpl* genes in mice. Consistent with the in vitro findings described above, both knockout mice displayed MK and platelet levels 5–15% that of littermate controls (25–27). The mean ploidy of the remaining few MKs was shifted to more immature values by two classes, and MK and platelet size were also smaller than that found in control animals. These data clearly indicate that thrombopoietin is the primary regulator of MK and platelet production. Moreover, the stage of development of the residual MK and platelets in the knockout animals correlates with the ploidy and morphology of the cells which we found to develop in the presence of IL-3 and IL-11 and the absence of thrombopoietin in vitro. Whether these or other cytokines are responsible for the residual thrombopoietin-independent platelet production identified in the knockout models is not yet certain, but this may be forthcoming by studying the effects of multiple cytokine knockout mice.

V.   THROMBOPOIETIN AND ERYTHROPOIESIS

Another aspect of thrombopoietin physiology now being explored is its lineage specificity. As noted above, prior to the cloning of the *tpo* gene, most investigators in the field believed the molecule to be specific for MK development. With the availability of the recombinant protein, this hypothesis could be explored. Several theoretical arguments and observations support the contention that the erythroid and megakaryocytic lineages are derived from a common lineage (28–31). On this basis, and the observation that erythropoietin affects megakaryopoiesis (22), we and others have begun to investigate whether thrombopoietin might act on erythropoiesis. In the presence of IL-3 and erythropoietin, but not in their absence, thrombopoietin augments the number of early blast-forming unit erythroid (BFU-E) progenitor cells that develop into colonies in semisolid cultures, and triples the generation of colony-forming unit erythroid (CFU-E) progenitors that arise in suspension cultures of murine marrow cells (17). Kobayashi and coworkers (32) showed that in the presence of erythropoietin, but not in its absence, thrombopoietin tripled the number of erythroid colonies that developed from purified, plucked immature BFU-E progeny derived from cord blood or marrow cells. These in vitro findings were mirrored by in vivo results; the administration of thrombopoietin to normal mice expanded the numbers of marrow and splenic BFU-E, and its application to myelosuppressed mice accelerated the recovery of both BFU-E and CFU-E in these organs (17). The erythroid effect in thrombopoietin-treated myelosuppressed mice lead to a more rapid recovery of peripheral blood reticulocyte and erythrocyte levels than in the control animals (17).

VI.   THROMBOPOIETIN AND STEM CELL BIOLOGY

There are several observations that point to a role for c-*mpl* in stem cell biology. Infection of mice with MPLV causes not only disorders of megakaryopoiesis but also induces derangements in erythropoiesis and myelopoiesis (13). c-*mpl* is expressed in a large number of fresh marrow samples from patients with all histological types of acute myelogenous leukemia (33,34). And using reverse transcriptase–polymerase chain reaction (RT-PCR) we have been able to detect c-*mpl* transcripts from very small numbers of purified hematopoietic stem cells (Fig. 2). Based on these results, the effects of thrombopoietin on hematopoietic stem cell development were investigated. Using highly selected cells [derived from lin⁻/Ly-6A/E⁺/c-kit⁺ marrow cells from 2-day post-5-FU 5-fluorouracil treated mice], Ku and coworkers (35) found that the addition of thrombopoietin to SCF resulted in greatly increased total numbers of culture-derived cells, including not only MK progenitors but also CFU–granulocyte-macrophage (GM) and CFU–granulocyte-erythroid-macrophage-megakaryocyte (GEMM). Similar findings have also been reported for highly purified human progenitor and stem cells (36,37). We utilized a previously published method to purify hematopoietic stem cells from murine marrow (38) and tested individual cells for their response to combinations of cytokines, including IL-3, SCF, and thrombopoietin. By itself, thrombopoietin was found to support the survival of 30–40% of these stem cells for 4–14 days compared to 0% for no growth factor and 60–70% for IL-3 or SCF alone. But unlike cultures containing either of these latter two cytokines, thrombopoietin-containing cultures contained only the initial cell; no proliferation occurred in the absence of additional cytokines. However, in the combined presence of either IL-3 plus thrombopoietin or SCF plus thrombopoietin, cells were found to undergo their first division earlier and to undergo more divisions compared to cultures containing only IL-3 or SCF (39).

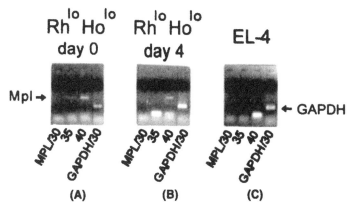

Figure 2 Reverse transcriptase-polymerase chain reaction (RT-PCR) of purified hematopoietic stem cells. Murine marrow cells were purified using a previously described procedure (38) that results in a population of cells, 10 of which will repopulate all aspects of hematopoiesis in 100% of recipient mice undergoing transplantation. The technique is based on low retention of rhodamine (Rh) and Hoechst (Ho) dyes. (A). RNA from 20 Rh-low, Ho-low cells was obtained, reverse transcribed, and amplified for 30, 35, or 40 cycles with murine c-*mpl*–specific oligodeoxynucleotide primers or with those for the housekeeping gene glyceraldehyde phosphate dehydrogenase (GAPD). An ethidium bromide–stained agarose gel is shown. (B). The same cells were cultured for 4 days in IL-3, IL-6, and stem cell factor (SCF) and the analysis repeated. (C). The murine T-cell line EL-4 served as a negative control for the mpl analysis.

Like the studies of Ku and colleagues (35), thrombopoietin was found to augment the output of all types of hematopoietic progenitor cells.

Two lines of evidence suggest that these in vitro effects on stem cells are important in vivo. First, the administration of thrombopoietin to normal mice and monkeys has been associated with expansion of all classes of hematopoietic progenitor cells and their more rapid recovery following myelosuppressive therapy (40–42). Second, genetic elimination of thrombopoietin or its receptor is associated with greatly reduced numbers of these same progenitor cell types (26–27). Taken together, the results from studies of erythroid progenitors and primitive hematopoietic cells strongly suggest that the hematological effects of thrombopoietin are not limited to the megakaryocytic lineage, and holds open the hope that its effects on hematological recovery following natural or iatrogenic states of marrow failure may be more widespread than initially anticipated.

VII. DOES THROMBOPOIETIN "STEAL" FROM OTHER HEMATOPOIETIC LINEAGES?

Several investigators have begun to explore the effects of thrombopoietin on hematological recovery following cytoreductive therapies. In mice, multiple studies have demonstrated that thrombopoietin alone accelerates platelet recovery following combined radiation and chemotherapy (43–45). Similar results have been reported for dogs and nonhuman primates. However, given the therapeutic benefits of G-CSF and GM-CSF administration in the same settings, it is unlikely that clinical trials of thrombopoietin will proceed without the use of one of the granulopoietic growth factors. Despite nearly two decades of study, one major area of controversy in the hematopoietic literature focuses on whether stimulation of one lineage is detrimental to the others (46,47). Put simply, do hematopoietic growth factors compete for multilineage progenitors? In order to determine whether thrombopoietin might interfere with the beneficial effects of G-CSF, or whether the granulopoietic hormone might hinder the response to thrombopoietin, the effects of the two hormones alone and together in mice treated with radiation and chemotherapy were studied (48). We found that the accelerated platelet recovery characteristic of thrombopoietin-treated animals was not impaired by the addition of G-CSF (actually, the modest rebound thrombocytosis following recovery was enhanced by the addition of G-CSF), and acceleration of neutrophil recovery in response to G-CSF was actually enhanced by the administration of both hormones. Thus, no evidence for competition for a limited pool of progenitors in chemotherapy/radiation–treated mice was garnered. Similar findings have been reported for the treatment of nonhuman primates in combination with G-CSF following radiation therapy (42).

VIII. PRECLINICAL TRIALS OF THROMBOPOIETIN IN STEM CELL TRANSPLANTATION

Preclinical studies investigating the effects of thrombopoietin on hematological recovery following marrow or stem cell transplantation have begun to appear. Fibbe and coworkers (49) found that the administration of thrombopoietin to lethally irradiated recipients of 1×10^5 transplanted murine marrow cells failed to augment platelet recovery compared to vehicle-treated controls. Interestingly, the administration of the hormone to the marrow donors resulted in accelerated platelet recovery in the transplant recipients whether the latter were given thrombopoietin or not. In contrast, Molineaux and colleagues (50) found that platelet recovery was accelerated if thrombopoietin was administered to lethally irradiated recipients of 1×10^6 murine marrow cells. The explanation for the discrepancy between these two results, other than possibly being due to differences in administered cell number, is not clear at present; however, clinical trials of thrombopoietin in the setting of stem cell transplantation have begun, the results of which could serve to settle this issue.

IX. THROMBOPOIETIN AND MATURE PLATELET FUNCTION

The effects of thrombopoietin on the function of mature platelets has come under intense study, a line of investigation prompted by the effects of GM-CSF and G-CSF on the function of their corresponding mature cells, neutrophils, and monocytes (51–55). Although little evidence suggests that thrombopoietin can act as a direct and independent platelet agonist, several ex vivo studies have appeared reporting synergistic effects on platelet aggregation or activation in the presence of adenosine diphosphate (ADP) and other classic platelet agonists (56–58). These effects to "prime" platelets to respond to subthreshold levels of other platelet agonists are inhibitable with prostaglandin blockade. The nature of thrombopoietin signaling in mature platelets has also been explored (59–62), and this has revealed mechanisms similar to those demonstrated in engineered and naturally occurring megakaryocytic cell lines and mature MKs (63–67). However, the physiological relevance of these findings is not revealed by in vitro studies. Two groups of investigators have attempted to address this potentially clinically important issue. Peng and colleagues (68) reported that in contrast to the proaggregatory effects of IL-6, the administration of thrombopoietin to dogs failed to alter platelet function as assessed by exteriorization of P-selectin in response to thrombin stimulation. In a more extensive study, Harker and coworkers (69) found that platelet deposition on an exteriorized vascular shunt was not out of proportion to the platelet count in thrombopoietin-treated dogs, although administration of the hormone was associated with in vitro evidence of primed platelets. It is thus fair to conclude from this study that as long as the platelet count does not become excessively increased, the administration of thrombopoietin is unlikely to trigger pathological thrombosis in patients who receive it. However, given this growing body of preclinical data, clinical trials of the agent should pay particular attention to this aspect of its safety. In this regard, as discussed below, the initial clinical experience has been favorable.

The in vitro effects of thrombopoietin have been carefully evaluated over the 6 years since its cloning. For the most part, results from in vivo studies have reflected those previously found in vitro. Despite these favorable results and the insights into normal MK and platelet development they provide, the utility of the hormone for improving hematopoiesis in patients will only come from carefully controlled clinical trials. The second half of this chapter will review our present understanding of the safety and utility of thrombopoietin and its derivative molecules in thrombocytopenic patients.

X. CLINICAL STUDIES

Clinical development commenced using two commercial preparations of the Mpl ligand. A truncated, pegylated form that contained the mpl receptor binding domain was developed by scientists at Amgen Inc., Thousand Oaks, CA (pegylated, recombinant human megakaryocyte growth and development factor; MGDF). Scientists at Genentech, Inc., South San Francisco, CA produced a recombinant form of full-length human thrombopoietin (rhTPO). Preliminary clinical studies have been reported using both of these materials and from several clinical groups (70–80). The first completed clinical reports utilized MGDF (81,82).

The initial study design for evaluation of MGDF was unusual for a phase I analysis and employed a double-blinded, randomized, placebo-controlled strategy. The placebo-controlled design was reasoned to be important given the thrombocytosis that occurs in normal individuals in response to venesection. This study design was used by both groups that initially examined the clinical action of MGDF (70,71,74,77). The effects of MGDF were examined both alone (81,82) and in patients undergoing chemotherapy for solid tumors (73,74,77).

Prior to any chemotherapy treatment, patients were randomly assigned (in the ratio of 3 : 1) to receive either MGDF at 0.03, 0.1, 0.3, or 1 μg/kg/day or a placebo. A minimum of three patients were enrolled in each cohort, and the study drug was given for a maximum of 10 days (81). Administration of MGDF was associated with a concentration-dependent increase in the platelet count (Fig. 3). The increase in the median platelet count was first evident at 10 days for the 0.3 μg/kg/day cohort and at 8 days for the 1 μg/kg/day cohort. After this, the platelet count continued to rise. The maximum platelet count occurred between days 12 and 18 and had returned to $<450 \times 10^9/L$ between days 22 and 30. Thus, unlike the action of G-CSF on neutrophil counts, the effect of MGDF was delayed, with maximum responses occurring up to more than 1 week after cessation of MGDF. For the two highest dose levels, the median increase in the platelet count was threefold. However, as with other growth factors, there was wide variation between different individuals. For example, at a dose of 0.3 μg/kg/day, the increase in the platelet count

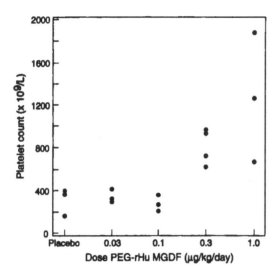

Figure 3 Dose-response platelet effects of megakaryocyte growth and development factor (MGDF). Maximum platelet counts ($\times$ 10^9/L) for individuals randomly assigned to receive MGDF at a dose of 0.03, 0.1, 0.3, or 1.0 μg/kg/day or placebo. Note the dose-related increase in platelet count (82).

ranged from 2.3- to 4.1-fold. At the 1 μg/kg/day dose, the increase was between 1.6- and 10-fold, with the maximum platelet count observed being 1876 $\times$ 10^9/L. Because of the degree of thrombocytosis observed at the 1 μg/kg/day dose, further escalation of MGDF was not examined.

For the two lowest dose cohorts of MGDF and also for the placebo cohort there was no significant increase in the median platelet count by day 12 of the study; the median increase in the platelet count was 1.2-fold. However, it was noteworthy that one individual in the placebo cohort had a two-fold increase in the platelet count by day 12. This was likely a response to the regular venesection (approximately 400 mL in 12 days) and illustrated the value of the placebo control when examining changes in platelet counts. It also highlights the variability between individuals in their response to endogenous thrombopoietin. The inability to detect an increase in the platelet count in the two lowest dose cohorts of MGDF was probably a consequence of the study design. Because no increase was detected by day 12, patients proceeded to treatment with chemotherapy. However, it is possible that a rise in the platelet count may have been detected had the study duration been longer. This notion is supported by the finding that the number of bone marrow MKs was increased by day 8 in all MGDF cohorts. Thus, a rise in bone marrow MKs was observed in individuals in whom no rise in platelet count was seen; confirming a biological effect of MGDF even at a dose of 0.03 μg/kg/day. The maximum increase in bone marrow MKs was approximately two-fold at the highest doses of MGDF. Although this was a relatively modest rise in bone marrow MKs, the double-blinded study design and the inclusion of a placebo cohort (in which no increase in bone marrow MKs was seen) validated this result.

The effect of MGDF on the blood was lineage specific; there was no change in other blood parameters. The total white cell count, neutrophil count, lymphocyte count, hematocrit, and hemoglobin remained unchanged (81). Similarly, the changes in the bone marrow were restricted to the MK lineage.

The initial evaluation of rhTPO was also performed both prior to and after chemotherapy, although a placebo-control group was not examined (80). The study design utilized patients with sarcomas, and initially a single dose of rhTPO was administered at doses of 0.3, 0.6, 1.2, or 2.4 µg/kg. This was associated with an up to 3.6-fold increase in the platelet count, with the maximum levels occurring around day 12 (range 10–15 days) (75,80). Subsequently, two doses of rhTPO were evaluated with an up to 4.4-fold platelet rise. These changes in the platelet count were also associated with an increase in bone marrow MKs (79).

XI. ASSAYS OF PLATELET PRODUCTION, TURNOVER, AND FUNCTION

To determine whether new platelet production could be detected in patients receiving MGDF, "reticulated platelets" (83,84) were quantitated (82). Platelets were stained for 1 h with thiazole orange using established techniques (83,84). This assay measures "new" platelets as defined by their ribonucleic acid (RNA) content, and requires rigorous attention to the experimental procedure. Patients who received placebo served as an additional control. The earliest increase in reticulated platelets was evident after 2–3 days of treatment with MGDF and preceded the rise in the platelet count by several days. Elevation of reticulated platelet levels was the earliest detectable effect of MGDF. In comparison, there was no increase above baseline values (less than approximately 4%) for patients who received placebo. However, given the small number of patients examined in this first clinical study and the controversial nature of this technique, this result remains to be confirmed in subsequent studies. However, this observation raises the possibility that assessment of reticulated platelets may serve as an early predictor of a response to MGDF. The rise in the platelet count in response to MGDF was associated with a reciprocal change in the mean platelet volume (MPV). A similar decrease in the size of platelets generated in response to MGDF was also seen in preclinical models (41,43). .

Plasma glycocalicin levels were also monitored as an indicator of platelet turnover (85,86). Plasma glycocalicin is generated by cleavage of the platelet surface protein glycoprotein Ib, and levels are increased in disorders of thrombocytosis and with impaired renal function. The rise in levels of plasma glycocalicin paralleled the increase in the platelet count but occurred 2–3 days later (82). Similarly, the decline in levels of glycocalicin was observed in parallel with, but 2–3 days after, the fall in the platelet count. In addition, there was a linear correlation between the platelet counts observed and the level of glycocalicin. This suggested that there was normal turnover of platelets generated in response to MGDF, with the increased levels of glycocalicin reflecting the increased platelet mass. Moreover, platelets generated in response to MGDF had a normal appearance under the light microscope and showed normal ultrastructure (82).

The expression of a variety of platelet surface markers was examined during administration of MGDF. Glycoprotein (GP) Ib (CD42) is a molecule that acts as a receptor for von Willebrand factor and thrombin, and it mediates the initial contact adhesion of platelets to blood vessels (87). On platelet activation, the majority of GP Ib becomes inaccessible owing to internalization. However, there was no change in platelet GP Ib expression following the administration of MGDF. Platelet aggregation is mediated by binding of fibrinogen and the von Willebrand factor to the β_3-integrin complex, GP IIb-IIIa (CD41/CD61). The number of copies of surface GP IIb-IIIa approximately doubles on platelet activation (87). In addition, platelet activation results in changes in the structure of the complex that can be detected by the monoclonal antibody D3GP3 (88,89). There was no change in the surface expression of CD41, CD61 and no change in expression detected using D3GP3 following administration of MGDF. Consistent with these findings, there was also no change in surface expression of P-selectin (CD62P), an α-granule membrane protein that is surface expressed on platelet activation (82). Thus, there was no evidence of platelet activation occurring in vivo in response to MGDF treatment.

Platelets generated in response to MGDF showed normal function in in vitro assays. Platelet aggregation responses to ristocetin, thrombin-receptor agonist peptide, collagen, and four concentrations of ADP were examined (Fig. 4). In addition, release of adenosine triphosphate (ATP) in response to these agents was documented. These studies were particularly important given the evidence demonstrating that the Mpl ligand enhances platelet aggregation or "primes" platelets in vitro. (59–62). At baseline there were no platelet function differences between the placebo cohort and patients randomized to receive MGDF, and there were no differences in the aggregation response or platelet ATP-release when cohorts were compared 24 h after administration of MGDF and on the final day of study drug (82). For patients in the 1 μg/kg/day cohort, these tests were also performed 1 h after administration of MGDF and were again unchanged. Although there was variability in the results for some individuals, these changes were not consistent between patients, were not sustained throughout the treatment period, and were similar to the variations observed in patients who received placebo. The lack of change in platelet function as assessed in platelet aggregation and ATP-release assays was consistent with the lack of change in platelet surface activation markers.

The platelets produced in response to MGDF also showed typical in vitro responses following administration of aspirin. One patient received 300 mg aspirin when the platelet count was >1700 × 10⁹/L. Following aspirin administration, there was ablation of platelet

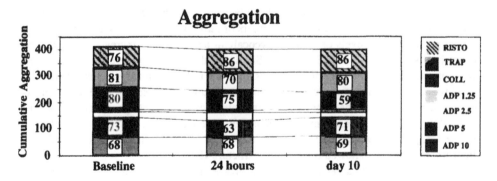

Figure 4 Platelet aggregation is unaltered following treatment with megakaryocyte growth and development factor (MGDF). Platelet aggregation was examined at baseline, after 24 hs of MGDF, and after 10 days of MGDF for one individual who received 10 days' treatment with 0.3 mg/kg/day MGDF. The platelet agonists examined were ristocetin (RISTO), thrombin-receptor agonist peptide (TRAP), collagen (COLL), and ADP at four concentrations (1.25, 2.5, 5.0, and 10.0 μmol/L). The percentage aggregation (if >20%) is shown as numerals for each agonist (82).

aggregation and ATP response to arachidonic acid and inhibition of ADP and collagen-induced responses. Thus, aspirin administration is a possible therapeutic option if deemed necessary for MGDF-induced thrombocytosis. This patient also underwent platelet pheresis when the count was >1800 × 10^9/L and continuing to rise. This procedure was without complication and the patient had no adverse clinical sequelae as a result of thrombocytosis. Taken together, all these results suggest that platelets generated in response to MGDF function normally, respond normally to aspirin, and show no evidence of activation in vivo.

XII. MOBILIZATION OF BLOOD PROGENITOR CELLS

Multiple cytokines have been shown to mobilize marrow progenitor cells into the peripheral blood. To test for an action of MGDF in this regard, we measured marrow and blood lineage-committed progenitor cell levels using established techniques (37,90). Although up to four-fold changes were observed in the frequency of bone marrow progenitor cells, these changes were within the error associated with this assay and were not consistent between different patient cohorts. Moreover, changes of similar magnitude were seen in patients who received placebo. Thus, we concluded that there was no change in the frequency of progenitor cells in the bone marrow after 8 days treatment with MGDF. This was the case for both early (day 14) and late (day 7) CFU-GMs for BFU-E and CFU-MKs. In contrast, levels of progenitor cells of all lineages increased in the blood (73; J. E. Rasko et al., unpublished data). The increase in day 14 and day 7 CFU-GMs, BFU-E, and CFU-MKs was only evident at the two highest doses of MGDF. The increase in day 14 CFU-GMs was a median of three-fold and seven-fold for the 0.3 and 1 µg/kg/day cohorts, respectively. The maximum increase observed was 15-fold. Similar changes were observed with BFU-E and CFU-MKs (median 4-fold increase; maximum 30-fold increase for CFU-MKs). There were no changes observed in the placebo cohort of patients; levels of blood progenitor cells remained constant during the period of study (J. E. Rasko et al., unpublished data). The magnitude of the increase in blood progenitor cell levels in response to MGDF was comparable to the increase initially reported for G-CSF–mobilized progenitor/stem cells (91). However, the kinetics of the response were markedly different. Levels of blood progenitor cells are maximal 5 or 6 days after commencing G-CSF treatment (91–93). Similar kinetics are also observed with GM-CSF alone or G-CSF when combined with SCF (94,95). However, maximum levels of progenitor cells following MGDF were seen at day 12. This suggests that mobilization in response to MGDF may occur via a different mechanism compared with, for example, G-CSF.

The results in the bone marrow described above appear to differ from those reported with rhTPO where a two- to four-fold increase in the frequency of CFU-GMs and BFU-E and an increase of >10% CFU-MKs was reported 7 days after a single dose of rhTPO (78). There was no evidence of a dose-response relationship. Changes in blood progenitor cells were also observed with a maximum of 5- to 9.5-fold increase in the frequency of CFU-GMs and BFU-E 7 days following an injection of rhTPO.

Although the changes in levels of blood CFU-GMs and BFU-E were not seen in primate studies (41), they are consistent with the reported action of the Mpl ligand on murine and human cells (26,27,35,36,37,39). Moreover, the human assays with MGDF were performed by investigators blinded to patient randomization and clinical data. In addition, the lack of change in the placebo cohort further validates this assay. Further studies are required to determine whether MGDF is comparable to other factors when used alone to mobilize progenitor cells. However, the mobilization response to MGDF suggests that this aspect of its function is worthy of further investigation, particularly in combination with G-CSF.

Pharmacokinetic studies with MGDF revealed that the levels progressively increased during MGDF administration (76). The levels observed were directly related to the dose administered and were, in general, inversely related to the platelet count. Following cessation of MGDF, levels returned to baseline over a 4-day period. The terminal half-life was approximately 40 hs. Pharmacokinetic analysis of rhTPO after a single dose showed a terminal half-life of between 18 and 32 hs and with maximum levels inversely related to the platelet count (80).

When administered alone, MGDF was very well tolerated (81). There was no fever, weight change, hypotension, or edema noted in any patient. There was no lethargy (although this was reported in the placebo cohort), headache (also reported the placebo cohort), or myalgia. One reaction at the local injection site was reported in both the placebo and the MGDF cohorts. There was one episode of superficial thrombophlebitis in a patient with adenocarcinoma of the colon given MGDF. The phlebitis resolved spontaneously. There was no evidence of deep venous thrombosis. Biochemical, renal, and liver function tests remained normal. There was no evidence of induction of an acute phase response; levels of fibrinogen were unchanged during and after administration of MGDF (81,82).

XIII. ACTIONS OF MPL LIGAND AFTER CHEMOTHERAPY

Following one course of MGDF administration, patients went on to receive chemotherapy with carboplatin 600 mg/m^2 and cyclophosphamide 1200 mg/m^2. This treatment schedule was chosen as earlier studies had indicated thrombocytopenia was a significant toxicity with this regimen. All patients received G-CSF (filgrastim, 5 µg/kg/day) after chemotherapy and were randomized to receive MGDF or placebo. The doses of MGDF were 0.03, 0.1, 0.3, and 1.0 µg/kg/day for those patients who had received MGDF prior to chemotherapy. For these patients, MGDF was administered for a maximum of 20 days after chemotherapy. For subsequent patients (dose levels 1, 3, 5 µg/kg/day), MGDF was given for a maximum of 7 days. A total of 41 patients completed the chemotherapy phase of this study. The patients were well matched in terms of age, gender, tumor-type, and prior treatment regimens (74; R. Basser et al., unpublished data). Analogous to the action of G-CSF on neutrophil recovery, MGDF acted significantly to shorten the time to the platelet nadir after chemotherapy. It also acted to hasten the platelet recovery in a dose-dependent manner. Although there was no significant difference in the depth of the platelet nadir for different patients cohorts, there was a significant advantage for MGDF versus placebo in terms of platelet count recovery to baseline. The chemotherapy was associated with significant neutropenia despite administration of G-CSF. There was no evidence of an effect of MGDF influencing neutrophil recovery. However, such an action of MGDF may have been masked because of the coadministration of G-CSF.

The action of MGDF was also examined after chemotherapy but without G-CSF (77). In that study, thrombocytopenia was less marked; however, MGDF also acted to speed platelet recovery compared with patients who received placebo. This work has formed the basis of ongoing studies that examine the action of MGDF in patients with acute myeloid leukemia, although this study is too early to evaluate (72).

As when MGDF was administered prior to chemotherapy, the administration of this factor after chemotherapy was well tolerated. There were no significant adverse events directly attributable to treatment with MGDF (74,77; R. Basser et al., unpublished data). In addition, platelet function after chemotherapy showed no differences compared with the placebo cohort and there were no changes in platelet surface marker characteristics.

Chemotherapy with doxorubicin (Adriamycin) and ifosfamide was used in patients with sarcoma to examine the action of rhTPO after chemotherapy (80). After the first and second cycles of chemotherapy, the platelet nadir and the duration of thrombocytopenia appeared to suggest an advantage for two doses of rhTPO versus a single dose (80). And like MGDF, rhTPO was well tolerated.

XIV. CONCLUSION

These early clinical studies of thrombopoietin have demonstrated its ability to elevate platelet counts in a "lineage-specific" or "lineage-dominant" manner. The platelets generated in response to MGDF show normal function, normal surface antigen expression, and normal turnover. The rise in the platelet count was preceded by an increase in reticulated platelets and was associated with increased bone marrow MKs (81,82). There was mobilization into the blood of progenitor cells of multiple hematopoietic lineages. After chemotherapy, administration of MGDF resulted in a hastening of platelet recovery with the suggestion that pretreatment with MGDF may hasten platelet recovery in subsequent cycles of chemotherapy. MGDF was well tolerated alone, and in combination with G-CSF, and was safely administered for up to 20 days. Further clinical assessment of this molecule in a variety of clinical contexts is ongoing.

Our understanding of MKs and platelet biology has progressed much since the cloning and characterization of thrombopoietin. One of the challenges yet facing us is to determine the optimal use of the hormone to ameliorate the thrombocytopenic complications of iatrogenic and natural states of marrow failure.

ACKNOWLEDGMENTS

The authors wish to thank Allan Dimaunahan and Zenaida Sisk for preparation of the manuscript, and all of the outstanding investigators who participated in the studies summarized here. The authors would also like to thank Catherine Carow for the studies illustrated in Figure 1 and Norma Fox for the data of Figure 2. Many of the clinical studies with MGDF reviewed here were performed at the Center for Developmental Cancer Therapeutics in Melbourne, Australia, and reflect the effort of many clinical and laboratory colleagues whose enthusiasm and dedication is gratefully acknowledged.

REFERENCES

1. Ogawa M. Differentiation and proliferation of hematopoietic stem cells. Blood 1993; 81:2844–2853.
2. Ikebuchi K, Clark SC, Ihle JN, Souza LM, Ogawa M. Granulocyte colony-stimulating factor enhances interleukin 3–dependent proliferation of multipotential hemopoietic progenitors. Proc Natl Acad Sci USA 1988; 85:3445–3449.
3. Kaushansky K, O'Hara PJ, Berkner K, Segal GM, Hagen FS, Adamson JW. Genomic cloning, characterization, and multilineage growth-promoting activity of human granulocyte-macrophage colony-stimulating factor. Proc Natl Acad Sci USA 1986; 83:3101–3105.

4. Robinson BE, McGrath HE, Quesenberry PJ. Recombinant murine granulocyte macrophage colony-stimulating factor has megakaryocyte colony-stimulating activity and augments megakaryocyte colony stimulation by interleukin 3. J Clin Invest 1987; 79:1648–1652.

5. Segal GM, Stueve T, Adamson JW. Analysis of murine megakaryocyte colony size and ploidy: effects of interleukin-3. J Cell Physiol 1988; 137:537–544.

6. Briddell RA, Bruno E, Cooper RJ, Brandt JE, Hoffman R. Effect of c-kit ligand on in vitro human megakaryocytopoiesis. Blood 1991; 78:2854–2859.

7. Avraham H, Vannier E, Cowley S, Jiang SX, Chi S, Dinarello CA, Zsebo KM, Groopman JE. Effects of the stem cell factor, c-kit ligand, on human megakaryocytic cells. Blood 1992; 79:365–371.

8. Ikebuchi K, Wong GG, Clark SC, Ihle JN, Hirai Y, Ogawa M. Interleukin 6 enhancement of interleukin 3-dependent proliferation of multipotential hemopoietic progenitors. Proc Natl Acad Sci USA 1987; 84:9035–9039.

9. Burstein SA, Mei RL, Henthorn J, Friese P, Turner K. Leukemia inhibitory factor and interleukin-11 promote maturation of murine and human megakaryocytes in vitro. J Cell Physiol 1992; 153:305–312.

10. Metcalf D, Waring P, Nicola NA. Actions of leukaemia inhibitory factor on megakaryocyte and platelet formation. Ciba Found Symp 1992; 167P174–82; discussion 182–7:174–182.

10a. Hodohara K, Fujii N, Yamamoto N, Kaushansky K. Stromal cell-derived factor-1 (SDF-1) acts together with thrombopoietin to enhance the development of megakaryocytic progenitor cells (CFU-MK). Blood 2000; 95(3):769–775.

11. McDonald TP. Thrombopoietin: its biology, purification, and characterization. Exp Hematol 1988; 16:201–205.

12. Hill RJ, Levin J. Regulators of thrombopoiesis: their biochemistry and physiology. Blood Cells 1989; 15:141–166.

13. Wendling F, Varlet P, Charon M, Tambourin P. MPLV: a retrovirus complex inducing an acute myeloproliferative leukemic disorder in adult mice. Virology 1986; 149:242–246.

14. Vigon I, Mornon JP, Cocault L, Mitjavila MT, Tambourin P, Gisselbrecht S, Souyri M. Molecular cloning and characterization of MPL, the human homolog of the v-mpl oncogene: identification of a member of the hematopoietic growth factor receptor superfamily. Proc Natl Acad Sci USA 1992; 89:5640–5644.

15. Methia N, Louache F, Vainchenker W, Wendling F. Oligodeoxynucleotides antisense to the proto-oncogene c-mpl specifically inhibit in vitro megakaryocytopoiesis. Blood 1993; 82:1395–1401.

16. Kaushansky K. Thrombopoietin: the primary regulator of platelet production (see comments). Blood 1995; 86:419–431.

17. Kaushansky K, Broudy VC, Grossmann A, Humes J, Lin N, Ren HP, Bailey MC, Papayannopoulou T, Forstrom JW, Sprugel KH. Thrombopoietin expands erythroid progenitors, increases red cell production, and enhances erythroid recovery after myelosuppressive therapy. J Clin Invest 1995; 96:1683–1687.

18. Kaushansky K, Broudy VC, Lin N, Jorgensen MJ, McCarty J, Fox N, Zucker FD, Lofton DC. Thrombopoietin, the Mpl ligand, is essential for full megakaryocyte development. Proc Natl Acad Sci USA 1995; 92:3234–3238.

19. Kaushansky K, Lok S, Holly RD, Broudy VC, Lin N, Bailey MC, Forstrom JW, Buddle M, Oort PJ, Hagen FS, Roth GJ, Papayannopoulou T, Foster DC. Promotion of megakaryocyte progenitor expansion and differentiation by the c-Mpl ligand thrombopoietin (see comments). Nature 1994; 369:568–571.

20. Debili N, Wendling F, Katz A, Guichard J, Breton GJ, Hunt P, Vainchenker W. The Mpl-ligand or thrombopoietin or megakaryocyte growth and differentiative factor has both direct proliferative and differentiative activities on human megakaryocyte progenitors. Blood 1995; 86:2516–2525.

21. Kato T, Horie K, Hagiwara T, Maeda E, Tsumura H, Ohashi H, Miyazaki H. GpIIb/IIIa+

subpopulation of rat megakaryocyte progenitor cells exhibits high responsiveness to human thrombopoietin. Exp Hematol 1996; 24:1209–1214.

22. Broudy VC, Lin NL, Kaushansky K. Thrombopoietin (c-mpl ligand) acts synergistically with erythropoietin, stem cell factor, and interleukin-11 to enhance murine megakaryocyte colony growth and increases megakaryocyte ploidy in vitro. Blood 1995; 85:1719–1726.

23. Broudy VC, Lin NL, Fox N, Taga T, Saito M, Kaushansky K. Thrombopoietin stimulates colony-forming unit-megakaryocyte proliferation and megakaryocyte maturation independently of cytokines that signal through the gp 130 receptor subunit. Blood 1996; 88:2026–2032.

24. Zucker FD, Kaushansky K. Effect of thrombopoietin on the development of megakaryocytes and platelets: an ultrastructural analysis. Blood 1996; 88:1632–1638.

25. Gurney AL, Carver MK, de-Sauvage FJ, Moore MW. Thrombocytopenia in c-mpl–deficient mice. Science 1994; 265:1445–1447.

26. Alexander WS, Roberts AW, Nicola NA, Li R, Metcalf D. Deficiencies in progenitor cells of multiple hematopoietic lineages and defective megakaryocytopoiesis in mice lacking the thrombopoietic receptor c-Mpl. Blood 1996; 87:2162–2170.

27. Solar GP, Kerr WG, Zeigler FC, Hess D, Donahue C, de Sauvage FJ, Eaton DL. Role of c-mpl in early hematopoiesis. Blood 1998; 92:4–10.

28. McDonald TP, Sullivan PS. Megakaryocytic and erythrocytic cell lines share a common precursor cell (see comments). Exp Hematol 1993; 21:1316–1320.

29. Hunt P. A bipotential megakaryocyte/erythrocyte progenitor cell: the link between erythropiesis and megakaryopoiesis becomes stronger (editorial; comment). J Lab Clin Med 1995; 125:303–304.

30. Papayannopoulou T, Brice M, Farrer D, Kaushansky K. Insights into the cellular mechanisms of erythropoietin-thrombopoietin synergy. Exp Hematol 1996; 24:660–669.

31. Debili N, Coulombel L, Croisille L, Katz A, Guichard J, Breton GJ, Vainchenker W. Characterization of a bipotent erythro-megakaryocytic progenitor in human bone marrow. Blood 1996; 88:1284–1296.

32. Kobayashi M, Laver JH, Kato T, Miyazaki H, Ogawa M. Recombinant human thrombopoietin (Mpl ligand) enhances proliferation of erythroid progenitors. Blood 1995; 86:2494–2499.

33. Vigon I, Dreyfus F, Melle J, Vigui, Ribrag V, Cocault L, Souyri M, Gisselbrecht S. Expression of the c-mpl proto-oncogene in human hematologic malignancies. Blood 1993; 82:877–883.

34. Matsumura I, Kanakura Y, Kato T, Ikeda H, Ishikawa J, Horikawa Y, Hashimoto K, Moriyama Y, Tsujimura T, Nishiura T, Miyazaki H, Matsuzawa Y. Growth response of acute myeloblastic leukemia cells to recombinant human thrombopoietin. Blood 1995; 86:703–709.

35. Ku H, Yonemura Y, Kaushansky K, Ogawa M. Thrombopoietin, the ligand for the Mpl receptor, synergizes with steel factor and other early acting cytokines in supporting proliferation of primitive hematopoietic progenitors of mice. Blood 1996; 87:4544–4551.

36. Kobayashi M, Laver JH, Kato T, Miyazaki H, Ogawa M. Thrombopoietin supports proliferation of human primitive hematopoietic cells in synergy with steel factor and/or interleukin-3. Blood 1996; 88:429–436.

37. Rasko JE, O'Flaherty E, Begley CG. Mpl ligand (MGDF) alone and in combination with stem cell factor (SCF) promotes proliferation and survival of human megakaryocyte, erythroid and granulocyte/macrophage progenitors. Stem Cells 1997; 15:33–42.

38. Wolf NS, Kon, Priestley GV, Bartelmez SH. In vivo and in vitro characterization of long-term repopulating primitive hematopoietic cells isolated by sequential Hoechst 33342-rhodamine 123 FACS selection. Exp Hematol 1993; 21:614–622.

39. Sitnicka E, Lin N, Priestley GV, Fox N, Broudy VC, Wolf NS, Kaushansky K. The effect of thrombopoietin on the proliferation and differentiation of murine hematopoietic stem cells. Blood 1996; 87:4998–5005.

40. Kaushansky K, Lin N, Grossmann A, Humes J, Sprugel KH, Broudy VC. Thrombopoietin

expands erythroid, granulocyte-macrophage, and megakaryocytic progenitor cells in normal and myelosuppressed mice. Exp Hematol 1996; 24:265–269.

41. Farese AM, Hunt P, Boone T, MacVittae TJ. Recombinant human megakaryocyte growth and development factor stimulates thrombocytosis in normal nonhuman primates. Blood 1995; 86: 54–59.

42. Farese AM, Hunt P, Grab LB, MacVittie TJ. Combined administration of recombinant human megakaryocyte growth and development factor and granulocyte colony-stimulating factor enhances multilineage hematopoietic reconstitution in nonhuman primates after radiation-induced marrow aplasia. J Clin Invest 1996; 97:2145–2151.

43. Ulich TR, del Castillo J, Yin S, Swift S, Padilla D, Senaldi G, Bennett L, Shutter J, Bogenberger J, Sun D, Samal B, Shimamoto G, Lee R, Steinbrink R, Boone T, Sheridan WT, Hunt P. Megakaryocyte growth and development factor ameliorates carboplatin-induced thrombocytopenia in mice. Blood 1995; 86:971–976.

44. Hokom MM, Lacey D, Kinstler OB, Choi E, Kaufman S, Faust J, Rowan C, Dwyer E, Nichol JL, Grasel T, Wilson J, Steinbrink R, Hecht R, Winters D, Boone T, Hunt P. Pegylated megakaryocyte growth and development factor abrogates the lethal thrombocytopenia associated with carboplatin and irradiation in mice. Blood 1995; 86:4486–4492.

45. Grossmann A, Lenox J, Ren HP, Humes JM, Forstrom JW, Kaushansky K, Sprugel KH. Thrombopoietin accelerates platelet, red blood cell, and neutrophil recovery in myelosuppressed mice. Exp Hematol 1996; 24:1238–1246.

46. McDonald TP, Clift RE, Cottrell MB. Large, chronic doses of erythropoietin cause thrombocytopenia in mice (see comments). Blood 1992; 80:352–358.

47. Locatelli F, Zecca M, Beguin Y, Giorgiani G, Ponchio L, De SP, Cazzola M. Accelerated erythroid repopulation with no stem-cell competition effect in children treated with recombinant human erythropoietin after allogeneic bone marrow transplantation. Br J Haematol 1993; 84:752–754.

48. Grossmann A, Lenox J, Deisher TA, Ren HP, Humes JM, Kaushansky K, Sprugel KH. Synergistic effects of thrombopoietin and granulocyte colony-stimulating factor on neutrophil recovery in myelosuppressed mice. Blood 1996; 88:3363–3370.

49. Fibbe WE, Heemskerk DP, Laterveer L, Pruijt JF, Foster D, Kaushansky K, Willemze R. Accelerated reconstitution of platelets and erythrocytes after syngeneic transplantation of bone marrow cells derived from thrombopoietin pretreated donor mice. Blood 1995; 86:3308–3313.

50. Molineux G, Hartley CA, McElroy P, McCrea C, McNiece IK. Megakaryocyte growth and development factor stimulates enhanced platelet recovery in mice after bone marrow transplantation. Blood 1996; 88:1509–1514.

51. Metcalf D, Begley CG, Johnson GR, Nicola NA, Vadas MA, Lopez AF, Williamson DJ, Wong GG, Clark SC, Wang EA. Biologic properties in vitro of a recombinant human granulocyte-macrophage colony-stimulating factor. Blood 1986; 67:37–45.

52. Begley CG, Lopez AF, Nicola NA, Warren DJ, Vadas MA, Sanderson CJ, Metcalf D. Purified colony-stimulating factors enhance the survival of human neutrophils and eosinophils in vitro: a rapid sensitive microassay for colony-stimulating factors. Blood 1986; 68:162–166.

53. Weisbart RH, Kwan L, Golde DW, Gasson JC. Human GM-CSF primes neutrophils for enhanced oxidative metabolism in response to the major physiological chemoattractants. Blood 1987; 69:18–21.

54. DiPersio JF, Billing P, Williams R, Gasson JC. Human granulocyte-macrophage colony-stimulating factor and other cytokines prime human neutrophils for enhanced arachidonic acid release and leukotriene B4 synthesis. J Immunol 1988; 140:4315–4322.

55. Weisbart RH, Kacena A, Schuh A, Golde DW. GM-CSF induces human neutrophil IgA-mediated phagocytosis by an IgA Fc receptor activation mechanism. Nature 1988; 332:647–648.

56. Chen J, Herceg HL, Groopman JE, Grabarek J. Regulation of platelet activation in vitro by the c-Mpl ligand, thrombopoietin. Blood 1995; 86:4054–4062.

57. Montrucchio G, Brizzi MF, Calosso G, Marengo S, Pegoraro L, Camussi G. Effects of recombinant human megakaryocyte growth and development factor on platelet activation. Blood 1996; 87:2762–2768.

58. Wun T, Paglieroni T, Hammond WP, Kaushansky K, Foster DC. Thrombopoietin is synergistic with other hematopoietic growth factors and physiologic platelet agonists for platelet activation in vitro. Am J Hematol 1997; 54:225–232.

59. Ezumi Y, Takayama H, Okuma M. Thrombopoietin, c-Mpl ligand, induces tyrosine phosphorylation of Tyk2, JAK2, and STAT3, and enhances agonists-induced aggregation in platelets in vitro. FEBS Lett 1995; 374:48–52.

60. Miyakawa Y, Oda A, Druker BJ, Kato T, Miyazaki H, Handa M, Ikeda Y. Recombinant thrombopoietin induces rapid protein tyrosine phosphorylation of Janus kinase 2 and Shc in human blood platelets. Blood 1995; 86:23–27.

61. Oda A, Miyakawa Y, Druker BJ, Ozaki K, Yabusaki K, Shirasawa Y, Handa M, Kato T, Miyazaki H, Shimosaka A, Ikeda Y. Thrombopoietin primes human platelet aggregation induced by shear stress and by multiple agonists. Blood 1996; 87:4664–4670.

62. Rodriguez-Linares, Watson SP. Thrombopoietin potentiates activation of human platelets in association with JAK2 and TYK2 phosphorylation. Biochem J 1996; 316P93–8:93–98.

63. Drachman J, Griffin JD, and Kaushansky K. Stimulation of tyrosine kinase activity by MPL-ligand (thrombopoietin). J Biol Chem 1995; 270:4979–82.

64. Pallard C, Gouilleux F, enit L, Cocault L, Souyri M, Levy D, Groner B, Gisselbrecht S, Dusanter Fl. Thrombopoietin activates a STAT5-like factor in hematopoietic cells. EMBO J 1995; 14:2847–2856.

65. Sattler M, Durstin MA, Frank DA, Okuda K, Kaushansky K, Salgia R, Griffin JD. The thrombopoietin receptor c-MPL activates JAK2 and TYK2 tyrosine kinases. Exp Hematol 1995; 23:1040–1048.

66. Tortolani PJ, Johnston JA, Bacon CM, McVicar DW, Shimosaka A, Linnekin D, Longo DL, O'Shea JJ. Thrombopoietin induces tyrosine phosphorylation and activation of the Janus kinase, JAK2. Blood 1995; 85:3444–3451.

67. Drachman JG, Sabath DF, Fox NE, Kaushansky K. Thrombopoietin signal transduction in purified murine megakaryocytes. Blood 1997; 89:483–492.

68. Peng J, Friese P, Wolf RF, Harrison P, Downs T, Lok S, Dale GL, Burstein SA. Relative reactivity of platelets from thrombopoietin- and interleukin-6-treated dogs. Blood 1996; 87: 4158–4163.

69. Harker LA, Marzec UM, Hunt P, Kelly AB, Tomer A, Cheung E, Hanson SR, Stead RB. Dose-response effects of pegylated human megakaryocyte growth and development factor on platelet production and function in nonhuman primates. Blood 1996; 88:511–521.

70. Basser R, Clarke K, Fox R, Green M, Cebon J, Marty J, Menchaca D, Tomita D, Begley G. Randomized, double-blind, placebo-controlled phase 1 trial of pegylated megakaryocyte growth and development factor (PEG-rHuMGDF) administered to patients with advanced cancer before and after chemotherapy—early results (abstr). Blood 1995; 86:257a.

71. Rasko JEJ, Basser R, O'Malley CJ, Mansfield R, Boyd J, Grigg A, McGrath K, Marty J, Sheridan W, Hussein S, Berndt MC, Begley CG. In vitro studies from a phase I randomized, blinded trial of pegylated megakaryocyte growth and development factor (PEG-rHuMGDF) (abstr). Blood 1995; 86:497a.

72. Archimbaud E, Ottmann O, Liu Yin JA, Lechner K, Dombret H, Sanz MA, Herrmann F, Gruss H, Fenaux P, Ganser A, Heil G, Kanz L, Brugger W, Sims T, Olsen K, Hoelzer D. A randomised, double-blind, placebo-controlled study using PEG-rHuMGDF as an adjunct to chemotherapy for adults with de novo acute myeloid leukemia (AML): early results (abstr). Blood 1996; 88:447a.

73. Basser R, Rasko J, Clarke K, Green M, Cebon J, Grigg A, Berndt M, Zalcberg J, Marty J, Menchaca D, Tomita D, Fox R, Begley G. Pegylated megakaryocyte growth and development

factor (PEG-rHuMGDF) enhances the mobilization of peripheral blood progenitor cells (PBPC) by chemotherapy and filgrastim (abstr). Blood 1996a; 88:641a.

74. Begley G, Basser R, Clarke K, Rasko J, Green M, Grigg A, Cebon J, Marty J, Menchaca D, Tomita D, Fox R. Randomised, double-blind placebo-controlled phase I trial of pegylated megakaryocyte growth and development factor (PEG-rHuMGDF) administered to patients with advanced cancer after chemotherapy (abstr). Proc Am Soc Clin Oncol 1996; 15:719a.

75. Bloedow D, Vadhan-Raj S, Paton V, Johnston T, Yang T, Senn T, Ashby M, Sims P. Pharmacokinetics of recombinant human thrombopoietin (rhTPO) after intravenous administration in cancer patients (abstr). Blood 1996; 88:351a.

76. de Boer R, Fox S, Hopkins W, Casper L, Cheung E, Roskos L, Basser R, Cebon J. Pharmacodynamics of pegylated megakaryocyte growth & development factor from a phase I study: effects of platelet count on serum levels & clearance (abstr). Exp Hematol 1996; 24:744a.

77. Fanucchi M, Glaspy J, Crawford J, Ozer H, Figlin R, Tomita D, Menchaca D, Harker L. Safety and biologic effects of pegylated megakaryocyte growth and development factor (PEG-rHuMGDF) in lung cancer patients receiving carboplatin and paclitaxel: randomised, placebo-controlled phase I study (abstr). Proc Am Soc Clin Onc 1996; 15:720a.

78. Murray LJ, Luens KM, Bruno E, Estrada MF, Cohen RL, Hellmann SD, Hoffman R, Vadhan-Raj S. Effects of thrombopoietin on megakaryocytes and progenitor cell populations in bone marrow and peripheral blood of sarcoma patients (abstr). Blood 1996; 88:351a.

79. Reddy SP, Bueso-Ramos C, Boiko I, Hittelman WN, Vadhan-Raj S. Effects of recombinant human thrombopoietin (rhTPO) on bone marrow megakaryocytes in humans (abstr). Blood 1996; 88:61a.

80. Vadhan-Raj S, Patel S, Broxmeyer HE, Bueso-Ramos C, Reddy SP, Papadopolous N, Burgess A, Johnston T, Yang T, Paton V, Hellmann S, Benjamin RS. Phase I-II investigation of recombinant human thrombopoietin (rhTPO) in patients with sarcoma receiving high dose chemotherapy (CT) with adriamycin (A) and ifosfamide (I) (abstr). Blood 1996; 8:448a.

81. Basser RL, Rasko JE, Clarke K, Cebon J, Green MD, Hussein S, Alt C, Menchaca D, Tomita D, Marty J, Fox RM, Begley CG. Thrombopoietic effects of pegylated recombinant human megakaryocyte growth and development factor (PEG-rHuMGDF) in patients with advanced cancer. Lancet 1996; 348:1279–1281.

82. O'Malley CJ, Rasko JE, Basser RL, McGrath KM, Cebon J, Grigg AP, Hopkins W, Cohen B, O'Byrne J, Green MD, Fox RM, Berndt MC, Begley CG. Administration of pegylated recombinant human megakaryocyte growth and development factor to humans stimulates the production of functional platelets that show no evidence of in vivo activation. Blood 1996; 88:3288–3298.

83. Romp KG, Peters WP, Hoffman M. Reticulated platelet counts in patients undergoing autologous bone marrow transplantation: an aid in assessing marrow recovery. Am J Hematol 1994; 46:319–324.

84. Dale GL, Friese P, Hynes LA, Burstein SA. Demonstration that thiazole-orange-positive platelets in the dog are less than 24 hours old. Blood 1995; 85:1822–1825.

85. Wilcox GR, Berndt MC, Mehrabani PA, Exner T, Trudinger BJ. An improved method for measuring plasma glycocalicin in the investigation of causes of thrombocytopenia. Platelets 1991; 2:45–50.

86. Beer JH, Buchi L, Steiner B. Glycocalicin: a new assay—the normal plasma levels and its potential usefulness in selected diseases. Blood 1994; 83:691–702.

87. Abrams C, Shattil SJ. Immunological detection of activated platelets in clinical disorders. Thromb Haemost 1991; 65:467–473.

88. Kouns WC, Wall CD, White MM, Fox CF, Jennings LK. A conformation-dependent epitope of human platelet glycoprotein IIIa. J Biol Chem 1990; 265:20594–20601.

89. Honda S, Tomiyama Y, Pelletier AJ, Annis D, Honda Y, Orchekowski R, Ruggeri Z, Kunicki TJ. Topography of ligand-induced binding sites, including a novel cation-sensitive epitope

(AP5) at the amino terminus, of the human integrin beta 3 subunit. J Biol Chem 1995; 270: 11947–11954.

90. Begley CG. Human progenitor cell assays. In: Morstyn G, Sheridan W, eds. Cell Therapy. Stem Cell Transplantation, Gene Therapy, and Immunotherapy. Cambridge, UK: Cambridge University Press, 1996: 59–74.

91. Dührsen U, Villeval JL, Boyd J, Kannourakis G, Morstyn G, Metcalf D. Effects of recombinant human granulocyte colony-stimulating factor on hematopoietic progenitor cells in cancer patients. Blood 1988; 72:2074–2081.

92. DeLuca E, Sheridan WP, Watson D, Szer J, Begley CG. Prior chemotherapy does not prevent effective mobilisation by G-CSF of peripheral blood progenitor cells. Br J Cancer 1992; 66: 893–899.

93. Sheridan WP, Begley CG, Juttner CA, Szer J, To LB, Maher D, McGrath KM, Morstyn G, Fox RM. Effect of peripheral-blood progenitor cells mobilised by filgrastim (G-CSF) on platelet recovery after high-dose chemotherapy (see comments). Lancet 1992; 339:640–644.

94. Villeval JL, Duhrsen U, Morstyn G, Metcalf D. Effect of recombinant human granulocyte-macrophage colony stimulating factor on progenitor cells in patients with advanced malignancies. Br J Haematol 1990; 74:36–44.

95. Basser R, Begley CG, Mansfield R, To B, Juttner C, Maher D, Fox J, Cebon J, Szer J, Grigg A, Clark K, Marty J, Menchaca D, Thomson B, Russell I, Collins J, Green M. Mobilization of PBPC by priming with stem cell factor (SCF) before filgrastim compared to concurrent administration (abstr). Blood 1995; 86:687a.

2

Preclinical Biology and Potential Clinical Utility of flt3 Ligand

DOUGLAS E. WILLIAMS

Immunex Corporation, Seattle, Washington

I. INTRODUCTION

The flt3 ligand (FL) is a growth and survival factor for hematopoietic stem and progenitor cells. Much of the biology of this molecule shows overlap with a related growth factor, stem cell factor (SCF). There are notable differences, however, including the narrow target cell spectrum of FL versus SCF, the low circulating levels of FL in normal individuals compared to nanogram/milliliter levels of SCF, and the absence of mast cell–associated toxicities with FL. In addition, FL is a potent growth factor for dendritic cells, natural killer cells, and B lymphocytes, but it has no direct erythroid-potentiating activity. Pharmacological administration of FL to experimental animals has demonstrated that it has potent effects on the mobilization of hematopoietic precursors and dendritic cells into the peripheral blood and profound effects on dendritic cell expansion which may allow FL to be used to promote antigen presentation in the tumor and infectious disease settings.

II. flt3 TYROSINE KINASE RECEPTOR

It has become abundantly clear over the last several years that the tyrosine kinase family of receptors plays an important role in the hematopoietic system. This realization has led several independent groups to pursue the identification of new members of this receptor class by various strategies. Rosnet and colleagues (1) used a probe encoding the catalytic domain of the c-fms tyrosine kinase receptor under low-stringency hybridization conditions to isolate complementary deoxyribonucleic acid (cDNA) clones from a mouse testis library. This resulted in the identification of a novel partial cDNA (fms-like tyrosine kinase receptor-3, flt3) and ultimately the human homologue. Matthews and his coworkers (2) took a different tack, using polymerase chain reaction (PCR) to identify a novel sequence they referred to as fetal liver tyrosine kinase-2 (flk2) receptor. As the name flk2 implies, these investigators used mouse fetal liver messenger ribonucleic acid (mRNA) as a source of RNA for their efforts. Small et al. (3) have also used the name stem cell tyrosine kinase receptor-1 (STK-1) to refer to the flt3/flk2 receptor. In this chapter, we will refer to the receptor as flt3.

The flt3 receptor appears to be derived from a common ancestral gene to c-*kit* and c-*fms*, since it shares a common intron/exon structure with these two important hematopoietic growth factor receptors (4). The fms, kit, and flt3 receptors posess five immunoglobulin-like domains in their extracellular regions. In addition they are all characterized by the presence of an unique insert of between 75 and 100 amino acids which splits the kinase region of the cytoplasmic portion of the receptor into two domains. The flt3 receptor has nine potential sites of N-linked glycosylation, at least one of which is utilized (5). The cell surface form of flt3 is approximately 160 kDa, arising from a 140-kDa precursor.

Within the hematopoietic hierarchy, flt3 expression is very restricted. It is not clear whether true pluripotent hematopoietic stem cells are flt3$^-$ or flt3 dim; however, it appears that activated cells which are very primitive in nature express flt3 (6). Within the blast cell compartment of murine bone marrow, only 30% express detectable flt3 (7), and within the human CD34$^+$ compartment, expression of flt3 occurs on a subpopulation of cells at low levels (8). Granulocyte-macrophage–committed precursor colony-forming units–granulocyte-macrophages (CFU-GMs) appear to lose expression of flt3 with progressive differentiation, whereas erythroid-committed precursors are devoid of detectable flt3 (9). Some morphologically recognizable monocytes in the bone marrow have been described as expressing flt3 (7), but these represent the only flt3$^+$-differentiated elements of the hematopoietic hierarchy identified to date. Within the megakaryocyte lineage, expression of flt3 is inferred on the megakaryocyte burst-forming unit (BFU-MK) but weak or absent on the megakaryocyte colony-forming unit (CFU-MK). Outside of the hematopoietic system, flt3 expression is rare, (10) having been described only in testis and brain in addition to the hematolymphoid organs. Tumor cells have not been exhaustively studied except for hematological tumors (11) (where expression of flt3 is common) but do not appear consistently to express flt3.

III. CLONING OF THE flt3L

Lyman et al. (12) and Hannum and coworkers (13) reported the cloning of a ligand for flt3. The flt3 ligand (FL) was isolated by using the extracellular ligand-binding domain of flt3. Lyman et al. (12) used a flt3-Fc fusion protein to screen for cell surface–bound ligand by flow cytometry. A murine T-cell clone was identified which expressed FL on the cell surface, a cDNA library was constructed using RNA from this cell line, and FL was isolated by expression cloning. A thymic stromal line was identified by Hannum and coworkers (13) which secreted FL. The protein was purified using a flt3 affinity column and N-terminal amino acid sequencing.

cDNA clones for FL reveal that the protein product is a type I membrane protein. Mouse and human cDNA clones show that FL is 72% identical at the amino acid level. The membrane-bound form of the molecule is biologically active, similar to stem cell factor (SCF), and a soluble molecule with full biological activity can be released by the actions of an as yet unidentified metalloproteinase enzyme (12). Metalloproteinases have also been implicated in the release of soluble SCF and colony-stimulating factor-1 (CSF-1), but whether the same protease is responsible for shedding of soluble forms of all three ligands is unknown. Cleavage of the membrane-bound FL to give rise to the soluble isoform occurs at a site proximal to the transmembrane region of the protein. It has also been shown that a naturally occurring soluble isoform can be transcribed in the mouse and human by alternate splicing of the sixth exon to introduce a stop codon upstream of the transmembrane region. An abundant message encoding an isoform unable to undergo proteolytic cleavage, and thereby membrane associated at all times, has also been identified in the mouse and is biologically active (14). Thus, FL can exist in soluble and cell-bound forms through a complex alternative splicing pathway (12,13,15).

Expression of FL transcripts and protein has been shown to be very widespread. Northern analysis of a number of human and murine tissues demonstrated the presence of FL transcripts, with the highest levels being seen in peripheral blood mononuclear cells, but they also are present in the heart, lung, liver, kidney, thymus, spleen, testis, brain, skeletal muscle, ovary, and intestine (12,13). Stromal cells express abundant FL, and mature hematopoietic cells such as monocytes, lymphocytes, and neutrophils also express FL. Reports have been published indicating that murine and human cell lines representing a variety of stages and lineages of hematopoiesis express FL. Thus, in contrast to the very restricted pattern of expression of the receptor, flt3, FL is ubiquitously expressed in hematopoietic and nonhematopoietic tissues (Table 1).

IV. BIOLOGICAL EFFECTS OF FL

Initial studies using recombinant human FL have helped to define the target cell spectrum for this growth factor in the hematopoietic hierarchy. FL by itself is a weak stimulus for clonogenic cell growth in vitro but it has been shown to synergize with numerous cytokines. One notable exception to the target cell spectrum of FL are clonogenic red cell precursors. FL fails to synergize with erythropoietin (EPO) to promote growth of burst-forming unit-erythroid (BFU-E) (16,17). Numerous reports have documented the effects of FL on colony-forming units–granulocyte-macrophage (CFU-GM), colony-forming units-granulocyte/erythroid/macrophage/megakaryocyte (CFU-GEMMs), and candidate stem cell populations from bone marrow, peripheral blood, cord blood, and mobilized or steady-state peripheral blood. Noteworthy among these reports are the studies by Gabbianelli et al. (9) and Petzer and coworkers (18,19) and their colleagues showing that FL could promote the expansion of primitive long-term culture-initiating cells (LTCICs) in vitro. LTCICs are thought to be related closely to pluripotent hematopoietic stem cells and suggests that FL is an important regulator of this cellular compartment. Studies carried out with mice with a deletion of the flt3 receptor have shown stem cell defects and further corroborate the importance of FL in maintaining the pool of primitive hematopoietic precursors (20). Further suggestions of the importance of FL on maintaining primitive hematopoietic pool size come from studies examining the levels of circulating FL in various clinical settings of impaired hematopoiesis (15,21). Recently published studies have shown a striking correlation between stem cell pool size, as measured by the in vitro clonogenic capacity of the marrow and elevations in FL levels in aplastic anemia patients (21). A similar correlation was observed in cancer patients receiving cytoreductive therapy between the degree of multilineage myelosuppression and circulating FL levels. This correlation has not been observed in settings where single hematopoietic lineages have been affected.

Table 1 Expression of flt3 and FL

	flt3	FL
	Activated	
	PHSC	
	CFU-BL	Monocytes
	HPP-CFC	
	LTCIC	Lymphocytes
	CFU-GEMM	
Cells	CFU-GM	Neutrophils
	CFU-DC	
	BFU-MK	Fibroblasts
	NK precursor	
	Pre–Pro-B cell	Stromal cells
	Pro-B cell	
	Pro-T cell	
	Thymus	PBMC
		Heart
		Lung
	Bone marrow	Liver
		Kidney
Tissues	Thymus	Thymus
		Spleen
	Brain	Testis
		Brain
	Fetal liver	Skeletal muscle
		Ovary
	Spleen	Intestine

PHSC, pluripotent hematopoietic stem cell; CFU-BL, colony-forming unit-BL; HPP-CFC, high proliferative potential colony-forming cell; LTCIC, Primitive long-term culture-initiating cells; CFU-GEMM, colony-forming unit- granulocyte/erythroid/macrophage/megakaryocyte; CFU-DC, colony-forming unit-DC; BFU-MK, burst-forming unit-megakaryocyte, NK, natural killer

It is also clear that FL is an important regulator of lymphoid development, particularly B lymphocytes and natural killer (NK) cells (8). The role of this growth factor in T lymphopoiesis is less well defined, although reports have been published showing that FL is capable of stimulating proliferation of day 14 fetal thymocytes (13). Further suggestive evidence of a role of FL in T-cell development is the expression of this cytokine in the thymic microenvironment (13). Confounding these data, however, is the lack of apparent T-cell defects in animals which have knockouts (KOs) in either the flt3 receptor or its ligand (8,20). It is clear that FL is important in the early stage of B-lymphocyte development, as expression of flt3 has been demonstrated on pre–pro-B cells with progressive loss as these cells mature to pre-B cells (22). We have observed that FL can enhance the proliferation of early B-lymphoid precursors in synergy with interleukin-7 (IL-7). Similar effects on human B-lymphoid precursors from fetal liver have been seen with FL in combination with IL-3 + IL-7 (23). It is also noteworthy that in flt3 receptor KO mice, there is a dramatic reduction in the pro–B- and pre–B-cell compartments (20), which has now been noted in the ligand KO mice as well (8) by both phenotypic and functional parameters. The ligand KO mice have also pointed out the need for this ligand in the development of the NK cell lineage (8). Animals which lack functional FL do not have detectable functional NK cells in their spleens in contrast to control animals. Furthermore, injection of FL is associated with the expansion of NK cells in vivo and supports the role of FL as a growth factor for the early stages of NK cell development.

Perhaps the most surprising biological activity of FL have been the effects observed on dendritic cells (DCs) (24). Pharmacological administration of FL results in profound increases in the size of the DC pool in various organs. Mobilization of DCs into the peripheral blood of experimental animals treated with FL has also been observed. This DC expansion is transient in nature and completely reversible within 1 week of cessation of treatment. Expansion is seen in all phenotypic subpopulations of DCs, including lymphoid and myeloid-derived DCs. DCs grown under the influence of in vivo FL administration are fully functional in their ability to present both alloantigens and peptide antigens such as keyhole limpet hemocyanin (KLH) (24). These DCs are capable of being pulsed with antigen ex vivo and injected into naive hosts and elicit an antigen-specific immune response against the peptide immunogen. A newly appreciated complexity of the DC pool has been made possible by the ability to propagate sufficient numbers to allow phenotypic and functional studies of this normally rare lineage(s) of cells. It has also been possible to examine the impact of expanding antigen-presenting cells in vivo to see if this can facilitate immune rejection of tumor cells. Studies in several model systems indicate that effective antitumor immunity can be achieved by this approach (25,26).

V. POTENTIAL CLINICAL UTILITY OF FL

Preclinical studies have shown in both primates and mice that FL administration, alone or in combination with granulocyte-macrophage colony-stimulating factor (GM-CSF) or granulocyte colony-stimulating factor (G-CSF) mobilizes large numbers of hematopoietic precursor cells into the peripheral blood (27–29). These cells have long-term, multilineage reconstitution potential in transplant studies. Primate studies with FL and GM-CSF or G-CSF indicated that the volumes of blood required to obtain a transplant dose of CD34+ cells could be significantly reduced (29). These observations have resulted in initiation of clinical studies to examine the utility of FL as a mobilizing agent for peripheral blood stem cells.

The FL may also be useful as a therapeutic agent to facilitate DC expansion to enhance tumor antigen presentation in vivo. Preclinical studies have shown that animals bearing modest tumor burdens can be rendered tumor free or show a reduction in the tumor growth rate when treated with FL alone (26). The mobilization of DCs into the peripheral blood also suggests that it may be possible to collect mobilized DCs in greater numbers for ex vivo antigen pulsing and reinfusion or as part of a cocktail of cytokines which could promote growth of DCs from CD34+ cells. In any event, FL is likely to become an important growth factor in any strategies involving manipulation of DCs for therapeutic purposes.

ACKNOWLEDGMENTS

The author wishes to acknowledge all of the collaborators at Immunex who have made contributions to this program. In particular, Stewart Lyman, Ken Brasel, Hilary McKenna, Eugene Maraskovsky, and David Lynch have contributed greatly.

REFERENCES

1. Rosnet O, Marchetto S, deLapeyriere O, Birnbaum D. Murine flt3, a gene encoding a novel tyrosine kinase receptor of the PDGFR/CSF1R family. Oncogene 1991; 6:1641–1650.

2. Matthews W, Jordan CT, Wiegand GW, Pardoll D, Lemischka IR. A receptor tyrosine kinase specific to hematopoietic stem and progenitor cell-enriched populations. Cell 1991; 65:1143–1152.

3. Small D, Levenstein M, Kim E, Carow C, Amin S, Rockwell P, Witte L, Burrow C, Ratajczak MZ, Gerwirtz AM, Civin CI. STK-1, the human homolog of flt3/flk2, is selectively expressed in CD34+ human bone marrow cells and is involved in the proliferation of early progenitor/stem cells. Proc Natl Acad Sci U.S.A. 1994; 91:459–463.

4. Agnès F, Shamoon B, Dina C, Rosnet O, Birnbaum D, Galibert F. Genomic structure of the downstream part of the human flt3 gene: exon/intron structure conservation among genes encoding receptor tyrosine kinases (RTK) of subclass III. Gene 1994; 145:283–288.

5. Lyman SD, James L, Zappone J, Sleath PR, Beckmann MP, Bird T. Characterization of the protein encoded by the flt3/flk2 receptor–like tyrosine kinase gene. Oncogene 1993; 8:815–822.

6. Zeigler FC, Bennett BD, Jordan CT, Spencer SD, Baumhueter S, Carroll KJ, Hooley J, Bauer K, Matthews W. Cellular and molecular characterization of the role of the flt3/flk2 receptor tyrosine kinase in hematopoietic stem cells. Blood 1994; 84:2422–2430.

7. Rask JEJ, Metcalf D, Rossner MT, Begley CG, Nicola NA. The flt3/flk2 ligand: receptor distribution and action on murine hemopoietic cell survival and proliferation. Leukemia 1995; 9:2058–2066.

8. McKenna HJ, Miller RE, Brasel KE, Maraskovsky E, Maliszewski C, Pulendran B, Lynch D, Teepe M, Roux ER, Smith J, Williams DE, Lyman SD, Peschon JJ, Stocking K. Targeted disruption of the flt3 ligand gene in mice affects multiple hematopoietic lineages, including natural killer cells, B lymphocytes, and dendritic cells. Blood 1996; 88:474a.

9. Gabbianelli M, Pelosi E, Montesoro E, Valtieri M, Luchetti L, Samoggia P, Vitelli L, Barberi T, Testa U, Lyman S, Peschle C. Multi-level effects of flt3 ligand on human hematopoiesis: expansion of putative stem cells and proliferation of granulomonocytic progenitors/monocytic precursors. Blood 1995; 86:1661–1670.

10. deLapeyriere O, Naquet P, Planche J, Marchetto S, Rottapel R, Gambarelli D, Rosnet O, Birnbaum D. Expression of flt3 tyrosine kinase receptor gene. In mouse hematopoietic and nervous tissues. Differentiation 1995; 58:351–359.

11. Brasel K, Escobar S, Anderberg R, deVries P, Gruss H-J, Lyman SD. Expression of the flt3 receptor and its ligand on hematopoietic cells. Leukemia 1995; 9:1212–1218.

12. Lyman SD, James L, VandenBos T, deVries P, Brasel K, Gliniak B, Hollingsworth LT, Picha KS, McKenna HJ, Splett RR, Fletcher FF, Maraskovsky E, Farrah T, Foxworthe D, Williams DE, Beckmann MP. Molecular cloning of a ligand for the flt3/flk2 tyrosine kinase receptor: A proliferative factor for primitive hematopoietic cells. Cell 1993; 75:1157–1167.

13. Hannum C, Culpepper J, Campbell D, McClanahan T, Zurawski S, Bazan JF, Kastelein R, Hudak S, Wagner J, Mattson J, Luh J, Duda G, Martina N, Peterson D, Menon S, Shanafelt A, Muench M, Kelner G, Namikawa R, Rennick D, Roncarolo M-G, Zlotnick A, Rosnet O, Dubreuil P, Birnbaum D, Lee F. Ligand for flt3 / flk2 receptor tyrosine kinase regulates growth of haematopoietic stem cells and is encoded by variant RNAs. Nature 1994; 368:643–648.

14. Lyman SD, James L, Escobar S, Downey H, de Vries P, Brasel K, Stocking K, Beckmann MP, Copeland NG, Cleveland LS, Jenkins NA, Belmont JW, Davison BL. Identification of soluble and membrane-bound isoforms of the murine flt3 ligand generated by alternative splicing of mRNAs. Oncogene 1995; 10:149–157.

15. Lyman SD, Seaberg M, Hanna R, Zappone J, Brasel K, Abkowitz JL, Prchal JT, Schultz JC, Shahidi NT. Plasma/serum levels of flt3 ligand are low in normal individuals and highly elevated in patients with Fanconi anemia and acquired aplastic anemia. Blood 1995; 86:4091–4096.

16. Broxmeyer HE, Lu L, Cooper S, Ruggieri L, Li ZH, Lyman SD. Flt3 ligand stimulates costimu-
    lates the growth of myeloid stem/progenitor cells. Exp Hematol 1995; 23:1121–1129.
17. McKenna HJ, deVries P, Brasel K, Lyman SD, Williams DE. Effect of flt3 ligand on the ex
    vivo expansion of human CD34$^+$ hematopoietic progenitor cells. Blood 1995; 86:3413–3420.
18. Petzer AL, Hogge DE, Landsdrop PM, Reid DS, Eaves CJ. Self-renewal of primitive human
    hematopoietic cells (long-term-culture-initiating cell) in vitro and their expansion in defined
    medium. Proc Natl Acad Sci U.S.A. 1996; 93:1470–1474.
19. Petzer AL, Zandstra PW, Piret JM, Eaves CJ. Differential cytokine effects on primitive
    (CD34$^+$ CD38$^-$) human hematopoietic cells: novel responses to flt3$^-$ ligand and thrombopoie-
    tin. J Exp Med 1996; 183:2551–2558.
20. Mackarehtschian K, Hardin JD, Moore KA, Boast S, Goff SP, Lemischka IR. Targeted disrup-
    tion of the flt3/flk2 gene leads to deficiencies in primitive hematopoietic progenitors. Immunity
    1995; 3:147–161.
21. Wodnar-Filipowicz A, Lyman SD, Gratwohl A, Tichelli A, Speck B, Nissen C. Flt3 ligand
    level reflects hematopoietic progenitor cell function in multilineage bone marrow failure.
    Blood 1996; 88:4493–4499.
22. Hunte BE, Hudak S, Cambell D, Xu Y, Rennick D. Flt3/flk2 ligand is a potent cofactor for
    the growth of primative B cell progenitors. J Immunol 1996; 156:489–496.
23. Namikawa R, Muench MO, deVries JE, Roncarolo MG. The flt3/flk2 ligand synergizes with
    interleukin-7 in promoting stromal-cell–independent expansion and differentiation of human
    fetal pro-B cells in vitro. Blood 1996; 87:1881–1890.
24. Maraskovsky E, Brasel K, Teepe M, Roux ER, Lyman SD, Shortman K, McKenna HJ. Dra-
    matic increase in the numbers of the functionally mature dendritic cells in flt3 ligand-treated
    mice: Multiple dendritic cell subpopulations identified. J Exp Med 1996; 184:1953–1962.
25. Chen K, Braun SE, Lyman SD, Broxmeyer HE, Cornetta K. Soluble and membrane bound
    isoforms of flt3-ligand induce antitumor immunity in vivo. Blood 1996; 88:274a.
26. Lynch DH, Andreasen A, Maraskovsky E, Whitmore J, Miller RE, Schuh JCL. Flt3 ligand
    induces tumor regression and anti-tumor immune responses in vivo. Nature Med 1997; 3:625–
    631.
27. Brasel K, McKenna HJ, Charrier K, Morrissey P, Williams DE, Lyman SD. Synergistic effects
    in vivo of flt3 ligand with GM-CSF or G-CSF in mobilization of colony forming cells in mice.
    Blood 1995; 86:499a.
28. Brasel K, McKenna HJ, Williams DE, Lyman SD. Flt3 ligand mobilized hematopoietic pro-
    genitor cells are capable of reconstituting multiple lineages in lethally irradiated recipient mice.
    Blood 1996; 88:601a.
29. Winton EF, Bucur SZ, Bond LD, Hegwood AJ, Hillyer CD, Holland HK, Williams DE, Mc-
    Clure HM, Troutt AB, Lyman SD. Recombinant human (rh) flt3 ligand plus rhGM-CSF or
    rhG-CSF causes a marked CD34$^+$ cell mobilization to blood in rhesus monkeys. Blood 1996;
    88:642a.

3

Stem Cell Factor

LEO LACERNA, JR. and WILLIAM P. SHERIDAN

Amgen Inc., Thousand Oaks, California

RUSSELL BASSER

Royal Melbourne Hospital, Melbourne, Australia

C. GLENN BEGLEY

Western Australia Institute for Medical Research, Perth, Australia

JEFFREY CRAWFORD

Duke University Medical Center, Durham, North Carolina

GEORGE DEMETRI

Dana-Farber Cancer Institute, Boston, Massachusetts

CRAIG H. MOSKOWITZ

Memorial Sloan-Kettering Cancer Center, New York, New York

GUIDO TRICOT

University of Arkansas for Medical Sciences, Little Rock, Arkansas

ANDREW WEAVER

Christie Hospital, Manchester, England

JOHN A. GLASPY

University of California School of Medicine, Los Angeles, California

I. INTRODUCTION

Efforts to understand mutations in inbred laboratory mice leading to abnormalities of coat color, hematopoiesis, and fertility began 4 decades ago and were ultimately explained after the characterization of stem cell factor (SCF) and its receptor, c-*kit*. The history, biochemistry, and preclinical biology of SCF have been described in an extensive review by Galli et al. (1) and elsewhere (2–6). (Note that reviews are frequently cited as references; reviews are indicated as such at the end of their citations in the reference list.)

The purpose of this chapter is to focus on clinical studies of patients undergoing transplantation of hematopoietic peripheral blood progenitor cells (PBPCs), and to relate these recent observations to preclinical findings and relevant clinical questions: Will SCF, when combined with filgrastim [granulocyte colony-stimulating factor (G-CSF)], be useful in PBPC transplantation? Will the combination mobilize increased numbers of PBPCs and improve the yield of leukapheresis? Will this facilitate multiple cycles of high-dose chemotherapy? Will SCF/filgrastim-mobilized PBPCs shorten the time to engraftment? Will adding SCF to filgrastim increase the number of patients who are candidates for PBPC transplantation?

II. BASIC BIOLOGY

Mutations at the white spotting (*W*) and steel (*Sl*) loci in mice can lead to similar phenotypic abnormalities in multiple tissues (1,7). Depending on their severity, the mutations can adversely affect hematopoiesis, gametogenesis, pigmentation, and tissue mast cells, with manifestations in both the developing and adult animal. If mutations are severe, the animals die in utero. With less severe mutations, the classic spectrum of phenotypic abnormalities may include macrocytic anemia, sterility, lack of pigmentation in the skin and coat hairs, and lack of tissue mast cells (1,4–6).

The results of transplantation, embryo fusion, and in vitro analyses indicate that the *W* defect is cell autonomous or intrinsic to the affected cell, whereas the *Sl* defect is attributable to the lack of a product secreted by cells in the microenvironment. Russell (7) hypothesized that the *W* locus might encode a receptor and the *Sl* locus might encode the corresponding ligand. Subsequent studies confirmed that the *W* locus coincides with the c-*kit* gene, which was previously described as a proto-oncogene encoding a tyrosine kinase receptor. The *Sl* locus encodes the corresponding ligand, which has multiple names, including SCF, c-*kit* ligand, Steel factor, and mast cell growth factor (1,5,6). This chapter uses the terms *SCF* for the ligand and c-*kit* for the receptor.

In mice, hematopoietic stem and progenitor cells, gametocytes, melanocytes, and mast cells express c-*kit*. Cells that are anatomically juxtaposed to the c-*kit*–expressing cells, such as bone marrow stromal cells, testicular Sertoli cells, and skin keratinocytes, express SCF. Although no single clinical condition corresponds with the full scope of abnormalities seen in mutant c-*kit* (*W*) and SCF (*Sl*) mice, defects in c-*kit* have been detected in humans with the piebald trait, which is manifested by patches of hypopigmented skin and hair (1).

The SCF gene is found on chromosome 10 in mice and on chromosome 12 in humans. SCF is initially expressed in two membrane-bound forms dictated by alternative messenger RNA splicing (1,4–6). The longer of these two forms, after removal of a 25–amino acid signal sequence, has 248 amino acids (SCF^{248}): 189 amino acids in an extracellular domain, 23 amino acids in a transmembrane domain, and 36 amino acids in a cytoplasmic domain. The extracellular domain of SCF^{248} has a proteolytic cleavage site after amino acid 165, which leads to release of a soluble molecule (SCF^{165}). The shorter of the two membrane-bound forms has 220 amino acids (SCF^{220}) and a smaller extracellular domain (161 amino acids); SCF^{220} essentially lacks 28 amino acids found in SCF^{248}, namely, amino acids 149 through 177, which are encoded by exon 6 of the SCF gene. Because this missing segment contains the proteolytic cleavage site, this shorter form tends to remain membrane bound.

SCF was purified in 1989–1990, and Zsebo and colleagues (8) first cloned the human gene. Native soluble SCF is a heavily glycosylated protein with a molecular weight of approximately 53 kDa in its homodimeric form, including the carbohydrate moieties (1,4–6). The sequence of amino acids is reasonably homologous among species, with, for example, approximately 83% homology between human and murine forms. When soluble SCF is produced by recombinant DNA technology in *Escherichia coli*, the resultant protein is a noncovalently associated homodimer with a molecular weight of 37 kDa. Each monomer consists of 166 amino acids. The primary differences between this form of recombinant SCF and native SCF are that the recombinant form is nonglycosylated and contains an additional amino acid [N-terminal methionine at position (-1)], hence, the designation recombinant methionyl human SCF (r-metHuSCF). Unless otherwise indicated, SCF will refer to r-metHuSCF for the remainder of this chapter.

III. PRECLINICAL STUDIES

The availability of recombinant forms of SCF triggered a series of in vitro and in vivo studies (1,4–6). In vitro, the hallmark of SCF action is pronounced synergy with later-acting hematopoietic factors, which, for example, promotes both the number and size of in vitro colonies derived from hematopoietic progenitors. The colony types generally reflect the lineage specificity of the later-acting factor(s) present, such as erythroid burst-forming units (BFU-Es) in the presence of SCF and erythropoietin. The in vitro effects of SCF on germ cells, melanocytes, and mast cells have also been studied. In vivo studies, first in experimental models and ultimately in humans, indicate that SCF, alone and in combination with other growth factors, promotes the survival and proliferation of primitive and more committed hematopoietic progenitor cells in a dose-related fashion. The following sections summarize representative preclinical studies.

A. Effects of SCF on Hematopoiesis in Animals

Species-specific SCF can increase the numbers of hematopoietic cells of multiple lineages in the peripheral blood in rodents (9–12), dogs (13), and baboons (14,15). The primary effects are dose related and include leukocytosis manifested as neutrophilia and marked increases in the number of primitive hematopoietic cells in both the bone marrow and peripheral blood. Rat SCF enhances the effect of filgrastim on leukocytosis in normal mice (9). Rat SCF also corrects the macrocytic anemia seen in *Sl* mutant mice (16) and has a radioprotective effect in mice (17). Human SCF reduces the duration of chemotherapy-induced neutropenia in monkeys (18).

In addition to its effects on hematopoiesis, human SCF expands the mast cell population in monkeys and baboons (19). The resulting mast cell hyperplasia is reversible after discontinuation of SCF and is not associated with obvious clinical evidence of mast cell activation (19).

B. Mobilizing Effects of SCF plus Filgrastim on PBPCs in Animals

Species-specific SCF combined with filgrastim increases PBPCs in rodents (9,20,21), dogs (22), and baboons (23). The doses of SCF used in these studies were low and, in fact, produced minimal effects if used alone.

When low-dose SCF is added to optimal doses of filgrastim, the combination is synergistic. PBPCs mobilized by SCF plus filgrastim rescue lethally irradiated animals, leading to complete restoration of bone marrow function.

Individual studies provide quantitative and qualitative insights regarding the synergistic activity of SCF combined with filgrastim. Compared with filgrastim 200 µg/kg alone, rat SCF 25 µg/kg plus filgrastim 200 µg/kg administered to splenectomized mice led to 1.5-fold increases in peripheral white blood cells (WBCs), fivefold increases in peripheral blood GM-CFCs, and twofold increases in peripheral blood high-proliferative–potential colony-forming cells (HPP-CFCs). Moreover, the combination is associated with more than fivefold increases in the number of cells with in vivo repopulating ability (20). Transplantation of PBPCs mobilized by the combination produces more rapid engraftment with fewer cells than transplantation of PBPCs mobilized by either hematopoietic growth factor alone (20). When lethally irradiated mice are transplanted with 5×10^6 peripheral blood low-density mononuclear cells (LDMNCs), the survival rate is higher if LDMNCs are obtained after treatment with the combination (80%) than if obtained after treatment with filgrastim alone (40%) (24).

Long-term hematopoietic reconstitution after transplantation with PBPCs mobilized by SCF plus filgrastim can be shown by serial transplantation. Transplantation of PBPCs mobilized by SCF plus filgrastim results in donor engraftment in 98% of primary recipients 11–14 months after transplantation (25). Six months after harvesting and transplanting bone marrow cells from primary recipients, donor engraftment can be demonstrated in 100% of the secondary recipients (25). Finally, 6 months after harvesting and transplanting bone marrow cells from the secondary recipients, donor engraftment can be demonstrated in 90% of tertiary recipients (25). These findings indicate that PBPCs mobilized by SCF plus filgrastim are not only transplantable but are also able to maintain hematopoiesis for more than 2 years. Furthermore, mobilized long-term reconstituting stem cells appear to resemble those residing in bone marrow.

In dogs, a 7-day course of canine SCF 25 µg/kg/day and canine G-CSF 10 µg/kg/day dramatically increases the numbers of hematopoietic progenitor cells and GM-CFCs in peripheral blood (22). Irradiated dogs can be rescued by transplantation of 1×10^8 peripheral blood mononuclear cells mobilized by the combination or by either hematopoietic growth factor alone (SCF alone administered at 200 µg/kg/day). In contrast, irradiation is uniformly lethal if donor animals are not pretreated with a hematopoietic growth factor. Importantly, the combination is associated with more rapid engraftment than either high-dose SCF (200 µg/kg/day) alone or G-CSF alone (22).

In baboons, combining low-dose SCF with filgrastim induces a more sustained increase in numbers of multilineage hematopoietic progenitors compared with either filgrastim alone or SCF alone (Fig. 1) (23). Increases in the numbers of GM-CFCs, BFU-Es, and MK-CFUs in the peripheral blood are evident after the second day of treatment, continue throughout a 14-day course, and are rapidly reversible after discontinuation. The synergy between SCF and filgrastim is dose and time dependent (23).

These findings prompted a study to evaluate the effects of PBPCs mobilized by SCF plus filgrastim in lethally irradiated baboons (26). Leukapheresis products contain 2-fold more mononuclear cells and 14-fold more progenitor cells if baboons are treated with the combination than if they receive filgrastim alone. After lethal irradiation, baboons achieve engraftment earlier if they are transplanted with cells mobilized by the combination than by filgrastim alone regardless of whether engraftment is defined as recovery of WBCs, neutrophils, or platelets. For example, the mean time to reach an absolute neutrophil count

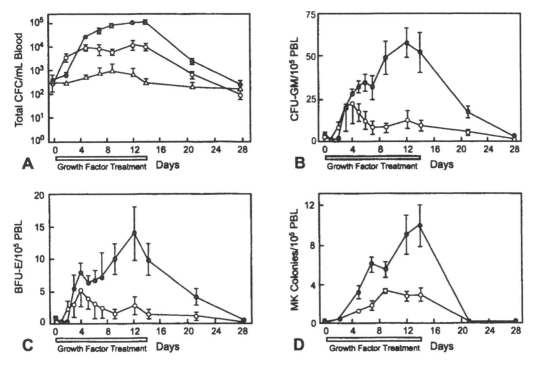

Figure 1   Changes in PBPCs in baboons during treatment with SCF 25 µg/kg/day (n = 4), fil-grastim 100 µg/kg/day (n = 6), or both (n = 9). CFC, colony-forming cell (CFU-GM plus BFU-E); CFU-GM, colony-forming units-granulocyte-macrophage; BFU-E, burst-forming units-erythroid; MK, megakaryocyte; PBL, peripheral blood lymphocyte. (From Ref. 23.)

(ANC) of 0.5×10^9/L is 12 days with cells mobilized by the combination versus 24 days with cells mobilized by filgrastim alone ($P < .05$) (26).

IV. CLINICAL STUDIES

During the past decade, it has become apparent that autologous PBPCs, when available in sufficient quantity, can be used effectively for transplantation and hematopoietic reconstitution after high-dose chemoradiotherapy in the treatment of various cancers (27). It has been found that the normally low numbers of PBPCs can be dramatically enhanced (reaching counts feasible for harvesting and transplantation) by the administration (alone and in combination) of agents such as chemotherapeutics, G-CSF, and GM-CSF. The multilineage hematopoietic engraftment after PBPC transplantation can be durable and, if anything, more rapid than that after bone marrow transplantation. In addition, the leukapheresis procedure(s) used for PBPC harvesting is less invasive to the patient than bone marrow harvesting.

The cell surface marker CD34 has emerged as the most adequate and reliable single indicator of the quantity and quality of desired cells in a human PBPC harvest. Generally speaking, "more is better" with regard to the CD34$^+$-cell number in a PBPC harvest. Transplantation of $\geq 5 \times 10^6$ CD34$^+$ cells per kilogram of body weight typically leads to rapid and durable ("optimal") engraftment, whereas $1–2 \times 10^6$ CD34$^+$ cells/kg is typically used as a lower limit of harvested cells required to proceed with high-dose chemoradiotherapy and PBPC transplantation (27–30).

The results of preclinical studies and of phase I clinical studies provided the basis for a series of additional clinical studies comparing the use of SCF in combination with filgrastim (±chemotherapeutics) to the use of filgrastim (±chemotherapeutics) alone for mobilization of PBPCs for harvesting and transplantation. The clinical studies have explored the ability of SCF plus filgrastim to enable mobilization of adequate or optimal levels of PBPCs harvested with a minimum number of leukaphereses. Phase I and clinical safety observations are summarized at the end of Section IV. This section focuses on biological findings in patients receiving SCF combined with filgrastim, beginning with an introduction to the clinical studies. This is followed by descriptions of the effects of SCF plus filgrastim on levels of peripheral blood leukocytes and on mobilization of PBPCs and of the effects of SCF/filgrastim–mobilized PBPC on engraftment.

A. Overview of SCF Studies in Humans

Table 1 summarizes the designs of studies in patients with breast cancer (29,31–33), non-Hodgkin's lymphoma (30,34), multiple myeloma (35,36), or ovarian carcinoma (37,38). Patients were randomized to receive filgrastim alone or filgrastim combined with sequentially escalating doses of SCF (5–30 µg/kg/day) in several of the studies. Based on these SCF dose-ranging studies, patients in subsequent studies were randomized to receive filgrastim alone or filgrastim combined with a fixed dose of SCF (20 µg/kg/day). In two of the studies, chemotherapy was used for mobilization along with the cytokine(s). The dose of filgrastim was fixed within any given study [10 or 12 µg/kg/day for studies with cytokine(s)-only mobilization, and 5 µg/kg/day for studies with chemotherapy plus cytokine(s) mobilization]. The cytokine(s) were administered subcutaneously for 5–13 days depending on the study and the patient. PBPCs were harvested using a predefined, fixed number of leukaphereses in the earlier studies or, in the later studies, using the number of leukaphereses (for any particular patient) required to obtain a predefined target quantity of harvested CD34$^+$ cells. Most patients had received previous, often extensive, chemotherapy; however, patients with previously untreated cancer were enrolled in two of the studies.

B. Effects of SCF plus Filgrastim on Peripheral Blood Leukocytes

As expected, administration of filgrastim alone or SCF plus filgrastim increases the number of peripheral WBCs, generally to peak levels on the order of $50–100 \times 10^9/L$ (29,31,33,34). Relative to the use of filgrastim alone, the use of SCF plus filgrastim appears to increase the peak WBC levels slightly (<1.5-fold depending on the SCF dose). There have been no clinical sequelae associated with leukocytosis, and the leukocytosis reverses after discontinuation of therapy (29,31,33,34). Administration of SCF plus filgrastim does not affect hemoglobin concentrations or platelet counts (29,34).

C. PBPC-Mobilizing Effects of SCF plus Filgrastim

The administration of SCF in combination with filgrastim during periods of up to 2 weeks has led to higher peak levels of PBPCs than administration of filgrastim alone. In addition, and of clinical relevance, the kinetics of PBPC mobilization with SCF plus filgrastim has differed from that for mobilization with filgrastim alone. Peak levels of PBPCs are reached

Table 1 Design of Randomized, Controlled Studies to Assess the Efficacy of SCF plus Filgrastim in PBPC Mobilization[a]

Refs.	Phase	Tumor	Prior chemoradiotherapy	Primary objectives	PBPC collection			No. of patients		r-metHuSCF plus filgrastim:filgrastim alone			
					Mobilization regimen	Doses of SCF (µg/kg/day)	Method	SCF plus G-CSF	G-CSF alone	Median CD34+ cells/kg (×10⁶) per leukapheresis	Proportion of patients reaching target of 5 × 10⁶ CD34+ cells/kg	Median no. of leukaphereses to reach 5 × 10⁶ CD34+ cells/kg	PBPC transplant method
34	I–II	Lymphoma (NHL)	Moderate/extensive	PBPC mobilization, hematopoietic reconstitution, and safety	Cytokines only (7 days)	5, 10, 15, 20	Three leukaphereses (last 3 days of cytokines)	18[c]	5[c]	0.59:0.09	11:0	≥4:≥4	Single transplant
31, 32	I–II	Breast (high-risk stage II/III)	None	PBPC mobilization, hematopoietic reconstitution, and safety	Cytokines only (7 days)	5, 10, 15	Three leukaphereses (last 3 days of cytokines)	44	18	6.69:3.81	97:83	1:2	Multiple cycles (3); high-dose chemotherapy
29	I–II	Breast (high-risk, stage II/III/IV)	Moderate	PBPC mobilization, hematopoietic reconstitution, and safety	Cytokines only (7, 10 or 13 days)	5, 10, 15, 20, 25, 30	Three leukaphereses (last 3 days of cytokines)	160	55	2.57:1.10	51:35	3:≥4	Single transplant
37, 38	I–II	Ovarian (stage Ic–V)	None	PBPC mobilization, hematopoietic reconstitution, and safety	Chemo plus cytokines	5, 10, 15, 20	One leukapheresis[d]	33	12	9.06:3.18	79:42	1:≥2	Multiple cycles (4)
36	II	Myeloma	Moderate	CS34+ cell mobilization to a target, and safety	Chemo plus cytokines	20	Target CS34+ 5 × 10⁶/kg[d,e]	55	47	9.42:2.5	85:77	1:2	Single transplant
30	II	Lymphoma (NHL, HD)	Extensive	CD34+ cell mobilization to a target, and safety	Cytokines only	20	Target CD34+ 5 × 10⁶/kg[f]	48	54	0.73:0.48	44:17	≥6:≥6	Single transplant
35	II	Myeloma	Extensive	CD34+ cell mobilization to a target, and safety	Cytokines only	20	Target CS34+ 10 × 10⁶/kg[e,f]	18	21	0.90:0.75	50:33	5:≥7	Two transplants
33	III	Breast (high-risk stage II/III/IV)	Moderate	CD34+ cell mobilization to a target, and safety	Cytokines only	20	Target CD34+ 5 × 10⁶/kg[f]	100	103	1.69:1.00	63:47	4:≥6	Single transplant

[a] SCF and filgrastim (G-CSF) administered subcutaneously in all studies.
[b] Only patients receiving 20 µg/kg/day and with fixed number of leukaphereses are included.
[c] Includes only patients defined as heavily pretreated.
[d] Leukaphereses initiated when WBCs reached ≥4 × 10⁹/L after the chemotherapy (cyclophosphamide)–induced nadir; cytokine(s) administration was started 2 days after the cyclophosphamide in the case of Weaver et al. (38) and 1 day after the cyclophosphamide in the case of Facon et al. (36).
[e] Maximum of four leukaphereses (36), five leukaphereses (30, 33), or six leukaphereses (35).
[f] Leukaphereses initiated on day 5 of cytokine administration.

within a few days (about day 5 to day 6) in each case and then begin to decline (despite continued cytokine administration). However, in the case of SCF plus filgrastim, the decline tends to be much more gradual, and PBPC levels remained elevated for at least a week after the cessation of treatment. These phenomena were apparent when blood aliquots taken from the peripheral circulation were analyzed (29,31,32), and since PBPC determinations made directly on whole blood aliquots correlate reasonably well with determinations made on leukapheresis products collected on a daily basis (e.g., see Ref. 32), the phenomena were also apparent when the latter were analyzed (33). Because of the higher peak levels of PBPCs and the more gradual decline from the peak, there is a larger window for collection and a larger "area under the curve" with SCF plus filgrastim.

In the ovarian cancer patient study (38) and one of the multiple myeloma studies (36), in which chemotherapy for mobilization was given 1 or 2 days before the start of daily filgrastim ± SCF for mobilization, peak PBPC counts were not reached until about 10–11 days (median) after the start of cytokines. This delayed kinetics of mobilization has been observed in other clinical studies using chemotherapy and G-CSF for mobilization (27,28), and it is most likely due to the myelosuppressive effects of the chemotherapy.

In certain of the SCF dose-ranging studies, the effects on PBPC levels in the blood and in leukapheresis products were generally dose responsive over the 5–30 µg/kg/day dose range that was studied (29,38) (Fig. 2). The results led to selection of 20 µg/kg/day for the fixed SCF–dose studies (see Table 1).

The extent of the increase in the peak peripheral blood CD34$^+$ cell levels, as measured in whole blood aliquots, has been about two- to threefold for SCF plus filgrastim administration versus administration of filgrastim alone. This was the case when no chemotherapy for mobilization was used (29) and also when chemotherapy was used along with the filgrastim ±SCF (38). Similar increases (three- to fivefold for SCF plus filgrastim vs filgrastim alone) have been seen using additional measures of PBPCs; that is, CFU-GMs and BFU-Es (31,38). The "day-of-start" criteria for daily leukaphereses, and the total number of leukaphereses carried out (e.g., predefined fixed number or variable number when leukapheresing to a target CD34$^+$ cell yield; see Table 1) have differed between studies. In general, for the combined total leukapheresis products (per patient) in studies which specified a predefined fixed number of leukaphereses, increases in CD34$^+$ cell yields for SCF plus filgrastim patient groups versus filgrastim-alone patient groups have been in the range of two- to threefold (29,31,32,38). For the combined total leukapheresis prod-

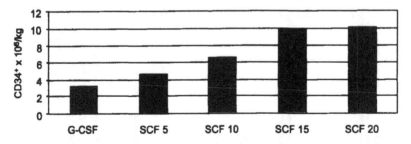

Figure 2 Median CD34$^+$ cells in the leukapheresis products obtained from 48 patients with ovarian cancer randomized to receive filgrastim (G-CSF) alone or in combination with sequentially escalating doses of SCF, each beginning 48 h after chemotherapy. Doses are in µg/kg/day. (From Ref. 38.)

ucts in studies which specified leukaphereses to a target CD34$^+$ cell yield, increases in CD34$^+$ cell yields for the SCF plus filgrastim groups versus the filgrastim-alone groups have been less; that is, in the range of 1.1- to 1.5-fold (30,33). This is at least partly because patients in the SCF plus filgrastim groups have generally required fewer leukaphereses to reach the specified target CD34$^+$ cell yields (as discussed below). For all studies, the median CD34$^+$ cells/kg per leukapheresis values are given in Table 1 for the SCF plus filgrastim groups versus the filgrastim-alone groups. The values generally ranged from 1.5- to 3-fold higher for the SCF plus filgrastim groups versus the corresponding filgrastim-alone groups.

The extent of prior chemotherapy and/or radiotherapy is well established as a risk factor for poor mobilization (27,28). Several of the SCF/filgrastim–mobilization studies were carried out in the settings of lymphoma (non-Hodgkin's lymphoma and Hodgkin's disease) or myeloma. Lymphoma and myeloma patients tend to have undergone considerable prior chemoradiotherapy before being considered for high-dose chemotherapy and transplantation, and this was the case for patients included in the lymphoma studies and one of the multiple myeloma studies with SCF/filgrastim. The other studies (ovarian cancer, breast cancer, and the second of the multiple myeloma studies) enrolled patients who had received moderate prior chemoradiotherapy or no prior chemoradiotherapy (see Table 1). In general, it can be seen in Table 1 that, overall, poorer efficacy of mobilization correlated with greater extent of prior chemoradiotherapy. This correlation was borne out by detailed statistical analyses within individual studies as well. However, regardless of the overall efficacy of mobilization within any given study population, there was benefit provided by the added use of SCF. Thus, patients receiving SCF with filgrastim generally yielded more CD34$^+$ cells (per leukapheresis and also for the total of all leukaphereses per patient; see above); were more likely to reach the "optimal" target of 5×10^6 CD34$^+$ cells/kg (see Table 1); were more likely to reach this optimal target with fewer leukaphereses (see Table 1); and also were more likely to yield the minimum number of CD34$^+$ cells ($1–2 \times 10^6$/kg) required to proceed to high-dose chemotherapy and transplantation (29,30). The last of these benefits, that is, an increased likelihood of yielding the minimum number of CD34$^+$ cells, may be particularly applicable to hard-to-mobilize patients [e.g., those with more extensive prior chemoradiotherapy (27,28,34)].

As discussed, when SCF is administered with filgrastim, there is generally a reduction in the number of (daily) leukaphereses needed to reach a CD34$^+$ cell target yield (e.g., 5×10^6/kg). This can result in greater convenience and safety to the patient and a reduction in medical costs.

In the phase III breast cancer study, tumor cell contamination in the bone marrow at baseline, in the peripheral blood during mobilization, and in the collected leukapheresis products was thoroughly compared for the SCF plus filgrastim group versus the filgrastim-alone group (33). For both groups, contamination in the bone marrow was most frequent. Frequency of contamination in the peripheral blood during mobilization and in the leukapheresis products was equivalently low for both groups. There was no indication that either treatment regimen led to mobilization of tumor cells from the bone marrow to the peripheral blood.

When filgrastim alone is used for mobilization, the dosing is typically about 10 μg/kg/day or about 5 μg/kg/day when chemotherapy for mobilization is used along with the filgrastim (27). All the SCF/filgrastim studies used filgrastim at these fixed doses (±SCF). Further clinical study of the mobilizing effects of higher doses of filgrastim alone (27,39), and of higher doses of filgrastim in combination with SCF, may be warranted. In a baboon model, SCF has enhanced the mobilizing effects of filgrastim over a range of filgrastim doses (23).

D. Mobilizing Effects of SCF plus Filgrastim on Very Primitive PBPCs

In one of the clinical studies that utilized chemotherapy along with the cytokine(s) for mobilization, the proportion of very primitive PBPCs in the leukapheresis products was measured by $CD34^+$ cell surface marker subset analysis and by in vitro functional analysis (37). The $CD33^-$ subset of $CD34^+$ cells ($CD34^+CD33^-$; CD33 = myeloid lineage differentiation marker) is considered to be more primitive than the $CD33^+$ subset ($CD34^+CD33^+$). For the filgrastim-alone group in the study by Weaver et al. (37), the median $CD34^+$ cell yield was 3.2×10^6/kg, whereas the median $CD34^+CD33^-$ cell subset yield was 0.084×10^6/kg; that is, only 2.6% of the $CD34^+$ cells were also $CD33^-$. For the groups receiving filgrastim plus dose-escalating SCF, there was a dose-dependent enhancement of $CD34^+$ cell yield with a much higher proportion (28–55%) of $CD34^+$ cells being $CD33^-$; for the group receiving filgrastim plus the highest dose of SCF (20 µg/kg/ day), the median $CD34^+$ cell yield was 10.1×10^6/kg and the median $CD34^+CD33^-$ cell subset yield was 5.55×10^6/kg; that is, 55% of the $CD34^+$ cells were also $CD33^-$. Thus, overall, the difference in $CD34^+CD33^-$ cell yield between the filgrastim-only group and the filgrastim/20 µg/kg/day SCF group was 66-fold. Moreover, there were SCF dose–dependent increases in the leukapheresis product frequency of long-term culture-initiating cells (LT-CICs), which are considered to be the most primitive of human progenitor cells definable in vitro (27,40). The median frequency of LT-CICs for the filgrastim/20 µg/ kg/day SCF group was 1 per 78 $CD34^+$ cells, whereas the median frequency for the filgrastim-alone group was 1 per 205 $CD34^+$ cells, such that the overall increase in the level of LT-CICs was 8.3-fold. It is reasonable to speculate that a higher level of more primitive progenitors provided in a transplant could be advantageous for long-term engraftment, but actual clinical benefit has yet to be established (27).

E. Effects of SCF plus Filgrastim on Engraftment in Humans

In all of the clinical studies, trilineage engraftment after the high-dose chemotherapy and transplantation has been rapid and durable. Engraftment to ANC $\geq 5 \times 10^9$/L and to platelets $\geq 20 \times 10^9$/L have typically occurred at day 10 (median) and at days 10–12 (median), respectively. There have been no statistically significant differences in median ANC or platelet engraftment times for SCF plus filgrastim groups versus filgrastim-alone groups except in the study of Shpall et al. (33), where ANC $\geq 5 \times 10^9$/L was reached at day 10 (median) for the SCF plus filgrastim group versus day 9 (median) for the filgrastim-alone group. In addition, there have been no statistically significant differences between treatment groups in red blood cell (RBC) or platelet transfusions posttransplant.

In general, all of the studies had aspects of their design and mobilization results that decreased the likelihood of observing differences between treatment groups in the rate of ANC or platelet engraftment. As discussed, numbers of $CD34^+$ cells collected and infused were generally higher in the SCF plus filgrastim groups than in the filgrastim-alone groups. However, the numbers were sufficiently high in all groups (including the

Table 2 Median CD34$^+$ Cells Collected and Infused

| Reference | Median CD34$^+$ cells collected ($\times 10^6$/kg) | | Proportion of collected CD34$^+$ cells infused per subsequent high-dose chemotherapy cycle |
	Filgrastim alone	SCF plus filgrastim	
34	3.0[a,b]	3.3[a,b]	All
31, 32	11.4	16.0[b]	0.33
29	3.2	7.9[b]	All
37,38	3.2	10.1[b]	0.25
36	8.2	12.4	All
30	2.4	3.6	All
35	3.9	4.9	0.50
33	4.8	5.3	All

[a] Includes patients not heavily pretreated and patients heavily pretreated, not just the latter as in Table 1.
[b] For studies with variable-dose SCF groups, values are given only for the SCF 20 µg/kg/day group [15 µg/kg/day in the case of Moskowitz et al. (34)]. Values for the other groups in these studies can be found in the cited references.

filgrastim-alone) (Table 2) that the observed rapid, and equivalent engraftment in all of these groups is not surprising. In particular, for the fixed SCF-dose studies whose design involved daily leukaphereses until a CD34$^+$ cell target yield was reached, major differences in CD34$^+$ cell yields between groups (Table 2) were not anticipated or observed, and likewise for engraftment rates.

Several of the study designs (see Table 2) prohibited patients who did not yield a minimum level of PBPCs ("mobilization failures") from proceeding to high-dose chemotherapy and transplantation. In two of the studies (30,32), there were tendencies toward greater frequency of mobilization failure in the filgrastim-alone groups than in the SCF plus filgrastim groups. These study results represent another factor that would lessen engraftment differences between the treatment groups.

Thus, the study designs were such that the rate of engraftment was not a major study endpoint. From the standpoint of engraftment, it becomes apparent that the use of SCF along with filgrastim for mobilization may be most applicable to patients who are at risk of poor mobilization [by criteria such as extent of prior chemoradiotherapy (e.g., see Ref. 34)] or who have failed to yield sufficient PBPCs after some other mobilization approach, such as filgrastim alone.

V. SAFETY

SCF used in combination with filgrastim has been generally well tolerated, given as specified in Table 1, and administered after the antiallergy premedication regimen described below. The premedications are thought to minimize the effects of the known action of SCF on mast cells. Because of the possibility of SCF-induced mast cell–mediated events, patients with asthma, severe allergy, or other significant IgE-mediated hypersensitivity have been excluded from the studies at screening.

The most common adverse event associated with SCF administration has been a skin reaction at the injection site, which occurs in nearly all patients. The local skin reactions have been mild to moderate and are manifested as edema or urticaria surrounded by a ring of erythema with or without pruritus. They generally appear within 24 h after the subcutaneous injection of SCF, persist for 24–48 h, and resolve spontaneously (see study references given in Table 1). The reactions appear to be mast cell mediated, since injection-site biopsies have shown mast cell degranulation (41). Mild, reversible (within months) injection-site hyperpigmentation results from the effects of SCF on melanocytes (see above and Refs. 41 and 42) and has been reported in a proportion of patients receiving SCF (<10%). Mild to moderate skin reactions distant from the injection site have been reported in about 20% of SCF-treated patients and have included rash, erythema, pruritus, and urticaria.

Serious but manageable systemic allergic-like reactions, probably mast cell mediated, and including respiratory and cutaneous symptoms, have occasionally been associated with SCF administration. The overall frequency of these allergic-like reactions has been about 3% in approximately 500 patients who have received SCF with premedications in the clinical studies. The frequency was substantially higher in initial phase I studies in which patients were neither consistently screened for atopy nor consistently premedicated. In phase I studies, 13 of 56 patients experienced moderate to severe multisystem allergic-like reactions, which were dose related and occurred primarily at 25 or 50 µg/kg/day (43,44). In subsequent phase II and phase III studies, a consistent premedication regimen (combinations of H1 and H2 antihistamines and albuterol with or without pseudoephedrine; albuterol and pseudoephedrine are β-agonists) has been used to minimize the risk of mast cell–mediated adverse events. As discussed, when the premedication regimen is given and when higher doses of SCF are avoided, systemic allergic-like reactions are infrequent.

Individual study references given in Table 1 provide detailed descriptions of the systemic allergic-like reactions that have occurred in the phase II and phase III studies. The reactions have typically involved skin symptoms (urticaria) and respiratory symptoms (throat tightness, dysphagia, and dyspnea). They have occurred at various points during the courses of SCF administration (i.e., not always after the first injection). In addition, they have usually been delayed in onset relative to SCF injection (usually within 10 h) and have resolved after treatment with additional antihistamines and/or steroids. Thus, the reactions have been manageable and, although they have had some features of anaphylactoid reactions, they have not been characterized by the progressive, life-threatening symptoms typical of anaphylaxis. Most of the patients experiencing the reactions have been withdrawn from further SCF treatment.

No specific adverse events have been attributed to SCF during the transplantation phases of the clinical studies. In two large studies, there were no differences in the overall and disease-free survival among patients receiving PBPCs mobilized by filgrastim alone versus those mobilized with SCF plus filgrastim after median follow-up periods of 23 months (29) and 100 days (33).

VI. OTHER POTENTIAL APPLICATIONS OF SCF RELATED TO CD34+ CELL COLLECTION AND MANIPULATION

There are continuing advances in the "ex vivo" manipulation of peripheral blood–derived hematopoietic stem/progenitor cells for transplantation and for other types of cell therapies. These include CD34+ cell selection and tumor cell purging (27). Other manipulations often use CD34+ cells as the starting population, such as ex vivo expansion to potentially increase the size of the graft; gene transfection/transduction for gene therapy; and immunomodulatory approaches such as generation of cytotoxic cells or antigen-presenting cells (e.g., dendritic cells) (27,45–48). Since many of these manipulations unavoidably lead to cell loss, the use of SCF for mobilization, by increasing the yields of harvested CD34[+] cells, can potentially increase the likelihood of successful outcomes. It has been shown that CD34[+] cells mobilized with filgrastim alone or with SCF plus filgrastim serve as equally good targets for retrovirally mediated gene transfection (49).

Moreover, several of the ex vivo manipulations themselves use SCF as a critical component. SCF is typically a component of ex vivo expansion conditions (4,6,21,45), including those that are the most beneficial so far reported for generating cells which reduce the time of ANC nadir and speed the time to engraftment after high-dose chemotherapy and transplantation (50–52). Similarly, SCF has been a component of the conditions that most efficiently promote retrovirally mediated gene transfection into hematopoietic stem/progenitor cells for gene therapy (2,4,6). Finally, SCF enhances, in some cases dramatically, the ex vivo generation of functional dendritic cells under conditions in which GM-CSF and tumor necrosis factor-α are the primary cytokines (47,48).

ACKNOWLEDGMENT

Drs. Keith E. Lanley and MaryAnn Foote assisted with the writing of this paper. The authors thank the phase III investigators whose work is reviewed in this updated paper: Dr. Patrick Stiff (Maywood, IL), Dr. Thiery Facon (Lille, France), Dr. Elizabeth J. Shpall (Denver, CO), and Dr. C. Fred LeMaistre (San Antonio, TX). The authors also thank the following staff at Amgen Inc. who were involved in the SCF clinical trials: Mark W. Davis, Melody R. Wyres, Stewart A. Turner, and William R.L. Parker.

REFERENCES

1. Galli SJ, Zsebo KM, Geissler EN. The kit ligand, stem cell factor. Adv Immunol 1994; 55: 1–96. (review)
2. McNiece IK, Briddell RA. Stem cell factor. J Leukoc Biol 1995; 57:14–22. (review)
3. Glaspy J. Clinical applications of stem cell factor. Curr Opin Hematol. 1996; 3:223–229. (review)
4. Broudy VC. Stem cell factor and hematopoiesis. Blood 1997; 90: 1345–1364. (review).
5. Besmer P. Kit-ligand–stem cell factor. In: Garland JM, Quesenberry PJ, Hilton DJ, eds. Colony-Stimulating Factors: Molecular and Cellular Biology. New York: Marcel Dekker, 1997: 369–404. (review)
6. Lyman SD, Jacobsen SE. c-kit Ligand and Flt3 ligand: stem/progenitor cell factors with overlapping yet distinct activities. Blood 1998; 91:1101–1134. (review)
7. Russell, ES. Hereditary anemias of the mouse: a review for geneticists. Adv Genet 1979; 20: 357–459. (review)
8. Zsebo KM, Williams DA, Geissler EN, et al. Stem cell factor is encoded at the S/locus of the mouse and is the ligand for the c-kit tyrosine kinase receptor. Cell 1990; 63:213–224.
9. Molineux G, Migdalska A, Szmitkowski M, Zsebo K, Dexter TM. The effects on hematopoiesis of recombinant stem cell factor (ligand for c-kit) administered in vivo to mice either alone or in combination with granulocyte colony-stimulating factor. Blood 1991; 78:961–966.
10. Ulich TR, del Castillo J, Yi ES, et al. Hematologic effects of stem cell factor in vivo and in vitro in rodents. Blood 1991; 78:645–650.
11. Bodine DM, Seidel NE, Zsebo KM, Orlic D. In vivo administration of stem cell factor to

mice increases the absolute number of pluripotent hematopoietic stem cells. Blood 1993; 82: 445–455.

12. Fleming WH, Alpern EJ, Uchida N, Ikuta K, Weissman IL. Steel factor influences the distribution and activity of murine hematopoietic stem cells in vivo. Proc Natl Acad Sci USA 1993; 90:3760–3764.

13. Schuening FG, Appelbaum FR, Deeg HJ, et al. Effects of recombinant canine stem cell factor, a c-kit ligand, and recombinant granulocyte colony-stimulating factor on hematopoietic recovery after otherwise lethal total body irradiation. Blood 1993; 81:20–26.

14. Andrews RG, Knitter GH, Bartelmez SH, et al. Recombinant human stem cell factor, a c-*kit* ligand, stimulates hematopoiesis in primates. Blood 1991; 78:1975–1980.

15. Andrews RG, Bartelmez SH, Knitter GH, et al. A c-*kit* ligand, recombinant human stem cell factor, mediates reversible expansion of multiple CD34+ colony-forming cell types in blood and marrow of baboons. Blood 1992; 80:920–927.

16. Zsebo KM, Wypych J, McNiece IK, et al. Identification, purification, and biological characterization of hematopoietic stem cell factor from Buffalo rat liver-conditioned medium. Cell 1990; 63:195–201.

17. Zsebo KM, Smith KA, Hartley CA, et al. Radioprotection of mice by recombinant rat stem cell factor. Proc. Natl. Acad. Sci. USA 1992; 89:9464–9468.

18. Monroy RL, Ganey IT, Davis TA, Perrin PJ, Zsebo K, Stead R. Enhancement of hematopoietic recovery using recombinant human stem cell factor (SCF) after high dose chemotherapy in nonhuman primates. Exp Hematol 1992; 20:242a. (abstract)

19. Galli SJ, Iemura A, Garlick DS, Gamba-Vitalo C, Zsebo KM, Andrews RG. Reversible expansion of primate mast cell populations in vivo by stem cell factor. J Clin Invest 1993; 91:148–152.

20. Briddell RA, Hartley CA, Smith KA, McNiece IK. Recombinant rat stem cell factor synergizes with recombinant human granulocyte colony-stimulating factor in vivo in mice to mobilize peripheral blood progenitor cells that have enhanced repopulating potential. Blood 1993; 82: 1720–1723.

21. McNiece IK, Briddell RA, Hartley CA, Smith KA, Andrews RG. Stem cell factor enhances in vivo effects of granulocyte colony stimulating factor for stimulating mobilization of peripheral blood progenitor cells. Stem Cells 1993; 11(suppl 2):36–41.

22. de Revel T, Appelbaum FR, Storb R, et al. Effects of granulocyte colony-stimulating factor and stem cell factor, alone and in combination, on the mobilization of peripheral blood cells that engraft lethally irradiated dogs. Blood 1994; 83:3795–3799.

23. Andrews RG, Briddell RA, Knitter GH, Rowley SD, Appelbaum FR, McNiece IK. In vivo synergy between recombinant human stem cell factor and recombinant human granulocyte colony-stimulating factor in baboons: enhanced circulation of progenitor cells. Blood 1994; 84:800–810.

24. Yan X-Q, Briddell RA, Hartley C, Stone G, Samal B, McNiece IK. Mobilization of long-term hematopoietic reconstituting cells in mice by the combination of stem cell factor plus granulocyte colony-stimulating factor. Blood 1994; 84:795–799.

25. Yan X-Q, Hartley C, McElroy P, Chang A, McCrea C, McNiece I. Peripheral blood progenitor cells mobilized by recombinant human granulocyte colony-stimulating factor plus recombinant rat stem cell factor contain long-term engrafting cells capable of cellular proliferation for more than two years as shown by serial transplantation in mice. Blood 1995; 85:2303–2307.

26. Andrews RG, Briddell RA, Knitter GH, Rowley SD, Appelbaum FR, McNiece IK. Rapid engraftment by peripheral blood progenitor cells mobilized by recombinant human stem cell factor and recombinant human granulocyte colony-stimulating factor in nonhuman primates. Blood 1995; 85:15–20.

27. To LB, Haylock DN, Simmons PJ, Juttner CA. The biology and clinical uses of blood stem cells. Blood 1997; 89:2233–2258. (review)

28. Demirer T, Buckner CD, Bensinger WI. Optimization of Peripheral Blood Stem Cell Mobiliation. Stem Cells 1996; 14:106–116. (review)
29. Glaspy JA, Shpall EJ, LeMaistre CF, et al. Peripheral blood progenitor cell mobilization utilizing stem cell factor in combination with filgrastim in breast cancer patients. Blood 1997; 90: 2939–2951.
30. Stiff P, Gingrich R, Luger S, et al. A randomized phase 2 study of PBPC mobilization by stem cell factor and filgrastim in heavily pretreated patients with Hodgkin's disease or non-Hodgkin's lymphoma. Submitted.
31. Begley CG, Basser R, Mansfield R, et al. Enhanced levels and enhanced clonogenic capacity of blood progenitor cells following administration of stem cell factor plus granulocyte colony-stimulating factor to humans. Blood 1997; 90:3378–3389.
32. Basser R, To LB, Begley CG, et al. Rapid hematopoietic recovery after multicycle high-dose chemotherapy: enhancement of filgrastim-induced progenitor-cell mobilization by recombinant human stem-cell mobilization. J Clin Oncol 1998; 16:1899–1908.
33. Shpall EJ, Wheeler CA, Turner SA, et al. A randomized phase 3 study of peripheral blood progenitor cell mobilization with stem cell factor and filgrastim in high-risk breast cancer patients. Blood 1999; 93:2491–2501.
34. Moskowitz CH, Stiff P, Gordon MS, et al. Recombinant methionyl human stem cell factor (r-metHuSCF) and filgrastim for PBPC mobilization and transplantation in non-Hodgkin's lymphoma patients—results of a phase I/II trial. Blood 1997; 89:3136–3147.
35. Tricot G, Jagannath S, Desikan KR, et al. Superior mobilization of peripheral blood progenitor cells (PBPC) using r-metHuSCF (SCF) and r-metHuG-CSF (filgrastim) in heavily pre-treated multiple myeloma (MM) patients (abstr). Blood 1996; 88:388a.
36. Facon T, Harousseau J, Maloisel F, et al. Stem cell factor in combination with filgrastim after chemotherapy improves peripheral blood progenitor cell yield and reduces apheresis requirements in multiple myeloma patients: a randomized, controlled trial. Blood 1999; 94:1218–1225.
37. Weaver A, Ryder D, Crowther D, Dexter TM, Testa NG. Increased numbers of long-term culture-initiating cells in the apheresis product of patients randomized to receive increasing doses of stem cell factor administered in combination with chemotherapy and a standard dose of granulocyte colony-stimulating factor. Blood 1996; 88:3323–3328.
38. Weaver A, Chang J, Wrigley E, et al. Randomized comparison of progenitor-cell mobilization using chemotherapy, stem-cell factor, and filgrastim or chemotherapy plus filgrastim alone in patients with ovarian cancer. J Clin Oncol 1998; 16:2601–2612.
39. Weaver CH, Birch R, Greco FA, et al. Mobilization and harvesting of peripheral blood stem cells: Randomized evaluations of different doses of filgrastim. Br J Haematol 1998; 100:338–347.
40. Sutherland HJ, Hogge DE, Lansdorp PM, Phillips GL, Eaves AC, Eaves CJ. Quantitation, mobilization, and clinical use of long-term culture-initiating cells in blood cell autografts. J Hematother 1995; 4:3–10. (review)
41. Costa JJ, Demetri GD, Harris TJ, et al. Recombinant human stem cell factor (Kit ligand) promotes human mast cell and melanocyte hyperplasia and functional activation in vivo. J Exp Med 1996; 183:2681–2684.
42. Grichnik JM, Crawford J, Jiminez F, et al. Human recombinant stem-cell factor induces melanocytic hyperplasia in susceptible patients. J Am Acad Dermatol 1995; 33:577–583.
43. Crawford J, Lau D, Erwin R, Rich W, McGuire B, Meyers F. A phase I trial of recombinant methionyl human stem cell factor (SCF) in patients (pts) with advanced non-small cell lung carcinoma (NSCLC) (abstr). Proc Am Soc Clin Oncol 1993; 12:135.
44. Demetri G, Costa J, Hayes D, et al. A phase I trial of recombinant methionyl human stem cell factor (SCF) in patients with advanced breast carcinoma pre- and post-chemotherapy (chemo) with cyclophosphamide (C) and doxorubicin (A) (abstr). Proc Am Soc Clin Oncol 1993; 12:142.

45. Lange W, Henschler R, Mertelsmann R. Biological and clinical advances in stem cell expansion. Leukemia 1996; 10:943–945.

46. Kohn DB. The current status of gene therapy using hematopoietic stem cells. Curr Opin Pediatr 1995; 7:56–63. (review)

47. Guillaume T, Rubinstein DB, Symann M. Immune reconstitution and immunotherapy after autologous hematopoietic stem cell transplantation. Blood 1998; 92:1471–1490.

48. Hart DNJ. Dendritic cells: Unique leukocyte populations which control the primary immune response. Blood 1997; 90:3245–3287. (review)

49. Elwood NJ, Zogos H, Wilson T, Begley CG. Retroviral transduction of human progenitor cells: Use of granulocyte colony-stimulating factor plus stem cell factor to mobilize progenitor cells in vivo and stimulation by Flt3/Flk-2 ligand in vitro. Blood 1996; 88:4452–4462.

50. Reiffers J, Caillot C, Dazey B, et al. Infusion of expanded CD34+ selected cells can abrogate post myeloablative chemotherapy neutropenia in patients with hematologic malignancies (abstr). Blood 1998; 92:126a.

51. McNiece I, Hami L, Jones R, et al. Transplantation of ex vivo expanded PBPC after high dose chemotherapy results in decreased neutropenia (abstr). Blood 1998; 92:126a–127a.

52. Andrews RG, Briddell RA, Gough M, McNiece IK. Expansion of G-CSF mobilized CD34+ peripheral blood cells (PBC) for 10 days in G-CSF, MGDF and SCF prior to transplantation decreased post-transplant neutropenia in baboons (abstr). Blood 1997; 90:92a.

4

Cytokine Modulation of Hematopoietic Stem Cell Phenotype

AHMAD-SAMER AL-HOMSI

University of Massachusetts Medical Center, Worcester, and Milford-Whitinsville Regional Hospital, Milford, Massachusetts

PETER J. QUESENBERRY

University of Massachusetts Medical Center, Worcester, Massachusetts

I. INTRODUCTION

The process of generation of mature and functional blood cells from common primitive and quiescent cells is a formidable task. Not only do trillions of cells need to be produced every day to replace the consumed ones, but also rapid changes in the rate of production have to be made constantly in adjustment to a variety of continuously arising needs.

Knowledge of the intricacy of the hematopoietic system led scientists long ago to surmise that factors capable of regulating the system existed. Although the experimental data are questionable, Paul Carnot, a Professor of Medicine at University of Paris, postulated in 1906 the existence of *hemopoietin* (1). Sixty years later, the development of new methodologies in hematopoietic cell cultures allowed for rapid development in our understanding of hematopoiesis. Today, more than 50 cytokines are known to play a role in a process of an ever-increasing complexity. In fact, the convenient concept of linear hierarchical proliferation and differentiation of stem cells into mature blood elements has been challenged recently in the light of knowledge derived from the study of cytokine signaling (2).

II. IDENTIFYING THE HEMATOPOIETIC STEM CELL

When transplanted into a myeloablated host, a hematopoietic stem cell (HPSC) is able to reconstitute and maintain blood cell production for an indefinite time. In other words,

Table 1 Phenotype
Characteristics of Hematopoietic
Stem Cells

Murine	Human
CD34$^{+/-}$	CD34$^{+/-}$
Lin$^-$	Lin$^-$
Sca-1$^+$	HLA-DR^{-a}
Thy1	c-kit$^+$
c-kit	Thy1$^+$
Rhodamine^{dull}	CD45RA^{low}
Hoechst^{dull}	CD71^{low}
Pyronin$^-$	CD59
	Rhodamine^{dull}
	Hoechst^{dull}

[a] Umbilical cord blood stem cells are
HLA-DR .
Source: Modified from Ref. 3.

Table 2 Hematopoietic Stem Cell Assays

Assay	Description	Comments
High proliferative potential colony-forming cell (HPP-CFC) assay	Formation of macroscopic colonies of more than 0.5 mm in semisolid culture in presence of multiple cytokines.	Measures very primitive, but hierarchically heterogeneous cells.
Colony-forming unit-blast (CFU-B1) assay	Formation of colonies of more than 25 blast-like cells in semisolid cultures in presence of multiple cytokines.	Target cells are similar to the more primitive HPP-CFC.
Long-term culture-initiating cell (LTCIC) assay	Formation of monocyte-granulocyte colonies in stroma-containing cultures.	May not be predictive of long-term hematopoiesis-reconstituting abilities. Suitable for frequency analysis when setup at limiting dilution.
Cobblestone area-forming cell (CAFC) assay	Generation of foci of phase dark cells in stroma-containing cultures.	Tested cells may be similar to LTCIC.
Colony-forming unit-spleen (CFU-S) assay[a]	Formation of hematopoietic colonies in the spleen of lethally irradiated mice.	Cells are hierarchically heterogeneous with the late-appearing colonies representing the least mature cells.

[a] Only applicable in mice; all other assays are applicable in murine and human species.

stemness of a HPSC implies the capability of self-maintenance, and under appropriate conditions, of proliferation and differentiation into committed cells that ultimately mature into functional elements.

A number of phenotypic markers have been identified as being characteristic of the most primitive HPSCs [reviewed in Ref. 3 (Table 1)]. No single marker, however, can precisely characterize HPSCs. Scientists had therefore to rely on the functional properties of these cells to identify them. Although the only gold standard assay for HPSCs is the measurement of their ability to reestablish long-term hematopoiesis in a myeloablated recipient, the impracticality of this kind of experiment has led to the development of a number of alternative in vitro and in vivo assays (3,5–8) (Table 2).

III. PROLIFERATION AND DIFFERENTIATION OF HPSCs

Throughout life, HPSCs give rise to transit progenitors which become progressively restricted to a single lineage. This progressive restriction is associated with the reduced capacity for further proliferation. Recognizable morphologically, the maturing cells lose specific surface markers while acquiring others. The whole process takes place under the control of microenviromental cells in intimate contact with the HPSCs and under command of the cytokines.

This ordered model of linear restriction of lineage presumes a high degree of concordance among daughter cells. However, experiments by Ogawa et al. suggest that daughter cells derived from a single cell can give rise, under a permissive combination of cytokines, to totally different lineages, implying that critical commitment decisions are made during one cell cycle transit (2). Our own work in transplantation models in nonmyeloablated and myeloablated mice show that bone marrow cells harvested 6 days after exposure to 5-fluorouracil acquire a long-term engraftment defect, which is reversible. In a similar vein, BALB/c or Ly5.1/Ly5.2 marrow cells exposed in vitro to a cytokine cocktail of stem cell factor (SCF), interleukin-3 (IL-3), IL-6, and IL-11 show a marked increase in progenitor cell number, in particular high proliferative potential colony-forming cells (HPP-CFCs), with progression from dormancy to a high proliferative state as demonstrated by in vitro killing with tritiated thymidine, an agent that selectively kills cells in S phase. At 48 hs, these cells appear to have maintained a normal short-term engraftment ability, but they have in essence lost their ability to function as long-term engraftable stem cells. However, evolving data suggest that this defect is also reversible and is not due to a terminal differentiation effect. These data suggest that regulation of primitive stem cells may be cell cycle rather than hierarchically based.

IV. BIOLOGY OF CYTOKINES

The cytokines are hormone-like peptides involved in the regulation of the production and function of blood cells (9). A large number of such biomolecules sharing some common features has been identified (Table 3).

A. Production

The cytokines are produced by a wide variety of cells, including mesenchymal cells such as fibroblasts and endothelial cells, monocytes, and granulocytes, mast cells, and T and B lymphocytes (4,9). Nonhematopoietic organs such as the liver and the kidneys also

Table 3 Cytokines and Their Predominant Action

Cytokine	Principal bioactivity
flt3 ligand	Costimulate multipotential HPSCs in combination with a number of cytokines, including SCF and Tpo. Stimulates generation of dendritic cells.
SCF	Similar to flt3 ligand. Enhances generation of mast cells.
Tpo	Major regulator of proliferation and differentiation of megakaryocytes. Costimulate multipotential HPSC in combination with SCF and IL-11. Promotes erythropoiesis in synergy with Epo.
IL-1	Costimulates early HPSCs in combination with other cytokines such as IL-3 (69–73). Induces production of IL-3, GM-, and G-CSF from different cell types (74–76). Regulates immune response (77,78).
IL-2	Inhibits myelo- and erythropoiesis (79,80). Stimulates T cell and immune response (81).
IL-3	Multilineage stimulator. Costimulates myelo-, erytho-, and megakaryopoiesis with different cytokines (82–84). Stimulates less mature megakaryocytes than Tpo (55). Does not promote full maturation of megakaryocytes (55). In vivo, increases blood monocytes and granulocytes (including eosinophils and platelets (85–87).
IL-4	Costimulates different types of colonies such as CFU-GM and CFU-E in combination with other cytokines (88). Stimulates B cells and dendritic cells and modulates immune response (89,91).
IL-5	Stimulates eosinophils production and activity (91). Stimulate B cells and enhances immune response (92).
IL-6	Stimulates megakaryopoiesis (93,94). Synergizes with IL-1, -2, -3, -4, GM-CSF and CSF-1 (23). Enhances plasma cell proliferation (95). Plays a role in the pathogenesis of Castelman's disease and in atrial myxoma (96).
IL-7	Induces in synergy with SCF pre–B-cell production (49).
IL-8	Stimulates production and function of neutrophils and acts as proinflammatory factor (97,98).
IL-9	Costimulates CFU-GM and CFU-Mix (99). With Epo, stimulates BFU-E. Synergizes with IL-3 to produce mast cells (100). Enhances T-cell production (101).
IL-10	Modulates immune cells (102). Inhibits cytokine production (103).
IL-11	Shares many activities with IL-6 (104,105). Increases neutrophils and platelets in blood in primates (106,107).
IL-12	Increases generation of immunocompetent cells (108,109).
IL-13	Enhances SCF-induced proliferation of Lin⁻ Sca⁺ bone marrow cells (110). Inhibits cytokine production by monocytes (111,112). Stimulates B cells and activates T cells (109,110).

IL-14	Acts as B-cell growth factor (113).
IL-15	Modulates T-cell activity (114).
IL-16	Acts as immunomodulators (115).
IL-17	Induces production of other cytokines such as IL-6, IL-8, and G-CSF and enhances the expression of adhesion molecules (116,117).
IL-18	Induces GM-CSF and interferon-γ production (118,119). Inhibits IL-10 production (118).
CSF-1	Enhances production and function of monocytes (12).
GM-CSF	Costimulates many types of progenitors, including early multipotential cells. Stimulates CFU-GM and induces maturation of bipotential mono- and granulocytic progenitors. Synergizes with IL-4 to produce dendritic cells from monocytes. In vivo, increases monocytes, neutrophils, and eosinophils.
G-CSF	Costimulates early progenitors in synergy with a number of cytokines. Promotes production and activity of neutrophils. In vivo, enhances neutrophil production and shortens time to neutrophils recovery after cytotoxic therapy.
Epo	Stimulates BFU-E and CFU-E (120,121). Stimulates CFU-MK (122). In vivo, promotes red blood cell production.
MIP-1α	Inhibits early multipotential colony formation, but enhances committed progenitors.
TGF-β1	Suppresses early multipotential progenitors, but may stimulate late progenitors.
MCAF	Similar to TGF-β1.
PF4	Similar to TGF-β1.
H-ferritin	Similar to TGF-β1.
TNF-α	Similar to TGF-β1 with more pronounced effects on BFU-E and CFU-E.
Activin	Enhances IL-3 and Epo stimulated BFU-E and CFU-E. Inhibits IL-3–stimulated CFU-GM.
Inhibin	Inhibits CFU-Mix, CFU-GM, and BFU-E.
Interferon-α, -β, -γ	Coinhibits CFU-Mix, CFU-GM, and BFU-E. Induces production of cytokines (60).
Prostaglandin E1 and E2	Suppress CFU-M with less or no activity on CFU-GM and CFU-G. Enhances BFU-E indirectly through CD8+ lymphocytes (60).
Peptide Glu-Glu-Asp-Asp-Lys	Inhibits CFU-S and CFU-GM (12,58).
N-acetyl-Ser-Asp-Lys-Pro	Inhibits CFU-S and other progenitors entry into cell cycling (12,58).
Leukemia inhibitory factor	Inhibits GM- and G-CSF–stimulated CFU-GM and CFU-G, respectively (123).

produce specific cytokines (9). The cytokines are produced locally by stromal cells or reach the bone marrow through the circulation. The locally assembled molecules may remain on the surface of the producing cell and act through cell to cell contact. Some of the extracellular matrix molecules such as heparan sulfate may also play a role in presenting the cytokines to the target cells (10).

B. Receptors

The cytokines exert their biological function by binding to specific receptors on the surface of the target cells. These receptors are expressed in low numbers that do not exceed a few hundred per cell (9,10). The multipotent cells possess receptors to most cytokines. On the other hand, the more mature cells have a distribution of receptors that matches the biological activity known to each cytokine (9).

Two major families of receptors have been recognized (11,13). The hematopoietic receptor family include receptors to erythropoietin (Epo), granulocyte-monocyte colony-stimulating factor (GM-CSF), granulocyte colony-stimulating factor (G-CSF), IL-2, IL-3, IL-4, IL-5, IL-6, IL-7, and IL-9. The extracellular binding domain of these receptors contain four conserved cyteine residues and a WS-X-WS motif (X is a variable nonconserved amino acid). Some also have an immunoglobulin-like structure. The cytoplasmic domain is variable and has no kinase activity. The receptors for GM-CSF, IL-3, and IL-5 contain a low-affinity α chain specific to each receptor and a high-affinity β chain shared by all three receptors. The common β chain may play a role in competitive binding to different ligands. The family of tyrosine kinase receptors represented by receptors for flt3 ligand, SCF (or c-kit ligand), colony-stimulating factor-1 (CSF-1), and thrombopoietin (Tpo) shows an immunoglobulin-like structure and 10 conserved cyteines in the extracellular domain and tyrosine kinase activity in the cytoplasmic domain. IL-1 and IL-8 receptors do not belong to any of the two families. The extracellular region of IL-1 receptor is entirely composed of an immunoglobulin-like structure, whereas IL-8 has seven membrane-spanning regions (13).

C. Biological Activity

Although each cytokine has its private ligand-specific receptor, the cytokines share public class-specific signal transducers (13). After dimerization of their receptor molecules, almost all the lymphohematopoietic cytokines trigger activation of a tyrosine kinase and promote phosphorylation of intracellular proteins. The receptors that belong to the hematopoietic receptor family, and therefore do not have an intrinsic enzymatic activity, induce protein phosphorylation through associated nonreceptor-type tyrosine kinase activities such as JAK2, Fes, and Lyn (13). Transcription factors are thereafter activated and transported to the nucleus where they activate target genes (13). Specific transcription factors may direct differentiation of hematopoietic cells toward a particular lineage. GATA-1 and SCL are examples of such transcription factors of which cytokine-mediated expression promotes erythroid differentiation (14). GATA-1 also influences megakaryocytic differentiation (15).

Other mechanisms by which cytokines regulate hematopoiesis include the modulation of cell cycling, potentiation of expression of receptors for other growth factors, and regulation of apoptosis. In in vitro assays, SCF reduces cell cycle time by decreasing the G1 phase, whereas IL-11 shortens all cell cycle phases without affecting the relative duration of each phase (16). Tpo has been shown to upregulate the transformation of p53 protein from the wild-type suppressor conformation to a promotor conformation. This upregulation was associated with downregulation of the protein products of p53 wild-type–enhancing genes without any change in the levels of *bcl-2* gene product (17). IL-3, however, was shown to play a role in *bcl-2* transcription maintenance in TF-1 cells through protein kinase C activation (18). On the other hand, CD-34$^+$ adult human bone marrow cells cultured in the presence of a combination SCF, IL-3, G-CSF, and Epo gradually became positive for Fas antigen, a surface molecule that mediates apoptosis. Increasing Fas antigen positivity was associated with loss of *bcl-2* expression, suggesting an intrinsic cell "suicide" program (19).

Recently, increasing attention has been paid to the regulation of adhesion molecules by the cytokines. Adhesion molecules allow physical contact between the hematopoietic cells and bone marrow microenviroment through binding with specific ligands. Studied in vitro, SCF, IL-3, and GM-CSF were shown to activate very late antigens 4 and 5 (VLA-4 and VLA-5), which are two adhesion molecules normally expressed on CD34$^+$ cells (20). This activation resulted in promoting the VLA-4 and VLA-5 ability to bind to fibronectin. Interestingly, a significant correlation between the mitogenic state of hematopoietic cells and their avidity to fibronectin was evident.

Furthermore, the combinations of cytokines with the most marked ability to enhance hematopoietic cell proliferation were the most efficient in stimulating their adhesion capability to fibronectin.

The fact that cytokines function through common signal tranducers explains in part the pleiotropy and redundancy of the cytokine network. As an example, IL-6 induces the acute phase response, stimulates osteoclasts, activates megakaryopoiesis, enhances plasma cell growth, and promotes protein synthesis in the liver. Yet, the same cytokine appears to be dispensable for the most part when tested in knockout mice, probably because other cytokines such as oncostatin M (OM) and IL-11 share most of its activity (13,21).

Another characteristic of cytokines is interdependency. Three forms of interaction between cytokines can be observed in simple cultures: synergy, recruitment, and mandatory double signaling (21). Synergy refers to a process by which a combination of cytokines induce the formation of *larger* colonies than achievable by using twice the concentration of either factor alone in simple cultures. An example of synergy is observed when SCF is combined with IL-6, GM-CSF, and G-CSF (22). Recruitment implies that a combination of cytokines results in an increase in the *number* of colonies by activation of additional clonogenic cells. This is illustrated by the addition of IL-6 to IL-3 to form multilineage colonies (23). Mandatory double signaling means that a given cytokine has no effect on its own unless other cytokines are present. Sorted CD34$^+$ cells, for instance, do not proliferate unless two or more cytokines are present. The synergistic interaction of cytokine on murine HPP-CFCs has been shown to occur at very low, subliminal levels if certain "anchor" factors, such as SCF, are kept at optimal concentration (24). IL-3 also has some anchoring activity, whereas GM-CSF and G-CSF have none.

V. EFFECTS OF CYTOKINES ON HPSCs

A large number of cytokines have now been identified and their effects on the HPSCs studied in vitro and some in vivo (Tables 3–6). In vitro experiments can be deceiving. Wrong functions may be ascribed to specific cytokines unless highly enriched target cells are used and serum-free conditions are employed in order to eliminate any colony-stimulating activity produced by accessory cells or contained in serum.

Table 4 Summary of Human Stroma-Free In Vitro Hematopoietic Cell Expansion Studies

Reference	Input	Cytokines	Test	Duration (days)	Fold-expansion
124	PB CD34$^+$	IL-1, -3, -6, SCF, Epo	TNC	12	30–110
			CFU	12	20–100
			LTCIC	12	>1
125	PB CD34$^+$	IL-1, -3, -6, SCF, Epo	TNC	16	76–995
			CFU	12–14	49–930
			CD34$^+$Lin$^-$	14	3–21
			4-HC resistant	24	>1
126	PB CD34$^+$	IL-1, -3, -6, SCF, GM-CSF, G-CSF	TNC	21	1324
			CFU-GM	14	66
127	PB CD34$^+$ or Lin$^-$	Il-3, -6, SCF, Epo	LTCIC	4	<1
128	PB CD34$^+$	PIXY321	TNC	12	7.4–207.0
			CFU	12	1.0–11.6
			CD34$^+$	12	6–64
129	PB CD34$^+$	IL-1, -3, SCF	TNC	14	223
			CFUGM	14	109
130	BM CD34$^+$/HLA-DR$^-$/CD15$^-$/Rh^{dull}	SCF, PIXY321	HPP-CFC	21	2
				28	5.5
129	BM CD34$^+$	IL-3, -6, SCF	TNC	14	59
			CFU-GM	14	
131	UCB CD34$^+$	IL-1, -3, SCF	LTCIC	7–14	15–20
132	UCB CD34$^+$/CD45-RA^{lo}/CD71^{lo}/Thy-1$^+$	IL-3, SCF, PIXY321, GMCSF, M-CFS, G-CSF, Epo	CFU	29	31000
			HPP-CFC	29	652
			CD34$^+$/Thy1$^+$	21	20

PB, peripheral blood; BM, bone marrow; TNC, total nucleated cells; Rh, rhodamine.
Source: Modified from Ref. 3.

A. flt3 Ligand

On its own, the flt3 ligand has minimal activity in agar cultures of murine or human bone marrow or umbilical cord blood enriched in CD34$^+$ cells, stimulating only dispersed colony-forming units granulocyte-monocyte (CFU-GM) but not HPP-CFC colonies, mixed colony-forming units (CFU-Mix), or burst-forming Unit-erythroid (BFU-E). However, in combination with other cytokines, such as SCF, IL-3, and GM-CSF, flt3 ligand has additive or more than additive effects. These effects remain apparent even on single cells in wells (25).

Several lines of evidence suggest that flt3 ligand acts on the early myeloid progenitors. First, flt3 ligand receptors are only detectable on CD34$^+$ but not CD34$^-$ human bone marrow cells (26). Second, in suspension cultures of CD34$^+$ column-separated umbilical cord blood cells, whereas SCF and GM-CSF/IL-3 fusion protein (PIXY321) favor the expansion of the more mature progenitors, the addition of flt3 ligand enhances the amplification of more immature progenitors (25). Third, flt3 ligand was the only cytokine to increase the number of long-term culture-initiating cells (LTCICs) above the input value after 10 days of liquid cultures of CD34$^+$/CD38$^-$ human bone marrow cells (27). Fourth, serum levels of flt3 ligand, but not of SCF, are elevated in patients with multilineage bone

Table 5 Summary of Studies of Murine Stroma-Free In Vitro Expansion of Hematopoietic Cells

Reference	Study	5-FU pretreatment	Duration of culture (days)	Cytokines	Outcome
133	Comparison of C to NC BM	Yes	7	IL-1 and -3	Accelerated hematological recovery. Maintained HPP-CFC at 5 and 10 weeks
134	Comparison of C to NC BM	Yes	7	IL-1 and SCF	Accelerated hematological recovery. Maintained of HPP-CFC at 40 weeks. Maintained reconstituting ability in secondary hosts.
135	Comparison of C and NC BM	Yes	3	IL-3 and -6 or IL-3 and SCF	Improved radioprotective ability. Maintained long-term reconstituting ability in *competitive, experiments*
136	Comparison of C to NC Lin⁻/Sca-1⁺/WGA⁺BM cells	No	14	IL-6, SCF, and Epo with or without IL-3	Maintained (but not increased) in vivo reconstituting ability
137–138	Comparison of C to NC BM	No	2	IL-3, -6, -11, and SCF	HPP-CFC expansion with impaired engraftment in *competitive transplant experiments*

C, cultured; BM, bone marrow; NC, noncultured; WGA, wheat germ agglutinin.
Source: Modified from Ref. 3.

Table 6   Summary of Stroma-Containing Ex Vivo Hematopoietic Cell Expansion Studies

Reference	Input	Cytokines	Readout	Duration	Fold-expansions	Comment
139	Human BM	IL-3, SCF, GM-CSF, Epo	TCN	14	10	
			CFU-GM	14	21	
			LTCIC	14	7.5	
140	Human CD34$^+$-enriched BM with preformed stroma	Il-3, SCF, GM-CSF, Epo	TNC	14	3	
			CFU-GM	14	5	
			LTCIC	14	3	
141	Human CD34$^+$-enriched UCB with stroma noncontat system	None	LTCIC	7	3.57	
		IL-3, MIP-1α	LTCIC	14	4	
				7	5.92	
				14	4.87	
142	Human CD34$^+$/Lin$^-$/Thy1$^+$-enriched BM with PMVEC	IL-3, -6, SCF, GM-CSF	CAFC	21	>1	No loss in capability of engraftment
			Scid-hu assay	21		

BM, bone marrow; PMVEC, porcine endothelial micovascular endothelial cell; Scid-hu assay; transplantation of hematopoietic progenitors into human fetal bone fragments of disparate HLA-type preimplanted into the mouse peritoneal cavity.
Source: Modified from Ref. 3.

marrow failure and correlate inversely with the colony-forming abilities of bone marrow precursors from these patients. The levels do not normalize after correction of a single lineage, such as after the transfusion of red blood cells (28).

The effect of flt3 ligand on adhesion molecules of hematopoietic cells were studied in suspension cultures of human umbilical cord blood CD34$^+$ cells. In a conditioned media from a human stromal cell line, flt3 ligand maintained CD31 [or platelet/endothelial cell adhesion molecule (PECAM)] and VLA-4 levels of expression, whereas increasing the lymphocyte function-associated (LFA) molecule level of expression (29). This maintenance of adhesion molecule expression may explain the preservation of engraftment ability of Ly5.1 *Sca-1$^+$/c-kit$^+$* bone marrow cells from 5-fluorouracil (5-FU)–treated mice into lethally irradiated Ly5.2 mice after in vitro expansion with flt3 ligand and IL-11 at days 7 or 21 (30).

In ex vivo expansion experiments, flt3 ligand was compared to SCF. Neither factor could alone support the proliferation of *Lin$^-$/Sca-1$^+$/c-kit$^+$* cells derived from 5-FU–treated mouse bone marrows in suspension cultures. Both factors were however synergistic with IL-11, enhancing the production of progenitors and of nucleated cells. Longer exposure to flt3 ligand was required. Again, no engraftment defect after incubation with cytokines was noted after transplantation into lethally radiated mice except for the cells exposed to SCF and IL-11 for 21 days (30). In a different set of experiments, flt3 ligand in combination with Tpo resulted in extensive expansion with little differentiation of CD34$^+$ umbilical cord blood cells cultured under stroma-free conditions. In stroma-free cultures of human CD34$^+$ umbilical cord blood cells, flt3 ligand in combination with Tpo induced a several thousand-fold expansion of both CD34$^+$/CD38$^-$ and CD34$^+$/CD38$^+$ populations after 20 weeks of culture. Furthermore, when the expanded cells were stimulated by IL-7, IL-11, and flt3 ligand, the percentage of CD2$^+$ and CD19$^+$ cells reached 33.8 and 3.7%, respectively, after 14 days, suggesting that T- and B-lymphocyte progenitors were also expanded (31).

The effects of flt3 ligand on generation of dendritic cells has also been studied both in vitro and in vivo. The addition of flt3 ligand to a combination of IL-4, GM-CSF, and tumor necrosis factor-α (TNF-α) to human CD34$^+$ bone marrow cell cultures enhanced the generation of dendritic cells (32). The injection of flt3 ligand subcutaneously into mice for 10 days resulted in a significant expansion of dendritic cells. Dendritic cells expressing class II major histocompatibility class (MHC) molecules, CD11c, CD86, and DEC205 constituted 30% of the treated mice spleen cells. The antigen-presenting efficiency of these cells was maintained (33).

Finally, flt3 ligand was demonstrated to downregulate B-lymphopoiesis in NOD/SCID mice engrafted with human CD34$^+$/CD38$^-$ bone marrow or umbilical cord blood cells. In fact, pretreatment of recipients with flt3 ligand shifted lineage distribution of the engrafting cells toward the myeloid lineage, as witnessed by reduction in the percentage of CD19-expressing cells (34).

B. SCF

Mice with mutations at either the dominant *W* or *Sl* loci encoding for the *c-kit* and SCF, respectively, display a similar phenotype characterized by a reduction in the number of hematopoietic stem cells with hypoplastic anemia and mast cell deficiency, a defect in germ cells with sterility, and a decrease in the melanocyte number with defective pigmentation (35,36). Transplantation of *Sl* mouse bone marrow into *W* recipients resulted in a normal hematological phenotype, leading to the hypothesis that c-*kit* is the receptor for SCF (37–39). Although the number of molecules per cell varies extensively according to the cell type, c-*kit* is now known to be expressed by most of the hematopoietic cells (40).

Similar to flt3 ligand, SCF plays a central role in the regulation of early hematopoiesis. In one series of experiments, SCF alone had no effect on HPP-CFCs from CD34$^+$/HLA-DR$^-$/CD15$^-$ human bone marrow cells. However, the addition of SCF to a combination of IL-3 and GM-CSF resulted in a 12-fold increase in the number of HPP-CFC–derived colonies. Moreover, SCF addition resulted in an increase in the number of erythroid elements in these colonies. Similar effects were observed on BFU-E, CFU-GM, and burst- and colony-forming unit-megakaryocyte (BFU-MK and CFU-MK) (41,42).

The action of SCF on adhesion molecules was studied using a myeloid cell line MOE7 and CD34$^+$ human umbilical cord blood cells. The adhesiveness of MOE7 cells to endothelial cells and to vascular cell adhesion molecule (VCAM-1)–expressing cells increased after exposure to SCF. This effect was mediated by VLA-4 and VLA-5 integrins and was transient. In fact, the opposite effect was noted if the exposure of cells extended beyond 24 h (43). In suspension cultures of human CD34$^+$ human umbilical cord blood cells, SCF was examined only as part of a combination of cytokines, including IL-1, IL-3, IL-6, GM-CSF, G-CSF, and Epo. The level of expression of PECAM and LFA of these cells dropped dramatically, whereas VLA-4 levels of expression did not change (29).

SCF has been studied extensively in ex vivo expansion experiments both in stroma-free and stroma-containing cultures (Table 4 and 5). Although it is difficult to draw conclusions on the role of any single cytokine, SCF was frequently represented in the most effective combinations.

In vivo, the effects of the administration of SCF were studied in patients with breast and non–small cell lung cancer (44,45). Patients were treated with subcutaneous injections for 14 days. Bone marrow CD34$^+$/HLA-DR$^-$/CD15$^-$ cells increased by 2.4-fold, whereas CD34$^+$/HLA-DR$^+$ cells increased by 3.7-fold. Pretreatment with SCF also resulted in the increased efficiency of HPP-CFC, CFU-Mix, BFU-E, CFU-GM, and CFU-MK.

Mast cells and lymphocytes are also targeted by SCF. The effects on mast cells are evident in mice and in humans and include promotion of the production and upregulation of function (46,47). Skin biopsies from patients pretreated with SCF showed doubling in the number of dermal mast cells (48). On the other hand, despite the lack of an obvious defect in Sl mice, SCF has been reported to be synergistic with IL-7 on the growth of pre–B-lymphocyte colonies in agar culture (49).

C. Tpo

Tpo, or c-mpl ligand, has been shown in several studies to play a pivotal role in the regulation of megakaryopoiesis. In vitro, Tpo promotes the proliferation and differentiation of immature megakaryocytes (50–53). Its augmenting effects on CFU-MK are synergistic when combined with SCF, IL-11, or Epo. On the other hand, these effects were only additive in combination with IL-3 and IL-6 (50). Compared to those generated in cultures containing IL-3, megakaryocytes produced in the presence of Tpo showed increased ploidy (50). In vivo, treatment of mice with Tpo resulted in a 20-fold expansion of megakaryocyte progenitors in the bone marrow with 5-fold increase in the number of platelets in blood (54).

Tpo is lineage predominant but not specific (55). Beside governing platelet production, Tpo has a noticable effect on the myeloid and erythroid lineages. When single adult bone marrow $CD34^+/Thy1^+/Lin^-$ cells were cultured in the presence of a murine stromal cell line, Tpo alone resulted in a plating efficiency of 63% with an average of 351 cells per 1 cell input (56). Although some cultures displayed megakaryocytic differentiation, about 75% of cultures exhibited blast cell outgrowths with myeloid, erythroid, and megakaryocytic potential, suggesting that a hierarchy exists among $CD34^+/Lin^-/Thy1^+$ cells and that the least mature cells can be expanded under the influence of Tpo while maintaining a multilineage differentiation potential. Similarily, Tpo acted synergistically with SCF and IL-3 to support the production of CFU-GM, CFU-E, and CFU-Mix in suspension cultures of $CD34^+/c-kit^{low}/CD38^{low}$ human bone marrow cells (57).

The effects of Tpo on erythropoiesis was tested in vitro and in vivo (54). In vitro, Tpo showed synergistic effects on BFU-E and CFU-E in combination with Epo and SCF or IL-3. In vivo, in mice treated with Tpo, BFU-E were significantly expanded in the bone marrow, whereas CFU-E redistributed from the marrow to the spleen. Furthermore, animals exposed to radiation therapy and carboplatin then treated with Tpo showed a 20% recovery of BFU-E and 60% recovery of CFU-E on day 13 compared to normal animals. The animals untreated with Tpo had almost undetectable levels of BFU-E and CFU-E at the same time point.

Interestingly, Tpo was shown to induce no significant changes in the level of expression of different adhesion molecules such as VLA-4, LFA-1, and ICAM-1 on the surface of megakaryocytes after exposure in vitro to different concentrations for 6 and 24 h (52).

D. Inhibitors

It is now well recognized that regulation of hematopoiesis requires not only stimulating but also inhibiting molecules. A number of suppressors acting mostly on the stem cell compartment have now been characterized and studied. These cytokines act mainly during S-phase of the cell cycle (12,58,59).

The effects of macrophage inflammatory protein-1α (MIP-1α), MIP-2β, transforming growth factor-$\beta1$ (TGF-$\beta1$), macrophage/chemotactic and activating factor (MCAF), platelet factor 4 (PF4), and H-ferritin have been studied at the level of single $CD34^{3+}$ bone marrow and umbilical cord blood cells (59). All these molecules had significant suppressive effect on HPP-CFCs, CFU-Mix, and CFU-GM assessed at day 14. Umbilical cord blood cells were, however, less sensitive to the effect of these cytokines. In a different series of experiments, MIP-1α and TGF-$\beta1$ showed no effect on the more committed CFU-M, CFU-G, and CFU-E stimulated by a single cytokine. Indeed, MIP-1α enhanced the activity of these progenitors (60). In concert with these experiments, TGF-$\beta1$ and MIP-1α demonstrated inhibitory activity on $CD34^+/CD38^-$ human bone marrow cells studied by means of a two-stage pre–Colony-forming cell (pre-CFC) assay. The effect was evident on the total cell number in the liquid phase as well as on the secondary colony-forming cells. TGF-$\beta1$ was the strongest acting between the two molecules. On the other hand, TGF-$\beta1$ had no effect on the more mature $CD34^+/CD38^+$ cells, whereas MIP-1α exhibited an enhancing activity (61). In keeping with these results, TGF-$\beta1$ had a negative effect on the fold-expansion and on the colony-forming activity of three different populations of umbilical cord blood: $CD34^+/CD45RA^{low}/CD71^{low}$ cells (primitive cells), $CD34^+/CD45RA^+/CD71^{low}$ cells (more mature cells and enriched for myeloid progenitors), and $CD34^+/CD45RA^{low}/CD71^+$ cells (also more mature but enriched for erythroid progenitors) (62). Its effects were particularly pronounced on the BFU-E of all three populations. The effects of MIP-1α were limited to the primitive population. TNF-α was similar to TGF-β1, although its action was more pronounced on the CFU-E than on BFU-E. Of note, the effects of these inhibitory molecules were studied in the last set of experiments in the presence of SCF, IL-3, IL-6, and Epo.

Activin and inhibin are two additional cytokines that have been implicated in the regulation of hematopoiesis. Activin has been known to enhance colony formation by IL-3 and Epo-stimulated human BFU-E and CFU-E (63,64). More recently, activin delayed colony formation by peripheral blood–derived CFU-GM stimulated by IL-3 but not by GM- or G-CSF (64). Inhibin, structurally related to activin protein, plays a negative regulation role that also does not seem to be limited to erythropoiesis (65). Injected intravenously into mice, inhibin significantly reduced the number of CFU-Mix in the bone marrow and CFU-Mix, BFU-E, and CFU-GM in the spleen.

E. GM-CSF and G-CSF

GM-CSF and G-CSF are among the most studied cytokines. Although they are mostly lineage specific acting on committed progenitors and mature cells, GM- and G-CSF are less specific when present at high concentrations or synergistically with other cytokines (66). For instance, GM-CSF stimulates not only CFU-GM, but also BFU-E and CFU-Mix in combination with Epo (67). Furthermore, when combined together, GM- and G-CSF can produce recruitment and proliferation of primitive multipotent stem cells with the formation of colonies containing mature monocytes and neutrophils (67). In vivo, both cytokines increase the neutrophil count and shorten the duration of neutropenia after cytotoxic treatments (67,68). GM-CSF also increases the number of monocytes and eosinophils (68).

The effect of cytokines on the differentiation commitment of HPSC can be best demonstrated in competitive development assays of maturing progenies where the lineage commitment of a specific progenitor is governed by the present cytokine. Bipotential mouse bone marrow cells stimulated by CSF-1, G-CSF, or both generate predominantly monocytic, granulocytic, or both types of colonies, respectively (66).

The phenotypic differences in the HPSCs mobilized by GM-, G-CSF, or both were recently studied by Ho et al. The CD34$^+$ percentage was highest in patients receiving G-CSF and lowest in patients treated with GM-CSF. On the other hand, the percentage of CD34$^+$/CD38$^-$ cells was highest in the group treated with GM-CSF alone. The cloning efficiency of the mobilized CD34$^+$ was two times higher when both cytokines were used as compared to when only G-CSF was administered, suggesting that a combination of GM- and G-CSF might be optimal for HPSC mobilization (69).

VI. CONCLUSION

The complexity of the cytokine network controlling blood production has tremendously increased over the last decade. With more than 50 interacting molecules, there is a huge number of possible outcomes where two or more molecules act additively, synergistically, or oppositely to influence survival, proliferation, and differentiation of the HPSCs.

Identification and cloning of these molecules has already had important clinical applications. Better understanding of this system will undoubtedly further serve the exciting field of stem cell therapy.

REFERENCES

1. Carnot P, Delandre G. Sur l'activite hemopoietique du serum au cours de la regeneration du sang. C Rendus Acad Sci Paris 1906; 143:384–386.
2. Ogawa M. Differentiation and proliferation of hematopoietic stem cells. Blood 1993; 81: 2844–2853.
3. Al-Homsi AS, Quesenberry PJ. Ex vivo expansion of hematopoietic stem and progenitor cells. In: Garland JM, Quesenberry PJ, Garland Hilton DJ, eds. Colony-Stimulating Factors. 2d ed. New York: Marcel Dekker 1997:533–546.
4. Gualtieri RJ, Shadduck RK, Baker DG, Quesenberry PJ. Hematopoietic regulatory factors produced in long-term murine bone marrow cultures and the effect of in vitro irradiation. Blood 1984; 64:516–525.
5. Gordon MY. Human hematopoietic stem cell assays. Blood Rev 1993; 7:190–197.
6. Sutherland HJ, Landsorp PM, Henkelman DH, Eaves AC, Eaves CJ. Functional characterization of individual human hematopoietic stem cells cultured at limiting dilution on supportive marrow stromal layers. Proc Natl Acad Sci USA 1990; 87:3584–3588.
7. DA Breems DA, Blokland EAW, Neben S, Plomarcher RE. Frequency analysis of human primitive hematopoietic stem cell subsets using cobblestone area-forming cell assay. Leukemia 1994; 8:1095–1104
8. Harrison DE. Evaluating functional abilities of primitive hematopopietic stem cell populations. Curr Top Microbiol Immunol 1992; 177:13–30.
9. Crosier PS, Clark SC. Basic biology of hematopoietic growth factors. Semin Oncol 1992; 19:349–361.
10. Chabannon C, Torok-Storb B. Stem cell–stromal interactions. Curr Top Microbiol Immunol 1992; 177:123–136.
11. Olsson I, Gullberg U, Lantz M, Richter J. The receptors for regulatory molecules of hematopoiesis. Eur J Haematol 1992; 48:1–9.
12. Quesenberry PJ. Hematopoietic stem cells, progenitor cells, and cytokines. In: Beutler E, Litchman MA, Coller BS, Kipps TJ, eds. Williams Hematology. 5th ed. New York: McGraw-Hill, 1996:211–228.
13. T Kishimoto, T Taga, S Akira: Cytokine signal transduction. Cell 1994; 76:253–262.
14. Whetton AD, Dexter TM. Influence of growth factors and substrates on differentiation of haematopoietic stem cells. Curr Opin Cell Biol 1993; 5:1044–1049.
15. Visvader JE, Elefanty AG, Strasser A, Adam JM: GATA-1 but not SCL induces megakaryocytic differentiation in an early myeloid line. EMBO J 1992; 11:4557–4564.
16. Tanaka R, Katayama N, Ohishi K, Mhmud N, Itoh R, Tanaka Y, Komada Y, Minami N, Sakurai M, Shirakawa S, Shiku H. Accelerated cell-cycling of hematopoietic progenitor cells by growth factors. Blood 1995; 86:73–79.
17. Ritchie A, Gaddy J, Braun S, Gotoh A, Broxmeyer HE. Thrombopoietin upregulates the promoter conformation of p53 in the human growth factor dependent cell line M07e: a potential mechanism for survival enhancing effects (abstr). Blood 1996; 88:1139.
18. Rinaud MS, Su K, Falk LA, Halder S, Mufson RA. Human interleukin-3 receptor modulates bcl-2 mRNA and protein levels through protein kinase C in TF-1 cells. Blood 1995; 86:80–88.
19. Takenaka K, Nagafuji K, Harada M, Mizuno S, Miyamoo T, Makino S, Goodo H, Okamura T, Niho Y. In vitro expansion of hematopoietic progenitor cells induces functional expression of Fas antigen (CD-95). Blood 1996; 88:2871–2877.

20. Levesque JP, Haylock DN, Simmons PJ. Cytokine regulation of proliferation and cell adhesion are correlated events in human CD-34$^+$ hemopoietic progenitors. Blood 1996; 88:1168–1176.

21. Metcalf D. Hematopoietic regulators: redundency or subtlety? Blood 1993; 82:3515–3523.

22. McNiece IK, Langley K, Zsebo KM. Recombinant human stem cell factor (rhSCF) synergises with GM-CSF, G-CSF, IL-3 and Epo to stimulate human progenitor cells of myeloid and erythroid lineages. Exp Hematol 1991; 19:226–230.

23. Bagby GC Jr, Segal G. Growth factors and the control of hematopoiesis. In: Hoffman R, Benz EJ, Jr, Shattil SJ, Furie B, Cohen HJ, Silberstein LE, eds. Hematology: Basic Principles and Practice. 2d ed. New York: Curchill Livingstone: 1995:207–241.

24. Lowry PA, Deacon DH, Whitfield P, McGrath HE, Quesenberry PJSCF. Induction of in vitro murine hematopoietic colony formation by "subliminal" cytokine combinations: the role of "anchor factors." Blood 1992; 80:663–669.

25. Broxmeyer HE, Lu L, Cooper S, Ruggieri L, Li ZH, Lyman SD. Flt3-ligand stimulates/costimulates the growth of myeloid stem/progenitor cells. Exp Hematol 1995; 23:1121–1129.

26. Lyman SD, Brasel K, Rousseau AM, Williams DE. The Flt3-ligand: a hematopoietic stem cell factor whose activities are distinct from steel factor. Stem Cells 1994; 12(suppl 1):99–110.

27. Petzer AL, Zandstra PW, Piret JM, Eaves CJ. Differential cytokine effects on primitive (CD-34$^+$ CD-38$^-$) human hematopoietic cells: novel responses to Flt3-ligand and thrombopoietin. J Exp Med 1996; 183:2551–2558.

28. Wondar-Filipowicz A, Lyman SD, Gratwohl A, Ticheeli A, Speck B, Nissen C. Flt3-ligand level reflects hematopoietic progenitor cell function in aplastic anemia and chemotherapy-induced bone marrow aplasia. Blood 1996; 88:4493–4499.

29. Reems JA. Differential modulation of adhesion receptors on human umbilical cord blood CD-34$^+$ cells after ex vivo expansion (abstr). Blood 1996; 88:1818.

30. Yonemura Y, Ku H, Lyman SD, Ogawa M. In vitro expansion of hematopoietic progenitors and maintenance of stem cells: comparison between Flt3/Flk2-ligand and kit-ligand. Blood 1997; 89:1915–1921.

31. Piacibello W, Sanvio F, Garetto L, Severino A, Ferrario J, Bergandi D, Aglietta M. The association of Flt3-ligand and thrombopoietin in stroma-free cultures allows extensive amplification and self renewal of primitive hematopoietic stem cells residing in the cord blood (abstr). Blood 1996; 88:1184.

32. Maraskovsky E, Roux E, Williams M, McKenna HJ, Brasel K, Lyman SD, Williams DE. The effect of Flt3-ligand and or/c-kit-ligand on the generation of dendritic cells from human CD-34$^+$ bone marrow (abstr). Blood 1996; 88:625.

33. Markavosky E, Brasel K, Pulendran B. Administration of Flt3-ligand results in the generation of large numbers of phenotypically distinct populations of dendritic cells in mice (abstr). Blood 1996; 88:626.

34. Kapp U, Bhatia M, Bonnet D, Murdoch B, Dick JE. Flt3-ligand downregulates B-lymphopoiesis in NOD/Scid mice engrafted with CD-34$^+$/CD-38$^-$ hematopoietic stem cells (abstr). Blood 1996; 88:170.

35. Russell ES. Hereditary anemia of the mouse: a review for geneticists. Adv Genet 1979; 20:357–459.

36. Mayer TC. A comparison of pigment cell development in albino, steel and dominant-spotting mutant mouse embryos. Dev Biol 1970; 23:297–309.

37. Russell ES. Proof of whole-cell implant in therapy of W-series anemia. Arch Biochem Biophys 1968; 125:594–597.

38. McCulloch EA, Siminovitch L, Till JE, Russell ES, Bernstein SE. Cellular basis of the genetically determined hemopoietic defect in anemic mice of genotype Sl/Sl^d. Blood 1964; 26:399–410.

39. Bernstein SE. Tissue transplantation as an analytic and therapeutic tool in hereditary anemias. Am J Surg 1970; 119:448–451.

40. Galli SJ, Zsebo KM, Geissler EN. Kit-ligand, stem cell factor. Adv Immunol 1994; 55:1–96.

41. Brandt J, Briddell RA, Srour EF, Leemhuis TB, Hoffman R. Role of c-kit–ligand in the expansion of human hematopoietic progenitor cells. Blood 1992; 79:634–641.

42. Hoffman R, Tong T, Brandt J, Traycoff C, Bruno E, McGuire BW, Gordon MS, McNiece I, Srour EF. The in vitro and in vivo effects of stem cell factor on human hematopoiesis. Stem Cells 1993; 11(suppl 2):76–82

43. Kovach NL, Lin N, Yednock T, Harlan, Broudy VC. Stem cell factor modulates avidity of alpha₄beta₅ and alpha₅beta₁ integrins expressed on hematopoietic cell lines. Blood 1995; 85:159–167.

44. Demetri G, Costa J, Hayes D, Sledge G, Galli S, Hoffman R, Merica E, Rich W, Harkins B, McGuire B, Gordon MS. A phase I trial of recombinant methionyl human stem cell factor (SCF) in patients with advanced breast carcinoma pre- and post-chemotherapy (chemo) with cyclophosphamide (C) and doxorubicin (A) (abstr). Proc ASCO 1993; 12:367.

45. Crawford J, Lau D, Erwin R, Rich W, McGuire B, Meyers F. A phase I trial of recombinant methionyl human stem cell factor (SCF) in patients (pts) with advanced non–small cell lung cancer (NSCLC) (abstr). Proc ASCO 1993; 12:338.

46. Kitamura Y, Go S. Decreased production of mast cells in Sl/Sl^d anemic mice. Blood 1978; 53:492–497.

47. Tsai M, Takeishi T, Thompson H, Langley KE, Zsebo KM, Metcalf DD, Geissler EN, Galli SJ. Induction of mast cell proliferation, maturation and heparin synthesis by rat c-kit-ligand, stem cell factor. Proc Natl Acad Sci USA 1991; 88:6382–6386.

48. Costa JJ, Demetri GD, Hayes DF, Merica EA, Menchaca DM, Galli SJ. Increased skin mast cells and urine methyl histamine in patients receiving recombinant methionyl human stem cell factor (abstr). Proc AACR 1993; 34:211.

49. McNiece IK, Langley KE, Zsebo KM. The role of recombinant stem cell factor in early B cell development. J Immunol 1991; 146:3785–3790.

50. Broudy VC, Lin NL, Kaushansky K. Thrombopoietin (c-mpl-ligand) acts synergistically with erythropoietin, stem cell factor, and interleukin-11 to enhance murine megakaryocyte colony growth and increases megakaryocyte ploidy in vitro. Blood 1995; 86:1719–1726.

51. Stinicka E, Lin N, Priestley GV, Fox N, Broudy VC, Wolf NS, Kaushansky K. The effect of thrombopoietin on the proliferation of murine hematopoietic stem cells. Blood 1996; 87:4998–5005.

52. Banu N, Wang J, Deng B, Groopman JE, Avraham H. Modulation of megakaryopoiesis by thrombopoietin: the c-mpl-ligand. Blood 1995; 86:1331–1338.

53. Ku H, Yonemura Y, Kaushansky K, Ogawa M. Thrombopoietin, the ligand for the mpl receptor synergizes with steel factor and other early acting cytokines in supporting proliferation of primitive hematopoietic progenitors of mice. Blood 1996; 87:4544–4551.

54. Kaushansky K, Broudy VC, Grossmann A, Humes J, Lin N, Ren HP, Baily MC, Papayannopoulou T, Forstorm JW, Sprugel KH. Thrombopoietin expands erythroid progenitors, increases red cell production and enhances erythroid recovery after myelosuppressive therapy. J Clin Invest 1995; 96:1683–1687.

55. Kaushansky K. Thrombopoietin: biological and preclinical properties. Leukemia 1996; 10(suppl 1):46–48.

56. Young JC, Bruno E, Luens KM, Spencer W, Backer M, Murray LJ. Thrombopoietin stimulates megakaryocytopoiesis, myelopoiesis, and expansion of CD-34⁺ progenitor cells from single CD-34⁺/Thy-1⁺/Lin⁺ primitive progenitor cells. Blood 1996; 88:1619–1631.

57. Kobayashi M, Laver JH, Kato T, Miyazaki H, Ogawa M. Thrombopoietin supports proliferation of human primitive hematopoietic cells in synergy with steel factor and/or interleukin-3. Blood 1996; 88:429–436.

58. Wright EG, Prangnell IB. Stem cell proliferation inhibitors. Baillieres Clin Hematol 1992; 5:723–739.
59. Lu L, Xiao M, Grisby S, Wang WX, Wu B, Shen RN, Broxmeyer HE. Comparative effects of suppressive cytokines on isolated single CD-34^{+++} stem/progenitor cells from human marrow and umbilical cord blood plated with and without serum. Exp Hematol 1993; 23: 1442–1446.
60. Broxmeyer HE. Suppressor cytokines and regulation of myelopoiesis. Am J Pediatr Hematol Oncol 1992; 14:22–30.
61. Van Ranst PCF, Snoeck HW, Lardon F, Lenjou M, Nijs G, Weekx SFA, Rodrigus I, Berneman ZN, Van Bockstaele DR. TGF-beta and MIP-1alpha exert their main inhibitory activity on very primitive CD-34^{++}/CD-38$^-$ cells but show opposite effects on more mature CD-34$^+$/CD-38$^+$ human hematopoietic progenitors. Exp Hematol 1996; 24:1509–1515.
62. Mayani H, Little MT, Dragowska W, Thornbury G, Lansdorp PM. Differential effects of the hematopoietic inhibitors MIP-1alpha, and TNF-alpha on cytokine-induced proliferation of subpopulations of CD-34$^+$ cells purified from cord blood and fetal liver. Exp Hematol 1993; 23:422–427.
63. Yu J, Shao LE, Vaughan J, Vale W, Yu AL. Characterization of the potentiation effect of activin on human erythoid colony formation in vitro. Blood 1989; 73:952–960.
64. Mizuguchi T, Kosaka M, Saito S. Activin A suppresses proliferation of interleukin-3–respon- sive granulocyte-macrophage colony-forming progenitors and stimulates proliferation and differentiation of interleukin-3–responsive erythroid burst-forming progenitors in the periph- eral blood. Blood 1993; 81:2891–2897.
65. Hangoc G, Carow CE, Scwall R, Mason AJ, Broxmeyer HE. Effects in vivo of recombinant human inhibin on myelopoiesis in mice. Exp Hematol 1992; 20:1243–1246.
66. Metcalf D and Nicola NA. Biological actions of the colony-stimulating factors in vitro. In: Metcalf D, Nicola NA, eds. The Hematopoietic Colony-Stimulating Factors. New York: Cambridge University Press 1995:109–165.
67. Demetri GD, Antman KHS. Granulocyte-macrophage colony-stimulating factor (GM-CSF): preclinical and clinical investigations. Semin Oncol 1992; 19:362–385
68. Glaspy JA, Golde DW. Granulocyte colony-stimulating factor (G-CSF): preclinical and clini- cal studies. Semin Oncol 1992; 19:386–394.
69. Ho AD, Young D, Maruyauma M, Corringham RET, Mason JR, Thompson P, Grenier K, Law P, Terastappen LWMM, Lane T. Pluripotent and lineage-committed CD-34$^+$ subsets in leukopheresis products mobilized by G-CSF, GM-CSF vs. a combination of both. Exp Hematol 1996; 24:1460–1468.
70. K Ikebuchi, J N Ihle, T Hirari, Wong GG, Clark SC, Ogawa M. Synergistic factors for stem cell proliferation: further studies of the target stem cells and mechanisms of stimulation by interleukin-1, interleukin-6, and granulocyte colony-stimulating factor. Blood 1988; 72: 2007–2014.
71. Hoang T, Haman A, Goncalves O, Letendre F, Mathieu M, Wong GG, Clark SC. Interleukin- 1 enhances growth factor–dependent proliferation of the clonogenic cells in acute myeloblas- tic leukemia and of normal human primitive hemopoietic precursors, J Exp Med 1988; 168: 463–474.
72. Zsebo KM, Wypych J, Yuschenkoff VN, Lu H, Hunt P, Dukes PP, Langley KE. Effects of hematopoietin-1 and interleukin-1 activities on early hematopoietic cells of the bone marrow. Blood 1988; 71:962–968.
73. Warren DJ, Moore MAS. Synergesim among interleukin-1, interleukin-3, and interleukin-5 in the production of eosinophils from primitive hemopoietic stem cells. J Immunol 1988; 140:94–99.
74. Kupper TS, Lee F, Birchall N, Clark SC, Dowers S. Interleukin-1 binds to specific receptors on human keratinocytes and induces granulocyte-macrophage colony-stimulating factor mRNA and protein. J Clin Invest 1988; 82:1787–1792.

75. Seelentag WK, Mermod JJ, Montesano R, Vassalli P. Additive effects of interleukin-1 and tumor necrosis factor-alpha on the accumulation of the three granulocytes and macrophage colony-stimulating factor mRNAs in human endothelial cells. EMBO J 1987; 6:2261–2265.

76. Herman F, Oster W, Muer SC, Lindemann A, Mertelsmann RH. Interleukin-1 stimulates T lymphocytes to produce granulocyte-monocyte colony-stimulating factor. J Clin Invest 1988; 81:1415–1418.

77. Dinarello CA. Interleukin-1 and the pathogenesis of the acute phase response. N Engl J Med 1984; 311:1413–1418.

78. Arend WP, Welgus HG, Eisenbery SP. Biologic properties of recombinant human monocyte-derived interleukin-1 receptor anragonist. J Clin Invest 1990; 85:1694–1697.

79. Naldini A, Fleischman WR, Ballas ZK, Klimpel KP, Klimpel GR. Interleukin-2 inhibits in vitro granulocyte-macrophage colony-formation. J Immunol 1987; 139:1880–1882.

80. Burdach SE, Levitt LJ. Receptor-specific inhibition of bone marrow erythropoiesis by recombinant DNA–derived interleukin-2. Blood 1987; 69:1368–1375.

81. Waldman TA, Goldman CK, Robb RJ, Deppper JM, Leonard WJ, Shrow SO, Bongiovanni KF, Korsmyer, SJ, Greene WC. Expression of interleukin-2 receptors on activated human B cells. J Exp Med 1984; 160:1450–1466.

82. Koike K, Ihle JN, Ogawa M. Selective culture of murine hemopoietic blast cell colonies based on cell cycle dormacy and requirement of low concentrations of interleukin-3. (abstr). Blood 1985; 66:168.

83. McNiece IK, Bertonello I, Kriegler AB, Quesenberry PJ. Colony-forming cells with high proliferative potential (HPP-CFC). Int J Cell Cloning 1990; 8:146–160.

84. Migliaccio G, Migliaccio AR, Visser JWM. Synergism between erythopoietin and interleukin-3 in the induction of hematopoietic stem cell proliferation and erythroid burst colony formation. Blood 1988; 72:944–951.

85. Ganser A, Lindeman A, Seipelt G, Ottmann OG, Eder M, Falk S, Herman F, Kaltwasser JP, Meusers P, Klausmann M, Frisch J, Achulz G, Mertelsmaa R, Hoezler D. Effects of recombinant human interleukin-3 in aplastic anemia. Blood 1990; 76:1287–1292.

86. Donahue RE, Seehra J, Metzger M, Lefebvre P, Rock B, Carbone S, Nathan PG, Garnick M, Sehgal PK, Laston D, La Vallie E, McCoy J, Shendel PF, Norton C, Turner K, Yang YC, Clark SC. Human IL-3 and GM-CSF act synergitically in stimulating hematopoiesis in primates. Science 1988; 241:1820–1823.

87. Kurzrock R, Talpaz M, Estrov Z, Rosenblum MG, Gutterman JU. Phase I study of recombinant human interleukin-3 in patients with bone marrow failure. J Clin Oncol 1991; 9:1241–1250.

88. Broxmeyer HE, Lu L, Cooper S, Tushinski R, Mochizuki D, Rubin BY, Gillis S, Williams DE. Synergistic effects of purified recombinant human and murine B cell growth factor-interleukin-4 on colony formation in vitro by hematopoietic progenitor cells. J Immunol 1988; 141:3852–3862.

89. Howard M, Farrar J, Hilfiker M, Johnson B, Takatsu K, Hamaoka T, Paul WE. Identification of a T cell–derived B cell growth factor distinct from interleukin-2. J Exp Med 1982; 155:914–923.

90. Vietta ES, Brooks K, Chen YW, Isakson P, Jone S, Layton J, Mishra GC, Pure E, Weiss E, Word C, Yuan D, Tucker P, Uhr JW, Krammer PH. T cell–derived lymphokines that induce IgM and IgG secretion in activated murine B cells. Immunol Rev 1984; 78:137–157.

91. Campbell HD, Tucker WQJ, Hort Y, Martinson ME, Mayo G, Clutterbuck EJ, Sanderson CJ, Young IG. Molecular cloning and expression of the gene encoding human eosinophil differentiation factor (interleukin-5). Proc Natl Acad Sci USA 1987; 84:6629–6633.

92. Takatsu K, Tominaga A, Mamaoka T. Antigen induced T cell replacing factor (TRF). I. Functional characterization of TRF-producing helper T cell subset and gentic studies on TRF production. J Immunol 1980; 124:2414–2422.

93. Quesenberry PJ, McGrath HE, Williams ME, Robinson BE, Deacon DH, Clark S, Urdal

D, McNiece IK. Multifactor stimulation of megakaryopoiesis: effects of interleukin-6. Exp Hematol 1991; 19:35–41.

94. Stahl CP, Zucker-Franklin D, Evatt BL, Winton EF. Effects of human interleukin-6 on megakaryocyte development and thrombocytopoiesis in primates. Blood 1991; 78:1467–1475.

95. Klein B, Zhang XG, Jourdan M, Content J, Hossiau UF, Arden L, Piechaczy M, Bataille R. Paracrine rather than autocrine regulation of myeloma cell growth and differentiation by interleukin-6. Blood 1989; 73:517–526.

96. Yoshizaki K, Matsuda T, Nishimoto N, Kuritani T, Taeho L, Aozasa K, Nakahata T, Kawai H, Tagoh H, Komori T, Krisimoto S, Hirano T, Kishimoto T. Pathogenic significance of interleukin-6 (IL-6/BSF-2) in Castleman's disease. Blood 1989; 74:1360–1367.

97. Kimberly JVZ, Fischer E, Hawes AS, Hebert CA, Terrell TG, Baker JB, Lowry SF, Moldawyer LL. Effects of intravenous IL-8 in nonhuman primates. J Immunol 1992; 148:1746–1752.

98. Oppenheim JJ, Zachariae COC, Mukaida N, Matsushima K. Properties of the novel proinflammatory super gene intercrine cytokine family. Annu Rev Immunol 1991; 9:617–648.

99. Holbrook ST, Ohls RK, Schibler KR, Yang YC, Christensen RD. Effect of interleukin-9 on clonogenic maturation and cell cycle status of fetal and adult hematopoietic progenitors. Blood 1991; 77:2129–2134.

100. Donahue RE, Yang YC, Clark SC. Human p40 T cell growth factor (interleukin-9) supports erythroid colony formation. Blood 1990; 75:2271–2275.

101. Van Snick J, Goethals A, Renauld JC, Van Roost E, Uyttenhove C, Rubira MR, Moritz RL, Simpson RJ. Cloning and characterization of a cDNA for a new mouse T cell growth factor (P40). J Exp Med 1989; 169:363–369.

102. Chen WF, Zlotnick A. IL-10: a novel cytotoxic T cell differentiation factor. J Immunol 1991; 147:528–534.

103. Fiorentino DF, Bond MW, Mosmann TR. Two types of mouse T helper cell. J Exp Med 1989; 170:2081–2095.

104. Musashi M, Yang YC, Paul SR. Direct and synergistic effects of interleukin-11 on murine hemopoiesis in culture. Proc Natl Acad Sci USA 1991; 88:765–769.

105. Musashi M, Clark SC, Sudo T, Urdal DL, Ogawa M. Synergistic interactions between interleukin-11 and interleukin-4 in support of proliferation of primitive hematopoietic progenitors of mice. Blood 1991; 78:1448–1451.

106. Goldman S, Loebelenz J, McCarthy K, Hayes L, Nebent T, Stoudemire JB, Schaub RG. Recombinant human interleukin-11 stimulates megakaryocytic maturation and increase in peripheral platelet number in vivo. Blood 1991; 78:132 (abstr).

107. Du XX, Neben T, Goldman S, Williams DA. Effects of recombinant human interleukin-11 on hematopoietic reconstitution in transplant mice: acceleration of peripheral blood neutrophils and platelets. Blood 1993; 81:27–34.

108. Kobayashi M, Fitz L, Ryan M, Hewick RM, Clark SC, Chan S, Loudon R, Sherman F, Perussia B, Trinchieri G. Identification and purification of natural killer cell stimulatory factor (NKSF), a cytokine with multiple biologic effects on human lymphocytes. J Exp Med 1989; 170:827–845.

109. Gately MK, Desai BB, Woltizky AG, Quinn PM, Dwyer CM, Padalski FJ, Familletti PC, Sinigaglla F, Chizonnite R, Gubler U, Stern AS. Regulation of human lymphocyte proliferation by a heterodimeric cytokine, IL-12 (cytotoxic lymphocyte maturation factor). J Immunol 1991; 147:874–882.

110. Jacobson SEW, Okkenhaug C, Veiby OP, Caput D, Ferrera P, Minty A. Interleukin-13: novel role in direct regulation of proliferation and differentiation of primitive hematopoietic progenitor cells. J Exp Med 1994; 180:75–82.

111. Minty A, Chalon P, Derocq JM, Dumont X, Guillemon JC, Kaghad M, Labit C, Leplatois P, Liauzum P, Miloux B, Minty C, Casellas P, Ioison G, Lupker J, Shire D, Ferrara P, Caput

D. Interleukin-13 is a new human lymphokine regulating inflammatory and immune responses. Nature 1993; 362:248–250.

112. McKenzie ANJ, Culpepper JA, De Waal Malefyt A, Briere F, Punnonen J, Aversa G, Sato A, Dang W, Cock BG, Menon S, De Vries JE, Banchereau J, Zurawski G. Interleukin-13, a novel T cell–derived cytokine that regulates human monocyte and B cell function. Proc Natl Acad Sci USA 1993; 90:3735–3739.

113. Ambrus JL, Pippin J, Joseph A, Xu C, Blumenthal D, Tamayo A, Claypool K, McCourt D, Srikiatchatochorn A. Identification of a cDNA for a human high-molecular-weight B cell growth factor. Proc Natl Acad Sci USA 1993; 90:6330–6334.

114. Agostini C, Trentin L, Sancetta R, Facco M, Tassinari C, Cerutti A, Bortolin M, Milani A, Siviero M, Zambello R, Semenzato G. Interleukin-15 triggers activation and growth of the CD-8 T cell pool in extravascular tissues of patients with acquired immunodeficiency syndrome. Blood 1997; 90:1115–1123.

115. Baier M, Bannert N, Werner A, Lang K, Kurth R. Molecular cloning, sequence, expression, and processing of the interleukin-16 precursor. Proc Natl Acad Sci USA 1997; 94:5273–5277.

116. Fossiez F, Djossou O, Chomarat P, Flores-Romo L, Ait-Yahia S, Maat C, Pin JJ, Garrone P, Garcia E, Saeland S, Blanchard D, Gaillar C, Das Marhaptra B, Rouvier E, Golstein P, Banchereau J, Lebecque S. T cell IL-17 induces stromal cells to produce proinfalmmatory and hematopoietic cytokines. J Exp Med 1996; 183:2593–2603.

117. Yao Z, Painter SL, Fanslow WC, Ulrich D, Macduff B, Spriggs MK, Armitage A. Human IL-17: a novel cytokine derived from T cells. J Immunol 1995; 155:5483–5486.

118. Micallef MJ, Ohtsuki T, Kohno K, Tanabe F, Ushio S, Namba M, Tanimoto T, Torigoe K, Fujii M, Ikeda M, Fukuda S, Kurimoto M. Interferon-gamma–inducing factor enhances T helper 1 cytokine production by stimulated human T cells: synergism with interleukin-12 for interferon-gamma production. Eur J Immunol 1996; 26:1647–1651.

119. Okamura H, Tsutsi H, Komatsu T, Yutsudo M, Hajura A, Tanimoto T, Torigoe K, Okura T, Nukada Y, Hattori K, Akita K, Namba M, Tanabe F, Konishi K, Fukuda F, Kurimoto M. Cloning of a new cytokine that induces INF-gamma production by T cells. Nature 1995; 378:88–91.

120. Sytkowski AJ, Feldman L, Zubrbuch DJ. Biological activity and structural stability of N-deglycosylated recombinant human erythropoietin. Biochem Biophys Res Commun 1991; 176:698–704.

121. Gregory CJ, Eaves AC. Three stages of erythropoietic progenitor differentiation by a number of physical and biological properties. Blood 1978; 51:527–537.

122. McDonald TP, Cottrell MB, Clift RE, Cullen WC, Lin FK. High doses of recombinant erythropoietin stimulate platelet production in mice. Exp Hematol 1987; 15:719–721.

123. Maekawa T, Metcalf D. Clonal suppression of HL60 and U937 cells by recombinant human leukemia inhibitory factor in combination with GM-CSF and G-CSF. Leukemia 1989; 3:270–276.

124. Henschler R, Brugger W, Luft T, Frey T, Mertelsmann R, Kanz L. Maintenance of transplantation potential in ex vivo expanded CD-34+–selected human peripheral blood progenitor cells. Blood 1994; 84:2898–2903.

125. Brugger W, Mocklin V, Heimfeld S, Berneson RJ, Mertelsmann R, Kanz L. Ex vivo expansion of enriched peripheral blood CD-34+ progenitor cells by stem cell factor, interleukin-1 beta (IL-1 beta), IL-6, IL-3, interferon-gamma, and erythropoietin. Blood 1993; 83:2579–2584.

126. Haylock DN, To LB, Dowse TL, Juttner CA, Simmons PJ. Ex vivo expansion and maturation of peripheral blood CD-34+ cells into myeloid lineage. Blood 1992; 80:1405–1412.

127. Dooley DC, Plunkett JM, Oppenlander BK, Novak FP. Expansion of myeloid progenitors is accompanied by rapid loss of long-term culture initiating cells during ex vivo cultivation of steady state peripheral blood (absrt). Exp Hematol 1994; 22:305.

128. Williams SW, Lee WJ, Bender JG, Zimmerman T, Swinney P, Blake M, Carreon J, Schilling M, Smith S, Williams DE, Oldham F, Van Epps D. Selection and expansion of peripheral blood CD-34$^+$ cells in autologous stem cell transplantation for breast cancer. Blood 1996; 87:1687–1691.

129. Moore MAS, Schneider JG, Shapiro F, Bengla C. Ex vivo expansion of CD-34$^+$ hematopoietic progenitors. In: Gross S, ed. Advances in Bone Marrow Purging and Processing. 4th International Symposium. New York: Wiley-Liss, 1994:217–228.

130. Srour EF, Brandt JE, Briddell RA, Grisby R, Leemhuis T, Hoffman R. Long term generation and expansion of human primitive hematopoietic progenitor cells in vitro. Blood 1992; 81: 661–669.

131. Moore MAS, Hoskins I. Ex vivo expansion of cord blood–derived stem cells and progenitors. Blood Cells 1994; 20:468–481.

132. Mayani H, Lansdorp PM. Thy-1 expression is linked to functional properties of primitive hematopoietic progenitor cells from human umbilical cord blood. Blood 1994; 83:2410–2417.

133. Muench MO, Moore MAS. Accelerated recovery of peripheral blood cell counts in mice transplanted with in vitro cytokine-expanded hematopoietic progenitors. Exp Hematol 1992; 20:611–618.

134. Muench MO, Firpo MT, Moore MAS. Bone marrow transplantation with interleukin-1 plus kit-ligand—ex vivo expanded bone marrow accelerates hematopoietic reconstitution in mice without the loss of stem cell lineage and proliferative potential. Blood 1993; 81:3463–3473.

135. Ruggieri L, Heimfeld S, Broxmeyer HE. Cytokine dependent ex vivo expansion of early subsets of CD-34$^+$ cord blood myeloid progenitors is enhanced by cord blood plasma, but expansion of the more mature subsets of progenitors is favored. Blood Cells 1994; 20:436–454.

136. Rebel VI, Dragowska W, Eaves CJ, Humphries RK, Lansdorp PM. Amplification of Sca-1$^+$/Lin$^-$/WGA$^+$ cells in serum-free cultures containing steel factor, interleukin-6, and erythropoietin with maintenance of cells with long term in vivo reconstitution potential. Blood 1994; 83:128–136.

137. Peters SO, Kittler EL, Ramshaw HS, Quesenberry PJ. Murine marrow cells expanded with IL-3, IL-6, IL-11, and SCF acquire an engraftment defect in normal hosts. Exp Hematol 1995; 23:461–469.

138. Peters SO, Kittler EL, Ramshaw HS, Quesenberry PJ. Ex vivo expansion of murine marrow cells with interleukin-3 (IL-3), IL-6, IL-11, and stem cell factor leads to impaired engraftment in irradiated hosts. Blood 1996; 87:30–37.

139. Koller MR, Emerson SG, Palsson BO. Large scale expansion of human stem and progenitor cells from bone marrow mononuclear cells in continuous perfusion cultures. Blood 1993; 82:378–384.

140. Koller MR, Palsson MA, Manchel I, Palsson B. Long term culture-initiating cell is dependent on frequent medium exchange combined with stromal and other accessory cell effects. Blood 1995; 86:1784–1793.

141. Han CS, Dugan MJ, Verfaillie CM, Wagner JE, McGlave PB. In vitro expansion of umbilical cord blood committed primitive progenitors (abstr) Exp Hematol 1994; 23:170.

142. Brandt J, Galy A, Luens K, Travis M, Davis T, Lee K, Bruno E, Chen R, Tushinski R, Hoffman R. Maintenance of human hematopoietic stem cells during ex vivo progenitor cell expansion on a porcine endothelial cell line (abstr). Exp Hematol 1996; 24:28.

5

Homing and Self-Renewal of Hematopoietic Stem Cells

ANTHONY D. HO, MICHAEL PUNZEL, and STEFAN FRUEHAUF

University of Heidelberg, Heidelberg, Germany

SHIANG HUANG and BERNHARD PALSSON

University of California, San Diego, La Jolla, California

I. INTRODUCTION

Hematopoietic stem cell (HSC) transplantation has been shown to be a lifesaving procedure for a variety of malignant and hereditary diseases. The success of transplantation, both allogeneic and autologous, hinges on the abilities of the HSC to "home" to the bone marrow. Once homed in the appropriate microenvironment, the HSCs proliferate and make sequential decisions to self-renew as well as to produce progenitors that ultimately give rise to the mature blood cells. Hence homing to the marrow on the one hand and the dual abilities of self-renewal and differentiation on the other represent unique properties of HSCs.

Considering the complex cascade of events that the HSCs have to go through to reach the microenvironment of the bone marrow, homing is a fascinating phenomenon. Adhesion molecules, a large number of chemokines and cytokines, stroma cells, and probably "accessory cells" functioning in a coordinated fashion are prerequisites. After being infused into the circulation of the recipient, the HSCs have to marginalize to the endothelial cells of the blood vessels in the appropriate environment; that is, the sinusoids of the bone marrow. After slowing down, rolling, and adhesion, they then migrate through the vessel wall to their specific niche in the bone marrow and finally get attached to stroma cells (Fig. 1). Once settled, they must be aroused from the quiescent state and start to divide in order to to make sequential decisions to self-renew as well as to differentiate.

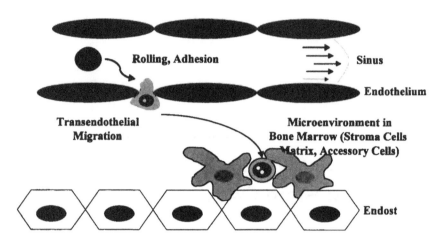

Figure 1 Homing of hematopoietic stem cells. For explanation see text.

Much research interest and efforts have thus far been devoted to identify, to acquire, and to multiply HSCs for transplantation and for gene therapy. Novel growth factors and cytokines have been discovered that stimulate various aspects of hematopoiesis. The approach to identify HSCs has included assays that provide a read-out of the growth potential of selected cell subsets. In vitro assays involved seeding of a particular subset of hematopoietic cells supposed to be enriched in HSCs onto a culture plate and performing a read-out after a defined period of between 14 days for in vitro "colony assays" and 4–6 weeks for "long-term" cultures. In vivo assays involved inoculation of HSCs into animals after irradiation and/or myeloablative chemotherapy and estimating the quantity of HSC candidates required to reconstitute marrow function after transplantation. Little interest has been devoted to the events that happen between seeding of HSCs and read-out.

This chapter will focus on the early events in homing and on the history of the first cell divisions of HSCs as well as on the relationship between divisional behavior to the long-term fate of the daughter cells. Our recently developed technology of automated fluorescence image cytometry (AFIC), combined with single cell culture, has provided a unique opportunity to study the early HSC behavior after being seeded.

II. METHODS FOR IDENTIFICATION OF HSC CANDIDATES

Several methods have been employed to separate the HSCs from the other cellular elements of the bone marrow or peripheral blood. Various properties such as size, buoyant density of the progenitor cells, and resistance to treatment with 5-fluorouracil have been exploited (1–3). The discovery of specific phenotypic markers and the development of fluorescence-activated cell sorting (FACS) technology have greatly facilitated the separation of subpopulations rich in HSCs. Cell selection is then based on phenotypic marker studies and on testing the sorted cells in clonogenic progenitor and in vivo reconstitution assays. The biological potentials of specific subsets are then tested in various clonogenic progenitor or in vivo reconstitution assays.

The development of monoclonal antibodies that recognize the surface molecule CD34 (4) has contributed significantly toward identification of HSCs. CD34 is a glycoprotein that is present on the membrane of 0.5% to several percentages of human bone marrow cells. Enriched fractions of CD34 cells contain virtually all hematopoietic progenitors that are clonogenic in vitro (5,6). However, with regard to phenotype and function, CD34 cells have been shown to be heterogeneous. Additional monoclonal antibodies have been used to subdivide the CD34$^+$ compartments, some of which are more enriched in stem cell candidates and others of lineage-committed progenitors (7–10). The primitive stem cells candidates are characterized by CD34$^+$/CD38$^-$ and can be further subclassified according to the presence or absence of additional surface membrane markers. The lineage-committed subsets are characterized by CD34$^+$/CD38$^+$ and the coexpression of one of the following antigens: CD7, CD10, CD16, CD33, CD61, CD64, or CD71 depending on the lineage commitment (7–12). It is controversial which CD34$^+$ subset represents the population with the highest self-renewal or multilineage potential and hence HSC candidates. Possible candidates include CD34$^+$/CD38$^-$ (7), CD34$^+$/HLA-DR$^-$ (13–16), CD34$^+$/CD38$^-$/HLA-DR$^+$ (9), CD34$^+$/Thy1$^+$/Lin$^-$ (16–17), or CD34$^+$/CD45RA^{low}/CD71^{low} (18). Among cell preparations derived from different sources, there are probably not only quantitative differences in the proportion of candidate stem cells versus lineage-committed progenitors but also significant functional differences among cells with the same phenotype (19).

In a murine model, the phenotype and function of HSCs has been characterized using competitive in vivo repopulation assays (20–22). Obviously such repopulation assays cannot be performed in humans, and surrogate in vitro assays have to be used to evaluate human HSC. Semisolid and liquid cultures of hematopoietic cells grown in the presence of various conditioned culture media or cytokines have been used broadly as surrogate tests for HSC activity.

For the precise correlation of phenotype and growth potential without interference from other cells, a single-cell suspension culture system has been developed (7). In this assay, cells were deposited using the automated cell deposition unit (ACDU) onto a 96-well plate. Each well contained a medium supplemented with recombinant human erythropoietin (rhEpo; Amgen, Thousand Oaks, CA), interleukin-3 (rhIL-3), rhIL-6, granulocyte-macrophage colony-stimulating factor (rhGM-CSF), basic fibroblast growth factor (rhbFGF), insulin-like growth factor-1 (rhIGF-1; Collaborative Research, Bedford, MA), and stem cell factor (rhSCF; Genzyme, Boston, MA). After 14 days of culture, colony efficiency and growth patterns were scored. Replating of the cell progeny was performed by dispersion of the cells into 8 wells of a 96-well flat-bottom plate in identical culture conditions. Growth was scored after an additional 14 days. Repetitive replating was performed if cells with dispersed and mixed growth pattern could be detected. With this single-cell liquid culture, we were able to define precisely the colony efficiency, the growth pattern, and the replating potential of each phenotype of CD34$^+$ cells. Colony efficiency (CE) is defined as the percentage of wells, each initially containing one single cell sorted into a 96-well plate, that develop into colonies after 14 days. Blast colony efficiency (BE) is defined as the percentage of colonies that show dispersed (blast colonies) and mixed growth pattern (blasts with clusters in between). The latter have the potential to give rise to further colonies when replated in a liquid culture system. Replating potential (RP) takes into consideration the percentages of cells that give rise to multiple generations and the number of generations that can be derived by replating the cells with a dispersed and mixed growth pattern derived from the corresponding phenotype. By applying this method, we have provided evidence that among the CD34$^+$ subpopulations derived from fetal bone marrow (FBM), the subset characterized by CD34$^+$/CD38$^-$/HLA-DR$^+$ gave rise to both myeloid and lymphoid precursors (7,9). Moreover, cells that grew in a dispersed growth pattern could give rise to up to four generations of colonies after repetitive replating (7,9,19). Further studies comparing CD34$^+$ subsets derived from fetal tissues, umbilical cord blood (UCB), adult bone marrow (ABM), and mobilized peripheral blood (MPB) have demonstrated that the single-sorted CD34$^+$/CD38$^-$/HLA-DR$^+$ cells from fetal liver gave rise to the highest number of cells with dispersed and mixed growth patterns and cells with the highest replating potential (19).

To maintain long-term growth and development of HSCs, the presence of stromal cells is essential. Stromal cells are derived from primary bone marrow cultures or from cloned stromal cell lines. These cells probably provide growth factors as well as other stimuli that are required to maintain hematopoiesis. The following in vitro assays, supported by the use of allogeneic bone marrow stromal cells, have been developed to enumerate HSC candidates and include long-term culture-initiating cell (LTCIC) assay (23), cobblestone area–forming cell (CAFC) assays (24), and extended LTC-IC (ELTCIC) assay (25). These methods enumerate primitive progenitors that can generate myeloid cells, but not cells with multilineage or self-renewal potential. Several groups have developed cultures that allow differentiation of single human CD34$^+$ Lin$^-$ cells into cells with myeloid, natural killer (NK), B-lymphoid, dendritic, and/or T-lymphoid phenotype demonstrating that a single cell can differentiate in vitro into multiple lineages (26–27). Recently, an even more primitive multilineage progenitor named myeloid-lymphoid–initiating cell (MLIC) has been described (28). This cell is capable of generating multiple secondary LTCICs as well as primitive lymphoid progenitors (NKICs) and is therefore closely related to the hematopoietic stem cell. The self-renewing capacity of the MLIC is currently being investigated. Thus, the in vitro read-out from the latter system provides a better estimation of more immature progenitors than LTCICs and may lead to the first in vitro assay for human HSCs.

Transplantation of human progenitors in xenogeneic transplant recipients, such as SCID mice (29–31), BNX mice (32,33), NOD-SCID mice (34–36), or fetal sheep, (37,38), allows detection of engrafting human cells. In vivo production of myeloid, NK, T-lymphoid, and B-lymphoid blood elements is seen for several months to years after transplantation. Through transplantation of limiting numbers of CD34$^+$ subpopulations, these xenotransplant models provide a semiquantitative assay for engrafting cells. However, such transplant models cannot prove that a single cell possesses both self-renewal and multilineage differentiation potentials that are characteristic of HSCs.

III. CHARACTERISTICS OF HSC CANDIDATES

Several studies have identified various phenotypes that are highly enriched for candidate stem cell populations. Some investigators have reported that adult bone marrow CD34 / Lin$^-$ cells which expressed low to undetectable levels of surface HLA-DR antigen contained primitive LTCICs and precursors which differentiated into lymphoid and myeloid cells in vitro (39–41). Others have shown that the CD34$^+$/Lin$^-$/HLA-DR^{low} cells retained a long-term repopulating ability in xenogeneic transplant models (42). Craig et al. reported that when CD34$^+$ cells derived from adult bone marrow were sorted on the basis of Thy1 expression, the majority of colony-forming progenitors in 14-day culture were recovered in the CD34$^+$/Thy1$^-$ fraction, whereas cells capable of producing myeloid colonies after 5–8 weeks of long-term culture (LTCICs) were recovered predominantly in the CD34 / Thy1$^+$ fraction (17). Uchida et al. reported that the dye rhodamine 123 was able to distinguish the primitive hematopoietic stem cells (which displayed a rapid efflux of Rh123) from committed progenitors among CD34$^+$/Thy1$^+$/Lin$^-$ cells (10). Leemhuis et al. used a combination of CD34, Hoechst 33342, and rhodamine 123 to distinguish primitive hemopoietic stem cells (43). They proposed that since Hoechst 33342 and rhodamine 123 (Rh123) both identify metabolically inactive cells, these two characteristics can be used in conjunction with CD34 antigen to isolate quiescent and metabolically inactive primitive hematopoietic progenitor cells. Hill et al. showed that CD59 identified a subset of CD34$^+$ bone marrow cells enriched for pluripotent stem cells (44). They reported that practically all CD34$^+$/Thy1$^+$/Lin$^-$ cells were found in the CD34$^+$/CD59^{high} population. Although virtually all primitive pluripotent stem cells were in the CD34$^+$/CD59^{high} subpopulation, the latter was again found to be heterogeneous. Young et al. used PKH26 to separate the CD34$^+$/Thy1$^+$/Lin$^-$ cells derived from ABM and MPB into PKH26 bright (<4 cell divisions) and PKH26 dim cells (bright >4 cell divisions) (45). They showed that single CD34$^+$/Lin$^-$/dye progenitors purified from bulk cultures could produce as many as 1000 CD34$^+$ progeny cells, which included multilineage colony-forming cells.

A combination of approaches might be necessary to identify the HSC candidates. We have demonstrated that the progenitors with the highest proliferative and replating potentials are found among CD34$^+$/CD38$^-$/HLA-DR$^+$ cells as compared to any other phenotypes from the same source (19). Our results are consistent with the report from Traycoff et al., who reported that in contrast to findings in adult bone marrow, where the LTCICs were shown to be found among CD34$^+$/HLA-DR$^-$ cells, the LTCICs appeared to be present among CD34$^+$/HLA-DR$^+$ cells in UCB (46). Hence, HSC candidates might be distributed among various phenotypes, depending on their ontogenic age. Using the combination of CD34, CD38, and CDw90 (Thy1), the cells demonstrating dispersed and mixed growth patterns from FLV and FBM seemed to be found predominantly in the CDw90$^-$ subsets. In UCB and MPB, the HSC candidates were found evenly distributed among CDw90$^+$ and CDw90$^-$ subsets (19). Whereas HSC candidates were found both among CD34$^+$/CD38$^-$/CDw90$^+$ and CD34$^+$/CD38$^-$/CDw90$^-$ subsets in the preparations from fetal tissues and UCB, they were found exclusively among CD34$^+$/CD38$^-$/CDw90$^+$ cells from MPB.

IV. VISUALIZATION OF CELL MOTION AND DIVISION

Visualization of cell motion and cell division by means of a time-lapse camera system represents a powerful tool to study the motion and divisional history of stem cells. Exciting discoveries in neural stem cell behavior have been made possible by imaging studies of neuroblast divisions and development.

Time-lapse measurements of cells in multiple microscope fields over long periods of time (hours to days) requires instrumentation that can operate in a fully automatic manner. We have established an automated fluorescence imaging cytometry (AFIC) system to monitor the behavior of HSCs after seeding onto in vitro cultures. The components of this operator-independent level of automation are autofocus, computerized microscope stage movement, and automated measurement/imaging system (47). The problem of image segmentation accuracy using real time methods was then approached by utilizing least squares designed filters for enhancing contrast (48). These filters were combined with automatic intensity thresholding for fully automated operation. Using this system, we have measured the motion of enriched CD34$^+$ cell populations at low and high densities. The preliminary data demonstrated the following: (1) CD34$^+$ cells have been observed to extend long, thin pseudopodia; (2) CD34$^+$ cells are motile exhibit directed motion; and (3) CD34$^+$ cells appeared to sense the presence of one another and communicate with one another (49).

In monitoring cell divisional history, images were acquired using an inverted fluorescent microscope (Nikon Diaphot 300, Nikon Inc., New York, NY) with a 4X objective such that an entire well of a Terasaki plate can be observed in a single image (1938 by

1523 µm) field of view. Illumination was provided by a 100-W mercury arc lamp which passed through a 41003 filter set (Chroma Technologies, Brattleboro, VT). Digitized images were acquired and stored on a SGI O_2 workstation (Silicon Graphics, Mountain View, CA). A motorized X, Y, Z stage (Ludl, Inc., Hawthorn, NY) moved the stage between wells so multiple images could be rapidly collected. All acquisition and processing functions were controlled by the Isee software (Inovision Corp., Durham, NC), which allowed the analysis of multiples from the list to create a composite image that showed changes in cell shape or position over time. Cells in a Terasaki plate can be simultaneously tracked in a single experiment and revisited at prescribed time intervals.

After the cells were deposited as single cells, the replication history of HSCs was monitored; initially every 3–12 hs for 7–10 days. The replication history of the HSCs was measured using the PKH membrane dyes, which were available in both green (PKH2) and red (PKH26) forms (50,51). These dyes consist of a fluorophore attached to an aliphatic carbon backbone which binds irreversibly to the lipid bilayer. With each cell division, the fluorescent intensity of the PKH dye is reduced by one half. Thus, one can determine, using the time-lapse camera system, the replication history of the daughter cells. We determined the kinetics of cell division by measuring the doubling times, and whether both daughters divided symmetrically, and under which conditions did the cells undergo asymmetrical division. The same plates were kept in culture for 10–14 days whenever possible and the colony efficiency and growth patterns were determined.

The mitosis index is defined as the number of single-sorted cells that have shown cell division after 8 days versus the total number of cells of the same phenotype deposited. Asymmetrical division is defined as the number of cells that demonstrated at least one asymmetrical division during the course of 8 days versus the total number of cells deposited. The asymmetrical division index (ADI) is defined as the number of cells that demonstrated at least one asymmetrical division during the course of 8 days divided by the number of dividing cells.

Using the AFIC system, we have monitored the divisional history of HSCs after seeding and correlated these data with the "long-term" outcome in vitro; that is, after 14-day cultures.

V. SELF-RENEWAL AND DIFFERENTIATION OF HSCs

HSCs are characterized by the dual abilities to self-renew and to differentiate into progenitors of all the mature blood cell lineages. These two features are especially evident after bone marrow transplantation and require that the HSCs undergo sequential decision processes and rounds of asymmetrical divisions to generate mature cells of the distinct blood lineages as well as cells to sustain long-term hematopoiesis (52). The two daughter cells from a HSC may be initially equivalent, but subsequent cell divisions must result in different fates of the progeny cells (53). It has therefore been suggested that the hallmark of a stem cell might be its ability to divide asymmetrically to produce a daughter cell identical to the mother and another cell committed to differentiation (54,55). Alternatively, a balance between symmetrical cell divisions that results in self-renewal versus that which results in differentiation might be able to maintain the stem cell pool and provide a source of multipotent progenitors. Even if the latter were true, asymmetrical division must have occurred during ontogenesis of these two populations, and further asymmetrical divisions must occur during their multilineage differentiation.

A central question in developmental biology is how a single cell can divide to produce two daughter cells that adopt distinct fates (55). Theoretically, daughter cells with different fates can arise by means of the following mechanisms. First, they may be different from each other at the time of cell division; that is, due to intrinsic factors. A parental factor, such as a transcription factor, may be distributed unevenly to the daughter cells. Second, the daughter cells may be similar at the time of cell division but become different on subsequent exposure to environmental signals such as a cytokine or contact with another cell; that is, due to extrinsic factors (53–55).

VI. MODEL FOR THE ASYMMETRICAL DIVISION OF STEM CELLS

Thus far, remarkably little is known if and how hematopoietic stem cells divide in a self-renewing, asymmetrical fashion. Recently, studies of asymmetrical division of neural stem cells in *Drosophila* and mammals have provided new insights into the mechanism of stem cell division and might serve as a model for hematopoietic reconstitution (54–57). These studies demonstrated that at least three types of asymmetrical divisions can be found in neural progenitors. (1) In *Drosophila*, neuroblasts (NBs) undergo a series of oriented asymmetrical divisions to renew themselves and produce smaller ganglion mother cells. (2) In the peripheral nervous system, a sensory organ precursor (SOP) responsible for forming external sensory organs (i.e., sensory bristles) generates an organ by dividing asymmetrically to form precursor cells to produce two outer support cells (a hair and a socket cell), a sensory neuron, and a sheath cell (54). (3) In the central nervous system, MP2 precursors are a pair of embryonic neural precursors that divide only once to produce two different postmitotic neurons (54). Recent genetic analysis has identified several proteins that differentially segregate during division and may be involved in determining the asymmetry of the division (53–58). These important cell fate determinants range from transcription factors (such as PROS) to modulations of cell-cell interactions (such as NUMB) and are asymmetrically localized during division of neuroblasts.

VII. DIVISIONS OF HSCs

In a series of experiments, Ogawa and his colleagues have reported disparate differentiation in paired hematopoietic progenitors (59–62). Initially in a murine model (59,60), later confirmed in the human HSC, (61,62), they demonstrated that when paired daughter cells from a single progenitor were cultured, about 20% of the progenitors divided asymmetrically, giving rise to different differentiation pathways. When mouse-derived primitive progenitors were cultured individually, asymmetrical divisions always involved multipotent progenitors (59,60). Symmetrical divisions involved both multipotent and monopotent progenitors and occurred in the rest. Similar results were observed in studies of human HSCs (61,62). Given these different types of evidence, Ogawa et al. suggested that stem cell differentiation is a stochastic process. Lansdorp et al. also described "asymmetry" of cell division of hematopoietic progenitors (63). In their studies, individually sorted human cord blood–derived primitive hematopoietic cells were allowed to undergo one division after which the two daughter cells were physically separated and cultured in either the same or different cytokine combinations. These investigators used cytokine combinations favoring erythropoiesis [mast cell growth factor (MGF) + interleukin-6 (IL-6) + interleukin-3 (IL-3) erythropoietin (Epo)] or myelopoiesis [MGF + IL-6 + fusion protein of IL-3 and GM-CSF + macrophage colony-stimulating factor (M-CSF) + granulocyte CSF (G-CSF)] in the culture media. Asymmetrical division was defined as a division that yields two daughter cells with distinct functional properties; that is, one of the daughter cells gave rise to erythroid and the other to myeloid or mixed colonies, corresponding to asymmetrical division of peripheral sensory organ progenitors described in neural stem cells (54). According to Lansdorp et al., asymmetrical divisions occurred in 3–17% of the cultured cells and lineage commitment did not seem to be influenced by cytokines. Based on all these observations, they also suggested that stem cell differentiation is a stochastic event. The fundamental question—if asymmetrical divisions of HSCs with one cell remaining quiescent and maintaining self-renewal capacity occur—was not addressed by these studies. With our present technology of AFIC, we have been able to visualize the behavior of dividing CD34$^+$/CD38$^-$ cells during the first rounds of cell divisions and to correlate this behavior with their corresponding fates in further cell culture. The focus was therefore on an earlier level in the hierarchy of HSC development, corresponding to the asymmetrical cell divisions of primitive neuroblasts (54). Recently, Brummendorf et al. linked cell division rate and asymmetrical cell divisions (55). They showed that the proliferative potential and cell cycle properties were unevenly distributed among daughter cells derived from single-sorted HSCs from fetal liver, and that expansion potential is associated with asymmetrical division.

VIII.   KINETICS AND SYMMETRY OF INITIAL MITOSIS OF CANDIDATE HSCs

Current evidence from the neural stem cell research supports the idea that asymmetrical divisions are defined mostly by cell-autonomous information, whereas extrinsic signal might also be involved initially in instructing the asymmetrical fates of daughter cells. To address this fundamental question in developmental biology, we have applied our AFIC system to observe directly the first divisions among primitive HSC candidates. Combined with our single-cell culture system, we can correlate the early replication behavior with

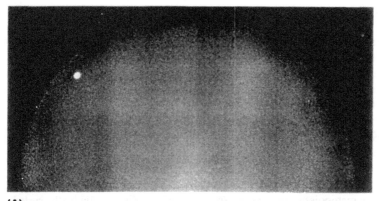

(A)

Figure 2   This figure is a summary of the divisional history of one single CD34$^+$/CD38$^-$ cell derived from a FLV sample, as monitored by our time-lapse camera system every 24 h over a period of 8 days. (A) In the first day, the image monitored confirmed that one single cell showing very bright fluorescence was deposited in the well. (B) After 24 h, two cells with bright fluorescence were observed. (C) Three days later (72 h), one bright cell was seen among 16–32 fluorescence dim or fluorescence-negative cells. (D) On the eighth day, the same bright cell was observed among thousands of fluorescence-negative cells, thus providing evidence that asymmetrical divisions occurred among CD34$^+$/CD38$^-$ cells derived from FLV.

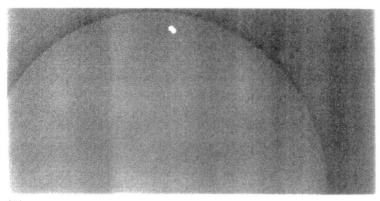

(B)

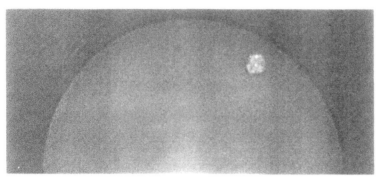

(C)

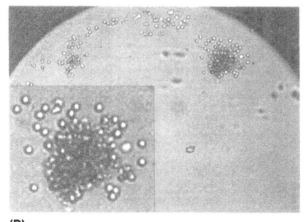

(D)

colony efficiency, growth pattern, and replating efficiency. Initially, we studied if asymmetrical division could be found among the first cell divisions of CD34$^+$/CD38$^+$ cells or CD34$^+$/CD38 cells derived from fetal liver. In the first series of experiments, we monitored the replication history of hematopoietic progenitors that were CD34$^+$. The cells were derived from fetal liver (FLV), umbilical cord blood (UCB), or from adult bone marrow (ABM). The whole CD34$^+$ population was stained in bulk with PKH26 for visualization in fluorescence light, followed by resorting as single cells in medium containing the above-described cytokine cocktail, and deposited onto a Terasaki plate. Image analysis included simultaneous assessment of cell number and fluorescence intensity in each of 72 wells at defined intervals; for example, every 3–12 h for 10 days. This enabled us to define precisely the replication history of each single CD34$^+$ cell. We found that the first division typically occurred at 36 h after being seeded. Following the first division, the subsequent doubling times was every 12 hs. With the AFIC system we observed 2 cells at 36–38 hours after seeding one CD34$^+$/CD38$^-$ cell derived from FLV, four cells at 48 hs, eight cells at 60 hs, and so forth. The majority (approximately 65–75%) of the CD34$^+$ cells showed synchronous and symmetrical divisions. However, about 30% of the single-sorted CD34$^+$ cells derived from FLV gave rise to a daughter cell that could remain quiescent for up to 8 days, whereas the other daughter cell multiplied exponentially. Such asynchronous divisions represented asymmetrical divisions with respect to the replication behavior of the two daughter cells.

We then focused our studies on CD34$^+$/CD38$^-$ cells derived from FLV, as our previous experiments indicated that this subset contained significantly higher frequencies of HSC candidates with self-renewal capacity (7,19). Preliminary experiments also demonstrated that $39.7 \pm 10.3\%$ (mean $\pm$ SD) of CD34$^+$/CD38$^-$ cells derived from FLV underwent asymmetrical divisions and was consistently and significantly higher than that of CD34$^+$/CD38$^+$ cells ($30.7 \pm 6.9\%$, paired t-test).

Figure 2 demonstrates the divisional history of one single CD34$^+$/CD38$^-$ cell that has divided asymmetrically as monitored by AFIC over a period of 8 days. The image confirmed that one single cell with very bright fluorescence was deposited in the well. After 36 hs, two cells with bright PKH26 fluorescence were observed. Seventy-two hours after culturing, one bright cell was observed among eight other cells with dim fluorescence. Whereas the one PKH26 bright cell remained quiescent, the other cells continued to divide symmetrically to give rise to 16, 32 cells, and so on, every 12 hs such that on the eighth

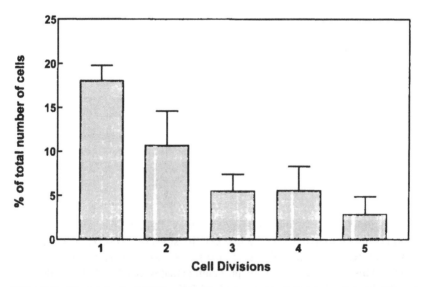

Figure 3 Percentages of HSC undergoing asymmetrical divisions after the first, second, third, and fifth division.

day, the same bright cell was observed among hundreds of fluorescence-negative cells. Other CD34$^+$/CD38$^-$ cells initially gave rise to two daughter cells that appeared equivalent after the first mitosis but then divided asymmetrically after the second division. We have analyzed the percentages of asymmetrical divisions found after the first, second, third, and up to the fifth cell division. The results are summarized in Figure 3.

IX. SYMMETRY OF DIVISION, ONTOGENIC AGE, AND REGULATORY MOLECULES

To examine the functional integrity of the quiescent cells with bright PKH26 fluorescence derived from asymmetrically divided HSCs, we separated the fluorescence bright cells from PKH26 dim cells at 32 + 1 to 64 + 1 cells stage (after 96–108 h). They were then replated as single cells in 96-well plates with medium containing the cytokine "cocktail." Culture of such cells for an additional 10–14 days showed that 60 ± 9.8% of the PKH26 bright cells (n = 137 cells from three different samples) give rise to colonies, whereas only 15.9 ± 11.1% of the PKH26 dim cells (n = 121 cells from three different samples) did so. Of the PKH26 bright cells, 15.8 ± 7.8% gave rise to colonies with dispersed growth pattern, which on replating gave rise to a third generation of colonies. Colonies with a dispersed growth pattern were observed in 2.5 ± 2.5% of the PKH26 dim cells; none of which showed replating potential.

To correlate the replication behavior of the CD34$^+$/CD38$^-$ cells in the first 8 days with the growth pattern of the corresponding single cell after culture, we have continued to incubate the plates for 10–14 days as previously described (19). Our hypothesis is that cells showing asymmetrical divisions would give rise to more blast colonies with dispersed and mixed growth patterns, whereas cells showing symmetrical divisions gave rise to more clusters. The median percentage of blast colonies (BCs) (which included wells with dispersed and mixed growth pattern) was 33.3% for cells showing asymmetrical divisions and 29.4% for cells showing symmetrical divisions. The median percentage of cluster colonies (CCs) was 35.3% for cells showing asymmetrical divisions and 43.5% for those with symmetrical divisions. The paired t-test confirmed a significant decrease of BCs in cells showing symmetrical divisions versus those showing asymmetrical divisions. This observation is compatible with that reported by Young et al. (45).

After establishing that asymmetrical divisions occurred among CD34$^+$/CD38$^-$ cells, we have determined the percentages of asymmetrical divisions among samples derived from different ontogenic ages. CD34$^+$/CD38$^-$ cells derived from FLV, UCB, or ABM were sorted, stained with PKH26, and deposited as single-sorted cells. Divisions were monitored every 12–24 h for up to 8 days. Mitotic rate, symmetry of the initial divisions, ADI, and colony efficiencies were documented. The data from at least five experiments are summarized in Figure 4. Whereas the mitotic rate, colony efficiency, and percentage of asymmetrical divisions all decreased with ontogenic age (i.e., from FLV, UCB, to ABM), the fraction of cells undergoing asymmetrical division among dividing cells (i.e., ADI) was consistently at 45% irrespective of ontogenic age.

We have then compared the effects of various regulatory molecules on symmetry of initial cell divisions. After single-cell sorting and deposition of CD34$^+$/CD38$^-$ cells derived from FLV, the cells were exposed to the regulatory molecules flt3 ligand (FL3), thrombopoietin (Tpo), rhSCF, a combination of the three, or to medium containing the above-described cocktail. Cell divisions were monitored every 6–12 h for up to 8 days. The results are summarized in Table 1. On monitoring the replication history, we observed

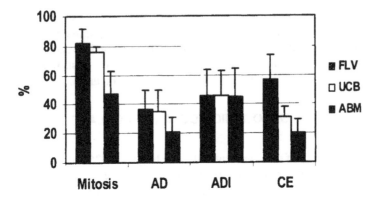

Figure 4 Changes in mitotic rate, percentages of asymmetric divisions (AD) among all cells plated, asymmetrical division index (ADI), and colony efficiency (CE) among CD34 /CD38⁻ cells derived from tissues of different ontogenic age. FLV = fetal liver, UCB = umbilical cord blood, ABM = adult bone marrow. Whereas there was a significant decrease in mitosis, AD, CE with ontogenic age, ADI remained constant at ~40%.

that with FL3, Tpo, or rhSCF, the time interval between exposure to cytokines and first mitosis was 48–50 h instead of 36–38 h. The mitotic rate, colony efficiency, and cells undergoing asymmetrical divisions decreased significantly on exposure to FL3, Tpo, or rhSCF as compared to the cocktail. With the exception of FL3, which induced a marginal decrease, ADI did not change significantly on exposure to different regulatory molecules or combinations thereof and has remained at about 40%. Thus, although divisional kinetics, mitotic rate, cloning efficiency, and asymmetrical divisions could be altered when using various regulatory molecules, the ADI was not altered significantly by Tpo or SCF.

Denkers et al. recently described a similar time-lapse recording system of human hematopoietic progenitors in culture (64). With this present technology, we were able to define retrospectively cells that gave rise to asymmetrical divisions, with one daughter cell that remained PKH26 bright and hence quiescent after mitosis and another that gave rise to multilineage progenitors, as shown in the formation of typical erythroid and myeloid clusters. When the PKH bright cells were replated onto fresh medium containing cytokine

Table 1 Regulatory Molecules on the Mitotic Rate, Colony Efficiency (CE), Asymmetrical Division, and Asymmetrical Division Index (ADI) of CD34 /CD38 Cells Derived from Fetal Liver.

Regulatory molecule	Mitotic rate (%)	CE (%)	Asymmetrical divisions (%)	ADI
FL3	48.9 ± 10.1[a]	9.2 ± 9.4[b]	16.9 ± 7.1[a]	33.3 ± 9.6[c]
Tpo	58.2 ± 4.4[a]	8.8 ± 0.9[b]	22.0 ± 5.1[c]	34.0 ± 7.4
SCF	64.5 ± 13.2[c]	29.6 ± 19.8[b]	29.5 ± 7.6[c]	46.1 ± 9.2
Cocktail	84.3 ± 3.5	68.2 ± 14.4	39.5 ± 7.6	46.9 ± 8.8

Results are shown in means ± SD.
[a] $P < .01$;
[b] $P < .001$ compared to cytokine cocktail;
[c] $P \leq .05$.

cocktail, each single-picked cell could give rise to colonies with dispersed and cluster growth patterns.

Using a different approach, Brummendorf et al. also drew similar conclusions from studies of single-sorted candidate HSCs from FLV (65). They reported that the results from culturing and replating of hematopoietic progeny cells from single-sorted HSCs were indicative of asymmetrical divisions in primitive hematopoietic cells. The proliferative potential and cell cycle properties were shown to be unevenly distributed among daughter cells derived from single-sorted HSCs from FLV. Judging from the continuous generation of functional heterogeneity among clonal progeny of HSCs, they also suggested that intrinsic control of stem cell fate is more likely than extrinsic.

X. CONCLUSION AND PERSPECTIVES

The fate of HSCs during the first hours and days after transplantation in vivo or after seeding onto culture plates in vitro has been largely unknown. Conventional stem cell assays have attempted to estimate their proliferative and differentiating potential by making use of their ability to form colonies after incubation for 14 days (67,68). Various modifications of long-term cultures (e.g., LTCICs) based on the use of a stromal feeder layer derived from bone marrow have been used to estimate the repopulating potential of stem cells, but such assays were not able to determine another dimension of stem cell activity—self-renewal capacity. Recent advances in the understanding of neural stem cell biology might serve as a model for HSC development. Based on these studies, a fundamental property of stem cell development seems to be asymmetrical division during which the generation of cell diversity requires daughter cells to adopt different pathways.

To follow the precise replication history and the fate of HSCs at a single-cell level, we have applied an AFIs to monitor directly early cell divisions. The following conclusions can be drawn from the use of this technology. First, we have confirmed that approximately 40% of the single-sorted CD34$^+$/CD38$^-$ cells derived from FLV gave rise to a daughter cell that remained quiescent for up to 8 days, whereas the other daughter cell proliferated exponentially. Such asynchronous divisions probably represented asymmetrical divisions and could be observed during the first and subsequent rounds of mitosis among CD34$^+$/CD38$^-$ cells. Second, the percentage of such asymmetrical divisions decreased with ontogenic age; that is, higher in CD34$^+$/CD38$^-$ cells derived from FLV than those from UCB or ABM. However, despite the fact that asymmetrical divisions, along with the mitotic rate and colony efficiency, decreased significantly with ontogenic age, the ADI; that is, the ratio of cells undergoing asymmetrical divisions versus dividing cells remained constant. Third, we have demonstrated that cells showing asynchronous or asymmetrical divisions gave rise to more blast colonies than those showing symmetrical divisions. Fourth, whereas significant changes in the mitotic rate, colony formation, and asymmetrical divisions were dependent on exposure to regulatory molecules, the ADI remained unchanged at approximately 40%. This interesting finding supports the notion that growth factors are probably not essential for determining the symmetry of divisions and hence the fate of the daughter cells.

Two mechanisms may be responsible for the adoption of different fates by the daughter cells. One, the intracellular or intrinsic mechanism involves an inherited determinant that is asymmetrically segregated into one daughter cell at the time of division (55,57,58). The other, extracellular or extrinsic mechanism, may result from communication of the daughter cells with each other or with surrounding cells (55). Current research indicates a stereotypic mechanism for the asymmetrical division of stem cells. Evidence from neural stem cell research supports the idea that asymmetrical divisions are defined mostly by cell-autonomous information, whereas extrinsic signal might also be involved initially in instructing the asymmetrical fates of daughter cells. Our observation of a fairly consistent ADI irrespective of ontogenic age or of exposure to regulatory molecules supports this hypothesis. The results indicate that, although the pattern of commitment can be skewed by extrinsic signaling, the proportion of asymmetrical divisions is probably under the control of intrinsic factors.

REFERENCES

1. Visser J, VanBekkum D. Purification of pluripotent hematopoietic stem cells. Exp Hematol 1990; 18:248–256.
2. Chen B, Galy A, Fraser C, Hill B. Delineation of the human hematolymphoid system.: Potential applications of defined cell populations in cellular therapy. Immunol Rev 1997; 157:41–51.
3. Hodgson GS, Bradley TR. Properties of hematopoietic stem cells surviving 5-fluorouracil treatment. Nature 1979; 281:381.
4. Civin CI, Strauss LC, Broval C, Fackler MJ, Schwartz JF, Shaper JH. Antigenic analysis of hematopoiesis. III. A hematopoietic progenitor cell surface antigen defined by a monoclonal antibody raised against KG-1a cells. J Immunol 1984; 133:157–165.
5. DiGiusto D, Chen S, Combs J, et al. Human fetal bone marrow early progenitors for T, B, and myeloid cells are found exclusively in the population expressing high levels of CD34. Blood 1994; 84:421–432.
6. Galy A, Webb S, Cen D, et al. Generation of T cells from cytokine-mobilized peripheral blood and adult bone marrow CD34$^+$ cells. Blood 1994; 84:104–110.
7. Terstappen LWMM, Huang S, Safford M, Lansdorp PM, Loken MR. Sequential generations of hematopoietic colonies derived from single nonlineage-committed CD34$^+$/CD38$^-$ progenitor cells. Blood 1991; 77:1218–1227.
8. Baum CM, Weissman IL, Tsukamoto AS, Buckle AM, Peault B. Isolation of a candidate human hematopoietic stem-cell population. Proc Natl Acad Sci USA 1992; 89:2804.
9. Huang S, Terstappen LW. Lymphoid and myeloid differentiation of single human CD34$^+$, HLA-DR$^+$, CD38$^-$ hematopoietic stem cells. Blood 1994; 83:1515–1526.
10. Uchida N, Combs J, Chen S, Zanjani E, Hoffman R, and Tsukamoto A. Primitive human hematopoietic cells displaying differential efflux of the Rhodamine 123 dye have distinct biological activities. Blood 1996; 88:1297–1305.
11. Ho AD, Young D, Maruyama M, Corringham RET, Mason JR, Thompson P, Grenier K, Law P, Terstappen LWMM, Lane T. Pluripotent and lineage-committed CD34$^+$ subsets in leukapheresis products mobilized by G-CSF, GM-CSF versus a combination of both. Exp Hematol 1996; 24:1460–1468.
12. Olweus J, Lund-Johansen F, Terstappen LW. CD64/fc gamma RI is a granulomonocytic lineage marker on CD34$^+$ hematopoietic progenitor cells. Blood 1995; 85:2402.
13. Sutherland HJ, Eaves CJ, Eaves AC, Dragowska W, Lansdorp PM. Characterization and partial purification of human marrow cells capable of initiating long term hematopoiesis in vitro. Blood 1989; 74:1563.
14. Verfaillie CM. Soluble factor(s) produced by human bone marrow stroma increase cytokine-induced proliferation and maturation of primitive hematopoietic progenitors while preventing their terminal differentiation. Blood 1993; 82:2045.
15. Verfaillie C, Blakolmer K, McGlave P.: Purified primitive human hematopoietic progenitor cells with long-term in vitro repopulating capacity adhere selectively to irradiated bone marrow stroma. J Exp Med 1990; 172:509.

16. Miller JS, Verfaillie CM. Ex vivo culture of CD34⁺Lin⁻DR⁻ cells in stroma derived soluble factors, MIP-la and IL-3 maintains not only myeloid but also lymphoid progenitors in a novel switch culture assay. Blood 1994; 84 (10 suppl 1):419a.

17. Craig W, Kay R, Cutler RL, Lansdorp PM. Expression of Thy-1 on human hematopoietic progenitor cells. J Exp Med 1993; 177:1331–1342.

18. Hoffman R. Human hematopoietic stem cells: Potential use as tumor-free autografts after high-dose myeloablative cancer therapy. Am J Med Sci 1995; 309:254.

19. Huang S, Law P, Young D, Ho AD. Candidate hematopoietic stem cells from fetal tissues, umbilical cord blood vs. adult bone marrow and mobilized peripheral blood. Exp Hematol 1998; 26:1162.

20. Spangrude GJ, Heimfeld S, Weissman IL: Purification and characterization of mouse hematopoietic stem cells. Science 1988; 241:58.

21. Spangrude GJ, Johnson JR. Resting and activated subsets of mouse multipotent hematopoietic stem cells. Proc Natl Acad Sci USA 1990; 87:7433.

22. Morrison SJ, Weissman IL. The long-term repopulating subset of hematopoietic stem cells is deterministic and isolatable by phenotype. Immunity 1994; 1:661.

23. Sutherland HJ, Lansdorp PM, Henkelman DH, Eaves AC, Eaves CJ. Functional characterization of individual hematopoietic stem cells cultured at limiting dilution on supportive marrow stroma layers. Proc Natl Acad Sci USA 1990; 87:3584.

24. Breems DA, Blokland EAW, Neben S, Ploemacher RE. Frequency analysis of human primitive haematopoietic stem cell subsets using a cobblestone area forming cell assay. Leukemia 1994; 8:1095.

25. Hao QL, Thiemann FT, Petersen D, Smogorzewska EM, Crooks GM. Extended long term culture reveals a highly quiescent and primitive human hematopoietic progenitor population. Blood 1996; 88:3306.

26. Hao QL, Smogorzewska EM, Barsky LW, Crooks GM. In vitro identification of single CD34+/CD38− cells with both lymphoid and myeloid potential. Blood 1998; 91:4145.

27. Miller JS, McCullar V, Punzel M, Lemischka IR, Moore KA. Single adult human CD34+/Lin−/CD38− progenitors give rise to NK cells, B-lineage cells, dendritic cells and myeloid cells. Blood 1999; 93:96.

28. Punzel M, Wissik SD, Miller JS, Moore KA, Lemischka IR, Verfaillie CM. The myeloid-lymphoid initiating cell (ML-IC) assay assesses the fate of multipotent human progenitors in vitro. Blood 1999; 93:3750.

29. McCune JM, Namikawa R, Kaneshima H, Schultz LD, Lieberman M, Weissman IL. The SCID-hu mouse: murine model for the analysis of human hematolymphoid differentiation and function. Science 1988; 24:1632.

30. Fraser CC, Kaneshima H, Hansteen G, Kilpatrick M, Hoffman R, Chen BP. Human allogeneic stem cell maintenance and differentiation in a long-term multilineage SCID-hu graft. Blood 1995; 86:1680.

31. Kollmann TR, Kim A, Zhuang X, Hachamovitch M, Goldstein H. Reconstitution of SCID mice with human lymphoid and myeloid cells after transplantation with human fetal bone marrow without the requirement for exogenous human cytokines. Proc Natl Acad Sci USA 1994; 91:8032.

32. Nolta JA, Smogorzewska EM, Kohn DB. Analysis of optimal conditions for retroviral mediated transduction of primitive human hematopoietic cells. Blood 1995; 86:101.

33. Nolta JA, Dao MA, Wells S, Smogorzewska EM, Kohn DB. Transduction of pluripotent human hematopoietic stem cells demonstrated by clonal analysis after engraftment in immune-deficient mice. Proc Natl Acad Sci USA 1996; 93:2414.

34. Larochelle A, Vormoor J, Hanenberg H, Wang JC, Bhatia M, Lapidot T, Moritz T, Murdoch B, Xiao XL, Kato I, Williams DA, Dick JE: Identification of primitive human hematopoietic cells capable of repopulating NOD/SCID mouse bone marrow: implications for gene therapy. Nature Med 1996; 2:1329.

35. Bhatia M, Wang JCY, Knapp U, Bonnet D, Dick JE: Purification of primitive human hemato-poietic cells capable of repopulating immune-deficient mice. Proc Natl Acad Sci USA 1997; 94:5320.

36. Cashman J, Bockhold K, Hogge DE, Eaves AC, Eaves CJ. Sustained proliferation, multilin-eage differentiation and maintenance of primitive human hematopoietic cells in NOD/SCID mice transplanted with human cord blood. Br J Haematol 1997; 98:1026.

37. Srour EF, Zanjani ED, Cornetta K, Traycoff CM, Flake AW, Hedrick M, Brandt JE, Leemhuis T, Hoffman R. Persistence of human multilineage, self-renewing lymphohematopoietic stem cells in chimeric sheep. Blood 1993; 82:3333.

38. Zanjani ED, Almeida-Porada G, Ascensao JL, MacKintosh FR, Flake AW. Transplantation of hematopoietic stem cells in utero. Stem Cells 1997; 15(suppl 1):79.

39. Weilbaecher K, Weissman I, Blume K, Heimfeld S. Culture of phenotypically defined hemato-poietic stem cells and other populations at limiting dilutions on Dexter monolayers. Blood 1991; 78:945.

40. Petzer AL, Hogge DE, Lansdorp PM, Reid DS, Eaves CJ. Self-renewal of primitive human hematopoietic cells (long-term culture-initiating cells) in vitro and their expansion in defined medium. Proc Natl Acad Sci USA 1996; 93:1470.

41. Gupta P, McCarthy JB, Verfaillie CM. Stromal fibroblast heparin sulfate is required for cytok-ine-mediated ex vivo maintenance of human long-term culture-initiating cells. Blood 1996; 87:3229.

42. Zanjani ED, Srour ED, Hoffman R. Retention of long-term repopulating ability of xenogeneic transplanted purified adult human bone marrow hematopoietic stem cells in sheep. J Lab Clin Med 1995; 126:24.

43. Leemhuis T, Yoder MC, Grigsby S, Aguero B, Eder P, Srour EF. Isolation of primitive human bone marrow hematopoietic progenitor cells using Hoechst 33342 and Rhodamine 123. Exp Hematol 1996; 24:1215–1224.

44. Hill B, Rozler E, Travis M, Chen S, Zannetino A, Galy A, Chen B, Hoffman R. High-level expression of a novel epitope of CD59 identifies a subset of CD34$^+$ bone marrow cells highly enriched for pluripotent stem cells. Exp Hematol 1996; 24:936–943.

45. Young JC, Varma A, DiGiusto D, Backer MP. Retention of quiescent hematopoietic cells with high proliferative potential during ex vivo stem cell culture. Blood 1996; 87:545–556.

46. Traycoff CM, Kosak ST, Grigsby S, and Srour EF. Evaluation of ex vivo expansion potential of cord blood and bone marrow hematopoietic progenitor cells using cell tracking and limiting dilution analysis. Blood 1995; 85:2059–2068.

47. Price JH, Gough DA. Comparison of digital autofocus functions for phase-contrast and fluo-rescent scanning microscopy. Cytometry 1994; 16:283–297.

48. Price JH, Hunter EA, Gough DA. Accuracy of least squares designed spatial FIR filtres for segmentation of images of fluorescence stained cell nuclei. Cytometry 1996; 26:4–10.

49. Francis K, Ramakrishna R, Holloway W, Palsson BO. Two new pseudopod morphologies displayed by the human hematopoietic KG1a progenitor cell line and by primary human CD34$^+$ cells. Blood 1998; 92:3616–3623.

50. Teare GF, Horan PK, Slezak SE, Smith C, Hay JB. Long-term tracking of lymphocytes in vivo: the migration of PKH-labeled lymphocytes. Cell Immunol 1991; 134:157–170.

51. Slezak SE, Horan PK. Fluorescent in vivo tracking of hematopoietic cells. Part I. Technical considerations. Blood 1989; 74:2172–2177.

52. Keller G: Clonal analysis of hematopoietic stem cell development in vivo. Curr Top Microbiol Immunol 1992; 177:41.

53. Horvitz HR, Herskowitz I. Mechanisms of asymmetric cell division: two Bs or not two Bs, that is the question. Cell 1992; 68:237.

54. Lin H, Schagat T: Neuroblasts: a model for the asymmetric division of stem cells. TIG 1997; 13(1):33.

55. Yuh NJ, Lily YJ. Asymmetric cell division. Nature 1998; 392:775.

56. Chang, F, Drubin DG. Cell division: why daughters cannot be like their mothers. Curr Biol 1996; 6:651.
57. Guo M, Jan LY, Jan YN. Control of daughter cell fates during asymmetric division: interaction of numb and notch. Neuron 1996; 17:27.
58. Chenn A, McConnel SK. Cleavage orientation and the asymmetric inheritance of Notch1 immunoreactivity in mammalian neurogenesis. Cell 1995; 82:631.
59. Suda J, Suda T, Ogawa M. Analysis of differentiation of mouse hemopoietic stem cells in culture by sequential replating of paired progenitors. Blood 1984; 64:393.
60. Suda T, Suda J, Ogawa M. Disparate differentiation in mouse hemopoietic colonies derived from paired progenitors. Proc Natl Acad Sci USA 1984; 81:2520.
61. Leary AG, Ogawa M, Strauss LC, Civin CI. Single cell origin of multilineage colonies in culture: evidence that differentiation of multipotent progenitors and restriction of proliferative potential of monopotent progenitors are stochastic processes. J Clin Invest 1984; 74:2193.
62. Leary AG, Strauss LC, Civin CI, Ogawa M. Disparate differentiation in hemopoietic colonies derived from human paired progenitors. Blood 1985; 66:327.
63. Mayani H, Dragowska W, Lansdorp PM. Lineage commitment in human hemopoiesis involves asymmetric cell division of multipotent progenitors and does not appear to be influenced by cytokines. J Cell Physiol 1993; 157:579.
64. Denkers IAM, Gragowska, W, Jaggi B, Palcic B, Lansdorp PM. Time lapse video recordings of highly purified human hematopoietic progenitor cells in culture. Stem Cells 1993; 11:243.
65. Brummendorf TH, Dragowska W, Mark J, Zijlmans JM, Thornbury G, Lansdorp PM. Asymmetric cells divisions sustain long-term hematopoiesis from single-sorted human fetal liver cells. J Exp Med 1998; 118:117.
66. Bradly TR, Robinson W, Metcalf D. Colony production in vitro by normal, polycythemic and anemic bone marrow. Nature 1967; 214:511.
67. Metcalf D: Hemopoietic Colonies. Berlin: Springer-Verlag, 1977:227.
68. Metcalf D: Lineage commitment and maturation in hematopoietic cells: the case for extrinsic regulation. Blood 1998; 92:345.
69. Enver T, Heyworth CM, Dexter TM: Do stem cells play dice? Blood 1998; 92:348.

6

Requirements for Hematopoietic Stem Cell Engraftment and Graft Engineering
Role of Facilitating Cells

MICHAEL NEIPP, CHRISTINA L. KAUFMAN, MARIANNE BERGHEIM,
BEATE G. EXNER, and SUZANNE T. ILDSTAD

Institute for Cellular Therapeutics, University of Louisville, Louisville, Kentucky

I. INTRODUCTION

Since the first successful bone marrow transplants were carried out almost 40 years ago, bone marrow transplantation (BMT) is now the preferred therapy in the treatment of a number of hematological malignancies (1). It was during the early period of BMT that the importance of histocompatibility antigens became evident. The establishment of human leukocyte antigen (HLA) typing has made the selection of major histocompatibility complex (MHC)–identical or MHC-compatible allogeneic donor/recipient pairs possible (2,3). In spite of these advances, there remain two major limitations to BMT for leukemia: (1) graft-versus-host disease (GVHD) and (2) failure of engraftment. In addition, the observation that the incidence of GVHD is highly correlated with the degree of genetic disparity between donor and recipient currently prohibits the expansion of the limited donor pool.

Bone marrow transplantation has the potential to cure a number of nonmalignant disorders, including autoimmune diseases, enzyme deficiencies, erythrocyte and platelet disorders, and immunodeficiency states, as well as to induce donor-specific tolerance for organs, tissues, and cellular grafts (Table 1). However, the morbidity and mortality associated with conventional BMT has currently limited the widespread clinical application of bone marrow chimerism for the treatment of nonmalignant diseases. In addition to GVHD

Table 1 Diseases Potentially Treatable with
Bone Marrow Chimerism

Nonmalignant hematological disorders
  Sickle cell disease
  Thalassemia
  Histiocytosis
  Wiskott-Aldrich syndrome
  Aplastic anemia
  Myelodysplastic syndrome
  Fanconi's anemia
Enzyme deficiencies
  Lysosomal storage diseases
    Mucopolysaccharidosis
      Hunter's disease
      Hurler's disease
    Glycogenosis
    Spingolipidosis
      Gaucher disease
      Leukodystrophy
      Krabbe's disease
  Hereditary immunodeficiency syndromes
    Severe combined immunodeficiency
        (SCID) syndrome
    Chronic granulomatous disease
    Adenosine deaminase (ADA) deficiency
Autoimmunity
  Type I diabetes mellitus
  Systemic lupus erythematosus
  Multiple sclerosis
  Rheumatoid arthritis
  Inflammatory bowel disease
  Psoriasis
  Scleroderma
Tolerance induction for solid organs and cellular
        transplants

---

and failure of engraftment, the morbidity and mortality associated with fully ablative host conditioning is significant. Methods to understand the mechanism for conditioning as well as the components essential for engraftment may allow the expansion of the use of BMT to nonmalignant disease states.

Until recently, it was presumed that complete cytoablation was required for engraftment of allogeneic bone marrow to occur. In the last decade, an understanding of components in the host critical for engraftment of allogeneic bone marrow have been identified. Various sublethal conditioning protocols utilizing monoclonal antibodies, total body irradiation (TBI), thymic irradiation, and immunosuppressive drugs have been used to achieve a state of stable mixed bone marrow chimerism (4–8). Studies to achieve engraftment with sublethal conditioning of the recipient are now under way in the clinic.

Owing to this progress, the prevention of GVHD is the last remaining limitation.

In experimental models, GVHD does not occur if highly purified hematopoietic stem cells (HSCs) are infused instead of whole bone marrow. This can be explained by the absence of effector cells for GVHD; namely, T and natural killer (NK) cells. However, as was observed in transplantation of T-cell–depleted marrow, the administration of highly purified HSCs across an MHC barrier is associated with poor engraftment (9–14). The observation that T cells or T-cell–like subpopulations are required to facilitate and secure the engraftment of HSCs across MHC barriers has been demonstrated in a number of animal models (15,16). Furthermore, donor CD8$^+$ T cells seem to be critical in preventing allogeneic marrow graft rejection (16).

We have phenotypically identified a cell population, separate from stem cells, that facilitates engraftment of highly purified stem cells in allogeneic recipients. The facilitating cell expresses some markers typical of lymphoid (CD8$^+$, CD3$^+$, and Thy1$^+$) as well as others typical of myeloid (class II$^{dim/intermediate}$, CD45R$^+$) lineage but is $\alpha\beta$TCR$^-$ and $\gamma\delta$TCR$^-$. Although highly purified HSCs fail to engraft in MHC-disparate recipients in a murine model, the addition of as few as 30,000 facilitating cells is sufficient to permit engraftment across MHC barriers without inducing GVHD (13). Until now, the BMT has controlled the clinician. Now, one can potentially engineer a bone marrow graft to contain only the desired cell types. The use of facilitating cells in human BMT may avoid GVHD yet enhance engraftment, and therefore expand the potential donor pool dramatically. The establishment of a minimal conditioning regimen in this context will make BMT a safe treatment for a number of diseases, including nonmalignant hematological and autoimmune diseases and the induction of donor-specific tolerance for solid organ and cellular grafts.

II. LIMITATIONS TO THE WIDESPREAD APPLICATION OF BONE MARROW TRANSPLANTATION

A. Graft-Versus-Host Disease

Three major limitations to the widespread application of BMT for malignant and nonmalignant diseases are (1) GVHD, (2) failure of engraftment, and (3) the shortage of compatible donors. GVHD is defined as a severe, potentially lethal disorder in which functional and mature donor cells as a part of the transplanted bone marrow graft detect antigens present on the surface of cells in the immunosuppressed host and initiate an immune response directed against the host (17,18). Mature T cells and especially the CD8$^+$ subset are the most important effector cells in GVHD (19,20). CD4$^+$ T cells also play a major role, especially in the presence of a disparity in class II between donor and recipient (21,22). Although $\alpha\beta$TCR$^+$ T cells clearly make up the majority of cells infiltrating GVHD lesions, it has been shown in experimental models that $\gamma\delta$TCR$^+$ T cells are also capable of mediating lethal GVHD (23). In transgenic mouse models where the majority of peripheral T cells express the $\gamma\delta$TCR and are specific for class Ib on C57BL/6 cells, the infusion of these T-cell–depleted bone marrow cells plus $\gamma\delta$TCR$^+$ lymph node cells into lethally irradiated (900 cGy) B6 mice resulted in the generation of lethal GVHD (23). Immunohistochemical analysis showed that $\gamma\delta$TCR$^+$ cells had infiltrated the target organs of GVHD, and that the lethal affect could be ameliorated by anti-$\gamma\delta$TCR–specific antibodies (23).

Natural killer cells also contribute to the development of GVHD (18,24). Ferrara and coworkers observed in a murine model that effector cells in the skin had a phenotype characteristic for NK cells (25). Administration of antiasalio GM1 [anti–NK-cell mono-clonal antibody (mAb)] prevented GVHD in irradiated mice reconstituted with a mixture of bone marrow and spleen cells from minor antigen disparate donors (26).

Two distinct forms of GVHD have been observed in humans and numerous animal models: acute and chronic GVHD (27). Acute GVHD develops usually within 10–60 days after BMT and is associated with an inflammatory destruction of all epithelial cell-bearing tissues, including skin, small bowel, liver, and host bone marrow (28). The onset of chronic GVHD occurs after day 70 of BMT and is mainly associated with progressive fibrosis and sclerosis of a wide variety of organs and tissues, including skin, liver, and gastrointesti-nal tract (27).

The frequency with which acute GVHD occurs is highly correlated with the degree of genetically determined histocompatibility differences between recipient and donor as well as the lack of functional T cells in the host to reject the graft (29–31). However, GVHD can also be observed in patients receiving bone marrow from genetically HLA-identical siblings due to disparities in minor antigens (32) and even in autologous BMT (18,33,34). The underlying immune process observed in autologous recipients can be ex-plained by an autoimmune-like mechanism of transplanted effector cells as a result of ineffective negative and positive selection of immature T cells in the thymus of these individuals due to damage caused by the anti-GVHD immunosuppressive regimen (18,33,35). In recipients of marrow grafts from HLA-identical siblings, the incidence of acute GVHD is approximately 30–50% (36,37). If the donor and the recipient are related but mismatched for only one of six HLA antigens (both alleles of HLA-A, HLA-B, and HLA-DR locus), the occurrence of acute GVHD increases to 65% and the mortality in those who develop GVHD reaches 50% (38). Most BMT centers therefore limit matching to HLA-identical donors or one antigen-disparate donor. The probability of patients wait-ing for BMT to have a matched sibling is low (39), and the trend toward smaller family size is further decreasing this probability (40). Owing to an increasing number of unrelated bone marrow donors registered in the National Marrow Donor Program (NMDP), the probability of finding an unrelated HLA-A, HLA-B, and HLA-DR phenotypically matched donor is currently more than 70% (41). However, the risk of developing acute GVHD after bone marrow transplantation approaches 80% in this group of patients (42). In 47% of recipient's, grades III and IV acute GVHD occurs (44). In another study, Hansen and colleagues report an incidence of grades I and II acute GVHD in 35% of recipients receiv-ing bone marrow from fully HLA-matched unrelated donors, whereas grades III and IV occur in 30 and 10%, respectively (37). The transplant-related mortality in these patients averages 20, 50, and greater than 90% in the presence of grade I/II, grade III, and grade IV acute GVHD, respectively (37). In patients where BMT had to be performed between haploidentical donors and recipients with two or more loci mismatched, acute GVHD occurs in almost 100% (30,36,43,44).

In addition to the prominent role of MHC antigens in the development of GVHD, Korngold found that a disparity of minor (non-MHC) histocompatibility antigens also increases the risk of GVHD in mice (45). In a recent report, minor histocompatibility antigens (HLA-C) have also been shown to initiate cytotoxic responses in humans receiv-ing HLA-C–mismatched marrow. Patients matched for HLA-C showed a significantly improved clinical outcome regarding the frequency and severity of GVHD as well as the incidence of graft rejection (46,47). Other minor histocompatibility antigens have recently been classified in humans (HA-1, HA-2, HA-3, HA-4, and HA-5), and comparative studies suggest that matching for these minor antigens can further reduce the risk of GVHD (48).

Therefore, acute GVHD is currently the major limitation in clinical BMT if unmanipulated marrow is transplanted. Even for those patients with HLA-identical related donor's, lethal complications due to GVHD have limited the success of BMT for hematological malignancies.

B. Failure of Engraftment

In most cases, failure of engraftment after complete ablation of the host hematopoietic system leads to a fatal outcome. Spontaneous repopulation of residual host stem cells does not usually occur, and a second graft will seldom be tolerated without additional very toxic conditioning (49,50). Conditioning of the recipient involves two components: cytoreduction, or the production of "space" in the microenvironment, and immunosuppression to prevent rejection of the graft. The rejection of bone marrow grafts has been attributed to residual host T cells or NK cells, both of which are relatively radio- and chemoresistant (51,52) or to antibody-mediated rejection (53,54). A second component to failure of engraftment may relate directly to the hematopoietic environment itself and a requirement for accessory cells to provide a niche or ligand for the donor stem cell. In general, marrow failure is uncommon after transplantation of unmanipulated genotypically identical marrow (1%) (50,55), but it can rise to as much as 10–30% of HLA-identical T-cell–depleted transplants (56), and up to 70% of T-cell–depleted HLA-nonidentical transplants (57). Although clearly influenced by MHC compatibility, graft failure has also occurred when HLA-identical twins were transplanted (58), suggesting that an abnormal microenvironment can also play a role in graft failure. Strategies to enhance engraftment by optimizing the composition of the donor marrow and conditioning the recipient may allow the more widespread application of BMT to nonmalignant disease.

III. REQUIREMENTS FOR ENGRAFTMENT OF ALLOGENEIC BONE MARROW

A. Graft Rejection in Patients Receiving T-Cell–Depleted Bone Marrow

Because T cells were recognized as important effector cells in GVHD, clinical trials in the 1970s and 1980s implemented protocols directed at aggressively depleting T cells from the donor bone marrow graft. Protocols for T-cell depletion included immunotoxins (59), E rosetting/lectin agglutination (60), counterflow elutriation (61), and treatment with different T-cell–directed mAbs plus complement-mediated lysis (62–66). Although a reduction in the incidence of GVHD was observed in most of these studies (62–68), many centers reported that T-cell depletion was associated with an increased risk of failure of engraftment (49,64,66,69–71). Some termed this phenomenon graft rejection. Variables including the presence or absence of GVHD, the genetic disparity between donor and recipient, the conditioning regimen, and the amount of T cells left behind after depletion may have affected the engraftment capacity of T-cell–depleted marrow. The number of residual T cells was inversely correlated with the incidence of graft failure (27). Different hypotheses emerged to explain the mechanism for T-cell depletion graft failure: donor T cells themselves or cytokines produced by T lymphocytes may be necessary for the engraftment of donor HSCs and progenitors. T cells of host origin may not be able to mediate this effect, because the number of functional T cells remaining in the host after myeloablation is not sufficient or because T cells must be completely MHC matched to the donor

HSCs (12–14). Alternatively, donor T cells may be required to eliminate residual cells in the host to allow for engraftment of the bone marrow graft. A final possibility is that accessory cells of donor origin, separate from the stem cell, are required for durable engraftment of the stem cell. Rather than preventing rejection of the stem cell, they may provide a ligand to which stem cells can anchor and engraft. Recent evidence from experimental (72) and clinical data (44) demonstrate that very high doses of T-cell–depleted bone marrow or mobilized peripheral blood stem cells can, at least partially, overcome the poor engraftment observed when T-cell–depleted marrow is infused at physiological doses. Whether this effect is a result of increased absolute numbers of T cells contaminating the graft or is attributed to the higher numbers of HSCs remains to be determined.

B. Requirements for Engraftment of Pluripotent Hematopoietic Stem Cells

1. Role of the Microenvironment

Bone marrow stem cells are thought to reside in hematopoietic niches. The hematopoietic microenvironment containing specific stromal and extracellular components influences HSC engraftment and subsequent function. The success of BMT is dependent on the homing of pluripotent HSCs to these niches. The observation that syngeneic bone marrow injected in nonablated recipients engrafted only at low levels drove the hypothesis that there are only a limited amount of niches for stem cells available in an individual and that these niches are virtually all occupied in unmanipulated animals (73–75). This is in accordance with the observation that cytoablative conditioning with irradiation and/or cytotoxic reagents is required to make space physically for the engraftment of bone marrow grafts in physiological doses (76).

The importance of the hematopoietic microenvironment on the regulation of hematopoiesis in vitro was studied in a mouse model by Dexter and coworkers (77) and later adapted for human cells by (78) using long-term marrow culture assays. Both found that bone marrow cultured under appropriate conditions gave rise to a complex layer containing stromal cells and other cellular components, including mononuclear phagocytic cells, endothelial cells, and adipocytes adherent on the bottom of the culture flask. This adherent cell layer seemed to imitate the microenvironment responsible for the regulation of hematopoiesis in vivo, including proliferation and differentiation of immature progenitors, and also the maintenance of the self-renewal capacity of primitive stem cells. Hematopoiesis as measured by the ability to produce granulocyte-macrophage progenitors could be maintained for more than 20 weeks in human cultures (78) and up to 1 year when bone marrow from mice was cultured under optimal conditions (79).

The importance of interactions between pluripotent stem cells and stromal cells in vivo was originally studied by Russell in an elegant model using SL/SL or "steel" mutant mice (80). Mice homozygous for the steel mutation have a defective stromal element and die in utero from anemia in spite of a fully competent HSC population (80). Mice with allelic forms of this mutation survive but suffer from severe anemia. All attempts to cure anemia in these mice by a BMT from a healthy donor failed, indicating that functional hematopoiesis is dependent on an intact microenvironment and that stromal cell/stem cell interactions may play an important role in the regulation of hematopoiesis.

2. Genetic Requirements for Stem Cell Engraftment

Technical progress in purifying HSCs has made it possible to study the genetic requirements for engraftment of highly purified HSCs. Unlike whole bone marrow, purified HSCs do not contain T cells capable of inducing GVHD. Surprisingly, purified HSCs suffer from the same limitations for engraftment observed in transplantation of T-cell–depleted bone marrow: Although purified HSCs engraft in recipients who are genetically identical or only minor antigen disparate, engraftment of physiological numbers of stem cells has not been reported to date in recipients with MHC class I and class II differences (12–14,81). El Badri and Good showed in a mouse model that wheat germ agglutinin–positive HSCs engraft when transplanted in syngeneic (B6 → B6) or minor antigen-disparate (BALB/c → DBA/2) recipients. Engrafted animals survived long term, and there were no signs of GVHD or immunodeficiency. In striking contrast, HSCs did not engraft when MHC-disparate strains were used (BALB/c → B6) as recipients (12).

Kaufman and colleagues reported that although 1000 highly purified stem cells (c-kit^+/SCA-1$^+$/lineage$^-$) routinely rescue syngeneic animals from aplasia induced by lethal TBI, even a 10-fold increase in the dose of HSCs did not result in engraftment when MHC-disparate recipients (B10.BR → B10) were used (13). These results indicate which cells and/or factors contained in whole bone marrow that are essential for engraftment of stem cells in MHC disparate, but not in syngeneic or minor antigen-disparate recipients, are lacking in highly purified HSCs.

IV. ROLE OF ACCESSORY CELLS IN ENGRAFTMENT

The role of accessory cells in bone marrow engraftment was studied by Lapidot and co-workers who demonstrated that as few as 8×10^4 donor-derived thymocytes facilitated engraftment of T-cell–depleted MHC-disparate bone marrow in irradiated mice (15). Engraftment was also enhanced when normal immunocompetent recipients received bone marrow from nude mice by adding thymocytes from genetically tolerant F1 animals. Bone marrow from nude mice alone did not engraft. The investigators therefore concluded that the facilitating effect observed in this experiment was not only generated by alloreactivity against residual host cells but also by interactions between stem cells, T cells, and stromal cells mediated by certain growth factors and cytokines (15). Based on these results, the same group showed 2 years later that this facilitating effect was attributed to the CD8$^+$CD4$^-$ subset of thymocytes but not to CD4$^+$CD8$^-$ thymocytes (82).

Martin developed a partial conditioning model in which transplantation of 5×10^6 T-cell–depleted bone marrow cells from B6C3 mice alone into sublethally (800 cGy) irradiated CB6 mice did not result in engraftment (16). As few as 0.5×10^5 CD8$^+$ donor T cells from pooled lymph nodes enriched by nylon wool and panning facilitated the engraftment of the T-cell–depleted bone marrow in all transplanted animals. In striking contrast, the same amount of CD4$^+$ donor cells could not mediate this facilitating effect. When the number of CD4$^+$ T cells was increased to 2.5×10^5 or more in order to titrate for a facilitating effect, all mice died within 39 days of transplant from severe GVHD. To address whether donor T cells highly enriched for CD4 could facilitate engraftment of allogeneic bone marrow without inducing GVHD, a model was used in which both rejection of allogeneic marrow and GVHD was caused by a disparity of MHC class I antigens (bm1 → B6.Ly5^a). Using this model, engraftment occurred in all of the transplanted animals when 2.5×10^5 CD8$^+$ donor T cells were added to the T-cell–depleted marrow, but only one out of five animals engrafted after receiving the same number of CD4$^+$ T cells. Even at a cell dose of 12.5×10^6 CD4$^+$, cellular rejection of the marrow graft was observed in two of five animals, indicating that the T-cell subpopulation enriched for CD8 was at least five times more effective in facilitating allogeneic bone marrow engraftment (16). Because GVHD is a potent spacemaker itself, an alternative hypothesis to the Martin model is that the mature CD8$^+$ T cells provide additional myeloablation at this threshold dose for conditioning. This unresolved question could be answered if the model were extended to use only purified donor stem cells as the source of marrow.

Failure of engraftment has also been reported from clinical studies in which patients with leukemia were transplanted with bone marrow aggressively depleted of CD8$^+$ cells from HLA-identical siblings (83). This depletion strategy surprisingly was associated with an incidence of failure of engraftment (11%) as high as that observed in marrow depleted of all T cells (83). When the marrow was less aggressively depleted, engraftment occurred more readily. Taken together these results indicate the existence of cells facilitating the engraftment of bone marrow which is at least in part removed by most T-cell–depleting procedures. There is also evidence that the CD8$^+$ population compared to the subset expressing CD4 mediates this effect to a remarkably higher extent. One question to be answered by the Martin studies is whether purified stem cells with CD8$^+$ lymph node lymphocytes would durably engraft, since in this sublethal model, one could argue that the role of the CD8$^+$ lymph node cells made space rather than facilitated engraftment of the stem cells (see below).

V. FACILITATING CELLS

Reconstitution of lethally irradiated mice with a mixture of 5×10^6 T-cell–depleted syngeneic plus 15×10^6 T-cell–depleted allogeneic bone marrow by rabbit anti–mouse brain (RAMB, which also reacts with mouse T cells) or Thy1.2 antibody plus complement results in engraftment of both syngeneic and allogeneic HSCs at a mean level of chimerism of 50% (Fig. 1b) (84–86). Administration of T-cell–depleted syngeneic bone marrow plus

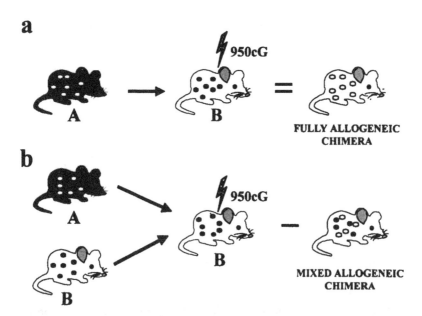

Figure 1 In fully allogeneic chimeras, the recipient hematopoietic environment is completely replaced by donor stem cells. In mixed chimeras, the host and donor hematopoietic stem cells coexist and function.

untreated allogeneic bone marrow enhanced the engraftment of the allogeneic marrow component significantly, with the level of donor chimerism approaching 100% (84).

To identify the phenotype of cell surface markers that accompany facilitation, CD8[+], Thy1.2[+], CD4[+], CD8[+] plus CD4[+], B220[+] B cells, NK cells, or Mac-1[+] cells were removed from the allogeneic bone marrow inoculum by treatment with mAbs and complement-mediated lysis. All animals transplanted with T-cell–depleted syngeneic and allogeneic marrow depleted of CD8[+], CD4[+], CD8[+]CD4[+], Mac-1[+], or B cells[+] (B220) engrafted as fully allogeneic chimeras, indicating that the facilitating cell population was Thy1.2[+] and RAMB reactive but did not express CD8, CD4, Mac-1, or B220 at a high density (13).

Cell sorting was utilized to characterize further the facilitating cell. The majority (57%) of lethally irradiated animals that received a mixture of 5×10^6 RAMB-treated syngeneic plus 5×10^6 RAMB-treated allogeneic bone marrow engrafted as fully synge-neic chimeras. The overall mean level of donor chimerism in animals that engrafted was 13%. Facilitation of the allogeneic marrow component, defined as a level of allogeneic chimerism of more than 95%, was achieved if MHC class II[dim/intermediate], CD8[+], CD45R[+], or CD45[+] allogeneic bone marrow cells were purified by cell sorting and coadministered at doses as low as 30,000 per animal with the syngeneic and allogeneic bone marrow inoculum (13).

In cell sorting, one of the most reliable phenotypic markers for graft facilitation was CD8[+] with a dim to intermediate level of expression (Fig. 2) (13,81,87). The disparity between the data from complement-mediated lysis and cell sorting with respect to CD8 is most likely explained by the level of antigenic expression. At best, one can achieve a 2-log depletion by antibody plus complement-mediated lysis (13). Moreover, cells ex-pressing an antigen brightly are most efficiently depleted. Finally, the facilitating cell effect requires very few cells. Therefore, if only a few facilitating cell escaped depletion, the fact that 15×10^6 CD8-depleted cells were given may have ensured that there were enough contaminating cells added back to mediate the observed facilitating effect.

The facilitating cell expresses a number of markers associated with T cells, including CD3ε, CD8αβ, CD5, and CD2, but it is negative for αβTCR as well as for γδTCR. More-

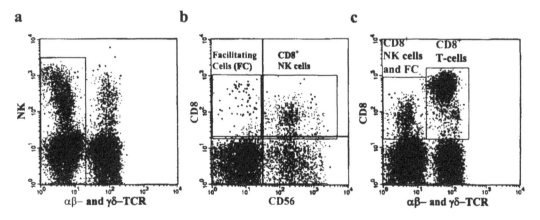

Figure 2 Three color flow cytometric analysis for facilitating cells. (a) CD56 bright/T-cell recep-tor (TCR)[+] cells are excluded. The FC population is within the box. (b) CD8[+]/CD56[+] NK cells are in right upper quadrant. CD8[+]FC are in the left upper quadrant. (c) CD8[+]/TCR[+]/T-cells are in upper right quadrant. CD8[+]/NK cells and FC are in left upper quadrant.

over, class II, which is not expressed on mouse T cells even during activation, is present on the facilitating cell, suggesting a possible nonlymphoid lineage derivation. The facilitating cell fraction (CD8$^+$/CD3$^+$/TCR$^-$) comprises less than 0.4% of total bone marrow cells. A phenotypically similar population of cells is present in human bone marrow (see Fig. 2).

To confirm that the facilitating cell by itself was sufficient to permit engraftment of highly purified HSCs in lethally irradiated MHC-disparate mice, a functional model of stem cell engraftment was established. One thousand stem cells rescued lethally conditioned (950 cGy) syngeneic recipients (B10.BR → B10.BR), but even a 10-fold increased amount of stem cells from MHC-disparate B10.BR mice failed to rescue allogeneic B10 mice (B10.BR → B10) from irradiation-induced aplasia (Fig. 3a,b). The addition of 30,000 facilitating cells to 10,000 allogeneic stem cells permitted engraftment in virtually all transplanted animals (Fig. 3c). All engrafted recipients survived long term without evidence of GVHD. The facilitating cell must be genetically matched to the HSCs, since MHC-disparate third-party facilitating cells do not facilitate stem cell engraftment in MHC-disparate recipients (Fig. 3d) (13).

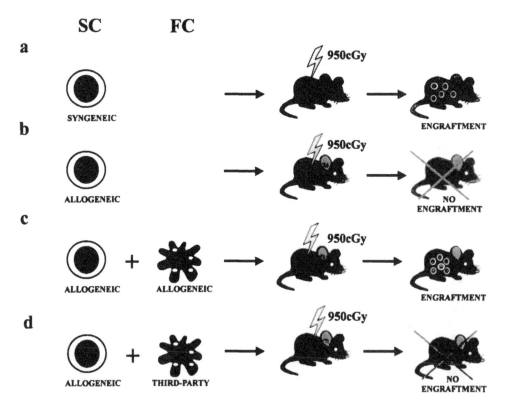

Figure 3 A mouse model was established to characterize which accessory cells in marrow allowed engraftment of highly purified stem cells in allogeneic recipients. While 1000 purified HSC engrafted in syngeneic recipients (a), they did not in allogeneic recipients (b). The addition of 30,000 FC to the HSC restored engraftment-potential (c) but only if the HSC and FC were genetically matched (d).

Gandy and Weissman recently reported that a bone marrow population which is CD8$^{dim/intermediate}$ but negative for the T-cell receptor facilitates engraftment of purified HSCs across allogeneic barriers without causing GVHD (81,87). Cells within this population, which express CD8 at a low level, and therefore stain dimly for this surface marker, were most important in mediating the facilitating effect, although CD8$^+$/TCR$^+$ T cells could also enhance the effect but to a lesser extent (87).

Facilitating cells are also required for the engraftment of purified fetal liver stem cells in MHC-disparate but not MHC-matched mice (88). Purified HSCs from the liver of 13- to 17-day-old fetuses were transplanted in adult syngeneic, minor antigen-disparate or MHC-disparate recipients. Although 2000–3000 fetal liver stem cells rescued lethally irradiated syngeneic and minor antigen-disparate recipients, even five times more fetal liver stem cells failed to engraft in MHC-disparate animals. However, the addition of 30,000 facilitating cells (CD8$^+$/αβTCR$^-$/γδTCR$^-$) MHC matched to the fetal stem cells resulted in durable engraftment of the allogeneic liver stem cells (88).

There are recent data suggesting that an accessory cell is also important for optimal engraftment of highly purified stem cells in nonablated syngeneic mice (76). When 2600–10,000 stem cells from male BALB/c mice were purified by cell sorting (lineage$^-$ and Rhodamine/Hoechst^{dull}) and injected in nonablated female BALB/c recipients, the level of engrafted (male) cells after injection of purified stem cells was significantly lower compared to recipients receiving whole bone marrow equivalents. The investigators conclude that cells and/or factors present in unmanipulated whole bone marrow are lacking when highly purified HSCs are transplanted into syngeneic recipients (76).

The role of facilitating cells on engraftment of allogeneic bone marrow was also studied in a rat model (88a). Lethally irradiated Wistar Furth rats reconstituted with 1×10^8 untreated bone marrow cells from ACI rats routinely developed severe GVHD. When the bone marrow was T-cell depleted using monoclonal antibodies directed against T-cell markers such as CD5 and CD3, which are also expressed on facilitating cells, the engraftment potential of T-cell–depleted marrow was limited. In fact, failure of engraftment was observed in up to 50% of recipients. In order to improve engraftment potential, a T-cell depletion protocol was employed using anti-αβTCR monoclonal antibody and ferromagnetic beads, since αβTCR is not expressed or only dimly expressed on facilitating cells. Following this T-cell depletion strategy, the facilitating cell population (CD8$^+$/αβTCR$^-$/NK3.2.3$^-$) was sustained and engraftment occurred in 100% of transplanted recipients. Moreover, high levels of donor chimerism ranging from 82% to 98% were detectable for more than 6 months. Thus, this study shows that facilitating cells are required to allow for reliable bone marrow engraftment in the allogeneic rat model (88a).

The precise definition of which cells are essential to engraftment in MHC-disparate recipients will allow the clinician to engineer a bone marrow graft to contain only those cells necessary for the desired outcome: engraftment without severe GVHD. As a result, the potential applications of BMT as a natural form of gene therapy are immense.

VI. BONE MARROW CHIMERISM AND TRANSPLANTATION TOLERANCE

The concept of hematopoietic chimerism was first described by Owen, who observed that genetically different freemartin cattle twins, which shared a common placental circulation, were red blood cell (RBC) chimeras (89). Billingham and Medawar observed that reciprocal skin grafts were accepted in genetically identical twins, whereas they were rejected in MHC-disparate donor/recipient combinations (90). The British Agriculture System commissioned their group to apply this technique to distinguish between monozygotic and dizygotic freemartin cattle twins early after birth, since the dizygotic cattle twins were of lower market value. Surprisingly, freemartin cattle did not reject skin grafts from their genetically disparate twin donor (91). The investigators hypothesized that the RBC chimerism reported by Owen was responsible for the actively acquired tolerance to donor skin (91). One year later, the same investigators demonstrated in a murine model that intraembryonical injection of a cell suspension containing hematopoietic-derived tissue from an allogeneic adult donor resulted in tolerance to subsequent donor-specific skin grafts (91). Since then, multiple investigators have studied the role of chimerism mainly in rodent models using a conditioning regimen based on irradiation, antibodies, and myeloablative chemotherapeutic agents (4,5,84,85,92–96). Lethal conditioning followed by infusion of allogeneic bone marrow usually resulted in fully allogeneic chimerism (see Fig. 1a). Although fully allogeneic chimerism induces donor-specific tolerance in vivo and in vitro, the complete replacement of the recipient's own immune system is associated with relative immunoincompetence for primary immune responses (84,97–99), and recipients were more likely to develop GVHD (45,94,100–102). This relative immunoincompetence in fully allogeneic chimeras can be explained by the following mechanism: T cells recognize antigens presented by antigen-presenting cells (APCs) in the context of self-MHC (103); a process which is now known as MHC restriction (104). In allogeneic chimeras, donor - cells mature in the host thymus and are restricted to host APCs. However, as a result of the lethal conditioning, there are no host APCs remaining in the periphery to present antigen properly to the donor T cells resulting in the observed immunoincompetence. As a result, primary immune responses, including antibody production and antiviral responses, are significantly impaired (97).

To overcome this limitation, in 1984, Ildstad and colleagues reconstituted lethally irradiated mice with a mixture of allogeneic and syngeneic bone marrow (see Fig. 1b) (105). In these recipients, both donor and host bone marrow components engrafted resulting in a state of mixed allogeneic chimerism (105). The presence of host-type APCs restored the immunoincompetence observed in fully allogeneic chimeras proven by normal survival of mixed allogeneic chimeras under conventional housing and even after challenge with viral infections to levels similar to that for normal mice (102).

The morbidity and mortality associated with lethal conditioning as applied in patients receiving a BMT for leukemia could not be accepted in the treatment of most of the nonmalignant diseases and the induction of tolerance for cellular and organ transplants. Until recently, it was accepted that complete recipient conditioning was essential to achieve durable engraftment. Considerable progress has now been made in the development of minimal conditioning approaches. These include TBI, the use of mAbs, irradiation of the thymus and secondary lymphatic organs, and immunosuppressive drugs to make "space" in the host microenvironment and to target cell populations in the host responsible for graft rejection (4–7,95,96,106,107).

One recently developed murine model allowed for stable donor chimerism at high levels, which was associated with tolerance to donor-specific skin grafts (5). The nonlethal conditioning in these experiments consisted of 300 cGy of TBI, 700 cGy thymic irradiation, and T-cell depletion of the host using mAbs against CD4 and CD8. Recipients were transplanted with $10-15 \times 10^6$ untreated bone marrow (5). Colson and coworkers reported that 700 cGy of TBI is required to achieve stable engraftment of allogeneic bone marrow in 100% of MHC-disparate or MHC-disparate plus minor antigen-disparate mice (6). Ad-

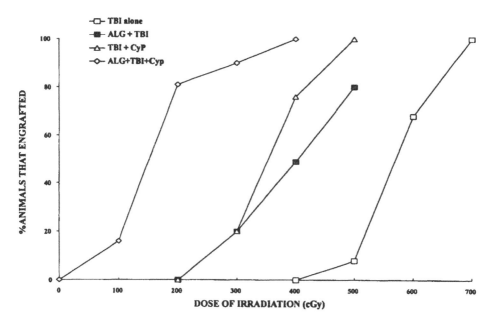

Figure 4 In the mouse, approximately 950 cGy of Total Body Irradiation (TBI) is considered fully ablative. The addition of ALG (□-□), cyclophosphamide (△-△), or both (◇-◇) allows a substantial reduction in the minimum TBI dose sufficient for durable engraftment.

ditional injection of a single dose of cyclophosphamide (200 mg/kg) intraperitoneally on day +2 reduced the dose of TBI required for engraftment to 500 cGy (Fig. 4). All animals reconstituted as mixed chimeras with a level of donor chimerism ranging from 60 to 99%. All cell lineages were present when chimeras were typed up to 18 months after transplantation (6). Bone marrow chimerism was associated with donor-specific tolerance in vitro and in vivo in these animals. This approach was nonlethal, since all animals conditioned with 500 cGy plus cyclophosphamide but not transplanted survived more than 30 weeks (6). Using this murine model, a further reduction of the TBI dose to 300 cGy was achieved when antilymphocyte globulin (1–2 mg/mouse) was injected 3 days prior to BMT (Fig. 4) (7). When the dose of donor cells was doubled to 30 × 10⁶, total cells, the irradiation dose was further reduced to 100 cGy of TBI in this model (7).

Allogeneic bone marrow chimerism was more recently achieved in MHC-disparate mice without the requirement for TBI (107). In this study, megadoses of allogeneic bone marrow (174 × 10⁶) divided into five doses were infused in B6 mice from day 0 through day 4. Recipients were additionally treated with anti-CD4 and anti-CD8 mAbs and 7 Gy of thymic irradiation. Stable multilineage chimerism was achieved in six of nine transplanted animals resulting in donor-specific tolerance to skin grafts (107).

In a dog model, it was recently reported that the administration of cyclosporine and mycophenolate mofetil in the peritransplant phase allows engraftment with a minimal TBI dose. Stable mixed hematopoietic chimerism was achieved in four of five dogs conditioned with 200 cGy TBI, cyclosporine (days-1–35) and mycophenolate mofetil (days 0–27) after transplantation with bone marrow from DLA-identical littermates (8).

The development of clinical protocols using nonlethal conditioning followed by transplantation of an engineered bone marrow graft, which facilitates engraftment without inducing GVHD, could prevent the current limitations in organ transplantation: acute and chronic rejection and the requirement of long-term immunosuppressive therapy in these patients.

VII. BONE MARROW CHIMERISM AS AN APPROACH FOR THE TREATMENT OF NONMALIGNANT DISEASES

A. Autoimmunity

Among over 50 disorders recognized at this time as having an autoimmune pathogenesis, there are a significant number of diseases which cannot be controlled by conventional long-term immunosuppressive therapy. Systemic lupus erythematosus (SLE) can be seen as the prototype of generalized autoimmune disease (108). In patients suffering from auto-immunity, not only end organ damage but also the risks of long-term drug therapy contribute to an increased mortality (109).

Numerous experimental models are available to study autoimmune diseases (110). These animal models include the nonobese diabetic (NOD) mouse, which develops insulinitis and diabetes, the mixed lymphocyte response (MLR) mouse, which suffers from SLE-like diseases, and the HLA-B27 transgenic rat, which develops chronic colitis and psoriasiform dermatitis (111). In mice, both type I diabetes (112–114) and SLE (115,116) can be cured by transplantation of allogeneic bone marrow. Conversely, the transplantation of bone marrow from disease-prone donors transfers autoimmunity to normal recipients (117).

The observation that human autoimmune diseases such as autoimmune thyroiditis and type I diabetes can be transferred by BMT to nonaffected individuals (118,119) indicates that autoimmunity is bone marrow related and suggests that BMT from disease-resistant donors could offer a treatment option in humans. A considerable number of cases have been reported in which BMT for hematopoietic indications have resulted in a cure or remission of various autoimmune diseases. These include "incidental" treatment of rheumatoid arthritis (120,121), psoriasis (122,123), and ulcerative colitis (123). A recent meeting in Basel, Switzerland, focused on the role of HSC therapy in autoimmune disease. Case reports were presented in which patients suffering from severe autoimmune diseases, including rheumatoid arthritis, multiple sclerosis, and SLE, were cured of their disease after lethal conditioning and transplantation with allogeneic bone marrow (124–126). In these patients, the morbidity and mortality associated with the lethal pretransplant conditioning was accepted because of the severity of their disease states.

It has been shown in experimental models using NOD mice that autoimmune diseases such as type I diabetes can also be cured by BMT using a more desirable, partial conditioning approach to achieve mixed chimerism (127). The combination of a nonlethal conditioning regimen together with a donor bone marrow cell processing, which allows for reduction of GVHD-inducing cells and enhancing the engraftment potential, could offer a safe treatment for many patients suffering from different autoimmune diseases (see Table 1). This could also lead to patient selection at an earlier stage of disease before end organ damage due to the autoimmune process or to drug-related side effects occurs.

B. Nonmalignant Hematological Disorders

Transplantation of allogenic bone marrow can be curative in several nonmalignant hematological disorders (see Table 1), including sickle cell disease (128), thalassemia (129,130), aplastic anemia (131), and the Wiskott-Aldrich syndrome (132,133). In most of these studies, complete ablation of the host was followed by transplantation of bone marrow from HLA-identical siblings to reduce the risk of GVHD and failure of engraftment (128–131,134). Although most of the transplanted patients engrafted as 100% donor, some recipients showed stable mixed chimerism. Even in those patients with less than 100% donor chimerism, symptoms of their disease disappeared (128).

C. Enzyme Deficiencies

Another group of diseases potentially treatable by BMT is lysosomal storage diseases, which develop on the basis of enzyme deficiencies. Whether these diseases should be treated by allogeneic BMT or gene therapy using autologous bone marrow is currently, being debated (135). However, numerous publications have shown that in diseases such as leukodystrophy (136–138), Hurler's disease (35,138–140), and Gaucher's disease (141), the progression of the underlying process is slowed or even stopped following allogeneic BMT. For other storage diseases such as Hunter's and Sanfilippo's diseases, allogeneic BMT is not recommended, at least in late-stage disease (138). Recent evidence suggests, however, that an earlier selection of patients in the presymptomatic phase could be more efficacious even in these diseases (138). This hypothesis is supported by an experimental study in which newborn and 6-week-old mice with mucopolysaccharidosis type VII were transplanted with syngeneic marrow from healthy animals. Bone marrow transplantation at birth was far more effective, since transplanted newborn mice had less lysosomal storage in the brain, and skeletal dysplasia was less severe compared to animals in which transplantation was delayed until 6 weeks of age (142).

Allogeneic BMT is the treatment of choice for patients with severe hereditary immunodeficiency syndromes (see Table 1) (143). The first successful allogeneic BMT was performed in a child with severe combined immunodeficient (SCID) syndrome in 1968 (144). Since then other hereditary immunodeficiencies such as adenosine deaminase (ADA) deficiency or chronic granulomatous disease have been successfully treated by allogeneic BMT (143,145–147).

VIII. CONCLUSION

Despite considerable progress in BMT in recent years, three major obstacles, GVHD, failure of engraftment, and the lack of compatible donors, remain limiting factors in the widespread clinical application of BMT. Since the incidence of GVHD is positively correlated with the grade of MHC and minor antigen disparities between donor and recipient, the donor pool is currently limited for the most part to related and unrelated donors with ≤ 1 HLA mismatch. The advantage of T-cell–depleted bone marrow to avoid GVHD and to expand the donor pool has been historically offset by an increased failure of engraftment even in HLA-identical donor/recipient pairs. The newly identified facilitating cell population, which has been shown to facilitate engraftment of T-cell–depleted MHC-disparate bone marrow as well as highly purified pluripotent HSCs may allow more widespread use of BMT. Until recently, the bone marrow graft has controlled the clinician in that nonspecific conditioning approaches and unmodified marrow have been required for successful engraftment. Now one can envision the application of graft engineering to tailor a bone marrow graft to contain only the desired cells (facilitating cells and HSCs for nonmalignant diseases, and facilitating cells and HSCs plus graft-versus-leukemia cells for malignancy) to optimize engraftment but minimize GVHD. Moreover, specific targeting of the host microenvironment to cytoreduce and remove the effector cells for graft rejection may permit conditioning in a focussed and specific fashion. As a result, BMT may be applied to induce tolerance for solid organs, cure disorders of RBCs, platelets, and granulocytes, reverse or slow the progress of autoimmunity, and treat enzyme deficiencies in the clinic.

ACKNOWLEDGMENTS

This work was supported by Deutsche Forschungsgemeinschaft (M.N.) and the National Institutes of Health grant DK 52294 (S.T.I.).

REFERENCES

1. Thomas ED, Lochte HL, Cannon JH, Sahler OD, Ferrebee JW. Supralethal whole body irradiation and isologous marrow transplantation in man. J Clin Invest 1959; 381:1709–1716.
2. Dausset J, Colombani J, Legrand L, Feingold N, Rapaport FT. Genetic and biological aspects of the HLA system of human histocompatibility. Blood 1970; 35:591–612.
3. Bach FH, Rood JJ. The major histocompatibility complex—genetics and biology (second of three parts). N Engl J Med 1976; 295:872–878.
4. Wood ML, Monoco AP. Models of specific unresponsiveness to tissue allografts in anti-lymphocyte serum (ALS) treated mice. Transplant Proc 1978; 10:379–387.
5. Sharabi Y, Sachs DH. Mixed chimerism and permanent specific transplantation tolerance induced by a nonlethal preparative regimen. J Exp Med 1989; 169:493–502.
6. Colson YL, Wren SM, Schuchert MJ, Patrene KD, Johnson PC, Boggs SS, et al. A nonlethal conditioning approach to achieve durable multilineage mixed chimerism and tolerance across major, minor, and hematopoietic histocompatibility barriers. J Immunol 1995; 155:4179–4188.
7. Colson YL, Li H, Boggs SS, Patrene KD, Johnson PC, Ildstad ST. Durable mixed allogeneic chimerism and tolerance by a nonlethal radiation-based cytoreductive approach. J Immunol 1996; 157:2820–2829.
8. Storb R, Yi C, Wagner JL, HJ D, RA N, Kiem HP, et al. Stable mixed hematopoietic chimerism in DLA-identical littermate dogs given sublethal total body irradiation before and pharmacological immunosuppression after marrow transplantation. Blood 1997; 89:3048–3054.
9. Smith LG, Weissman IL, Heimfeld S. Clonal analysis of hematopoietic stem-cell differentiation in vivo. Proc Natl Acad Sci USA 1991; 88:2788–2792.
10. Sprangrude GJ, Smith L, Uchida N, Ikuta K, Heimfeld S, Friedman J, Weissman IL. Mouse hematopoietic stem cells. Blood 1991; 78:1395–1402.
11. Andrews RG, Bryant EM, Bartelmez SH, Muirhead DY, Knitter GH, Bensinger W, Strong DM, Bernstein. ID. CD34+ marrow cells, devoid of T and B lymphocytes, reconstitute stable lymphopoiesis and myelopoiesis in lethally irradiated allogeneic baboons. Blood 1992; 80:1693–1701.
12. El Badri NS, Good RA. Lymphohemopoietic reconstitution using wheat germ agglutinin-positive hemopoietic stem cell transplantation within but not across the major histocompatibility antigen barriers. Proc Nat Acad Sci USA 1993; 90:6681–6685.
13. Kaufman CL, Colson YL, Wren SM, Watkins SL, Simmons RL, Ildstad ST. Phenotypic characterization of a novel bone-marrow derived cell that facilitates engraftment of allogeneic bone marrow stem cells. Blood 1994; 84:2436–2446.
14. Shizuru JA, Jerabek L, Edwards CT, Weissman IL. Transplantation of purified hematopoietic stem cells: requirements for overcoming the barriers of allogeneic engraftment. Biol Blood Marrow Transplant 1996; 2:3–14.

15. Lapidot T, Lubin I, Terenzi A, Faktorowich Y, Erlich P, Reisner Y. Enhancement of bone marrow allografts from nude mice into mismatched recipients by T cells void of graft-versus-host activity. Proc Natl Acad Sci USA 1990; 87:4595–4599.

16. Martin PJ. Donor CD8 cells prevent allogeneic marrow graft rejection in mice: potential implications for marrow transplantation in humans. J Exp Med 1993; 178:703–712.

17. Korngold R, Sprent J. GVHD after bone marrow transplantation across minor histocompatibility barriers in mice: prevention by removing mature T cells from marrow. J Exp Med 1978; 148:1687.

18. Ferrara J, Deeg HJ. Graft-versus-host disease. N Engl J Med 1991; 324:667–674.

19. Takata M, Imai T, Hirone T. Immunoelectron microscopy of acute graft versus host disease of the skin after allogeneic bone marrow transplantation. J Clin Pathol 1993; 46:801–805.

20. Favre A, Cerri A, Bacigalupo A, Lanino E, Berti E, Grossi CE. Immunohistochemical study of skin lesions in acute and chronic graft versus host disease following bone marrow transplantation. Am J Surg Pathol 1997; 21:23–34.

21. Sakamoto H, Michaelson J, Jones WK, Bhan AK, Abhyankar S, Silverstein M, Golan, DE, Burakoff SJ, Ferrara JL. Lymphocytes with a CD4$^+$ CD8$^-$ CD3$^-$ phenotype are effectors of experimental cutaneous graft-versus-host disease. Proc Natl Acad Sci USA 1991; 88: 10890–10894.

22. Truitt RL, Atasoylu AA. Contribution of CD4$^+$ and CD8$^+$ T cells to graft-vs-host disease and graft-vs-leukemia reactivity after transplantation of MHC-compatible bone marrow. Bone Marrow Transplant 1991; 8:51.

23. Blazar BR, Taylor PA, Panoskaltsis-Mortari A, Barrett TA, Bluestone JA, Vallera DA. Lethal murine graft-versus-host disease induced by donor gamma/delta expressing T cells with specificity for host nonclassical major histocompatibility complex class Ib antigens. Blood 1996; 87:827–837.

24. Vallera DA, Blazar BR. T cell depletion for graft-versus-host disease prophylaxis. A perspective on engraftment in mice and humans. Transplantation 1989; 47:751–760.

25. Ferrara J, Mauch P, Murphy G, Burakoff SJ. Bone marrow transplantation: the genetic and cellular basis of resistance to engraftment and acute graft-versus-host disease. Surv Immunol Res 1985; 4:253–263.

26. Charley MR, Mikhael A, Bennett M, Gilliam JN, Sontheimer RD. Prevention of lethal, minor-determinate graft-host disease in mice by the in vivo administration of anti-asialo GM1$^+$. J Immunol 1983; 131:2101.

27. Martin PJ, Hansen JA, Storb R, Thomas ED. Human marrow transplantation: an immunological perspective. Adv Immunol 1987; 40:379–438.

28. Glucksberg H, Storb R, Fefer A, Buckner CD, Neiman PE, Clift RA, Lerner KG, Thomas ED. Clinical manifestations of graft-versus-host disease in human recipients of marrow from HLA–matched sibling donors. Transplantation 1974; 18:295–304.

29. Billingham RE. The biology of graft-versus-host reactions. Harvey Lect 1966; 62:21–78.

30. Beatty PG, Clift RA, Mickelson EM, Nisperos BB, Flournoy N, Martin PJ, Sanders JE, Stewart P, Bruckner CD, Storb R, Thomas ED, Hansen JA. Marrow transplantation from related donors other than HLA-identical siblings. N Engl J Med 1985; 313:765–771.

31. Gale RP, Reisner Y. Graft rejection and graft-versus-host disease: mirror images. Lancet 1986; 1:1468–1470.

32. Rappeport J, Mihm M, Reinherz E, Lopansri S, Parkman R. Acute graft-versus-host disease in recipients of bone-marrow transplants from identical twin donors. Lancet 1979; 2:717–720.

33. Hess AD, Jones RC, Santos GW. Autologous graft-vs-host disease: mechanisms and potential therapeutic effect. Bone Marrow Transplant 1993; 12(suppl 3):S65–S69.

34. Prud'homme GJ, Vanier LE. Cyclosporine, tolerance, and autoimmunity. Clin Immunol Immunopathol 1993; 66:185–192.

35. Peters C, Balthazor M, Shapiro EG, King RJ, Kollman C, Hegland JD, Henlee-Downey J,

Trigg ME, Cowan MJ, Sanders J, Bunin N, Weinstein H, Lenarsk C, Falk P, Harris R, Bowen T, Williams TE, Grayson GH, Warkentin P, Sender L, Cool VA, Crittenden M, Packman S, Kaplan P, Lockman LA. Outcome of unrelated donor bone marrow transplantation in 40 children with Hurler syndrome. Blood 1996; 87:4894–4902.

36. Armitage JO. Medical progress: bone marrow transplantation. N Engl J Med 1994; 330:827–838.

37. Hansen JA, Anasetti C, Martin PJ, Mickelson EM, Petersdorf E, Thomas ED. Allogeneic marrow transplantation: the Seattle experience. Clin Transpl 1993; 193–209.

38. Kernan N, Bartsch G, Ash R, Champlin RJ, Filipovich AH, Gajewski JL, Hansen JA, Henslee-Downey J, McCullough J, McGlave P, Perkins HA, Phillips GL, Sanders J, Stroncek D, Thomas ED, Blume KG. Analysis of 462 Transplantations from unrelated donors facilitated by The National Marrow Donor Program. N Engl J Med 1993; 328:593–602.

39. Beatty PG, Dahlberg S, Mickelson EM, Nisperos B, Opelz G, Martin PJ, Hansen JA. Probability of finding HLA-matched unrelated marrow donors. Transplantation 1988; 45:714–718.

40. Anasetti C, Etzioni R, Petersdorf EW, Martin PJ, Hansen JA. Marrow transplantation from unrelated volunteer donors. Ann Rev Med 1995; 46:169–179.

41. Beatty PG, Kollman C, Howe CW. Unrelated-donor marrow transplants: the experience of the National Marrow Donor Program. Clin Transplant 1995; 271–277.

42. Sierra J, Storer B, Hansen JA, Bjerke JW, Martin PJ, Petersdor EW, Appelbaum FR, Bryant E, Chauncey TR, Sale G, Sanders JE, Storb R, Sullivan KM, Anasetti C. Transplantation of marrow cells from unrelated donors for treatment of high-risk acute leukemia: the effect of leukemic burden, donor HLA-matching, and marrow cell dose. Blood 1997; 89:4226–4235.

43. Anasetti C, Amos D, Beatty PG, Appelbaum FR, Bensinger W, Buckner CD, Clift R, Doney K, Martin PJ, Mickelson E, Nisperos B, O'Qigley J, Ramberg R, Sanders JE, Stewart P, Storb R, Sullivan KM, Witherspoon RP, Thomas ED, Hansen JA. Effect of HLA compatibility on engraftment of bone marrow transplants in patients with leukemia or lymphoma. N Engl J Med 1989; 320:197–204.

44. Aversa F, Tabilio A, Adelmo T, Velardi A, Falzetti F, Giannoni C, Iacucci R, Zei T, Martelli MP, Gambelunghe C, Rosetti M, Caputo P, Latini P, Aristei C, Raymondi C, Reisner Y, Martelli MF. Successful engraftment of T-cell-depleted halpoidentical "three-loci" incompatible transplants in leukemia patients by addition of recombinant human granulocyte colony-stimulating factor-mobilized peripheral blood progenitor cells to bone marrow inoculum. Blood 1994; 84:3948–3955.

45. Korngold R, Sprent J. Lethal GVHD after bone marrow transplantation across minor histocompatability barriers in mice: prevention by removing mature T cells from marrow. J Exp Med 1978; 148:1687–1698.

46. Bishara A, Amar A, Brautbar C, Condiotti R, Lazarovitz V, Nagler A. The putative role of HLA-C recognition in graft versus host disease (GVHD) and graft rejection after unrelated bone marrow transplantation (BMT). Exp Hematol 1995; 23:1667–1675.

47. Nagler A, Brautbar C, Slavin S, Bishara A. Bone marrow transplantation using unrelated and family related donors: the impact of HLA-C disparity. Bone Marrow Transplant 1996; 18:891–897.

48. Goulmy E, Schipper R, Pool J, Blokland E, Falkenburg JH, Vossen J, Grathwohl A, Vogelsang GB, Van Houwelingen HC, Van Rood JJ. Mismatches of minor histocompatibility antigens between HLA-identical donors and recipients and the development of graft-versus-host disease after bone marrow transplantation. N Engl J Med 1996; 334:281–285.

49. Martin PJ, Hansen JA, Torok-Storb B, Durnam D, Przepiorka D, O'Quigley J, Sanders J, Sullivan KM, Witherspoon RP, Deeg HJ, Appelbaum FR, Stewart P, Weiden P, Doney K, Buckner CD, Clift R, Storb R, Thomas ED. Graft failure in patients receiving T cell–depleted HLA-identical allogeneic marrow transplants. Bone Marrow Transplant 1988; 3:445–456.

50. Kernan NA, Bordignon C, Heller G, Cunningham I, Castro-Malaspina H, Shank B, Flomenberg N, Burns J, Yang SY, Black P, Collins NH, O'Reilly RJ. Graft failure after T-cell–

depleted human leukocyte antigen identical marrow transplants for leukemia: I. Analysis of risk factors and results of secondary transplants. Blood 1989; 74:2227–2236.

51. Bunjes D, Heit W, Arnold R, Schmeiser T, Wiesneth M, Carbonell F, Porzsolt F, Raghava-char A, Heimpel H. Evidence for the involvement of host-derived OKT8-positive T cells in the rejection of T-depleted, HLA-identical bone marrow grafts. Transplantation 1987; 43: 501–505.

52. Nakamura H, Gress RE. Graft rejection by cytolytic T cells. Transplantation 1990; 49:4538.

53. Barge AJ, Johnson G, Witherspoon R, Torok-Storb B. Antibody-mediated marrow failure after allogeneic bone marrow transplantation. Blood 1989; 74:1477–1480.

54. Klumpp TR, Herman JH, Mangan KF, Macdonald JS. Graft failure following neutrophil-specific alloantigen mismatched allogeneic BMT. Bone Marrow Transplant 1993; 11:243–245.

55. Champlin RE, Horowitz MM, Van Bekkum DW, Camitta BM, Elfenbein GE, Gale RP, Good RA, Rimm AA, Rozman C. Graft failure following bone marrow transplantation for severe aplastic anemia: risk factors and treatment results. Blood 1989; 73:606–613.

56. Wagner JE, Santos GW, Noga SJ, Rowley SD, Davis J, Vogelsang GB, Farmer ER, Zehn-bauer BA, Saral R, Donnenberg AD. Bone marrow graft engineering by counterflow centrifu-gal elutriation: results of a phase I-II clinical trial. Blood 1990; 75:1370–1377.

57. O'Reilly RJ, Keever CA, Small TN, Brochstein J. The use of HLA-non-identical T-cell–depleted marrow transplants for correction of severe combined immunodeficiency disease. Immunodeficiency Rev 1989; 1:273–309.

58. Appelbaum FR, Cheever MA, Fefer A, Storb R, Thomas ED. Recurrence of aplastic anemia following cyclophosphamide and syngeneic bone marrow transplantation: evidence for two mechanisms of graft failure. Blood 1985; 65:553–556.

59. Vallera DA, Ash RC, Zanjani ED, Kersey JH, LeBien TW, Beverley PC, Nevile DM, Youle RJ. Anti–T-cell reagents for human bone marrow transplantation: ricin linked to three mono-clonal antibodies. Science 1983; 222:512–515.

60. Reisner Y, Kapoor N, O'Reilly RJ, Good RA. Allogeneic bone marrow transplantation using stem cells fractionated by lectins: VI, in vitro analysis of human and monkey bone marrow cells fractionated by sheep red blood cells and soybean agglutinin. Lancet 1980; 2:1320–1324.

61. DeWitte T, Hoogenhout J, De Pauw B, Holdrinet R, Janssen J, Wessels J, van Daal W, Hustinx T, Haanen C. Depletion of donor lymphocytes by counterflow centrifugation suc-cessfully prevents graft-versus-host disease in matched allogeneic marrow transplantation. Blood 1986; 67:1302–1308.

62. Hale G, Bright S, Chumbley G, Hoang T, Metcalf D, Munro AJ, Waldmann H. Removal of T cells from bone marrow for transplantation: a monoclonal antilymphocyte antibody that fixes human complement. Blood 1983; 62:873–882.

63. Prentice H, Janossy G, Price-Jones L. Depletion of T lymphocytes in donor marrow prevents significant graft-versus-host disease in matched allogeneic leukemic marrow transplant recip-ients. Lancet 1984; 1:472.

64. Waldmann H, Hale G, Cividalli G, Weiss L, Weshler Z, Samuel S, Manor D, Brautbar C, Rachmilewitz EA, Slavin S. Elimination of graft-versus-host disease by in vitro depletion of alloreactive lymphocytes with a monoclonal rat anti-human lymphocyte antibody (Cam-path-1). Lancet 1984; 2:483–486.

65. Herve P, Flesch M, Cahn JY, Racadot E, Plouvier E, Lamy B, Rozenbaum A, Noir A, Des Floris RL, Peters A. Removal of marrow T cells with OKT3-OKT11 monoclonal antibodies and complement to prevent acute graft-versus-host disease. A pilot study in ten patients. Transplantation 1985; 39:138–143.

66. Martin P, Hansen J, Buckner C, Sanders J, Deeg H, Stewart P, Appelbaum FR, Clift R, Ferger A, Witherspoon RP. Effects of in vitro depletion of T cells in HLA-identical allogeneic marrow grafts. Blood 1985; 66:664–672.

67. Kernan NA, Collins NH, Juliano L, Cartagena T, Dupont B, O'Reilly RJ. Clonable T lympho-cytes in T cell–depleted bone marrow transplants correlate with development of graft-v-host disease. Blood 1986; 68:770–773.

68. Ash RC, Casper JT, Chitambar CR, Hansen R, Bunin N, Truitt RL, Lawton C, Murray K, Hunter J, Baxter-Lowe LA. Successful allogeneic transplantation of T-cell depleted bone marrow from closely HLA-matched unrelated donors. N Engl J Med 1990; 322:485–494.

69. O'Reilly RJ, Collins NH, Kernan N, Brochstein J, Dinsmore R, Kirkpatrick D. Transplanta-tion of marrow-depleted T cells by soybean lectin agglutination and E-rosette depletion: major histocompatability complex-related graft resistance in leukemic transplant recipients. Transplant Proc 1985; 17:455–459.

70. Patterson J, Prentice HG, Brenner MK, Gilmore M, Janossy G, Ivory K, Skeggs D, Morgan H, Lord J, Blacklock HA, Hoffbrand AV, Apperley JF, Goldman JM, Burnett A, Gribben J, Alcorn M, Pearson C, McVickers I, Hann IM, Reid C, Wardle D, Gravett PJ, Bacigalupo A, Robertson AG. Graft rejection following HLA-matched T lymphocyte depleted bone marrow transplantation. B J Haematol 1986; 63:221–230.

71. Maraninchi D, Gluckman E, Blaise D, Guyotat D, Rio B, Pico J, Leblonde V, Michallet M, Dreyfus F, Ifrah N, Bordigoni A. Impact of T-cell depletion on outcome of allogeneic bone marrow transplantation for standard risk leukemias. Lancet 1987; 2:175–178.

72. Bachar-Lustig E, Rachamim N, Li HW, Lan F, Reisner Y. Megadose of T cell-depleted bone marrow overcomes MHC barriers in sublethally irradiated mice. Nature Med 1995; 1:1268–1273.

73. Micklem HS, Clarke CM, Evans EP, Ford CE. Fate of chromosome-marked mouse bone marrow cells transfused into normal syngeneic recipients. Transplantation 1968; 6:299

74. Takada Y, Takada A. Proliferation of donor hematopoietic cells in irradiated and unirradiated host mice. Transplantation 1971; 12:334–338.

75. Takada A, Takada Y, Ambrus JL. Proliferation of donor spleen and bone-marrow cells in the spleens and bone marrows of unirradiated and irradiated adult mice. Proc Soc Exp Biol Med 1971; 136:222–226.

76. Nilsson SK, Doone MS, Tiarks CY, Weier HU, Quesenberry PJ. Potential and distribution of transplanted hematopoietic stem cells in a nonablated mouse model. Blood 1997; 89:4013–4020.

77. Dexter TM, Allen TD, Lajtha LG. Conditions controlling the proliferation of haemopoietic stem cells in vitro. J Cell Physiol 1977; 91:335–344.

78. Gartner S, Kaplan HS. Long-term culture of human bone marrow cells. Proc Natl Acad Sci USA 1980; 77:4756–4759.

79. Sakakeeny MA, Greenberger JS. Granulopoiesis longevity in continuous bone marrow cul-tures and factor-dependent cell line generation: significant variation among 28 inbred mouse strains and outbred stocks. J Natl Cancer Inst 1982; 68:305–317.

80. Russell ES. Hereditary anemias of the mouse: a review for geneticists. Adv Genet 1979; 20:357–459.

81. Aguila HL, Akashi K, Domen J, Gandy KL, Lagasse E, Mebius RE, Morrison SJ, Shizuru J, Strober S, Uchida N, Wright DE, Weissman IL. From stem cells to lymphocytes: biology and transplantation. Immunol Rev 1997; 157:13–40.

82. Lapidot T, Faktorowich T, Lubin I, Reisnet Y. Enhancement of T-cell–depleted bone marrow allografts in the absence of graft-versus-host disease is mediated by CD8$^+$ CD4$^-$ and not by CD8$^-$ CD4+ thymocytes. Blood 1992; 80:2406–2411.

83. Champlin R, Ho W, Gajewski J, Feig S, Burnison M, Holley G, Greenberg P, Lee K, Schmid I, Giorgi J. Selective depletion of CD8$^+$ lymphocytes for prevention of graft-versus-host disease after allogeneic bone marrow transplantation. Blood 1990; 76:418–423.

84. Ildstad ST, Wren SM, Bluestone JA, Barbieri SA, Stephany D, Sachs DH. Effect of selective T cell depletion of host and/or donor bone marrow on lymphopoietic repopulation, tolerance,

and graft-vs-host disease in mixed allogeneic chimeras (B10+B10.D2 → B10). J Immunol 1986; 136:28–33.

85. Sykes M, Sheard M, Sachs DH. Effects of T-cell depletion in radiation bone marrow chimeras. I. Evidence for a donor cell population which increase allogeneic chimerism but which lacks the potential to produce GVHD. J Immunol 1988; 141:2282–2288.

86. Sykes M, Chester CH, Sundt TM, Romick ML, Hoyes KA, Sachs DH. Effect of T-cell depletion in radiation bone marrow chimeras. III. Characterization of allogeneic bone marrow cell populations that increase allogeneic chimerism independently of graft versus host disease in mixed marrow recipients. J Immunol 1989; 143:3503–3511.

87. Gandy KL, Weissman IL. Characterization of the CD8$^+$ subpopulations of whole bone marrow that facilitate hematopoietic stem cells across allogeneic barriers. Blood 1996; 1(suppl): 88:594a

88. Gaines BA, Colson YL, Kaufman CL, Ildstad ST. Facilitating cells enable engraftment of purified fetal liver stem cells in allogeneic recipients. Exp Hematol 1996; 24:902–913.

88a. Neipp M, Exner BG, Maru D, Haber M, Gammie JS, Pham SM, Ildstad ST. T-cell depletion of allogeneic bone marrow using anti-αβTCR monoclonal antibody: prevention of graft-versus-host disease without affecting engraftment potential. Exp Hematol 1999; 27(5):860–867.

89. Owen RD. Immunogenetic consequences of vascular anastomoses between bovine twins. Science 1945; 102:400–401.

90. Billingham RE, Medawar PB. The technique of free skin grafting in mammals. J Exp Biol 1951; 28:385–402.

91. Billingham RE, Lampkin HG, Medawar PB, Williams HL. Tolerance of homografts, twin diagnosis and the freemartin conditions in cattle. Heredity 1952; 6:201.

92. Rapaport FT, Watanabe K, Cannon FD, Mollen N, Blumenstock D, Ferrebee JW. Histocompatibility studies in a closely bred colony of dogs. J Exp Med 1972; 136:1080–1097.

93. Slavin S, Strober S, Fukes Z, Kaplan HS. Induction of specific tissue transplantation tolerance using fractionated total lymphoid irradiation in adult mice. Long-term survival of allogeneic bone marrow and skin grafts. J Exp Med 1977; 146:34–48.

94. Ildstad ST, Wren SM, Bluestone JA, Barbieri SA, Sachs DH. Characterization of mixed allogeneic chimeras: immunocompetence, in vitro reactivity and genetic specificity of tolerance. J Exp Med 1985; 162:231–244.

95. Cobbold SP, Martin G, Qin S, Waldmann H. Monoclonal antibodies to promote marrow engraftment and tissue graft tolerance. Nature 1986; 323:164–166.

96. Mayumi H, Himeno K, Tanaka K, Tokuda N, Fan JL, Nomoto K. Drug-induced tolerance to allografts in mice. IX. Establishment of complete chimerism by allogeneic spleen cell transplantation from donors made tolerant to H-2-identical recipients. Transplantation 1986; 42:417–422.

97. Zinkernagel RM, Althage A, Callahan G, Welsh RM. On the immunoincompetence of H-2 incompatible irradiated bone marrow chimeras. J Immunol 1980; 124:2356–2365.

98. Singer A, Hatchcock KS, Hodes RJ. Self recognition in allogeneic thymic chimeras: self recognition by T helper cells from the thymus engrafted nude mice is restricted to their thymic H-2 haplotype. J Exp Med 1981; 339:343

99. Rayfield LS, Brent L. Tolerance, immunocompetence, and secondary disease in fully allogeneic radiation chimeras. Transplantation 1983; 36:183–189.

100. Matzinger P, Mirkwood G. In a fully H-2 incompatible chimera, T cells of donor origin can respond to minor histocompatibility antigens in association with either donor or host H-2 type. J Exp Med 1978; 148:84–92.

101. Vallera DA, Soderling CB, Carlson G, Kersey JH. Bone marrow transplantation across major histocompatibility barriers in mice. Effect of elimination of T cells from donor grafts by treatment with monoclonal Thy-1.2 plus complement or antibody alone. Transplantation 1981; 31:218–222.

102. Ruedi E, Sykes M, Ildstad ST, Chester CH, Althage A, Hengartner H, Sachs DH, Zinkernagel RM. Antiviral T cell competence and restriction specificity of mixed allogeneic (P1 + P2 → P1) irradiation chimeras. Cell Immunol 1989; 121:185–195.

103. Singer A, Hathcock KS, Hodes RJ. Cellular and genetic control of antibody responses. VIII. MHC restricted recognition of accessory cells, not B cells, by parent-specific subpopulations of normal F1 T helper cells. J Immunol 1980; 124:1079–1085.

104. Doherty PC, Blanden RV, Zinkernagel RM. Specificity of virus-immune effector T-cells for H-2K and H-2D compatible interactions: implications for H-antigen diversity. Transplant Rev 1976; 29:89–124.

105. Ildstad ST, Sachs DH. Reconstitution with syngeneic plus allogeneic or xenogeneic bone marrow leads to specific acceptance of allografts or xenografts. Nature 1984; 307:168–170.

106. Tomita Y, Khan A, Sykes M. Mechanism by which additional monoclonal antibody (mAB) injections overcome the requirement for thymic irradiation to achieve mixed chimerism in mice receiving bone marrow transplantation after conditioning with anti–T cell mABs and 3-GY whole body irradiation. Transplantation 1996; 61:477–485.

107. Sykes M, Szot GL, Swenson KA, Pearson DA. Induction of high levels of allogeneic hemato-poietic reconstitution and donor-specific tolerance without myelosuppressive conditioning. Nature Med 1997; 3:783–787.

108. Steinberg AD, Krieg AM, Gourley MF, Klinman DM. Theoretical and experimental ap-proaches to generalized autoimmunity. Immunol Rev 1990; 118:129–163.

109. Urowitz MB, Gladman DD. Late mortality in SLE—"the price we pay for control." J Rheu-matal 1980; 7:412–416.

110. Bernard CCA, Mandel TA, Mackay IR. Experimental models of human autoimmune dis-eases: overview and prototypes. In: Mackay IR, Rose N, eds. The Autoimmune Disease II. San Diego/Toronto: Academic Press, 1992:47–106.

111. Hammer RE, Richardson JA, Simmons WA, White AL, Breban M, Taurog JD. High preva-lence of colorectal cancer in HLA-B27 transgenic F344 rats with chronic inflammatory bowel disease. J Invest Med 1995; 43:262–268.

112. Ikehara S, Good RA, Nakamure T, Sekita K, Inoue S, Oo MM, Muso E, Ogawa K, Hamas-hima Y. Rationale for bone marrow transplantation in the treatment of autoimmune disease. Proc Natl Acad Sci USA 1985; 82:2483–2487.

113. Ikehara S, Ohtsuki H, Good RA, Asamoto H, Nakamura T, Sekita K, Muso E, Tochino Y, Ida T, Kuzuya H, Imura H, Hamashima Y. Prevention of type I diabetes in nonobese diabetic mice by allogeneic bone marrow transplantation. Proc Natl Acad Sci USA 1985; 82:7743–7747.

114. Van Bekkum DW. BMT in experimental autoimmune diseases. Bone Marrow Transplant 1993; 11:183–187.

115. Levite M, Zinger H, Zisman E, Reisner Y, Mozes E. Beneficial effects of bone marrow transplantation on the serological manifestations and kidney pathology of experimental sys-temic lupus erythematosus. Cell Immunol 1995; 162:138–145.

116. Nishioka N, Toki J, Cherry, Sugiura K, Than S, Yasumizu R, Inaba M, Nishimura M, Ikehara S. Repair mechanism of lupus nephritis in (NZB × NZW)F1 mice by allogeneic bone marrow transplantation. Immunobiology 1995; 192:279–296.

117. LaFace DM, Peck AB. Reciprocal allogeneic bone marrow transplantation between NOD mice and diabetes-nonsusceptible mice associated with transfer and prevention of autoim-mune diabetes. Diabetes 1989; 38:894–901.

118. Lampeter EF, Homberg M, Quabeck K, Schaefer UW, Wernet P, Bertrams J, Grosse-Wilde H, Gries FA, Kolb H. Transfer of insulin-dependent diabetes between HLA-identical sibling by bone marrow transplantation. Lancet 1993; 341:1243–1244.

119. Vialettes B, Maraninchi D, San Marco MP, Birg F, Stoppa AM, Mattei-Zevaco C, Thivolet C, Hermitte L, Vague P, Mercier P. Autoimmune polyendocrine failure—type 1 (insulin-

dependent) diabetes mellitus and hypothyroidism—after allogeneic bone marrow transplantation in a patient with lymphoblastic leukaemia. Diabetologia 1993; 36:541–546.

120. Jacobs P, Vincent MD, Martell RW. Prolonged remission of severe refractory rheumatoid arthritis following allogeneic bone marrow transplantation for drug-induced aplastic anemia. Bone Marrow Transplant 1986; 1986:237–239.

121. Lowenthal RM, Cohen ML, Atkinson K, Biggs JC. Apparent cure of rheumatoid arthritis by bone marrow transplantation. J Rheumatol 1993; 20:137–140.

122. Eedy DJ, Burrows D, Bridges JM, Jones FG. Clearance of severe psoriasis after allogeneic bone marrow transplantation. Br Med J 1990; 300:908

123. Yin JL, Lowitt SN. Resolution of immune-mediated diseases following allogeneic bone marrow transplantation for leukaemia. Bone Marrow Transplant 1992; 9:31–33.

124. Cottler-Fox M, Khan M, Sensenbrenner LL. Resolution of hypogammaglobulinemia, psoriatic skin lesions and arthritis in a patient with Fanconi's anemia after allogeneic blood stem cell transplantation. Meeting September 16–28, 1996, Basel, Switzerland. International Meeting: Hematopoietic stem cell therapy in autoimmune disease, 1996:19

125. MacAllistar L, Beatty PG. Allogeneic marrow transplant for chronic myelogenous leukemia in a patient who also has multiple sclerosis. International Meeting: Hematopoietic stem cell therapy in autoimmune disease. 1996; September 16–28, 1996, Basel, Switzerland, 15 Abstract.

126. Snowden JA, Lowenthal RM, Francis H, Kearney P, Brooks P, Atkinson K, Biggs JC. Does over a decade of remission from rheumatoid arthritis (RA) after bone marrow transplantation (BMT) represent a cure? Long term follow up of two Australian cases. International Meeting: Hematopoietic stem cell therapy in autoimmune disease, 1996; September 16–28, 1996, Basel, Switzerland, 6 Abstract.

127. Li H, Kaufman CL, Boggs SS, Johnson PC, Patrene KD, Ildstad ST. Mixed allogeneic chimerism induced by a sublethal approach prevents autoimmune diabetes and reverses insulitis in non-obese diabetic (NOD) mice. J Immunol 1996; 156:380–388.

128. Walters MC, Patience M, Leisenring W, Eckman JR, Scott JP, Mentzer, Davies SC, Ohene-Frempong K, Bernaudin F, Matthews DC, Storb R, Sullivan KM. Bone marrow transplantation for sickle cell disease. N Engl J Med 1996; 335:369–376.

129. Lucarelli G, Galimberti M, Polchi P, Angelucci E, Baronciani D, Giardini C, Politi P, Durazzi SM. Bone Marrow Transplantation in Patients with Thalassemia. N Engl J Med 1990; 322: 417–421.

130. Walters MC, Sullivan KM, O'Reilly RJ, Boulad F, Brockstein J, Blume K, Amyson M, Johnson FL, Klemperer M, Graham-Pole J. Bone marrow transplantation for thalassemia. The USA experience. Am J Pediatr Hematol Oncol 1994; 16:11–17.

131. Camitta BM, Storb R, Thomas ED. Aplastic anemia (first of two parts): pathogenesis, diagnosis, treatment, and prognosis. N Engl J Med 1982; 306:645–652.

132. Parkman R, Rappeport J, Geha R, Belli J, Cassady R, Levey R, Nathan DG, Rosen FS. Complete correction of the Wiskott-Aldrich syndrome by allogeneic bone-marrow transplantation. N Engl J Med 1978; 298:921–927.

133. O'Reilly RJ, Brochstein J, Dinsmore R, Kirkpatrick D. Marrow transplantation for congenital disorders. Semin Hematol 1984; 21:188–221.

134. Camitta BM, Storb R, Thomas ED. Aplastic anemia (second of two parts): pathogenesis, diagnosis, treatment, and prognosis. N Engl J Med 1982; 306:712–718.

135. Roberts I. Bone marrow transplantation in children: current results and controversies. Meeting, Hilton Head Island, SC, March 1994. Bone Marrow Transplant 1994; 14:197–199.

136. Bayever E, Ladisch S, Philippart M, Brill N, Nuwer M, Sparkes RS, Feig SA. Bone marrow transplantation for metachromatic leucodystrophy. Lancet 1985; 2:471–473.

137. Lipton M, Lockman LA, Ramsay NK, Kersey JH, Jacobson RI, Krivit W. Bone marrow transplantation in metachromatic leukodystrophy. Birth Defects: Original Article Series 1986; 22:57–67.

138. Shapiro EG, Lockman LA, Balthazor M, Krivit W. Neuropsychological outcomes of several storage diseases with and without bone marrow transplantation. J Inherit Metab Dis 1995; 18:413–429.

139. Whitley CB, Ramsay NK, Kersey JH, Krivit W. Bone marrow transplantation for Hurler syndrome: assessment of metabolic correction. Birth Defects: Original Article Series 1986; 22:7–24.

140. Whitley CB, Belani KG, Chang PN, Summers CG, Blazar BR, Tsai MY, Latchaw RE, Ramsay NK, Dersey JH. Long-term outcome of Hurler syndrome following bone marrow transplantation. Am J Med Genet 1993; 46:209–218.

141. Ringden O, Groth CG, Erikson A, Granqvist S, Mansson JE, Sparrelid E. Ten years' experience of bone marrow transplantation for Gaucher disease. Transplantation 1995; 59:864–870.

142. Sands MS, Vogler C, Torrey A, Levy B, Gwynn B, Grubb J, Sly WS, Birkenmeier EH. Murine mucopolysaccharidosis type VII: long term therapeutic effects of enzyme replacement and enzyme replacement followed by bone marrow transplantation. J Clin Invest 1997; 99:1596–1605.

143. Good RA. Bone marrow transplantation for immunodeficiency diseases. Am J Med Sci 1987; 294:68–74.

144. Gatti RA, Meuwissen HJ, Allen HD, Hong R, Good RA. Immunological reconstitution of sex-linked lymphopenic immunological deficiency. Lancet 1968; 2:1366–1369.

145. Chen SH, Ochs HD, Scott CR, Giblett ER, Tingle AJ. Adenosine deaminase deficiency: disappearance of adenine deoxynucleotides from a patient's erythrocytes after successful marrow transplantation. J Clin Invest 1978; 62:1386–1389.

146. Silber GM, Winkelstein JA, Moen RC, Horowitz SD, Trigg M, Hong R. Reconstitution of T- and B-cell function after T-lymphocyte-depleted haploidentical bone marrow transplantation in severe combined immunodeficiency due to adenosine deaminase deficiency. Clin Immunol Immunopathol 1987; 44:317–320.

147. Bluetters-Sawatzki R, Friedrich W, Ebell W, Vetter U, Stoess H, Goldmann SF, Kleihauer E. HLA-haploidentical bone marrow transplantation in three infants with adenosine deaminase deficiency: stable immunological reconstitution and reversal of skeletal abnormalities. Eur J Pediatr 1989; 149:104–109.

7

Ins and Outs of Hematopoietic Stem Cells
Regulation by Genes and Stromal Cells

CHRISTA E. MÜLLER-SIEBURG*

Medical Biology Institute, La Jolla, California

RAJEEV SONI

Medical Biology Institute and LIDAK Pharmaceuticals, La Jolla, California

I. INTRODUCTION

Since many terms in the field of stem cell biology can be ambiguous, we here define our use of terminology:

Primitiveness: a quality that reflects the position of a stem cell in the developmental hierarchy; a very primitive stem cell is thought to have extensive proliferative capacity which is reflected in the repopulation kinetics; for example, long-term repopulation with late onset characterizes a primitive stem cell. Less primitive stem cells repopulate faster but have less differentiation capacity.

Proliferation: Division of a stem cell that can lead to differentiation or persistence or expansion.

Persistence: If a stem cell receives a signal that prevents differentiation or death, it will retain its repopulation capacity; that is, state of primitiveness.

Maintenance: Keeping the level of stem cells constant through persistence or a balance of loss and expansion.

Expansion: If after a division, both daughter cells receive signals permitting persistence, more stem cells are found than before.

Many hematopoietic cells are short-lived and are constantly replenished through a differentiation cascade from precursors and stem cells. Thus, stem cells, the ultimate source

---

* *Current affiliation*: Sidney Kimmel Cancer Center, San Diego, California.

of all hematopoietic cells, are believed to self-renew to avoid depleting the compartment through differentiation. Self-renewal, defined as producing unaltered copies of the same cell (1), signifies that the daughter cells are genetically and functionally identical to the parental stem cells. Owing to our incomplete understanding of the molecular biology of stem cells, the exact and complete identity of two cells is difficult to verify. Nevertheless, hypotheses have been formulated that range from "a stem cell is defined by self-renewal and therefore all stem cells must self-renew" (1) to "stem cells lose repopulation capacity every time they divide and therefore do not self-renew" (2–5). Data supporting these views have been published (reviewed in Refs. 6–10). The ultimate goal of self-renewal is the maintenance of the stem cell pool, and most of the available evidence indicates that the size of the stem cell compartment is stable and tightly regulated. Thus, although the mysteries of self-renewal remain to be elucidated, a look at the mechanisms that control the size of the stem cell pool may help us understand what regulates stem cell proliferation, differentiation, and maintenance. We review here data that collectively suggest that the regulation of the size of the stem cell compartment is controlled through an interplay of extrinsic and intrinsic events. An understanding of the regulation of the stem cell is dependent on the resolution of the analysis tools available to detect these cells. Thus, we begin with a brief discussion of the parameters detected by the different stem cell assays.

II. FUNCTIONAL PROPERTIES OF A STEM CELL

A. Stem Cells Are Repopulating Units

A discussion about stem cells should be prefaced by a definition of stem cells. This is necessitated by the inherent limitations of our current methods to analyze stem cells. Stem cells are exceedingly rare, which prevents their direct examination. Moreover, markers or characteristics that are unique to stem cells have not been defined. Thus, stem cells are measured indirectly as repopulating units. Indeed, all stem cell assays, both in vivo and in vitro use the ability to differentiate to generate mature hematopoietic cells as a hallmark for stem cell activity. Because of the enormous amplification achieved during differentiation, the progeny of a stem cell can be readily detected. The presence of differentiated progeny is then taken as a sign that a stem cell did exist at the beginning of the experiment.

B. Limitation of Repopulation Systems

As with any indirect detection system, there are several caveats to each type repopulation assays. All repopulation assays assume a direct and reproducible correlation of stem cell numbers with the number of mature cells generated. This is the very definition of a repopulating unit. However, this assumption may not be entirely justified. By their very nature, stem cell assays fail to detect quiescent stem cells that do not generate mature cells in an assay. In certain conditions, such cells can be revealed, and quiescent stem cells have been detected after retransplantation of marked stem cells (11,12) and in blastocyst aggregation chimeras (13). These data suggest that quiescent stem cells are common and, by extension, that most assays underestimate the number of stem cells.

The outcome of a repopulation assay is also influenced by the fitness of the progeny. Defective or hyperproliferative progeny can lead to misrepresentation of mature cells in the periphery and thereby bias estimates of stem cell numbers or stem cell behavior. This is particularly evident when mutant mice are examined. For example, mice with the WW mutation appear to have normal numbers of stem cells; however, the mutation results in a diminished ability to sustain precursors and mature cells (14,15). Consequently, these mice were falsely believed to have a defect in stem cells. Even in normal strains of mice, peripheral repopulation does not necessarily reflect the number of stem cells. That was shown clearly in aggregation chimeras between the strains DAB/2 and C57BL/6 (13). In some of these chimeras, contribution by the parental DBA/2 is very low and the periphery is dominated by cells derived from the C57BL/6 strain. However, after transplanting the chimeric bone marrow, both DAB/2 and C57BL/6 stem cells repopulated the secondary hosts to roughly the same extent. Thus, comparison of stem cells from different sources is not straightforward. Collectively, the data raise the disturbing specter that even our best and most stringent stem cell assays fail to detect selectively certain subsets of stem cells. One way of addressing this dilemma is to measure a number of parameters that together define stem cell behavior.

C. Parameters Defining Repopulating Units

There are least three parameters that together define the properties of a repopulating unit: (1) differentiation capacity or clone size, that is, how many mature cells are generated in the host; (2) duration of repopulation; that is, the time during which a stem cell clone contributes to mature cells in the periphery; and (3) strength; that is, the ability of a stem cell to repopulate in competition with other stem cells. As summarized in Table 1, all stem cell assays detect only a subset of these parameters. For example: the in vitro assay that measures long-term culture-initiating cells (LTCICs) readily measures clone size and persistency of repopulation and allows quantification of stem cells (16–18). However, the LTCIC assay fails to reveal the whole extent of the differentiation capacity by being limited to myeloid differentiation and does not measure the strength of a stem cell. The

Table 1 Parameters Detected by Different Stem Cell Assays

| | Assay system | | |
Parameter	Competitive repopulation	Noncompetitive repopulation[a]	LTCIC
Differentiation capacity	Y	Y	N
Clone size of individual Stem cells	N	Y[b]	Y
Strength	Y	N	N
Duration of repopulation	Y	Y	Y
Quantitative	Y	Y[b]	Y
Genetic restrictions[c]	Y	Y	Y
Influenced by seeding Efficiency or homing Ability	Y	Y	N

LTCIC, long-term culture-initiating cells.

[a] Noncompetitive repopulation assays refer here to assays where the stem cell parameters are tested in the presence of a source of radioprotecting cells. Radioprotection is provided by a stem cell–deleted or "compromised" source of cells. These assays are sometimes falsely referred to as competitive repopulation assays.

[b] Only when done in limiting dilution.

[c] Refers to the necessity to match transplantation antigens in host and donor.

in vivo noncompetitive repopulation assays in lethally irradiated or nonirradiated hosts detect differentiation capacity, clone size, and persistence but fail to measure stem cell strength. Unless these assays are done in limiting dilution (19), they do not quantify stem cells. This is also true for repopulation assays that use a source of compromised stem cells for radioprotection (20). The in vivo competitive repopulation assay (21) is geared to detect the strength of a stem cell and measures differentiation capacity and persistence. However, this assay is less well suited to detect clone sizes. Thus, each assay system detects different properties of stem cells, revealing facets of the complete picture of stem cell behavior. This, compounded by the tendency of each investigator to set different thresholds for the lowest level of repopulation that is considered positive, can account for the marked differences in the frequency of stem cells estimated in the bone marrow even in the same strain of mice (19,21–24).

To gauge accurately the composition of the stem cell pool, it would be important to measure all parameters listed here. Of course, financial and time constrains prevent such an extensive analysis, leaving us with tantalizing glimpses rather than complete understanding. Nevertheless, the available data collectively make it possible to infer mechanisms that regulate the maintenance of the stem cell pool. Recent data indicate that the stem cell pool is controlled by both intrinsic and extrinsic regulatory events.

III. INTRINSIC REGULATION OF STEM CELL MAINTENANCE

Intrinsic regulation refers to cell-autonomous events independent of the microenvironment of the stem cell and includes developmental changes, allelic effects, and/or regulation of gene expression. The data summarized below show that intrinsic events determine the differentiation capacity and strength of stem cells and play a major role in stem cell maintenance.

A. Developmental Changes

That intrinsic events play a role in regulating stem cell behavior is obvious when stem cells from fetal, adult, and old animals or humans are compared. Fetal stem cells have a much larger proliferation and differentiation capacity than stem cells from adult tissues shown both in vivo and in vitro (25–28). The basis for this increased proliferative capacity of fetal stem cell is not well understood. There is recent evidence that fetal stem cells interact more efficiently with the fetal than with the adult environment. Stem cells from yolk sac cannot repopulate adult hosts. This led to the hypothesis that yolk sac does not contain definitive stem cells (29). However, when yolk sac stem cells are injected into a fetus, these cells will contribute to long-term definitive repopulation (30,31). Thus, the intrinsic difference of a stem cell may require a matching extrinsic signal.

There is also evidence that the function of stem cells is changed in the old animal. Stem cells isolated from old individuals had shorter telomeres than stem cells from young humans (32,33). This indicates that the genetic make-up of stem cells changes during aging. This is particularly surprising because telomerase activity has been demonstrated in hematopoietic stem cells (34,35). Telomerase is found preferentially in cells that show extensive expansion capacity, including gonads and tumor cells (36–38). Thus, even though the presence of telomerase activity in hematopoietic stem cells supports the interpretation that stem cells can self-renew, the shorted telomeres show that stem cells change during development.

There is additional evidence that aging changes stem cells intrinsically. Several groups reported that the frequency of stem cells is higher in the bone marrow of old than of young mice (39,40). However, four times as many cells were needed from old mice compared to young ones for reconstitution of irradiated recipients (40). Both sources of stem cells had similar abilities to differentiate in vitro in response to stromal cells, indicating comparative differentiation capacity. This suggests that the stem cells from old mice are impaired in their ability to home in vivo to the appropriate hematopoietic niches. The genetic mechanisms that are responsible for these developmental changes remain to be identified.

B. Allelic Differences Affecting the Stem Cell Pool

Several groups have taken advantage of the power of mouse genetics to analyze the behavior of stem cells in vivo. That intrinsic mechanisms play a role in regulating the size of the stem cell pool was demonstrated using a LTCIC-based system for the detection of stem cells (43). In this series of experiments, Müller-Sieburg and Riblet (43) demonstrated that the frequency of LTCICs differed significantly in strains of inbred mice. The strain C57BL/6 showed the lowest levels with about 2 LTCICs per 10^5 marrow cells, whereas DBA/2 mice showed the highest levels, containing an 11-fold higher frequency of LTCICs (about 28 per 10^5 marrow cells). BALB/c and CBA mice showed intermediate levels of LTCICs. Interestingly, the strains FvB and 129 also showed elevated levels of LTCICs. These mice are frequently used to generate transgenic or null mutation mice. Thus, great care should be taken to assure that the engineered mice are compared to the same stain when assessing stem cell function.

The difference in LTCIC levels was preserved regardless of the genotype of the stromal cell lines used. This suggest that the stem cell frequency (Scfr) genes regulate the size of the stem cell pool intrinsically. The genes controlling the size of the stem cell pool were mapped by measuring LTCIC levels in the bone marrow of C57BL/6 × DBA/2 recombinant inbred (BXD RI) strains (43). LTCIC levels showed a broad distribution indicative of multigenic control. Statistical analysis indicated that at least four genes are involved in regulating the LTCIC frequency. Three loci that contributed to the difference in stem cell levels were mapped: two to chromosome 1 near Acrg and Adprp, respectively, and one locus to chromosome 11 near histone 3 (Hist3) protein. The location of the loci on chromosome 1 near Adprp was independently confirmed with a congenic mouse, B6.C-H-25, which carries a 20-centimorgan part of BALB/c on chromosome 1. LTCIC levels in H-25 congenic mice were found to be intermediate between BALB/c and C57BL/6. Current efforts are directed toward fine-mapping the genes on chromosome 1.

After the initial description of genetic loci that control the size of the stem cell pool, the finding was corroborated by others (44). This group also used an LTCIC assay (44). More recently, Weissman and coworkers identified a similar genetic polymorphism in the size of the stem cell pool in AKR and C57BL/6 mice. AKR mice showed approximately a fivefold higher number of repopulating stem cells than C57BL/6 mice, and mapping efforts are in progress (I. L. Weissman, personal communication). Thus, differences in the frequency of stem cells in inbred strains of mice can be detected both on the level of in vivo repopulating stem cells and in vitro LTCIC. The combined assays allow the conclusion that the stem cells differ in number but not clone size. However, so far, there is little information on their competitive strengths.

In contrast to stem cells, the frequency of mature cells and the myeloid precursor compartment did not differ significantly between the DBA/2 and C57BL/6 strains of mice (41,43; C. E. Müller-Sieburg, unpublished observation). In addition, all strains of mice tested are healthy with no overt deficiencies in hematopoiesis. Clearly, C57BL/6 mice, with the lowest frequency of stem cells, have sufficient stem cells for life-long hematopoiesis. Indeed, this strain of mice lives on average longer than other strains (45). Thus, it seems likely that the other strains have an excess of stem cells. The size of the stem cell pool is likely to be a balance between differentiation, persistence, and expansion (10). The DBA/2 alleles of the *Scfr* genes could lead to increased proliferation, prolonged persistence, or decreased differentiation of stem cells. Recent data (45a) show that the LTCIC compartments of the DBA/2 and C57BL/6 mice do not differ in their cycling status, suggesting that differences in stem cell proliferation are unlikely to account for the markedly dissimilar stem cell numbers.

Whatever the mechanism is that causes most of the strains to have high numbers of stem cells, it is tempting to speculate that the allelic forms of the *Scfr* genes will be predictor of stem cell number and thus may be useful for evaluating cell sources in clinical stem cell transplantation. In support of this hypothesis are data that indicate that the outbred human population shows a similar continuum of LTCIC frequencies with differences up to 100-fold in individual donors (46). So far, no correlation of LTCIC levels with age or medical history of the subjects has been found (46). This suggests that the size of the stem cell pool in humans is regulated by genes similar to the *Scfr* genes identified in the mouse. Indeed, the region on mouse chromosome 1 that contains the *Scfr-1* gene is syntentic to human chromosome arm 1q. Thus, it is likely that the human homologue of the mouse stem cell regulatory gene will also reside on human 1q.

C. Intrinsic Regulation of Stem Cell Behavior by Transcription Factors

Another approach to identify intrinsic regulators for stem cell behavior has been to look for genes expressed specifically in immature cells in vivo and cell lines in vitro. A variety of transcriptional regulators have been identified, most of which appear to be important in differentiation events. For example, knockout mutations of the *Ikaros* gene resulted in mice that did not develop lymphoid cells (47). The *SCL/tal-1* gene was identified through cloning of chromosomal translocation breakpoints in human T-cell leukemias (48). The gene product is broadly expressed in immature and mature cells and knockout mice die in utero (reviewed in Ref. 49). Homozygous null mutations in embryonic stem cells rendered the progeny incapable of giving rise to hematopoietic cells in chimeric mice (50). This suggests that the *SCL/tal-1* gene plays a role in the ontogeny of the hematopoietic system.

Another transcription factor, the homeobox gene *HOXB4* is an important regulator of stem cell proliferation. Sauvageau and coworkers (51) reported that murine bone marrow cells, transduced with a retroviral construct carrying *HOXB4*, have considerably more repopulating capacity than control cells. Myeloid and lymphoid precursors were also increased, suggesting that *HOXB4* causes enhancement of the proliferative capacity in all hematopoietic precursor compartments. More importantly, serial transplantation experiments showed that *HOXB4*-transduced stem cells retained about 100-fold more repopulating units in the primary hosts than control cells even though the absolute number of repopulating units was decreased by transplantation in both control and transfected cells. This suggests that *HOXB4* causes increased persistence and/or proliferation of stem cells. Interestingly, *HOXB4* overexpression did not change the behavior of undifferentiated embryonic stem (ES) cells (52) but enhanced the generation of erythroid and mixed colony progenitors from differentiating ES cells. This suggests that *HOXB4* is an intrinsic regulator of proliferation and/or persistence in early stages of hematopoietic stem cell development, which is consistent with its expression pattern in normal cells (53).

Collectively, the data indicate a strong component of intrinsic regulation of all aspects of stem cell behavior and particularly in regulating the size of the stem cell compartment. Most of the genes involved have yet to be identified and characterized. It is difficult to isolate bone marrow stem cells of sufficient purity and quantity to permit molecular studies. Therefore, differentiation systems of ES cells have been established to identify genes that regulate stem cell proliferation and differentiation. ES cells can be induced to differentiate by withdrawal of leukemia inhibitory factor (LIF) (54,55). The embryonic bodies that appear in these cultures contain erythroid islands, a site of hematopoietic development. Several reports suggest that stem cell activity is found in this system (54,56). Thus, it is likely that the ES cell system will be useful for identification of further intrinsic regulators of stem cells.

IV. EXTRINSIC REGULATION OF STEM CELL MAINTENANCE

All stem cells, regardless of their intrinsic state, need extrinsic signals for their survival, proliferation, and differentiation, (reviewed in Refs. 57–59). In vivo, the microenvironment provides these signals in the form of cellular interactions, or secreted molecules. Molecules secreted into the extracellular space that impact on stem cells include cytokines, hormones, and extracellular matrix (ECM) molecules. The interaction of stem cells with the ECM and cytokines have been extensively reviewed (60, 61; see also other chapters this book). We shall focus here on the role of stromal cells in regulating stem cell maintenance.

A. Stromal Cells Are Functionally Heterogeneous

That the cellular microenvironment plays an important role in controlling stem cell differentiation and proliferation has been appreciated for several decades. Trentin (62) hypothesized that an inductive microenvironment directs the differentiation of stem cells toward the different hematopoietic lineages. This hypothesis was extended to provide a model of stem cell proliferation and account for the heterogeneity within the stem cell compartment. Weissman (7) and Wineman et al. (63,64) postulated that the microenvironment is organized into discrete niches comprising functionally different types of stromal cells. These stromal cell niches would selectively enable the proliferation of stem cells that differ in primitiveness. Rare niches would allow the proliferation of very primitive stem cells. Once these niches are filled, any surplus stem cell would have to leave and would encounter other, more frequent stromal cell niches that support less primitive stem cells (7). This model accounts for the observation that primitive stem cells are very rare, whereas less primitive stem cells are increasingly more frequent.

Data by Wineman and coworkers (63,64) support this hypothesis. They analyzed a large panel of developmentally matched stromal cells for the ability to maintain repopulating stem cells. The lines were isolated from murine fetal liver and immortalized with a retroviral construct encoding a temperature-sensitive simian virus (SV40) T antigen. SV40 T antigen–transduced cells establish lines with a roughly 10-fold higher frequency than primary cells (C. E. Müller-Sieburg, unpublished observation). Thus, SV40 T antigen assists in revealing at least part of the stromal cell heterogeneity found in vivo. Individual cloned stromal cells were seeded in vitro with a source of stem cells, cultures were maintained for 3 weeks, and thereafter the stem cell content in the cultures was measured in an in vivo competitive repopulation assay.

Most lines in this panel failed to support any stem cells in culture. From the 16 stromal cell lines in this series, only one could maintain input levels of long-term repopulating stem cells. The level of stem cells retained in these cultures were identical to those originally seeded. Similarly, the competitive strength of the cultured stem cells was indistinguishable from that of freshly explanted bone marrow stem cells. The kinetic of repopulation indicates that this stromal cell line, CFC034, maintains both primitive and less primitive stem cells. This pattern of support is very similar to that of the marrow-derived stromal cell line S17 (63). Six additional stromal cell lines in this panel were capable of supporting repopulating stem cells. The stem cells cultured on these lines gave rise to multilineage repopulation in the irradiated host early after transplantation. However, the stem cells ceased to contribute to the periphery over time, suggesting that these stem cells were less primitive. Whether this less primitive status is a reflection of limited differentiation capacity or reduced proliferation capacity of the stem cells remains to be determined.

One stromal cell line, 2012, originally comprised two morphologically different adherent cell types, a small slow-growing cell and a large fibroblastoid cell type that grew rapidly. Despite this heterogeneity, the line was likely monoclonal, because the parental line and its subclones showed the same integration sites for the retroviral construct (64). The line 2012, consisting of this cell mixture, was capable of supporting high levels of stem cells. Stem cells cultured on the line 2012 showed a delayed onset of repopulation; early after transplantation, few donor-type cells were seen; however, donor-type repopulation increased steadily over the 7 months of the experiment. This distinct kinetic of repopulation suggest that the line 2012 maintained preferentially very primitive stem cells. When the line 2012 was reexamined, the morphological heterogeneity was lost and the fibroblastoid cell type dominated the cultures. Simultaneously, the line lost the ability to maintain high levels of stem cells. However, subclones of the line 2012 retained the ability to support a lower level of stem cells with a delayed onset of repopulation. Thus, the ability to maintain high levels of stem cells was separable from the retention of preferentially primitive cells by subcloning. By extension, this suggests that different stromal cells with different molecular programs are responsible for regulating stem cell numbers and stem cell primitiveness. Indeed, the molecular analysis of stromal cell programs has allowed isolation of a delta-like molecule that selectively acts on less primitive, short-term repopulating stem cells (65). This supports the interpretation that distinct stromal cell–derived molecules will extrinsically regulate distinct parameters of stem cell behavior.

An equally exhaustive analysis of stromal function in the human system has not been performed so far. However, the data from several reports together indicate that human stem cells interact similarly with stromal cells as do mouse stem cells. Traditionally, it has been difficult to derive long-term human stromal cell lines (reviewed in Ref. 59). Thus, a number of groups have explored mouse stem cells as a support for human stem cells. These experiments show that rare mouse stromal cell lines support human stem cells (66–68). In our experience, those mouse stromal cell lines that maintain mouse stem cells well will also support human stem cells (A.D. Ho and C.E. Müller-Sieburg, unpublished observation). Roecklein and coworkers described an ingenious method to establish human stromal cell lines (69). They took advantage of a retroviral construct that encodes the human papilloma virus E6/E7 genes. The E6/E7 proteins prevent the cell cycle arrest by interfering with the tumor-suppressor proteins p53 and Rb. Cell cycle arrest caused by senescence had been the major stumbling block in establishing human stromal cell lines (reviewed in Ref. 59). A limited analysis of the support capacity of these human E6/E7 immortalized stromal cell lines (69) suggested that supportive stromal cell lines are as infrequent in the human as in the mouse system. Undoubtedly, this improved method of generating human stromal cell lines will make the human microenvironment more accessible to analysis.

Collectively, these data, particularly from the mouse system, show that stromal cells, as represented by stromal cell lines, are markedly heterogeneous in their ability to interact with stem cells. Heterogeneity was seen in both the number of repopulating units sustained and the type of stem cells supported. These different stromal cells were responsible for selectively maintaining different types and different numbers of stem cells during the culture period. These data are consistent with the interpretation that functionally different stromal cells form niches that are responsible for stem cell persistence and differentiation. Thus, stromal cells provide important extrinsic signals for the maintenance of the stem cell pool.

B. Mechanisms of Extrinsic Stem Cell Support

We do not know how the stromal cell lines selectively maintain primitive and less primitive stem cells and what accounts for the failure of many lines to support stem cells. We do know, however, that the ability of the stromal cell lines to support stem cells was not correlated with how well these lines supported mature cells (64). Thus, the failure of most stromal cells to maintain primitive stem cells is not due to broadly inhibitory stromal cell products. By extension, the lack of correlation suggests that stem cell maintenance requires molecules different from those necessary for the support of their differentiated progeny. This interpretation was supported by the results of an extensive reverse transcriptase-polymerase chain reaction (RT-PCR) analysis of the cytokines made by the different stromal cell lines. The stromal cell lines within the panel varied little in cytokine production, at least on the RNA level. All stromal cell lines tested produced readily detectable levels of c-kit ligand and flk2 ligand, suggesting that these cytokines are not primarily responsible for stem cell maintenance. Moreover, there is no obvious correlation of the patterns of cytokine transcription and stem cell support. Thus, it is likely that stromal cells regulate stem cells by still unidentified molecules or interactions.

A limited functional analysis supports this view. The stromal cell line S17 maintains input levels of repopulating stem cells (63). Blocking monoclonal antibodies (mAbs) that specifically blocked the function of cytokines or their receptors [c-kit ligand, c-fms, interleukin (IL)-6, LIF] did not change the maintenance of stem cells (63; C.E. Müller-Sieburg, unpublished observation). Similar results with c-kit–specific mAb have been reported by Kodama and colleagues on the stromal cell line PA6 (70). Thus, the functional studies agree with the PCR analysis, both indicating that these cytokines are not the "active ingredient" in stromal cell support of primitive stem cells. Gupta and coworkers (71) identified a high molecular weight heparan sulfate proteoglycan purified from stroma-conditioned supernatant, which together with the cytokines c-kit, MIP-1a, IL-6, granulocyte colony-stimulating factor (G-CSF), granulocyte-macrophage colony-stimulating factor (GM-CSF), and LIF can substitute for stromal cells in supporting human LTCIC. The low level of recovery of LTCICs in this system suggests that additional molecules are needed. These molecules are likely to be found on the cell surface of stromal cells.

Verfaillie (72) reported that human LTCICs are maintained more efficiently in non-contact than in direct-contact cultures. Stem cells were separated from stromal cells by a semipermeable membrane that allowed the stromal cell conditioned supernatant to pass freely but inhibited direct contact to the stroma. However, the yield of LTCICs after all culture conditions was low, and the murine stromal cell line, M2-10B4, used in these studies can be categorized as a line that supports limited numbers of less primitive stem cells (68). On the stromal cell line S17, an efficient supporter of stem cells, direct contact of stem cells and stromal cells was necessary for maintenance. Repopulating stem cells did not survive when separated by a membrane from the stroma even though good hematopoiesis was found on the membranes (64). Similar data have been reported in both the mouse and the human system (73,74). These studies used stromal cell lines that support high numbers of repopulating stem cells. Thus, the distinguishing factor appears that those stromal cell lines that are designed to interact with primitive stem cells do so by direct cell contact. This indicates that an important "active ingredient" made by stromal cells is membrane associated. Such molecules could be membrane forms of cytokines, adhesion molecules, and/or ECM molecules.

C. Models of Stem Cell Maintenance

On the experience gained in the analysis of stromal cell-stem cell interactions, we hypothesized (10) that stem cells will differentiate unless they encounter certain, yet unidentified, signals from the microenvironment. We have named these molecules "guardian molecules." This model assumes that stem cells are constantly exposed to cytokines that promote activation and differentiation. Stem cells will proliferate on stimulation with activating factors and differentiate. However, if appropriate guardian molecules are present, proliferating stem cells will receive a negative signal, which reinstates the resting state thereby preventing differentiation. This molecule is likely to be present on the cell surface of stromal cells. Our model predicts persistence or expansion of primitive stem cells if, and only if, guardian molecules are present in sufficient concentration in vivo and in vitro. This model makes the testable prediction that the extent of stem cell proliferation will be unaffected by inhibiting access to these guardian molecules; however, persistence and expansion of stem cells should be severely reduced.

This model would predict that the stromal cell lines that maintain high levels of stem cells express high levels of guardian molecules and thereby retain the primitiveness of the cultured stem cells. So far, the best results with stem cells from marrow has been maintenance of stem cells; the number of repopulating units seeded initially equaled the number retrieved after several weeks of stromal cell coculture. It is possible that the stem cells originally seeded remain in the resting state and never divide. However, there is evidence that stem cells proliferate in long-term stromal cell supported cultures. Fraser et al. (20) initiated cultures with retrovirally marked stem cells. After in vivo transplantation, the clonal make-up of the progeny showed that a subset of stem cells proliferated in stromal cell supported cultures, whereas most stem cells were lost. Similar conclusions were drawn from a series of replating experiments. Highly purified human stem cells were seeded into noncontact cultures. Several weeks later, nonadherent cells were replated onto fresh stroma to measure LTCIC content (75). About 16% of LTCICs originally seeded gave rise to LTCICs revealed in the secondary cultures. Both studies were performed with stromal cells that were suboptimal for stem cell support. Whether the stromal cell lines that support high levels of stem cells permit more stem cells to proliferate or more stem cells to persist remains to be addressed. Regardless of the mechanism, these data show clearly that selected stromal cell elements in the microenvironment can directly influence the size of the stem cell pool by regulating the maintenance of stem cells.

V. CONCLUSION

Both intrinsic and extrinsic events regulate the size of the stem cell pool. The microenvironment provides necessary signals without which stem cells lose their stemness. However, stem cells must be intrinsically ready to react to the stimuli provided. The available data suggest that this intrinsic readiness is not only a function of the developmental stage but also of inherited traits that vary markedly between different mice and perhaps humans. Stem cell transplantation is used routinely as a curative treatment of many diseases. This is a remarkable case where medicine has surged forward with great success even though many of the issues about stem cell proliferation remain to be resolved. Nevertheless, it is likely that a better understanding of the ins and outs of stem cell regulation will improve the judicious application of stem cell therapy. Whether cytokine mobilization could lead to problems for the donor in the future, finding improved methods for in vitro manipulation and expansion of repopulating stem cells, enhanced repopulation of normal and manipulated stem cells are areas that will likely benefit from an increased understanding of stem cell biology.

ACKNOWLEDGMENT

Work cited from our laboratory was supported in part by grant DK48015 from the National Institutes of Health, Bethesda, MD.

REFERENCES

1. Lajtha LG. Stem cell concepts. Differentiation 1979; 14:23–34.
2. Kay HEM. How many cell-generations? Lancet 1965; 2:418–419.
3. Rosendaal M, Hodgson GS, Bradley TR. Haemopoietic stem cells are organised for use on the basis of their generation-age. Nature 1976; 264:68–69.
4. Rosendaal M, Hodgson GS, Bradley TR. Organization of haemopoietic stem cells: the generation-age hypothesis. Cell Tiss Kinet 1979; 12:17–29.
5. Hellman S, Botnick LE, Hannon EC, Vigneulle RM. Proliferative capacity of murine hematopoietic stem cells. Proc Natl Acad Sci USA 1978; 75:490–494.
6. Spangrude GJ, Smith L, Uchida N, Ikuta K, Heimfeld S, Friedman J, Weissman IL. Mouse hematopoietic stem cells. Blood 1991; 78:1395–13402.
7. Weissman IL. Developmental switches in the immune system. Cell 1994; 76:207–218.
8. Moore MA. Clinical implications of positive and negative haematopoietic stem cell regulators. Blood 1991; 78:1–19.
9. Morrison SJ, Shah NM, Anderson DJ. Regulatory mechanisms in stem cell biology. Cell 1997; 88:287–298.
10. Müller-Sieburg CE, Deryugina E. The stromal cells' guide to the stem cell universe. Stem Cells 1995; 13:477–486.
11. Keller G. Clonal analysis of hematopietic stem cell development in vivo. Curr Top Microbiol Immunol 1992; 177:41–57.
12. Lemischka IR. What we have learned from retroviral marking of hematopoietic stem cells. Curr Top Microbiol Immunol 1992; 177:59–71.
13. Van Zant G, Micus KS, Thompson BP, Fleischman RA, Perkins S. Stem cell quiescence/activation is reversible by serial transplantation and is independent of stromal cell genotype in mouse aggregation chimeras. Exp Hematol 1992; 20:470–475.
14. Barker JE, McFarland EC. Hemopoietic precursor cell defects in nonanemic but stem cell-deficient W44/W44 mice. J Cell Physiol 1988; 135:533–8.

15. Nakano T, Waki N, Asai H, Kitamura Y. Different repopulation profile between erythroid and nonerythroid progenitor cells in genetically anemic W/Wv mice after bone marrow transplantation. Blood 1998; 1989 74:1552–1556.

16. Ploemacher RE, Van der Sluijs JP, Voerman JSA, Brons NHC. An in vitro limiting-dilution assay of long-term repopulating hematopoietic stem cells in the mouse. Blood 1989; 74:2755–2763.

17. Sutherland HJ, Eaves CJ, Eaves AC, Dragowska W, Lansdorp PM. Characterization and partial purification of human marrow cells capable of initiating long-term hematopoiesis in vitro, Blood 1989; 74:1563–1570.

18. Weilbaecher K, Weissman IL, Blume K, Heimfeld S. Culture of phenotypically defined hematopietic stem cells and other progenitors at limiting dilution on Dexter monolayers. Blood 1991; 78:945–952.

19. Trevisan M, Yan XQ, Iscove NN. Cycle initiation and colony formation in culture by murine marrow cells with long-term reconstituting potential in vivo. Blood 1996; 88:4149–4158.

20. Fraser CC, Szilvassy SJ, Eaves CJ, Humphries RK. Proliferation of totipotent hematopoietic stem cells in vitro with retention of long-term competitive in vivo reconstituting ability. Proc Natl Acad Sci USA 1992; 89:1968–1972.

21. Harrison DE. Evaluating functional abilities of primitive hematopoietic stem cell populations. Curr Tops Microbiol Immunol 1992; 177:13–30.

22. Boggs DR, Saxe DF, Boggs SS. Aging and hematopoiesis II. The ability of bone marrow cells from young and aged mice to cure and maintain cure in W/W. Transplantation 1984; 37:300–306.

23. Müller-Sieburg CE, Townsend K, Weissman IL, Rennick D. Proliferation and differentiation of highly enriched mouse hematopoietic stem cells in response to defined growth factors. J Exp Med 1988; 167:1825–1840.

24. Smith LG, Weissman IL, Heimfeld S. Clonal analysis of hematopoietic stem-cell differentiation in vivo. Proc Natl Acad Sci USA 1991; 88:2788–2792.

25. Lansdorp PM, Dragowska W. Maintenance of hematopoiesis in serum-free bone marrow cultures involves sequential recruitment of quiescent progenitors. Exp Hematol 1993; 21:1321–1327.

26. Harrison DE, Zhong RK, Jordan CT, Lemischka IR, Astle CM. Relative to adult marrow, fetal liver repopulates nearly five times more effectively long-term than short-term. Exp Hematol 1997; 25:293–297.

27. Berger CN, Sturm KS. Estimation of the number of hematopoietic precursor cells during fetal mouse development by covariance analysis. Blood 1996; 88:2502–2509.

28. Lu L, Shen RN, Broxmeyer HE. Stem cells from bone marrow, umbilical cord blood and peripheral blood for clinical application: current status and future application. Cri Rev Oncol Hematol 1996; 22:61–78.

29. Muller AM, Medvinsky A, Strouboulis J, Grosveld F, Dzierzak E. Development of hematopoietic stem cell activity in the mouse embryo. Immunity 1994; 1:291–301.

30. Yoder MC, Hiatt K, Dutt P, Mukherjee P, Bodine DM, Orlic D. Characterization of definitive lymphohematopoietic stem cells in the day 9 murine yolk sac. Immunity 1997; 7:335–344.

31. Yoder MC, Hiatt K. Engraftment of embryonic hematopoietic cells in conditioned newborn recipients. Blood 1997; 89:2176–83.

32. Vaziri H, Dragowska W, Allsopp RC, Thomas TE, Harley CB, Lansdorp PM. Evidence for a mitotic clock in human hematopoietic stem cells: loss of telomeric DNA with age. Proc Natl Acad Sci USA 1994; 91:9857–9860.

33. Lansdorp PM. Telomere length and proliferation potential of hematopoietic stem cells. J Cell Sci 1995; 108:1–6.

34. Chiu CP, Dragowska W, Kim NW, Vaziri H, Yui J, Thomas TE, Harley CB, Lansdorp PM. Differential expression of telomerase activity in hematopoietic progenitors from adult human bone marrow. Stem Cells 1996; 14:239–248.

35. Morrison SJ, Prowse KR, Ho P, Weissman IL. Telomerase activity in hematopoietic cells is associated with self-renewal potential. Immunity 1996; 5:207–216.

36. Kim NW, Piatyszek MA, Prowse KR, Harley CB, West MD, Ho PL, Coviello GM, Wright WE, Weinrich SL, Shay JW. Specific association of human telomerase activity with immortal cells and cancer. Science 1994; 266:2011–2015.

37. Prowse KR, Greider CW. Developmental and tissue-specific regulation of mouse telomerase and telomere length. Proc Natl Acad Sci USA 1995; 92:4818–4822.

38. Shay JW, Wright WE. Telomerase activity in human cancer. Curr Opin Oncol 1996; 8:66–71.

39. Harrison DE, Astle CM, Stone M. Numbers and functions of transplantable primitive immuno-hematopoietic stem cells: effects of age. J Immunol 1989; 142:3833–3840.

40. Morrison SJ, Wandycz AM, Akashi K, Globerson A, Weissman IL. The aging of hematopoietic stem cells. Nature Med 1996; 2:1011–1016.

41. Van Zant G, Eldridge PW, Behringer RR, Dewey MJ. Genetic control of hematopoietic kinetics revealed by analyses of allophenic mice and stem cell suicide. Cell 1983; 35:639–465.

42. Van Zant G, Holland BP, Eldridge PW, Chen JJ. Genotype-restricted growth and aging patterns in hematopoietic stem cell populations of allophenic mice. J Exp Med 1990; 171:1547–1565.

43. Müller-Sieburg CE, Riblet R. Genetic control of the frequency of hematopoietic stem cells in mice: mapping of a candidate locus to chromosome 1. J Exp Med 1996; 183:1141–1150.

44. de Haan G, Nijhof W, Van Zant G. Mouse strain-dependent changes in frequency and proliferation of hematopoietic stem cells during aging: correlation between lifespan and cycling activity. Blood 1997; 89:1543–1550.

45. Green MC, Witham BA. Handbook on Genticall Standardized Jax Mice. 4th ed. Bar Harbor, ME: The Jackson Laboratory, 1991.

45a. Müller-Sieburg CE, Cho RH, Sieburg HB, Kupriyanov S, Riblet R. Genetic control of hematopoietic stem cell frequency in mice is mostly cell autonomous. Blood 2000, in press.

46. Koller MR, Manchel I, Brott DA, Palsson BO. Donor-to-donor variability in the expansion potential of human bone marrow cells is reduced by accessory cells but not by soluble growth factors. Exp Hematol 1996; 24:1484–1493.

47. Georgopoulos K, Bigby M, Wang JH, Molnar A, Wu P, Winandy S, Sharpe A. The Ikaros gene is required for the development of all lymphoid lineages. Cell 1994; 79:143–156.

48. Begley CG, Aplan PD, Davey MP, Nakahara K, Tchorz K, Kurtzberg J, Hershfield MS, Haynes BF, Cohen DI, Waldmann TA, Kirsch IR. Chromosomal translocation in a human leukemic stem cell line disrupts the T-cell antigen receptor d-chain diversity region and results in a previously unreported fusion transcript. Proc Natl Acad Sci USA 1989; 86:2031–2035.

49. Shivdasani RA, Orkin SH. The transcriptional control of hematopoiesis. Blood 1996; 87:4025–4039.

50. Porcher C, Swat W, Rockwell K, Fujiwara Y, Alt FW, Orkin SH. The T cell leukemia onco-protein SCL/tal-1 is essential for development of all hematopoietic lineages. Cell 1996; 86:47–57.

51. Sauvageau G, Thorsteinsdottir U, Eaves CJ, Lawrence HJ, Largman C, Lansdorp PM, Humphries RK. Overexpression of HOXB4 in hematopoietic cells causes the selective expansion of more primitive populations in vitro and in vivo. Genes Dev 1995; 9:1753–1765.

52. Helgason CD, Sauvageau G, Lawrence HJ, Largman C, Humphries RK. Overexpression of HOXB4 enhances the hematopoietic potential of embryonic stem cells differentiated in vitro. Blood 1996; 87:2740–9.

53. Lawrence HJ, Sauvageau G, Humphries RK, Largman C. The role of HOX homeobox genes in normal and leukemic hematopoiesis. Stem Cells 1996; 14:281–291.

54. Wiles MV, Keller G. Multiple hematopietic lineages develop from embryonic stem cells in culture. Development 1991; 111:259–267.

55. Chen U. Differentiation of mouse embryonic stem cells to lympho-hematopoietic lineages in vitro. Dev Immunol 1992; 2:29–50.

56. Nakano T, Kodama H, Honjo T. Generation of lymphohematopoietic cells from embryonic stem cells in culture. Science 1994; 265:1098–1101.

57. Dorshkind K. Regulation of hemopoiesis by bone marrow stromal cells and their products. Ann Rev Immunol 1990; 8:111–137.

58. Eaves CJ, Cashman JD, Sutherland HJ, Otsuka T, Humphries RK, Hogge DE, Lansdorp PM, Eaves AC. Molecular analysis of primitive hematopoietic cell proliferation control mechanisms. Ann NY Acad Sci 1991; 628:298–306.

59. Deryugina EI, Müller-Sieburg CE. Stromal cells in long-term cultures: keys to the elucidation of hematopoietic development? Crit Rev Immunol 1993; 13:115–150.

60. Long MW. Blood cell cytoadhesion molecules. Exp Hematol 1992; 20:288–301.

61. Moore MA, Schneider JG, Shapiro F, Bengala C. Ex vivo expansion of CD34+ hematopoietic progenitors. Prog Clin Biol Res 1994; 389:217–228.

62. Trentin JJ. Determination of bone marrow stem cell differentiation by stromal hemopoietic inductive microenvironments (HIM). Am J Pathol 1971; 65:621–628.

63. Wineman JP, Nishikawa S, Müller-Sieburg CE. Maintenance of high levels of pluripotent hematopoietic stem cells in vitro: effect of stromal cells and c-kit. Blood 1993; 81:365–372.

64. Wineman J, Moore K, Lemischka I, Müller-Sieburg CE. Functional heterogeneity of the hematopoietic microenvironment: rare stromal elements maintain long-term repopulating stem cells. Blood 1996; 87:4082–90.

65. Moore KA, Pytowski B, Witte L, Hicklin D, Lemischka IR. Hematopoietic activity of a stromal cell transmembrane protein containing epidermal growth factor-like repeat motifs. Proc Natl Acad Sci USA 1997; 94:4011–4016.

66. Baum CM, Weissman IL, Tsukamoto A, Buckle SAM, Peault B. Isolation of a candidate human hematopoietic stem-cell population. Proc Natl Acad Sci USA 1992; 89:2804–2808.

67. Issaad C, Croisille L, Katz A, Vainchenker W, Coulombel L. A murine stromal cell line allows the proliferation of very primitive human CD34++/CD38−progenitor cells in long-term cultures and semisolid assays. Blood 1993; 81:2916–2924.

68. Hogge DE, Lansdorp PM, Reid D, Gerhard B, Eaves CJ. Enhanced detection, maintenance, and differentiation of primitive human hematopoietic cells in cultures containing murine fibroblasts engineered to produce human steel factor, interleukin-3, and granulocyte colony-stimulating factor. Blood 1996; 88:3765–3773.

69. Roecklein BA, Torok-Storb B. Functionally distinct human marrow stromal cell lines immortalized by transduction with the human papilloma virus E6/E7 genes. Blood 1995; 85:997–1005.

70. Kodama H, Nose M, Yamaguchi Y, Tsunoda J, Suda T, Nishikawa S, Nishikawa SI. In vitro proliferation of primitive haemopoietic stem cells supported by stromal cells: Evidence for the presence of a mechanism(s) other than that involving c-kit receptor and its ligand. J Exp Med 1992; 176:351–361.

71. Gupta P, McCarthy JB, Verfaillie CM. Stromal fibroblast heparan sulfate is required for cytokine-mediated ex vivo maintenance of human long-term culture-initiating cells. Blood 1996; 87:3229–3236.

72. Verfaillie CM. Direct contact between human primitive hematopoietic progenitors and bone marrow stroma is not required for long-term in vitro hematopoiesis. Blood 1992; 79:2821–2826.

73. Thiemann FT, Moore KA, Smogorzewska EM, Lemischka IR, Crooks. The murine stromal cell line AFT024 acts specifically on human CD34+CD38−progenitors to maintain primitive function and immunophenotype in vitro. Exp Hematol 1998; 26:612–629.

74. Jiang H, Sugimoto K, Sawada H, Takashita E, Tohma M, Gonda H, Mori KJ. Mutual education between hematopoietic cells and bone marrow stromal cells through direct cell-to-cell contact: factors that determine the growth of bone marrow stroma-dependent leukemic (HB-1) cells. Blood 1998; 92:834–841.

75. Verfaillie CM, Miller JS. A novel single-cell proliferation assay shows that long-term culture-initiating cell (LTC-IC) maintenance over time results from the extensive proliferation of a small fraction of LTC-IC. Blood 1995; 86:2137–2145.

8

Cell Signaling by Adhesion Receptors in Normal and Leukemic Hematopoiesis

CATHERINE M. VERFAILLIE, YUEHUA JIANG, and ROBERT C. H. ZHAO

University of Minnesota, Minneapolis, Minnesota

FELIPE PROSPER

Hospital Clinico Universitario, Valencia, Spain

RAVI BHATIA

City of Hope National Medical Center, Duarte, California

I. INTRODUCTION

Hematopoiesis is a complex process in which hematopoietic stem cells can self-replicate but also differentiate into myeloid and lymphoid lineage-committed progenitors. These committed progenitors undergo further multiplications before they terminally differentiate into mature blood elements. The process of myelopoiesis, B lymphopoiesis, T lymphopoiesis, and natural killer cell generation occurs in close proximity with a permissive microenvironment, which in adult life is provided in the bone marrow (Fig 1). The factors responsible and necessary for an orderly hematopoietic process, in which progenitors remain either quiescent or proliferate, differentiate, and mature are not yet understood. The marrow microenvironment is a complex organ in which so-termed stromal cells are responsible for providing most, if not all, factors required for the orderly development of the stem cell. Stromal cells are both mesenchymal and hematopoietic in origin, and they include osteoblasts, fibroblasts, adipocytes, myocytes, endothelial cells, dendritic cells, and macrophages. These cells are responsible for the production and deposition of a complex extracellular matrix (ECM) and the local production and concentration of hematopoietic cytok-

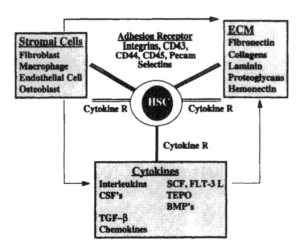

Figure 1   Schematic representation of stem and progenitor cell interactions with the marrow microenvironment. Hemopoietic stem and progenitor cells are localized within the bone marrow microenvironment where they are subject to interactions with growth-promoting and growth-inhibitory cytokines as well as with extracellular matrix components and stromal cell adhesive ligands.

ines. Hematopoietic cells interact through specific cell surface–expressed receptors with either immobilized or secreted growth-promoting/inhibitory cytokines and with adhesive ligands present on stromal cells or ECM components. It is believed that the concerted action of all these interactions results in ordered, normal hematopoiesis.

II.   ROLE OF ADHESIVE INTERACTIONS IN HEMATOPOIESIS

A.   Localization in and Homing to the Marrow Microenvironment

Multiple studies have demonstrated that undifferentiated and lineage-committed progenitors from normal marrow adhere in a lineage-specific and differentiation stage–specific manner to several ECM components, including heparan sulfate (1), thrombospondin (2), and fibronectin (3–5). We and others have demonstrated that primitive progenitors, functionally defined as long-term culture-initiating cells (LTCICs) and more mature colony-forming cells (CFCs) adhere to vascular cell adhesion molecule (V-CAM) and fibronectin present in stroma (3–6) through the $\alpha_4\beta_1$- and $\alpha_5\beta_1$-integrins (see Fig. 1). CD34$^+$ cells also express CD44, which supports adhesion to hyaluronate (7) and fibronectin (6). In addition, progenitors express β_2-integrins (8,9) and selectins (8,9), both of which may allow them to interact with endothelial cells (10). Progenitors express in addition mucins, such as CD34 (11,12), CD43 (13,14), and CD164 (15), the role of which is less clear even though there is mounting evidence that both CD43 and CD164 may play a role in regulation of progenitor survival and growth (13–15).

Several in vivo studies have demonstrated a dominant role for the β_1-integrin family in the homing and retention of stem cells in the marrow microenvironment. Engraftment of murine or baboon stem cells can be inhibited by anti-α_4 antibodies (16,17). Likewise, homing of human stem cells to a xenogeneic ovine marrow microenvironment can be inhibited by antihuman α_4 antibodies (18). Intravenous administration of anti-$\alpha4$ antibodies in baboons or mice results in peripheralization of colony-forming unit granulocyte-macrophage (CFU-GM) and stem cells (19–20). β_1-Defective embryonic stem cells can not successfully compete with wild-type stem cells in competitive engraftment experiments owing to their inability to migrate to the fetal liver (21). All these studies indicate that β_1-dependent interactions are needed to localize stem cells in the marrow and to allow their migration and adhesion to the marrow. In vitro, CFCs and LTCICs adhere to marrow stroma (3,22,23) at least in part through β1-integrins. Further, LTCICs and CFCs adhere to fibronectin and VCAM (4–6) (Fig. 2).

B. Regulation of Progenitor Growth

As has been shown in other biological systems, integrin-mediated interactions between progenitors and fibronectin or other stromal components may directly affect progenitor proliferation and/or differentiation (Fig. 3). In a series of experiments, our laboratory has shown that coculture of normal $CD34^+$ progenitors under physiological cytokine conditions with stromal ECM, more specifically fibronectin, inhibits proliferation of CFCs and LTCICs (22–27). That this is mediated through engagement of β_1-integrins was shown in studies in which the integrins were engaged by adhesion-blocking anti–β_1-integrin antibodies (25,26) (Fig. 3).

Integrins are a family of divalent cation-dependent cell surface glycoproteins responsible for both cell–ECM adhesion and cell–cell adhesion events (Fig. 4). Integrins are heterodimeric as a result of the noncovalent association between an α and β subunit. Integrins have a large, heterodimeric extracellular domain responsible for ligand recognition and binding. Ligand specificity is dictated mostly by the α chain. Integrins have a small membrane-spanning domain and an intracellular domain. The intracellular domain of the β_1 subunit has a dual role in that it initiates signal transduction cascades leading to alterations in cell proliferation and survival following binding of the integrin to its ligand (outside-in) and is responsible for affinity modulation of the integrin in response to signals provided to the cells through, for example, cytokine or other adhesion receptors (inside-out) (28,29).

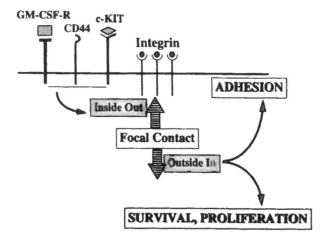

Figure 2   One view of the hemopoietic system is that adhesion receptors such as the $\alpha_4\beta_1$-integrin is not only responsible for localizing hemopoietic progenitors in the bone marrow microenvironment and to allow homing and engraftment of hemopoietic cells in the bone marrow microenvironment, but also to regulate progenitor proliferation.

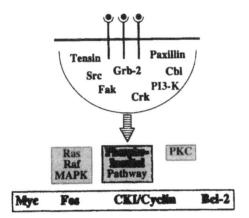

Survival, Differentiation, Proliferation

Figure 3 Engagement of integrins on normal progenitors under physiological conditions inhibits proliferation. $\alpha_4\beta_1$- and $\alpha_5\beta_1$-integrins on normal CD34$^+$ progenitors can form caps in the presence of an intact actin cytoskeleton. These integrins are responsible for the adhesion of progenitors to fibronectin or stromal extracellular matrix. In addition, engagement of integrins results in inhibition of proliferation of CD34$^+$ cells as a result of downregulation of Cdk-2 activity caused by upregulation of p27^{kip}. Which components are present in integrin-dependent focal adhesions in CD34$^+$ cells and which signal pathways are responsible for transferring growth inhibitory signals are unknown.

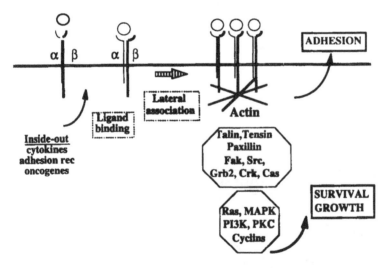

Figure 4 Schematic representation of integrin function: Integrins are transmembrane receptors which connect the extracellular matrix to the actin cytoskeleton within the cell. When present in a high-affinity state, an integrin binds to its extracellular matrix or cell surface–expressed ligand. The affinity state of integrins is modulated by cytokines, other adhesion receptors, and oncogenes. Following binding to the receptor, integrins laterally associate, which requires an intact actin cytoskeleton. Integrins are then localized in focal contacts or focal adhesions. These focal contacts consist of signal and adapter molecules including Fak, Src, Grb-2, Crk, Cas, paxillin, talin, and tensin, which activate a number of signal pathways required for induction of firm adhesion as well as for the regulation of cell survival and growth.

The presence of an adhesion receptor on the cell surface does not necessarily indicate that the receptor has functional significance. Certain integrins are constitutively expressed on the cell surface in an nonfunctional or low-affinity state, but they can be switched to a functional high-affinity state by specific activation signals. Stimulation of cells through other cell surface receptors or through cytokines or activating antibodies may alter the affinity state of integrins enabling more avid binding to the adhesive ligands (28–31).

Integrins colocalize with α-actinin, talin, vinculin, and F-actin in focal contacts (32,33). Members of the Rho family, including Rho and Rac, influence the formation and dynamic stability of actin-based cytoskeletal structures. Talin as well as the β_1-integrin itself bind to the focal adhesion kinase (Fak) (34). Thus, engagement of integrins results in the recruitment of Fak to focal contacts and its autophosphorylation. This creates a binding site for the SH2 domain of c-*Src*, which phosphorylates Fak further, creating binding sites for a number of SH2 containing adaptor proteins, such as paxillin, Crk, Grb-2, and the p85 subunit of phosphatidyl inositol-3 kinase (PI3-kinase). Since Grb2 (35) and Crk (36) can both lead to activation of the Ras/mitogen–activated protein kinase (MAPK) pathway, stimulation through integrins may alter cell proliferation much like stimulation of cytokine receptors. Activation of PI3-kinase not only affects cell proliferation and survival, but also plays a role in cell motility and adhesion (37). Thus, although the exact mechanism(s) through which engagement of integrins affects cell proliferation, differentiation or survival is not known, integrins can activate the Ras/MAPK pathway (38), which leads to the increased expression of c-*myc* and c-*fos* (39), activate PI3-kinase (37), and thus affect cell proliferation and survival, induce immediate-early inflammatory response genes (40), and alter levels of cyclins (41).

How these in vitro observations relate to the assembly of focal contacts that allow adhesion, migration or integrin-dependent signaling that affects proliferation and/or differentiation of hematopoietic cells is still unknown (see Fig. 3). As has been demonstrated for most biological systems, preliminary studies from our laboratory demonstrate that integrin engagement on CD34$^+$ cells results in the phosphorylation of Fak (manuscript in preparation), and that integrin-mediated alterations in progenitor proliferation depend on reorganization of the cytoskeleton (25,26). Further, engagement of integrins on normal hematopoietic progenitors results in elevated levels of the cyclin kinase inhibitor p27^{kip} with associated decreased cyclin-dependent kinase (cdk)-2 activity and decreases in cyclin-E and proliferation cell nuclear antigen (PCNA) protein levels (manuscript in preparation). However, the exact nature of intracellular structural and signal molecules involved in focal contact formation leading to adhesion, migration, and growth inhibition observed in the hematopoietic system after engagement of integrins is still unknown.

C. Conclusion

These studies from our laboratory and that of many others support a model of hematopoiesis in which β_1-integrin adhesion receptors are not only responsible for localizing progenitors in the marrow microenvironment and for homing of progenitors to the marrow microenvironment, but also to regulate (inhibit) progenitor growth under physiological conditions (see Fig. 2). This leads to the following questions: (1) Are there signals that can override the adhesion mediated proliferation inhibition? (2) If β_1-dependent adhesion causes inhibition of progenitor proliferation, then cells that are present under pathological conditions in a nonadherent state (outside of the marrow microenvironment) should be in S-phase.

III. EFFECT OF CYTOKINES ON ADHESION RECEPTOR FUNCTION

A number of recent studies have examined the effect of cytokines on integrin-mediated adhesion of hematopoietic progenitors (Fig. 5). Several groups have shown that high concentrations (nanogram/milliliter) of growth-promoting cytokines such as interleukin (IL)–3, granulocyte-macrophage (GM)–colony-stimulating factor (CSF), and stem cell factor (SCF) increase, at least short term, the adhesive capacity of serum- and cytokine-starved CD34+ cells and colony-forming cells (CFCs) (42,43). IL-3 and SCF did not upregulate adhesion when cells were previously exposed to protein kinase-C (PKC) inhibitors or tyrosine kinase inhibitors, respectively (42). Studies from our group show that pharmacological concentrations (nanogram/milliliter) of cytokines may not affect adhesion of human CD34+ CFCs maintained under physiological conditions (i.e., in the presence of serum and picogram amounts of cytokines) (44,44a). Thus, the effect of cytokines on integrin-mediated adhesion depends on the environment in which this is tested.

Of interest, we have also shown that culture of CD34+ cells on fibronectin or engagement of β_1-integrins on CD34+ cells with adhesion-blocking antibodies in the presence of high concentrations (ng/mL) of certain cytokines, including IL-3, GM-CSF, SCF, and fetal liver tyrosine, kinase-3 (flt3) ligand (FL) does not inhibit CD34+ cell proliferation. Thus, certain cytokines can override the proliferation inhibition resulting from β_1-integrin engagement. Like integrin receptors, cytokine receptors activate the Ras/MAPK pathway, PI3-kinase, and PKC (45). Further, cytokines recruit and/or phosphorylate Fak, paxillin, Grb2, and Crk (35,36,45). Since integrin-mediated signaling depends on the assembly of focal contacts in which most of these signal/adaptor proteins participate, it is possible that phosphorylation/recruitment of one or more focal contact–associated molecules by the cytokine receptor may prevent their participation in the integrin-mediated signaling cascade. Like in other biological systems, the final result of integrin-mediated signals in hematopoiesis also depends on other external signals to which the progenitors are subjected.

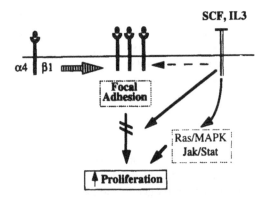

Figure 5 Combined stimulation of progenitor cells with cytokines and adhesive ligands results in alterations in adhesion and proliferation. Depending on external circumstances, growth factor stimulation increases adhesion through integrins or does not affect the adhesive ability of integrins. Likewise, under certain circumstances cytokines will or will not override growth inhibition mediated by integrin receptors.

IV. CHRONIC MYELOGENOUS LEUKEMIA: A DISEASE CHARACTERIZED BY ABNORMAL INTEGRIN-MEDIATED INTERACTIONS

Chronic myelogenous leukemia (CML) is a malignant disease of the pluripotent hematopoietic stem cell characterized by the Philadelphia chromosome (Ph) and a rearrangement between the *Bcr* gene (breakpoint cluster region) and the *Abl* gene. Clinically, CML is characterized by a massive expansion of immature progenitors and precursors which leave the marrow microenvironment prematurely (46). Although normal progenitors coexist with the malignant clone in CML, their growth seems to be inhibited, possibly as a result of abnormalities inherent to the CML marrow microenvironment (47). We and others have demonstrated that, compared to normal progenitors, Ph[+] CML long-term culture-initiating cells (LTCICs) and CFC adhere significantly less to stroma or fibronectin (26,31,48–50). Furthermore, Ph[+] CFCs and LTCICs are not subject to normal growth-inhibitory signals when present in contact with stroma, fibronectin, or following integrin engagement with anti-integrin antibodies (26,31). However, Ph[+] progenitors express normal numbers of $\alpha_4\beta_1$ and $\alpha_5\beta_1$ (48,49) adhesion receptors, suggesting that these receptors may either be structurally or functionally abnormal. Treatment of CML CD34[+] cells with interferon-α (IFN-α) restores adhesion and also adhesion-mediated proliferation inhibition (26,49,50). If this in vitro effect of IFN-α contributes to the hematological response seen in >80% of patients treated in vivo with IFN-α still needs to be determined (51). We have also shown that antisense oligodeoxy-nucleotides against the *Bcr/Abl* oncoprotein restore adhesion and growth-inhibitory signaling through β_1-integrins on CML CD34[+] cells (52). This suggests that presence of *Bcr/Abl* is responsible for the defective integrin function in CML which may contribute to the massive uncontrolled expansion of the Ph[+] clone seen in CML (Fig. 6).

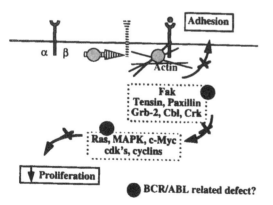

Figure 6   In CML, integrins present on hemopoietic cells are functionally and/or structurally defective. Adhesion through integrins does not occur and engagement of integrins does not transfer growth-inhibitory signals to CML progenitors. Although the mechanism through which the *Bcr/ Abl* oncoprotein causes these defects is not completely understood, it is clear that *Bcr/Abl* can bind to the actin cytoskeleton, recruit, and activate a number of signal and adapter proteins, including Fak, tensin, paxillin, Grb₂, Cbl, and Crkl, and can directly activate the Ras/MAPK pathway and affect Cdks and cyclins.

Why integrins are present in a low-affinity state on the majority of CML but not NL progenitors is currently unknown. The *Bcr/Abl* mRNA encodes for the $P210_{Bcr/Abl}$ tyrosine kinase which is located in the cytoplasm rather than the nucleus where $p145_{Abl}$ can be found (53). Although the exact mechanism underlying the clinical phenotype of CML is not completely understood, the presence of the $P210_{Bcr/Abl}$ oncoprotein is necessary and sufficient for malignant transformation of stem cells (54,56). $P210_{Bcr/Abl}$ has, in comparison with $p145_{Abl}$, increased tyrosine kinase activity resulting in autophosphorylation of the oncoprotein (57). This allows recruitment of the adaptor protein, Grb2, to the phosphorylated Y177 (58), which then leads to complex formation with son of sevenless (Sos) and activation of Ras. Activation of the Ras pathway may also be due to $P210_{Bcr/Abl}$–dependent phosphorylation of additional adaptor proteins such as Crkl and Cbl (58,59). This results in growth factor independence and malignant transformation. Aside from activating the Ras pathway, $P210_{Bcr/Abl}$ phosphorylates and activates a number of other intracellular proteins, including Fak (62), paxillin (61), Crkl (58), signal transducer and activator of transcription (Stat)-1 and Stat-5 (62), Cbl (58,59), and PI3-kinase (63). Finally, $P210_{Bcr/Abl}$ binds significantly more to F-actin (64); an observation that has been associated with transformation. Since integrin-mediated signaling requires recruitment and activation of, for example, Fak and paxillin (27–29), one might speculate that chronic phosphorylation of either of these molecules may result in their inability to participate in the integrin-mediated signaling cascade. In addition, since integrin stimulation may affect cell proliferation through activation of the Ras/MAPK pathway (38), and alternatively, since activation of Ras/MAPK may alter the type of focal contact assembled after engagement of integrins (65), it is possible that activation of Ras by $P210^{Bcr/Abl}$ may affect both integrin-mediated adhesion and signaling in CML. In addition, binding of *Bcr/Abl* to F-actin may interfere with the lateral association of integrins in the cell membrane and thus prevent integrins to localize to focal adhesions where they both transfer outside-in and accept inside-out signals.

Thus, in CML, integrin function is defective resulting in the inability of *Bcr/Abl*–containing CD34$^+$ cells, CFCs, and LTCICs to adhere to the marrow microenvironment and fibronectin. This is associated with increased proliferation of CML progenitors compared with that of normal CD34$^+$ cells. Thus, the CML model confirms our working hypothesis that integrins play not only a role in the localization of CD34$^+$ progenitors in the marrow, but also in regulating the proliferation of progenitors.

V. CONCLUSION

Our view of the hematopoietic process is that adhesion receptors, such as β_1-integrins, are important not only to localize progenitors and stem cells in the marrow microenvironment, but that these receptors also serve to regulate progenitor growth. Signals through adhesion receptors are integrated with other signals provided, for instance, by cytokine-receptor interactions, to initiate or inhibit cell proliferation. Although not covered in this chapter, there is also evidence that adhesion receptors may help protect progenitor and stem cells from apoptotic cell death.

Additional studies will be needed to identify structural and signal molecules associated with β_1-integrins in membrane-associated focal contact complexes that induce adhesion or migration and that transfer growth regulatory signals in normal hematopoietic progenitors. Such studies will provide significant new insights into mechanisms involved not only in survival, proliferation, and differentiation of normal progenitors, but also in mobilization and engraftment of normal hematopoietic progenitors. Such studies will also lead to a better understanding of abnormal hematopoietic processes characterized by increased or decreased circulation and expansion of progenitors which may ultimately provide us with novel therapies for such disorders.

REFERENCES

1. Bruno E, Luikart SD, Long MW, Hoffman R. Marrow-derived heparan sulfate proteoglycan mediates the adhesion of hematopoietic progenitor cells to cytokines. Exp Hematol 1995; 23: 1212–1217.
2. Long MW, Dixit VM. Thrombospondin functions as a cytoadhesion molecule for human hematopoietic progenitor cells. Blood 1990; 75:2311–2318.
3. Teixidó J, Hemler ME, Greenberger JS, Anklesaria P. Role of β1 and β2 integrins in the adhesion of human CD34^{hi} stem cells to bone marrow stroma. J Clin Invest 1992; 90:358–367.
4. Verfaillie CM, McCarthy JB, McGlave PB. Differentiation of primitive human multipotent hematopoietic progenitors into single lineage clonogenic progenitors is accompanied by alterations in their interaction with fibronectin. J Exp Med 1991; 174:693–703.
5. Verfaillie CM, Benis A, Iida G, McGlave PB, McCarthy J. Adhesion of committed human hematopoietic progenitors to synthetic peptides in the C-terminal heparin-binding domain of fibronectin: cooperation between the integrin α4β1 and the CD44 adhesion receptor. Blood 1994; 84:1802–1812.
6. Simmons PJ, Masinovsky B, Longenecker BM, Berenson R, Torok-Storb B, Gallatin WM. Vascular cell adhesion molecule-1 expressed by bone marrow stromal cells mediates the binding of hematopoietic progenitor cells. Blood 1992; 80:388–395.
7. Ghaffari S, Dougherty GJ, Landsdorp PM, Eaves AC, Eaves JC. Differentiation associated changes in CD44 isoform expression during normal hematopoiesis and their alteration in chronic myeloid leukemia. Blood 1995; 86:2976.
8. Mohle R, Murea S, Kirsch M, Haas R: Differential expression of L-selectin, VLA-4, and LFA-1 on CD34+ progenitor cells from bone marrow and peripheral blood during G-CSF-enhanced recovery. Exp Hematol 1995; 23:1535.
9. Dercksen MW, Gerritsen WR, Rodenhuis S, Dirkson MKA, Slaper-Cortenbach ICM, Schaasberg WP, Pinedo HM, von dem Borne AEG, van der Schoot CE. Expression of adhesion molecules on CD34+ cells: CD34+ L-selectin+ cells predict a rapid platelet recovery after peripheral blood stem cell transplantation. Blood 1995; 85:3313.
10. Kansas GS. Selectins and their ligands: current concepts and controversies. Blood 1996; 88: 3259.
11. Healy L, May G, Gale K, Grosveld F, Greaves M, Enver T. The stem cell antigen CD34 functions as a regulator of hemopoietic cell adhesion. Proc Natl Acad Sci USA 1995; 92: 12240.
12. Cheng J, Baumhueter S, Cacalano G, et al. Hematopoietic defects in mice lacking the sialomucin CD34. Blood 1996; 87:479.
13. Bazil V, Brandt J, Tsukamoto A, Hoffman R. Apoptosis of human hematopoietic progenitor cells induced by crosslinking of surface CD43, the major sialoglycoprotein of leukocytes. Blood 1995; 86:502.
14. Bazil V, Brandt J, Chen S, et al. A monoclonal antibody recognizing CD43 (leukosialin) initiates apoptosis of human hematopoietic progenitor cells but not stem cells. Blood 1996; 87: 1272.

15. Watt SM, Buhring HJ, Chan JHY, et al. The sialomucin CD164, a negative regulator of hema-
    poiesis is expressed by CD34+ and erythroid subsets and is located on chromosome 6q21.
    Exp Hematol 1997; 25:52a.

16. Williams DA, Rios M, Stephens C, Patel VP. Fibronectin and VLA-4 in hematopoietic stem
    cell–microenvironment interactions. Nature 1991; 352:438–441.

17. Papayannopoulou T, Craddock C, Nakamoto B, Priestley GV, Wolf SN. The VLA4/VCAM
    adhesion pathway defines contrasting mechanisms of lodging of transplanted murine hemato-
    poietic progenitors between bone marrow and spleen. Proc Natl Acad Sci USA 1995; 92:
    9647–9651.

18. Zanjani E, Papayanopoulou T. Human CD34+ cells transplanted in utero in sheep fetuses
    treated with anti-human VLA₄ remain "homeless" and persist in circulation. Blood 1994;
    84(suppl 1):1962a.

19. Papayannopoulou T, Nakamato B. Systemic treatment of primates with anti-VLA4 leads to
    an immediate egress of hemopoietic progenitors to periphery. Proc Natl Acad Sci USA 1993;
    90:9374–9378.

20. Craddock CF, Nakamoto B, Andrews RG, Priestley GV, Papayannopoulou T. Antibodies to
    VLA4 integrin mobilize long-term repopulating cells and augment cytokine-induced mobiliza-
    tion in primates and mice. Blood 1997; 90:4779–4788.

21. Hirsch E, Iglesias A, Potocnik AJ, Hartmann U, Fässler R. Impaired migration but not differen-
    tiation of hematopoietic stem cells in the absence of β1 integrins. Nature 1996; 380:171–175.

22. Hurley RW, McCarthy JB, Verfaillie CM. Direct adhesion to bone marrow stroma via fibro-
    nectin receptors inhibits hematopoietic progenitor proliferation. J Clin Invest 1995; 96:511–
    519.

23. Verfaillie C, Blakolmer K, McGlave P. Purified primitive hematopoietic progenitor cells with
    long-term in vitro repopulating capacity adhere selectively to irradiated bone marrow stroma.
    J Exp Med 1990; 172:509–520.

24. Verfaillie CM, Catanzarro P. Development of a novel single LTC-IC proliferation assay that
    can determine the fate of LTC-IC over time. Leukemia 1996; 10:498–504.

25. Hurley R, McCarthy JB, Verfaillie CM. Clustering of integrins results in proliferation inhibi-
    tion of committed hematopoietic progenitors through mechanisms involving the cell cytoskele-
    ton. Exp Hematol 1997;

26. Bhatia R, McCarthy JB, Verfaillie CM. Interferon-α restores normal β1-integrin mediated
    negative regulation of chronic myelogenous leukemia progenitor proliferation. Blood 1996;
    87:3883–3891.

27. Verfaillie CM. Direct contact between progenitors and stroma is not required for human in
    vitro hematopoiesis. Blood 1992; 79:2821–2826.

28. EA Clark, Brugge JS. Integrins and signal transduction pathways: the road taken. Science
    1995; 268:233–239.

29. Schwartz MA, Schaller MD, Ginsberg MH: Biol Integrins: emerging paradigms of signal trans-
    duction. Annu Rev Cell Dev 1995; 11:549–599.

30. Kovach NL, Carlos TM, Yee E, Harlan JM. A monoclonal antibody to β₁ integrin [CD29]
    stimulates VLA-dependent adherence of leukocytes to human umbilical vein endothelial cells
    and matrix components. J Cell Biol 1992; 116:499–509.

31. Lundell BI, McCarthy JB, Kovach NL, Verfaillie CM. Adhesion to fibronectin (FN) induced
    by the activating anti-integrin-β1 antibody, 8a2, restores adhesion mediated inhibition of CML
    progenitor proliferation. Blood 1996; 87:2450–2458.

32. Zigmond SH: Signal transduction and actin filament organization. Curr Opin Cell Biol 1996;
    8:66–73.

33. Craig SW, Johnson RP. Assembly of focal adhesions: progress, paradigms, and portents. Curr
    Opin Cell Biol 1996; 8:74–85.

34. Schaller MD, Parsons JT. Focal adhesion kinase and associated proteins. Curr Opin Cell Biol
    1994; 6:705–710.

35. Saxton TM, van Oostveen I, Bowtell D, Aebersold R, Gold MR. B cell antigen receptor cross-linking induces phosphorylation of the p21ras oncoprotein activators SHC and mSOS1 as well as assembly of complexes containing SHC, GRB-2, mSOS1, and a 145-kDa tyrosine-phosphorylated protein. J Immunol 1994; 153:623–636.

36. Teng KK, Lander H, Fajardo JE, Hanafusa H, Hempstead BL, Birge RB. v-Crk modulation of growth factor-induced PC12 cell differentiation involves the Src homology 2 domain of v-Crk and sustained activation of the Ras/mitogen-activated protein kinase pathway. J Biol Chem 1995; 270:20677–20685.

37. Carpenter CL, Cantley LC: Phosphoinositide kinases. Curr Opin Cell Biol 1996; 8:153–158.

38. Schlaepfer DD, Hanks SK, Hunter T, van der Geer P. Integrin-mediated signal transduction linked to Ras pathway by GRB2 binding to focal adhesion kinase. Nature 1994; 372:786–789.

39. Shaw RJ, Doherty DE, Ritter AG, Benedict SH, Clark RAF. Adherence dependent increase in human monocyte PDGF(B) mRNA is associated with increases in c-fos, c-jun and EGR2 mRNA. J Cell Biol 1990; 111:2139.

40. Yurochko AD, Liu DY, Eierman D, Haskill S. Integrins as a primary signal transduction molecule regulating monocyte immediate-early gene induction. Proc Natl Acad Sci USA 1992; 89: 9034–9038.

41. Zhu X, Ohtsubo M, Böhmer RM, Roberts JM, Assosian RK. Adhesion-dependent cell cycle progression linked to the expression of cyclin D1, activation of cyclin E-cdk2, and phosphorylation of the retinoblastoma protein. J Cell Biol 1996; 133:391–403.

42. Levesque JP, Leavesley DI, Niutta S, Vadas M, Simmons PJ. Cytokines increase human hemopoietic cell adhesiveness by activation of very late antigen (VLA)-4 and VLA-5 integrins. J Exp Med 1995; 181:1805–15.

43. Kovach NL, Lin N, Yednock T, Harlan JM, Broudy VC. Stem cell factor modulates avidity of alpha 4 beta 1 and alpha 5 beta 1 integrins expressed on hematopoietic cell lines. Blood 1995; 85:159–67.

44. Hurley R, Verfaillie CM. Cytokine/integrin mediated regulation of progenitor growth. Blood 1995; 86:2874a.

44a. Jiang Y, Prosper F, Verfaillie CM. Opposing effects of engagement of integrins and stimulation of cytokine receptors on cell cycle progression of normal human hematopoietic progenitors. Blood 2000; 95:846–854.

45. Ihle JN, Witthuhn BA, Quelle FW, Yamamoto K, Silvennoinen O. Signaling through the hematopoietic cytokine receptors. Annu Rev Immunol 1995; 13:369–398.

46. Kantarjian HM, Giles FJ, O'Brien SM, Talpaz M. Clinical course and therapy of chronic myelogenous leukemia with interferon-alpha and chemotherapy. Hematol Oncol Clin North Am 1998; 12:31–80.

47. Bhatia R, McGlave PB, Dewald GW, Blazar BR, Verfaillie CM. Abnormal function of the bone marrow microenvironment in chronic myelogenous leukemia: role of malignant stromal macrophages. Blood 1995; 85:3636–3645.

48. Verfaillie CM, McCarthy JB, McGlave PB. Mechanisms underlying abnormal trafficking of malignant progenitors in chronic myelogenous leukemia. Decreased adhesion to stroma and fibronectin but increased adhesion to the basement membrane components laminin and collagen type IV. J Clin Invest 1992; 90:1232–1241.

49. Bhatia R, Wayner E, McGlave P, Verfaillie CM. Interferon-α restores adhesion of malignant progenitors in CML by restoring β1 integrin function. J Clin Invest 1994; 94:384–391.

50. Bhatia R, McGlave PB, Verfaillie CM. Interferon-α treatment of normal bone marrow stroma results in enhanced adhesion of CML hematopoietic progenitors via mechanisms involving MIP-1α. J Clin Invest 1995; 96:931–939.

51. Inteferon alfa versus chemotherapy for chronic myeloid leukemia: a meta-analysis of seven randomized trials: Chronic Myeloid Leukemia Trialists' Collaborative Group. J Natl Cancer Inst 1997; 89:1616–1620.

52. Bhatia R, Verfaillie CM. Inhibition of BCR-ABL expression with antisense oligodeoxynucleo-tides restores beta1 integrin-mediated adhesion and proliferation inhibition in chronic myelo-genous leukemia hematopoietic progenitors. Blood 1998; 91:3414–3422.

53. Dhut S, Champlin T, Young BD. BCR-ABL and BCR proteins: biochemical characterization and localization. Leukemia 1990; 4:745–750.

54. Daley GQ, Van Etten RA, Baltimore D. Induction of chronic myelogenous leukemia in mice by the P210$^{bcr/abl}$ gene of the Philadelphia chromosome. Science 1990; 247:824–829.

55. Gishizky ML, Witte ON. Initiation of dysregulated growth of multipotent progenitor cells by bcr-abl in vitro. Science 1992; 256:836–839.

56. Honda H, Oda H, Suzuki T, Takahashi T, Witte ON, Ozawa K, Ishikawa T, Yazaki Y, Hi-rai H. Development of acute lymphoblastic leukemia and myeloproliferative disorder in transgenic mice expressing p210bcr/abl: a novel transgenic model for human Ph1-positive leukemias. Blood 1998; 91:2067–2075.

57. Pendergast AM, Quilliam LA, Cripe LD, Bassing CH, Dai Z, Li N, Batzer A, Rabun KM, Der CJ, Schlessinger J. BCR-ABL-Induced oncogenesis is mediated by direct interaction with the SH2 domain of the GRB-2 adaptor protein. Cell 1993; 75:175–185.

58. Oda T, Heaney C, Hagopian JR, Okuda K, Griffin JD, Druker BJ. Crkl is the major tyrosine-phosphorylated protein in neutrophils from patients with chronic myelogenous leukemia. J Biol Chem 1994; 269:22925–22928.

59. Salgia R, Brunkhorst B, Pisick E, Li JL, Lo SH, Chen LB, Griffin JD: Increased tyrosine phosphorylation of focal adhesion proteins in myeloid cell lines expressing p210BCR/ABL. Oncogene 1995; 11:1149–1155.

60. Gotoh A, Miyazawa K, Ohyashiki K, Tauchi T, Boswell HS, Broxmeyer HE, Toyama K. Tyrosine phosphorylation and activation of focal adhesion kinase (p125FAK) by BCR-ABL oncoprotein. Exp Hematol 1995;

61. Salgia R, Li JL, Lo SH, Brunkhorst B, Kansas GS. Sobhany ES, Sun Y, Pisick E, Hallek M, Ernst T. Molecular cloning of human paxillin, a focal adhesion protein phosphorylated by P210BCR/ABL. J Biol Chem 1995; 270:5039–5047.

62. Ilaria RL Jr, Van Etten RA. Constitutive activation of stat family members in BA/F3 cells transformed by P210 BCR/ABL. Blood 1995; 86(suppl):264a.

63. Skorski T, Kanakaraj P, Nieborowska-Skorska M, Ratajczak MZ, Wen SC, Zon G, Gewirtz AM, Perussia B, Calabretta B. Phosphatidylinositol-3 kinase activity is regulated by BCR/ABL and is required for the growth of Philadelphia chromosome-positive cells. Blood 1995; 86:726–736.

64. McWhirter JR, Wang JY. An actin-binding function contributes to transformation by the bcr/abl oncoprotein in Philadelphia chromosome positive human leukemias. EMBO J 1993; 12:1533–46.

65. Zhang Z, Vuori K, Wang H-G, Reed JC, Ruoslahti E: Integrin activation by R-ras. Cell 1996; 85:61–69.

9

Detection of Infrequent Cells in Blood and Bone Marrow by Flow Cytometry

LEON W. M. M. TERSTAPPEN

Immunicon Corporation, Huntingdon Valley, Pennsylvania

I. INTRODUCTION

Peripheral blood and bone marrow are composed of heterogeneous cell mixtures. Traditionally, the composition of blood cells has been performed by microscopic examination of cytochemically stained cell smears. This technique, however, is subjective and nucleated cells which appear at a frequency below 5% may be overlooked. The introduction of flow cytometry to discriminate between cell populations has significantly improved the ability to identify accurately and enumerate cell populations which cannot be distinguished by morphological features (1). A further improvement of the sensitivity of flow cytometric examination of heterogeneous cell mixtures has been obtained by multidimensional analysis of the data (2). Cell populations are identified by the simultaneous assessment of light-scattering and fluorescence parameters. Light-scattering parameters measure cell size and cell granularity. Fluorescence parameters can be used to assess cell surface antigens, intracellular antigens, deoxyribonucleic acid (DNA), ribonucleic acid (RNA), and protein content. By choosing an unique set of lineage-specific and or lineage-associated monoclonal antibodies, this technique has enabled the assignment of clusters of cells in bone marrow to a specific lineage and a maturational stage (3–6). Although cells can be identified in frequencies as low as $1/10^5$ to $1/10^6$, the practical detection limit of multidimensional flow cytometry to identify cells is $1/10^4$ (7,8). The ability reliably to detect infrequent cell populations such as hematopoietic progenitor cells, hematopoietic stem cells, and micrometastases in peripheral blood is becoming increasingly significant in the management of patients with cancer (9–14). In this chapter, various approaches are described which enable the enumeration of infrequent cell types by flow cytometry.

II. FLOW CYTOMETRIC ANALYSIS OF WHOLE BLOOD AND BONE MARROW

Examination of the different nucleated cell types by flow cytometry has been facilitated by procedures which eliminate the erythrocytes present in more then 1000-fold excess over leukocytes. The identification of leukocytes in the presence of erythrocytes by flow cytometry is already infrequent cell detection (frequency 0.1%). Erythrocyte-lysing procedures and density separations are therefore commonly used to study leukocytes in blood and bone marrow, and frequencies of cell populations are traditionally given as a percentage of leukocytes. The sample preparation procedures, however, introduce various artifacts in that some cell populations are more likely to be damaged then others. For instance, nucleated erythrocytes are more susceptible to the lysing agents then lymphocytes, and lysing procedures are therefore not suitable when the objective is to obtain an accurate distribution of the cells within the erythroid lineage.

Multidimensional flow cytometric analysis can be used to identify the major cell populations in whole blood or bone marrow. By simultaneous analysis of light-scatter and fluorescence parameters of individual cells passing through the laser beam, a multidimensional space is created in which the cells with dissimilar properties emerge in different locations. These static flow cytometric images of hematopoiesis are then used to reconstruct in vivo maturational pathways by detection of gradual changes in the expression of lineage-specific or lineage-associated cell surface antigens. An example is illustrated in Figure 1.

Figure 1 shows the flow cytometric analysis of a normal peripheral blood and adult bone marrow sample. The samples were stained with nucleic acid dyes (Thiazole Orange and SYIII8) and the monoclonal antibodies CD71 conjugated to phycoerthrin (PE), and CD45 conjugated with a phycoerythrin CY5 tandem (15). Before introduction of the samples in the flow cytometer, the samples were diluted 10-fold with phosphate-buffered saline (PBS) with a known amount of fluorescent beads which permit the determination of the sample volume analyzed (7,16). Without the dilution the cell concentration is too high, which results in multiple cell appearing in the measurement orifice, thereby preventing the discrimination of the cells from each other.

Panels A and B in Figure 1 show the position of 10,000 cells in the correlative display of the nucleic acid dyes and the transferrin receptor of blood and blood marrow, respectively. Erythrocytes (Ery) are depicted as small gray dots and do not stain. Mature reticulocytes (MRet) are depicted as small light gray dots and stain dimly with the nucleic acid dyes (RNA) but not with CD71. Immature reticulocytes (ImRet) stain with both the nucleic acid dye and CD71 and are depicted as black square dots in panels A and B and as small black dots in panels C,D,E and F and. Nucleated erythrocytes (Nuc Ery) are depicted as gray square dots and are only observed in the bone marrow sample and stain brightly with the nucleic acid dyes (RNA+DNA) and CD71 but lack CD45 (panel F). Leukocytes (Leuk) are depicted as small gray squares in panels A and B and stain brightly with the nucleic acid dyes (RNA+DNA), express CD45, and the majority lack CD71. Platelets (Plat) are depicted as small dark gray dots in Panels A and B, do not stain, and are discriminated from the erythrocytes by lower signals in forward and orthogonal light-scatter signals (not shown). As illustrated in panels A and B, these cell populations can be clearly distinguished from each other despite the large difference in frequency. Comparison between blood and bone marrow shows a larger frequency of the leukocytes in bone marrow as well as the presence of the nucleated erythrocytes. Within the erythrocyte

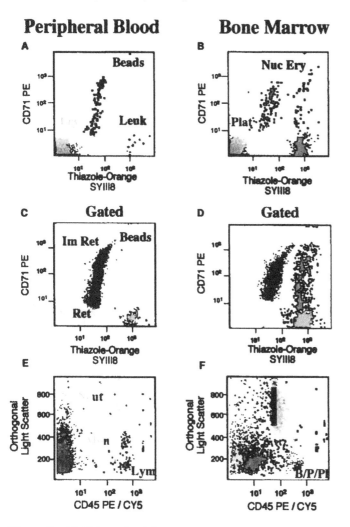

Figure 1 Multidimensional flow cytometric analysis of a whole peripheral blood (panels A, C, and E) and whole bone marrow sample (panels B, D, and F). Samples were stained with CD71 phycoerythrin (PE), CD45 PE/Cy5, and nucleic acid dye. Before analysis samples were diluted with phosphate-buffered saline (PBS) and a known number of fluorescent beads were added. Erythrocytes (Ery) are depicted as small gray dots in panels A and B, mature reticulocytes (Mret) are depicted as small light gray dots, immature reticulocytes (Im Ret) are depicted as black squares, nucleated erytrocytes (Nuc Ery) are depicted as gray squares, platelets (Plat) in panels A and B are depicted as small dark gray dots, leukocytes in panels A and B are depicted as gray crosses, and beads, depicted black, are present at the top of both panels. In panels C, D, E and F, neutrophils (Neut) are small gray dots, monocytes (Mono) are light gray crosses, lymphocytes (Lym) are depicted as dark gray crosses, and the cluster of cells depicted as light gray squares contain basophils, progenitor cells, and plasma cells.

lineage, different maturational stages can be observed. The earliest identifiable erythroid-committed cells in this analysis are the square gray depicted dots with the lowest CD71 density. Increasing densities of CD71 indicate further maturation of the cells. The loss of the nucleus can be observed by the gap between the bright CD71$^+$ square gray and bright CD71$^+$ black dots. Gradual loss of CD71 of the black-colored reticulocytes illustrates further maturation. This gradual loss is followed by the complete loss of CD71 for the mature reticulocytes and the loss of RNA for the erythrocytes thereafter. A maturational pathway can thus be identified and objective criteria can be made to designate different maturational stages.

Differentiation between the leukocytes can be obtained with the same sample, however, the sample acquisition time has to be extended and a threshold or gate has to be used to eliminate erythrocytes from the analysis. Panels C and D show the same measurement as panels A and B, only now the erythrocytes are not included in the measurement. In Panels E and F the correlative display of the human leukocyte antigen (CD45) and orthogonal light scatter of the blood and bone marrow is shown. Based on differential expression of CD45 and light-scatter characteristics, the leukocytes are differentiated into neutrophils (Neut) depicted as small gray dots, lymphocytes (Lym) depicted as dark gray crosses, and monocytes (Mono) depicted as gray crosses. Leukocytes expressing CD71 (associated with proliferative stages) can be discriminated from the CD71 expressing nucleated erythrocytes by the expression of CD45. The cells depicted as square gray dots contain basophils, plasma cells, and progenitor cells (B/P/PI) (panel F) (7,17–19). In normal peripheral blood, basophils are more frequent as compared to plasma cells or progenitor cells (CD34$^+$ cells), and the square gray dots are predominantly basophils, whereas the progenitor cells are the dominant population in normal bone marrow. Careful analysis of light-scatter parameters shows a slightly larger orthogonal light scatter of basophils as compared with progenitor cells and a slightly larger forward light scatter of plasma cells (17–19). The positions of these cell populations in the multidimensional space created by these parameters are too close to accurately distinguish these cell populations when not present in the same range of frequencies. Mobilization of progenitor cells by growth factors or chemotherapy results in a relative increase in progenitor cells. A reliable discrimination of the progenitor cells from the basophils becomes difficult if not impossible without the introduction of other parameters such as CD34 expression. It is thus important to choose a combination of parameters which places the cell population to be enumerated in a unique position. Replacement of the CD71PE by CD34PE provides such a combination when CD34$^+$ cells are the target cell population (7). The combination of parameters shown in Figure 1 is more suitable for enumeration of nucleated erythrocytes, and through acquisition of a larger number of nucleated cells one is able to identify nucleated erythrocytes in peripheral blood (19,20). Identification of these cells can be rightfully designated as rare event detection.

III. CONSIDERATIONS FOR ENUMERATION OF INFREQUENT CELL TYPES

Figure 2 shows the different cell types in peripheral blood as they are present per volume unit as well as their frequency as a function of the number of leukocytes. Although it is possible to detect and enumerate cell types by flow cytometry which are present in frequencies as low as 1 in 10^7, the time needed to perform such an analysis becomes practically unacceptable when no preenrichment procedures are used (8).

Figure 3 shows the acquisition time needed when a sample flow rate of 1 μL/s is used to process different blood volumes. For example, if CD34$^+$ cells are present in a

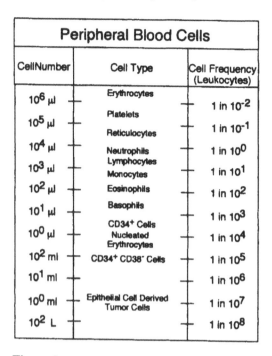

Figure 2   The presence of different cell types in peripheral blood.

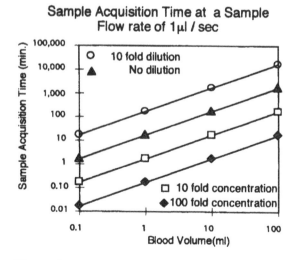

Figure 3   The time needed to acquire samples on a flow cytometer with a flow rate of 1 μL/s as a function of blood volume. Time is indicated for a 10-fold dilution, no blood dilution, 10-fold concentration, and 100-fold concentration.

frequency of 1/µL of blood, 100 µL of blood has to be analyzed to obtain 100 CD34$^+$ cells, and at best, a coefficient of variation of $1/\sqrt{100} \times 100 = 10\%$ can be obtained. The 10-fold dilution of the blood sample necessary to either lyse the erythrocytes in the sample or reduce the cell concentration (erythrocytes) before analysis results in a sample acquisition time of 16.7 mins. The need for standardized and accurate procedures for progenitor cell enumeration (CD34$^+$ cells) in peripheral blood, leukapheresis products, and bone marrow of patients has become increasingly important for the assessment of the quality of the grafts used for transplantation. A variety of procedures have been described to mobilize progenitor cells into the peripheral blood (21–23). Increases in relative and absolute numbers of CD34$^+$ cells can be measured reliably although active discussions are still taking place on which procedures are acceptable (24). As described above, the analysis of 100 µL of blood is sufficient to obtain a reasonable CD34$^+$ count, and the increase in CD34$^+$ cells in patient samples increases the precision of these counts. However, for measurements of subsets of CD34$^+$ cells, this blood volume is not sufficient and analysis of at least 1 mL of blood is needed. To determine subsets within the CD34$^+$ cell population, larger blood volumes will have to be processed and acquisition times increase proportionally (Fig. 3). For research purposes, erythrocyte lysing-procedures and density separations are most often used to concentrate the cells; however, a drawback is that the results are no longer quantitative.

IV. ANALYZING SUBSETS WITHIN THE CD34$^+$, CD38 CELL POPULATION

Identification of the pluripotent progenitor cells within the CD34$^+$ cell fraction has been established on samples with larger numbers of CD34$^+$ cells, such as bone marrow. In fetal bone marrow, there is an abundance of CD34$^+$ cells, as is illustrated in Figure 4A, which shows the correlated expression of CD34 and CD38 on an erythrocyte-lysed fetal bone marrow sample. The black depicted CD34$^+$ cells comprise 19.9% of the fetal bone marrow cells, which greatly facilitates the analysis of differentiation stages within the CD34$^+$ cell population. Figure 4B shows the correlated expression of CD38 and human leukocyte antigen (HLA) DR of only CD34$^+$ cells. The CD38^{2+} cells depicted as small black and gray dots are all lineage committed, whereas the CD38$^{-/dim}$ larger square dots contain the more primitive hematopoietic cells (5,25–29). Increase of the CD38 antigen density is correlated with differentiation of the progenitor cells (5). The cells with no CD38 expression are more primitive than the cells that dimly express CD38; the fluorochrome used for the assessment of CD38 is therefore of importance. The use of fluorescein isothiocyanate (FITC) conjugates instead of phycoerthrin conjugates of the CD38 antibody would have resulted in the inability to distinguish the cells depicted as black squares from the cells depicted as dark gray squares, and thus a less precise definition of the differentiation stage of the progenitor cells. Cell culture of single sorted CD34$^+$, CD38$^-$, HLA-DR$^-$ and CD34$^+$, CD38$^-$, HLA-DR$^+$ cells have shown that the majority of hematopoietic progenitors are confined within the black square CD34$^+$, CD38$^-$, HLA-DR$^+$ cells, whereas cells within the light gray squares CD34$^+$, CD38$^-$, HLA-DR$^-$ cell population expanded in a variety of stromal cell lineages and only few cells within this cell population had the ability to expand in the hematopoietic cell lineages (26,30).

To examine whether the heterogeneity within the CD34$^+$, CD38$^-$, HLA-DR$^-$ cell population could be traced back to differences in cell surface antigen expression, four color experiments were performed in which bone marrow cells were stained with CD34, CD38, HLA-DR and a fourth cell surface antigen. Light-scatter parameters, CD34, CD38

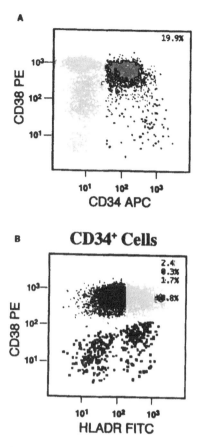

Figure 4 Flow cytometric analysis of an erythrocyte-lysed fetal bone marrow sample stained with CD34 allophycocyanine (APC), CD38 PE, and HLA-DR fluorescein isothiocyanate (FITC). Panel A shows the correlative display of CD34 APC and CD38 PE of the sample. The CD34$^+$ cells are depicted in black and all other cells are depicted in gray. Panel B shows the correlative display of CD38PE and HLA-DR FITC. The CD38^{2+}, HLA-DR$^{-\rightarrow+}$ cells are depicted as small black dots, the CD38^{2+} HLA-DR$^{2+\rightarrow3+}$ cells are depicted as small gray dots, the CD38$^{-\rightarrow+}$ HLA-DR$^{-\rightarrow+}$ cells are depicted as light gray squares, the CD38$^+$, HLA-DR^{2+} cells are depicted as dark gray squares, and the CD38$^-$, HLA-DR^{2+} cells are depicted as black squares.

and HLA-DR expression were used to identify the primitive progenitor cells and the expression of the fourth antigen was then examined on these primitive progenitor cells (30–32). A small percentage of the cells within the CD34$^+$, CD38$^-$, HLA-DR$^-$ expressed CD50 (ICAM-3) and all CD34$^+$, CD38$^-$, HLA-DR$^+$ cells expressed CD50. Cell culture of single-sorted cells showed that all hematopoietic cell growth was confined to cells that expressed CD50, whereas all stromal cell growth was confined to cells which did not express CD50 (30). The better definition of the cell surface profile of a homogeneous population of hematopoietic pluripotent progenitor cells is CD34$^+$, CD38$^-$, CD50$^+$, whereas that of CD34$^+$ cells of the stromal cell lineage is CD34$^+$, CD38$^-$, CD50$^-$.

Figure 5 shows a schematic representation of the expression of the cell surface antigens CD13, CD33, CD34, CD38, CD49b, CD49d, CD50, CD90w and HLA-DR on human

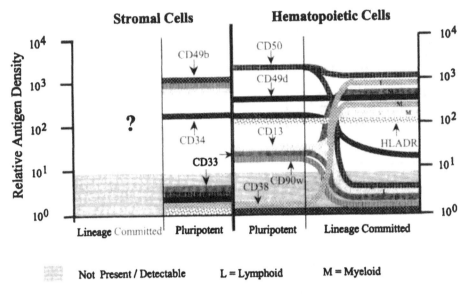

Figure 5   Schematic representation of the CD13, CD33, CD34, CD38, CD49b, CD49d, CD50, CD90w, and HLA-DR antigens during early hematopoietic and stromal cell differentiation.

progenitor cells defined as cells which express CD34. The vertical axis shows the relative antigen density and is correlated with the position of the cells on flow cytometric list mode acquisition. The flow cytometer was set such that cells with no detectable staining appear in the first decade and are colored gray. The horizontal axis shows the stromal cell progenitors and hematopoietic cell progenitors. The hematopoietic progenitor cells are subdivided into pluripotent progenitors and lineage-committed cells. A change in expression upon lymphoid commitment is indicated by the letter L, whereas myeloid commitment is indicated by the letter M in the bars. For cells of the stromal cell lineage, little is known about a potential hierarchy in differentiation into the various cell lineages and a question mark is more appropriate at this time. Although the frequency of CD34$^+$ cells in fetal bone marrow is relatively high, the frequency of CD34$^+$, CD38$^-$, CD50$^-$, HLA-DR$^-$ cells is low and decreases during gestation. Although the number of hematopoietic progenitor cells increases with the increase of the total bone marrow cells the stromal progenitor cell number as defined by clonogenic CD34$^+$, CD38$^-$, HLA-DR$^-$, CD50$^-$ cells remains constant (33). It is thus not surprising that in adult bone marrow the search for cells with this phenotype and the stromal cell growth patterns has not been successful. Large volumes of adult bone marrow will have to be processed and preenrichment procedures for CD34$^+$, CD38$^-$ cells will be necessary to obtain a sufficient number of cells to study stromal cell progenitor cells with this phenotype.

V.   SAMPLE PREPARATION FOR RARE CELL ANALYSIS

Conditions needed to detect infrequent/rare cells by flow cytometry are (1) enough sample has to be available for analysis; (2) the sample volume needs to be analyzed by the flow cytometer in a reasonable amount of time; (3) the parameters have to be chosen such that the target cell population of interest is located in a unique position; and (4) the frequency of the target cells should be larger then 1 in 10^5 cells. The current sample preparation procedures in which blood samples are incubated with fluorescently labeled antibodies followed by the addition of an erythrocyte-lysing agent dilutes the sample 10-fold and is thus not suitable for detection of rare cells. Reduction of the sample volume and an increase in cell concentration in research laboratories is achieved by density separations or NH_4Cl lysing procedures. These procedures lead to variable cell loses and are difficult to standardize between laboratories. Moreover, no significant enrichment of the target cells is obtained.

The use of immunospecific sample preparation procedures which immobilize monoclonal antibodies on a solid support, such as magnetic beads or ferrofluids, are being used

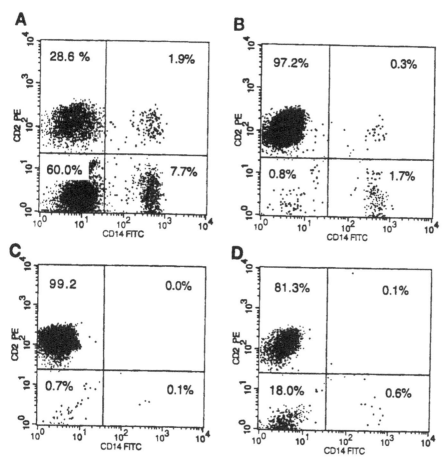

Figure 6 Flow cytometric analysis of immunospecific ferrofluid selected cells from 1 mL of peripheral blood. Samples were incubated simultaneously with the immunospecific ferrofluid and the fluorescently labeled antibodies. Panel A shows the correlative expression of CD2 PE and CD14 fluorescein isothiocyanate (FITC) of cells selected with CD45-specific ferrofluid. Panel B shows the correlative expression of CD2 PE and CD14 FITC of cells selected with CD4-specific ferrofluid. Panel C shows the correlative expression of CD2 PE and CD14 FITC of cells selected with CD8 specific ferrofluid. Panel D shows the correlative expression of CD2 PE and CD14 FITC of cells selected with CD25-specific ferrofluid.

to obtain an enrichment of target cells as well as a sample volume reduction (34). The presence of nanometer-sized colloids (ferrofluids) on the cell surface is compatible with flow cytometric analysis in contrast with that of the larger micrometer-sized particles which need to be detached from the cell surface before flow cytometric analysis. Until recently, separation of cells coated with ferrofluids needed high magnetic gradients achieved by internal magnetic devices such as steel wool columns placed between two opposing magnets (35,36). The immunospecific cells selected by such procedure need to be eluted from the columns and blood samples need to be diluted to avoid nonspecific trapping and clogging of the columns. Density separations or erythrocyte-lysing procedures of the starting cell preparation are therefore recommended.

Improvements of the magnetic properties of ferrofluids permit the separation of immunospecific ferrofluid-coated cells in open-field magnetic devices (37,38). Fluorescent-labeled and ferrofluid-labeled antibodies can be added to a Vacutainer (Becton Dickinson, Rutherford, NJ) of blood, incubated and placed in a magnetic field. After separation, the blood can be removed from the Vacutainer and the target cells present on the wall of the Vacutainer can be resuspended in the desired volume and analyzed by flow cytometry. This procedure is a departure from the traditional erthrocyte blood sample preparation procedures used in hematological analyzers and flow cytometers in that only the cells of interest are analyzed and variable amounts of blood can be analyzed. An example of the flow cytometric analysis of cells prepared through this procedure is shown in Figure 6. Four 1-mL blood samples were incubated with CD2 PE [T lymphocytes and natural killer (NK) cells], CD14 FITC (monocytes), and CD45-labeled ferrofluid (FF), CD4 FF, CD8 FF, and CD25 FF, respectively. After magnetic separation, the blood was discarded and the cells collected at the wall of the vessel were resuspended in 300 µL of an isotonic solution, and 10,000 cells were acquired on a flow cytometer using a threshold on forward light scatter. The correlative displays of CD14 FITC and CD2 PE of the CD45 FF, CD4 FF, CD8 FF, and CD25 FF selected cells are shown in Figure 6A, B–D, respectively. Figure 6A shows the selected $CD45^+$ cells comprising $CD2^+$ T lymphocytes and NK cells (28.5%), $CD14^+$ monocytes (7.7%), and the $CD2^-$, $CD14^-$ granulocytes and B-lymphocytes (60.0%). Figure 6B shows the $CD4^+$ cells comprising $CD2^+$ T lymphocytes (97.2%) and $CD14^+$ monocytes (1.7%). Figure 6C shows the $CD8^+$ cells comprising of $CD2^+$ lymphocytes (99.2%). Figure 6D shows the $CD25^+$ cells comprising $CD2^+$ lymphocytes (81.3%) and $CD2^-$, $CD14^-$ cells bearing CD25 (18.0%). This sample preparation procedure thus permits the selection of only target cells for analysis and no centrifugation steps are necessary to reduce the volume for flow cytometric analysis.

VI. RARE CELL ANALYSIS

Ferromagnetic whole blood cell selection has the potential to become a quantitative sample preparation technology for flow cytometric analysis of rare cells. Target cells indeed need to be recovered by these procedures; however, whether this recovery is 25, 50, 75, or 100% is not as important as the level of carryover of nontarget cells or nonspecific selection of nontarget cells [nonspecific binding (NSB)]. Figure 7 shows the effect of 1, 0.1, 0.01, and 0.001% nontarget cell carryover on target cell frequency obtained after the enrichment procedure. It is clear from Figure 7 that a nonspecific binding of 1% is not sufficient when the target cell frequency is below 1 in 10^5 cells, and preferably the carryover of nontarget cells should be as low as 0.01% to enable flow cytometric detection. Figure 7B shows that the number of target cells and nontarget cells present in the sample at different NSB

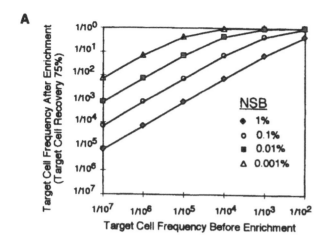

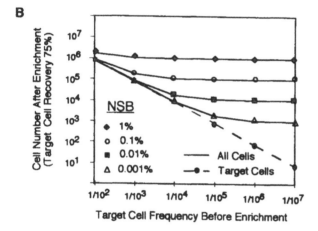

Figure 7 The effect on the target cell frequency before and after sample preparation at 1, 0.1, 0.01, and 0.001% nontarget cell carryover of the sample preparation procedure, panel A. The effect on the cell number after sample preparation at 1, 0.1, 0.01, and 0.001% nontarget cell carryover of the sample preparation procedure, panel B. 10^8 Cells were processed and the recovery of target cells was set at 75%.

levels in case the starting cell number is 10^8 cells. The low number of target cells will require the assessment of a combination of parameters, which places the target cells in a position in the multidimensional space which is truly unique, since one has to assign 1–10 events as truly being the rare cell(s). An application in the need for rare cell detection is the identification of tumor cells in peripheral blood or in the autologous grafts of patients (9,11–13). The sensitivity of the techniques used are reported to be around 1 cell in 5×10^5. Reporting sensitivity in this manner has resolved from the techniques used to detect the target cells rather than the information the clinician is interested in; that is, tumor cell load per volume unit.

In model systems in which epithelium-derived tumor cell lines are spiked into peripheral blood and samples are processed immunomagnetically and analyzed by flow cytometry, the recovery of the tumor cells is more than 50% with a nontarget cell carryover of less then 0.01%. Moreover, the target cell recovery is consistent over a large target cell frequency range as illustrated in Figure 8. Figure 8 shows the recovery of cells from the breast cancer line SKBR-3 spiked at different spike levels into 5 mL of blood of normal donors. To demonstrate that tumor cells can be detected even at levels as low as 1 tumor cell per mL of blood, 0 and 20 SKBR-3 cells were spiked into 20 mL of blood of 10 normal donors. The blood was processed with the immunomagnetic sample preparation methodology and analyzed by flow cytometry. Whereas no tumor cells were detected in the samples with no tumor cells spiked, tumor cells were clearly detected in all spiked samples. The data show that, in model systems, sensitivities of one epithelial cell/milliliter of blood can be achieved. The limitation that remains is that only a fraction of the peripheral blood or autologous graft can be used to screen for the presence of potential tumor cells.

To illustrate the flow cytometric analysis of ferrofluid-selected epithelial cells from 20 mL of blood from a normal donor, a patient with known metastatic breast cancer and a patient with metastatic colon cancer are shown in Figure 8A–C, respectively. Ferrofluid that is coupled to monoclonal antibodies specific for epithelial cells is added to the peripheral blood. After incubation, the blood is placed in a magnetic field and separated for 10 mins. The blood is aspirated and discarded leaving the magnetically captured cells collected at the wall of vessel. The vessel is taken out of the magnetic field and the captured cells are resuspended using a volume of 2 mL and transferred to a 12 × 75 mm vessel used for flow cytometric analysis. This vessel is placed in a magnetic field and after 5 mins of separation the volume is aspirated and discarded. The separated cells are resuspended in 200 μL containing a nucleic acid dye, a pan-leukocyte antibody coupled to PerCP, and a phycoerthrin-coupled antibody specific for epithelial cells and incubated 15 mins. Excess fluorochromes can be removed by an additional magnetic separation and the sample can be analyzed by flow cytometry. The 20-mL blood volume is thus reduced to a volume desired for flow cytometric analysis without the need of centrifugation. Epithelial cells

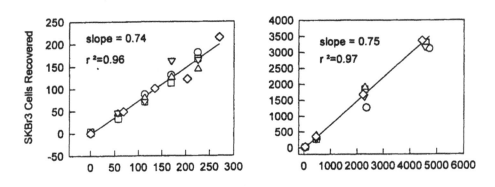

Figure 8   To peripheral blood of five normal donors, SKBR-3 cells were spiked at a frequency of 1000 cells/mL of blood. 5 mL of blood with no tumor cells, 0.5 mL of spiked blood mixed with 4.5 mL of unspiked blood, 2.5 mL of spiked blood mixed with 2.5 mL of unspiked blood, and 5 mL of spiked blood were processed by the immunomagnetic sample preparation procedure and analyzed by flow cytometry. The number of spiked cells in 5 mL of blood is plotted against the number of cells identified by the flow cytometer in panel B. Panel A shows the results of a similar experiment only the number of cells spiked is lower.

are characterized by typical light-scatter characteristics, nucleic acid content, the absence of CD45, and the presence of the epithelial cell marker. The number of epithelial cells identified is then equivalent to the number present in the blood volume. In Figure 9, panels A and B, the light-scattering characteristics and immunofluorescence staining with CD45 PerCP and anti-epithelial cell PE of the contents of 20 mL blood after the immunomagnetic

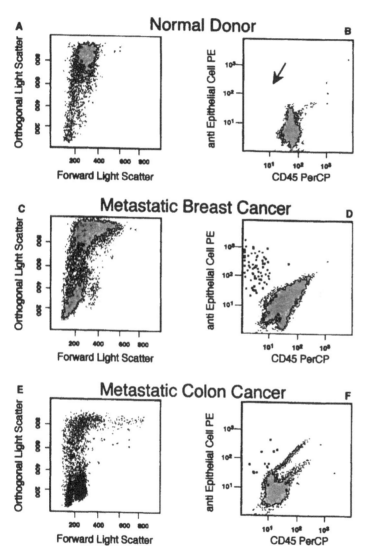

Figure 9   Flow cytometric analysis of epithelial cell–specific ferrofluid selected cells from 20 mL peripheral blood of a normal donor, panels A and B. A patient with breast cancer and bone metastasis, panels C and D. A patient with colon cancer and liver metastasis, panels E and F. After selection the cells were stained with an epithelial cell–specific phycoerythin (PE) conjugated monoclonal antibody, CD45 PerCP, and a nucleic acid dye. All events staining with the nucleic acid dye and not present in the region were epithelial cells are expected are depicted as small gray dots, and events present in the region were epithelial cells are expected are depicted as larger black squares.

sample preparation are shown. The location for potential epithelial cells is indicated with an arrow and no events are observed. All events present in the sample and analyzed by the flow cytometer are depicted as small gray dots. In panels C and D, an identical analysis is shown of a patient with metastatic breast cancer. Seventy events present in the region typical for epithelial cells are depicted as large black square dots and all other events are depicted as small gray dots. These results show that at least 70 epithelial cells were present in the 20 mL of blood processed. In panels E and F, the analysis is shown of a patient with metastatic colon cancer. Twelve events were present in the region typical for epithelial cells and are depicted as large black square dots and all other events are depicted as small gray dots. At least 12 epithelial cells were present in the 20 mL of blood. Immunocytochemistry analysis of 2×10^6 cells of both patients showed two and zero epithelial cells, respectively.

The combination of immunomagnetic sample preparation and flow cytometric analysis shows that this technology can identify rare cells even at frequencies below one cell per 1 mL of blood. The choice of the reagents used to select and identify the target cells is of importance for the sensitivity of the technique and determines the broadness of its applicability. In a recent study, the assay combining immunomagnetic enrichment with multiparameter flowcytometry was applied on peripheral blood (10–20 mL) from 30 patients with carcinoma of the breast before therapeutic intervention and 13 controls (39). In 13 of 14 patients with the tumor confined to the breast, cells classified as nucleic acid[+], leukocyte[-] (CD45) and epithelial cell[+] (cytokeratin) were found. Significantly larger numbers were found in patients with distant metastasis. In eight breast cancer patients with distant metastasis followed over a period of 1–10 months, a good correlation between disease activity or treatment response and the cell number was found. The assay may indeed be helpful in early detection, in monitoring, and in prognostification of the disease.

REFERENCES

1. Shapiro HM. Practical Flow Cytometry. 3d ed. New York: Wiley-Liss, 1995.
2. Terstappen LWMM, Loken MR. 5 Dimensional flow cytometry as a new approach for blood and bone marrow differentials. Cytometry 9:548–556.
3. Loken MR, Shah VO, Datilio KL, Civin CI. Flow cytometric analysis of human bone marrow: II. Normal B lymphoid development. Blood 1987; 70:1316–1324.
4. Terstappen LWMM, Safford M, Loken MR. Flow cytometric analysis of human bone marrow: III. Neutrophil development. Leukemia 1990; 4:657–663.
5. Terstappen LWMM, Huang S, Safford M, Lansdorp PM, Loken MR. Sequential generations of hematopoietic colonies derived from single non lineage committed progenitor cells. Blood 1991; 77:1218–1227.
6. Terstappen LWMM, Huang S, Picker LJ. Flow cytometric assessment of human T-cell differentiation in thymus and bone marrow. Blood 1992; 79:666–677.
7. Chen CH, Lin W, Shye S, Kibler R, Grenier K, Recktenwald D, Terstappen LWMM. Automated enumeration of CD34[+] cell in peripheral blood and bone marrow. Hematother 1994; 3:3–13.
8. Gross HJ, Verwer B, Houck D, Hoffman RA, Recktenwald D. Model study detecting breast cancer cells in peripheral blood mononuclear cells at frequencies as low as 10[-7]. Proc Natl Acad Sci. USA 1995; 92:537–543.
9. Brener MK, Rill DR, Moen RC. Gene-marking to trace the origin of relapse after bone marrow transplantation. Lancet 1993; 341:85–89.
10. Ross AA, Cooper BW, Lazarus HM, Mackay W, Moss TJ, Ciobanu N, Tallman MS, Kennedy

MJ, Davidson NE, Sweet D, Winter C, Akard L, Jansen J, Copelan E, Meagher RC, Herzig RH, Klumpp TR, Kahn DG, Warner NE. Detection and viability of tumor cells in peripheral blood stem cell collections from breast cancer patients using immunohistochemical and clonogenic assay techniques. Blood 1993; 82:2605–2610.

11. Brugger W, Bross K, Glatt M, Weber F, Mertelsman R, Kanz L. Mobilization of tumor cells and hematopoietic progenitor calls into peripheral blood of patients with solid tumors. Blood 1994; 83:636–640.

12. Braun S, Pantel K. Biological characteristics of micrometastatis carcinoma cells in bone marrow. Curr Top Microbiol Immunol 1996; 213:163–177.

13. Brockstein BE, Ross AA, Moss TJ, Kahn DG, Hollingsworth K, Williams SF. Tumor cell contamination of bone marrow harvest products: Clinical consequences in a cohort of advanced stage breast cancer patients undergoing high dose chemotherapy. J Hematother 1996; 5: 617–624.

14. Pelkey TJ, Frierson HF, Bruns DE. Molecular and immunological detection of circulating tumor cells and micrometastases from solid tumors. Clin Chem 1996; 42:1369–1381.

15. Chen CH, Terstappen LWMM. Multi-parameter cell differential analysis-using thiazole orange and labeled anti-CD45 and anti-CD71 antibodies used for analysis cells in blood and bone marrow samples. European Patent Application No: 552707, 1993.

16. Stewart CC, Steinkamp JA. Quantitation of cell concentration using the flow cytometer. Cytometry 1982; 2:238–243.

17. Terstappen LWMM, Hollander Z, Meiners H, Loken MR. Quantitative comparison of myeloid antigens on five lineages of mature peripheral blood cells. J Leukoc Biol 1990; 48:138–148.

18. Terstappen LWMM, Johnsen S, Segers-Nolten I, Loken MR. Identification and characterization of normal human plasma cells by high resolution flow cytometry. Blood 1990; 76:1739–1747.

19. Terstappen LWMM, Levin J. Bone marrow differential counts obtained by multidimensional flow cytometry. Blood Cells 1992; 18:311–330.

20. Terstappen LWMM, Johnson D, Mickaels RA, Chen J, Olds G, Hawkins JT, Loken MR, Levin J. Multidimensional flow cytometric blood cell differentiation without erythrocyte lysis. Blood Cells 1991; 17:585–602.

21. Siena S, Bregni M, Brandon M, Bell B, Bonadonna G, Gianni AAM. Circulation of CD34⁺ hematopoeitic stem cells in the peripheral blood of high dose cyclophosphamide-treated patients: enhancement by intravenous recombinant human granulocyte-colony stimulating factor. Blood 1989; 74:1905–1914.

22. To LB, Sheppard KM, Haylock DN, Dyson PG, Charles P, Thorp DL, Dale BM, Dart GW, Roberts MM, Sage RE, Juttner CA. Single high doses of cyclophosphamide enable the collection of high numbers of hemopoietic stem cells from peripheral blood. Exp Hematol 1992; 8:442–449.

23. Lane TA, Law P, Maruyama M, Young D, Butgess J, Mullen M, Mealiffe M, Terstappen LWMM, Hardwick A, Moubayed M, Oldham F, Corringham RET, and Ho AD. Harvesting and enrichment of hematopoietic stem cells mobilized into the peripheral blood of normal donors by G-CSF or GM-CSF. Blood 1995; 85:275–282.

24. Sutherland DR, Anderson L, Keeney M, Nayar R, Chin-Yee I. The ISHAGE guidelines for CD34⁺ cell determination by flow cytometry. J Hematother 1996; 3:210–213.

25. Issaad C, Croisille L, Katz A, Vainchenker W, Coulombel L. A murine stromal cell line allows the proliferation of very primitive human CD34⁺⁺/CD38⁻ progenitor cells in long term cultures and semisolid assays. Blood 1993; 81:2916–2924.

26. Huang S, Terstappen LWMM. Lymphoid and myeloid differentiation of single human CD34⁺, HLA-DR⁺, CD38⁻ hematopoietic stem cells. Blood 1994; 83:1515–1526.

27. Olweus J, Lund-Johansen F, Hoffman R, Terstappen LWMM. Changes in surface expression of cytokine receptors during lineage commitment of early hematopoietic progenitor cells. In: Schlossman SF, Boumsell L, Gilks W, Harlan JM, Kishimoto T, Morimot C, Ritz J, Shaw S,

Silverstein RL, Springer TA, Tedder TF, Todd RF, eds. Leukocyte Typing V: White Cell Differentiation Antigens. London: Oxford University Press, 1995:1943–1945.

28. Civin CI, Almeida-Porada G, Lee MJ, Terstappen LWMM, Zanjani ED. Sustained, retransplantable, multilineage engraftment of highly purified adult human bone marrow stem cells in vivo. Blood 1996; 88:4102–4109.

29. Hao Q, Thiemann FT, Petersen D, Smogorzewska EM, Crooks GM. Extended long-term culture reveals a highly quiescent and primitive human hematopoietic progenitor population. Blood 1996; 88:3306–3313.

30. Waller EK, Olweus J, Lund-Johansen F, Huang S, Nguyen M, Guo GR, Terstappen LWMM. The "common stem cell" hypothesis reevaluated: Human fetal bone marrow contains separate populations of hematopoietic and stromal progenitors. Blood 1995; 85:2422–2435.

31. Olweus J, Lund-Johansen F, Terstappen LWMM. Cell surface antigen expression during early hematopoietic cell differentiation in adult and fetal bone marrow. Immunomethods 1994; 5: 179–188.

32. Olweus J, Lund-Johansen F, Hoffman R, Terstappen LWMM. Changes in surface expression of cell adhesion molecules during lineage commitment of early hematopoietic progenitor cells. In: Schlossman SF, Boumsell L, Gilks W, Harlan JM, Kishimoto T, Morimoto C, Ritz J, Shaw S, Silverstein RL, Springer TA, Tedder TF, Todd RF, eds. Leukocyte Typing V: White Cell Differentiation Antigens. London: Oxford University Press, 1995; 1677–1679.

33. Waller EK, Huang S, Terstappen LWMM. Changes in growth properties of $CD34^+$, $CD38^-$ bone marrow progenitors during fetal development. Blood 1995; 86:710–718.

34. Ugelstad J, Berge A, Ellingsen T, Schmid R, Nilsen TN, Mork PC, Stenstad P, Hornes E, Olsvik O. Preparation and application of new monosized polymer particles. Prog Polym Sci 1992; 17:87–161.

35. Miltenyi S. Methods and materials for improved high gradient magnetic separation of biological materials. United States Patent. No. 5,411,863, 1995.

36. Miltenyi S, Radbruch A, Weichel W, Muller W, Gottlinger C, Meyer KL. Metal matrices for use in high gradient magnetic separation of biological materials and method for coating the same. United States Patent. No. 5,385,707, 1995.

37. Liberti PA, Feeley BP, Gohel DI. Apparatus for magnetic separation featuring external magnetic means. United States Patent. No. 5,186,827, 1993.

38. Liberti PA, Piccoli SP. Process of making resuspendable coated magnetic particles. United States Patent. No. 5,512,332, 1996.

39. Racila E, Euhus D, Weiss AJ, Rao C, McConnell J, Terstappen LWMM, Uhr JW. Detection and Characterization of Carcinoma Cells in the Blood. Proc Natl Acad Sci USA 1998; 95: 4589–4594.

10

Human/Sheep Hematopoietic Chimeras

GRAÇA ALMEIDA-PORADA, CHRISTOPHER D. PORADA, NAM D. TRAN, JOÃO L. ASCENSAO, and ESMAIL D. ZANJANI

Department of Veterans Affairs Medical Center and University of Nevada School of Medicine, Reno, Nevada

I. INTRODUCTION

Autologous or allogeneic hematopoietic stem cell (HSC) transplantation has been used successfully in the treatment of congenital and acquired immunodeficiencies, hematological and metabolic disorders, and neoplasias of children and adult patients (1–5). Historically, the bone marrow has represented the main source of HSCs in pediatric and adult individuals. However, in many cases, a matched marrow donor cannot be found, thus limiting the applicability of this life-saving procedure (6–7). This and the fact that the use of allogeneic HSCs frequently results in graft-versus-host disease (GVHD) have led to a search for alternative sources of HSCs for use in human transplantations. Three sources of human HSCs have been identified: fetal liver, cord blood, and peripheral blood. Of these, cord blood and peripheral blood are considered to be practical sources of HSCs, especially since methods exist which can mobilize significant numbers of stem/progenitor cells into the circulation (8–12). Cord blood is not only a rich source of HSCs, but its use in children with malignant and nonmalignant diseases has been associated with a relatively low incidence of GVHD (8,10,11). Acute GVHD appears to be due to hoste, reactive donor T lymphocytes (13,14). Depletion of T cells from the donor's graft can significantly decrease the incidence of GVHD (15–18). However, in most instances, this has led to an increasing number of graft rejections, leukemic relapses, and mixed chimerisms (17). To circumvent these difficulties and to devise better therapeutic strategies of HSC transplantation, considerable effort has been devoted to the isolation and characterization of stem/progenitor cell populations.

The purification and characterization of human HSCs has been difficult. Primitive HSCs are rare cells (estimated to comprise about 0.01% of marrow nucleated cells) and lack identifiable morphological characteristics (19–30). Therefore, the purification strategies used have relied on certain immunological, physical, and functional properties with particular emphasis on preserving the biological functions of HSCs that by definition include self-renewal as well as multilineage differentiation in vivo (31).

A variety of assay systems have been devised to monitor the functional properties of isolated/processed HSCs. The in vitro assays have been pivotal in detailing the many facets of the proliferation and differentiation of stem/progenitor cells and identifying and delineating the critical roles played by the many regulatory cytokines in these processes (32). However, the long-term in vivo repopulating ability of HSCs is universally accepted to represent the ultimate test by which the potential of these cells can be adequately assessed (31). It was the availability of a specific and sensitive in vivo HSC assay that permitted the successful characterization and phenotyping of mouse HSCs (33). In vivo hematopoietic reconstitution as well as gene marking experiments using highly purified preparations of HSCs led to the critical observation that relatively few HSCs may be adequate for long-term hematopoietic reconstitution (34–40). It is likely that highly purified HSCs from different human sources will bring about long-term hematopoietic reconstitution in humans as well.

It has long been known that the human HSC (and its progenies) express the CD34 cell surface antigen (19,20); several groups have used the expression, or lack thereof, of specific surface markers, light scatter properties, cell cycle status, and uptake of rhodamine 123 by HSCs to characterize further the human HSC (24,27,30,41,42). Based on a variety of in vitro assays, human primitive HSCs isolated from a number of tissue sources do not appear to express markers associated with mature lineages such as, but not limited to, CD7, CD10, CD14, CD15, CD16, CD,19, CD20, CD33, CD71, and glycophorin A. In addition, other markers such as CD38, human leukocyte antigen-DR (HLA-DR), and CD45RA have been proven to be useful in removing non-HSC populations (24,26,28). Antibodies to a number of other antigens, including Thy1 and c-Kit as well as antigen density levels of CD34 have been utilized to characterize further the human HSC (28,30,43–45). Recent observations by a number of investigators have supported the presence of a CD34$^-$ cell population that is markedly enriched for a long-term reconstituting capacity and may represent a more primitive precursor to the CD34$^+$ cell (46–51). Although this cell population was first characterized in rodents (52–54), a growing body of evidence now supports the existence of a similar population of cells in other species, including macaques and humans (46–48,55). Other studies have shown that immature HSCs isolated from adult marrow, cord blood, and fetal liver differ in their ability to produce hematopoietic progenitors in cytokine-supplemented suspension cultures in vitro, and that the proliferative capacity of these HSCs decrease markedly with age (56,57). These studies indicate the existence of significant ontogeny-related functional differences between HSCs (56). These types of information, if confirmed by in vivo evaluations, can be used to considerable advantage in clinical transplant settings.

To overcome the lack of appropriate in vivo assays for human HSCs, a number of investigators have developed xenogeneic systems utilizing immunodeficient mice in which to test the in vivo behavior of these cells (58–64). However, the relatively small size of the mouse and transient nature of human cell engraftment/expression, often lineage-restricted in many of the models, make the long-term in vivo study of human HSCs difficult.

We have developed a biologically relevant large animal model of human hematopoiesis in sheep by taking advantage of the permissive environment of the early gestational age fetus. The immunological naivete and available hematopoietic sites in the sheep fetuses have permitted the long-term engraftment and multilineage expression of human HSCs (65,66). The human/sheep xenograft has allowed the long-term evaluation of the in vivo proliferative/differentiation potential of human HSCs from fetal, pediatric, and adult sources and appears to represent a biologically relevant model for the in vivo assay of human HSCs.

II. HUMAN/SHEEP XENOGRAFT MODEL

The clinical application of HSC transplantation involves the administration of a source of HSCs after overcoming the immunological barriers that prevent the homing, engraftment, and proliferation of allogeneic or xenogeneic donor HSCs in host bone marrow. The strategies employed such lethal doses of ionizing radiation and/or chemotherapy they often result in depletion of preexisting HSCs. We have used a radically different approach by transplanting human HSCs into early gestational age fetuses to establish successfully a large animal model of human hematopoiesis in sheep.

Normal fetal development offers a unique "window of opportunity" to engraft donor HSCs into early gestational age recipients. There is a period in early immunological development, prior to thymic processing of mature lymphocytes, during which the fetus is tolerant of foreign antigen. Exposure to antigen during this period results in sustained tolerance which can be permanent if the presence of antigen is maintained (67–72). Cellular (T-cell) tolerance appears to be secondary to apoptosis of reactive lymphocytes in the thymus, whereas the mechanism of B-lymphocyte tolerance (peripheral tolerance) appears to involve both clonal deletion and clonal suppression (73–75). The end result is an immune system which is specifically tolerant of transplanted cells. In sheep, immune capability develops sometimes between days 67–77 of gestation. In the sheep fetus, prolonged survival of allogeneic skin grafts occurs before 67 days of gestation, whereas grafts placed after 77 days of gestation are rejected vigorously (67). We have restricted ourselves to using fetuses that are 50–60 days old at the time of donor cell infusion.

Engraftment of donor HSCs is also facilitated by the fact that during this same period of fetal development, expansion of the fetal marrow compartment and normal HSC migration patterns from liver to the bone marrow contribute to the receptivity of the marrow environment to circulating HSCs (76). Donor cells transplanted during this stage may home to a "relatively empty" and "naturally primed" marrow, thus facilitating the establishment of donor hematopoiesis which we have found to persist for long periods with multilineage expression of human cells. Because human HSCs persist in the human/ sheep chimeras for long periods with multilineage expression (77–79), and retain their biological responsiveness to human cytokines (66,77,80), it is possible to develop definitive information about the in vivo proliferative/differentiation potential of the transplanted human HSCs. This is facilitated by the fact that the large size of the sheep permits the evaluation of donor cell activity in the same chimeric animal for several years (78,79,81,82).

III. STUDIES WITH HUMAN FETAL LIVER CELLS

Prior studies showed that fetal liver–derived sheep HSCs transplanted into unrelated preimmune fetal recipients contributed to long-term multilineage lymphohematopoietic chi-

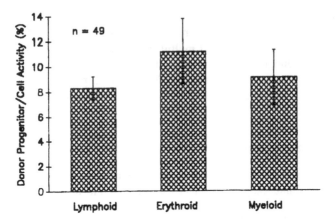

Figure 1 Multilineage expression of donor (sheep) hematopoietic cells in chimeric sheep follow-ing transplantation of sheep fetal liver cells in utero. In each case the sex of the donor was different from the recipient. Identification of donor cells/progenitors was achieved by karyotyping of cells (lymphoid) and progenitor-derived myeloid and erythroid hematopoietic colonies. In some experi-ments transplantation of cells from donors homozygous for type AA hemoglobin into preimmune type BB fetal sheep permitted the determination of donor erythroid cell activity by hemoglobin isoelectric focusing (97). Each value represents mean $\pm$ 1 standard error of the mean (SEM) of results obtained from quadruplicate determinations of peripheral blood (lymphoid) and bone mar-row-derived myeloid and erythroid cells from 49 different chimeric sheep at 2.2 years of age (about 29 months post-transplant).

merism for several years after birth without development of GVHD (65,66,83,84) (Fig. 1). With this information as the background, we expanded our studies to using cells ob-tained from livers of early gestational age human fetuses into preimmune fetal sheep. As reported earlier (77), we achieved long-term engraftment and expression of human cells in a significant number of these recipients. Engrafted cells were not only retained, but

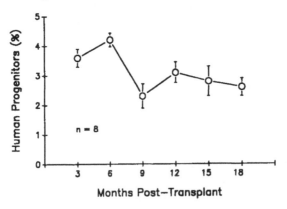

Figure 2 Persistence of donor (human) hematopoietic progenitors in chimeric sheep following transplantation of human fetal liver cells in utero. Each value represents mean $\pm$ 1 SEM of results obtained from quadruplicate determinations of bone marrow-derived hematopoietic colonies from eight different chimeric sheep. Values were derived by karyotype analyses of colony forming units-Mix (CFU-Mix), burst forming units-erythroid (BFU-E), and colony forming units-granulocyte mac-rophage (CFU-GM) derived colonies on day 19 of incubation. (See legends to Figure 4 for detail.)

Table 1 Isolation of Human Cells from Bone Marrow of Primary Sheep Recipients 3.5 Years After Transplantation of Human Fetal Liver Cells in Utero

	No. of cells obtained[a]	% Total
BMNCs[b]	1.91×10^9	—
CD45+ cells[c]	6.3×10^7	3.3
Sorted cells[d]	2.9×10^7	1.5

[a] Because of its large size, highly significant numbers of human cells can be obtained from marrow mononuclear cells by "priming." In other studies, this procedure has been repeated at least three times in the same animal.

[b] Bone marrow mononuclear cells (BMNCs) were obtained from three different chimeric sheep at 3.6, 3.2, and 3.4 years posttransplant.

[c] Represents the sum of CD45+ cells obtained in all bone marrow preparations.

[d] CD45+ cells were sorted from the all bone marrow using a panning technique, only 46% of CD45+ cells present were recovered (85).

they were capable of multilineage differentiation into cells bearing human cell surface markers, human karyotype (77), and an in vivo response to human-specific growth factors (77,80). Long-term persistence (several years) of the human cells (documented by karyotype analysis) was seen in at least 40% of these animals (Fig. 2). Although the persistence of human cells in these animals for long periods suggested that the engraftment involved

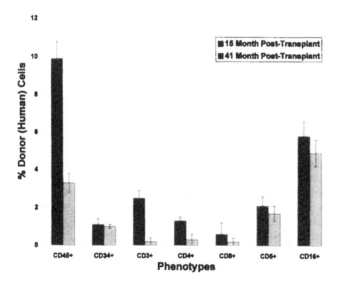

Figure 3 Long-term expression of human multilineage hematopoietic cell differentiation markers in sheep bone marrow. All bone marrow cells at a concentration of 10^6 were stained with the above monoclonal antibodies and analyzed by flow cytometry. Each value represents mean ± 1 SEM of results from two separate sheep (77).

a multipotential self-renewing human HSC, more definitive evidence was obtained by secondary transplantation into appropriate fetal sheep recipients (85). Human cells were isolated from bone marrow of primary chimeric hosts at about 3.5 years posttransplant (Table 1) and transplanted into normal preimmune fetal sheep recipients. Long-term donor cell engraftment was demonstrated in two of six secondary recipients (see Fig. 4) (85).

In both the primary and secondary chimeric recipients, human HSC engraftment was accompanied by multilineage human cell expression, primarily in bone marrow (Figs. 3 and 4). This was demonstrated by the presence of colony-forming cells and by flow cytometric analysis of specific human cell surface markers (Fig. 4) (85). The low level of human cell activity in these animals is likely a reflection of the fact that although the host (sheep) environment can support the proliferation of human HSCs, it does not provide significant support for the differentiation of human cells (77,84,86).

Normal hematopoiesis is dependent on cell–cell interactions and regulatory factors that may be species restricted. Little is known about the regulation of xenogeneic HSC activity in a genetically widely disparate microenvironment. Sheep phytohemagglutinin lymphocyte conditioned media (PHA-LCM) (a source of ovine hematopoietic growth fac-

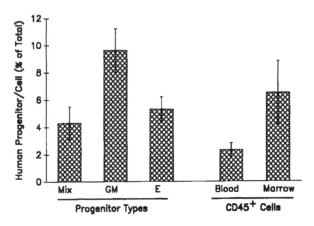

Figure 4 Relative distribution of donor (human) progenitors/cells in bone marrow of secondary recipient sheep at 24 weeks after transplantation. The progenitor values represent the percentage of total numbers of colonies enumerated. Bone marrow cells were cultured in multiple methylcellulose plates as previously described (77). Total colony numbers were enumerated on days 9 and 19 of incubation; all three progenitor types colony forming units-Mix (CFU-Mix), colony forming units-granulocyte macrophage (CFU-GM), burst forming units-erythroid (BFU-E) were detected on both days. On day 19, colonies were removed from the plate and individually processed for karyotyping. In experiments where the majority of plucked day 19 colonies exhibit an evaluable metaphase, nearly all are of human origin. However in general only 45% to 63% of the removed colonies can be successfully karyotyped. The values presented here were derived from the successfully karyotyped colonies and we believe, therefore, that they are underestimates. The relative percentages of human colonies were determined by the following formula: Percent human colonies = number of human colonies on day 19 × 100/total number of colonies on day 9. Values for CD45+ cells represent the frequency of human cells detected by flow cytometry after labeling with a monoclonal antibody-recognizing human CD45 antigen. The human cell expression in these animals was multilineage as detected flow cytometrically after labeling with antibodies recognizing the different CD antigens (79).

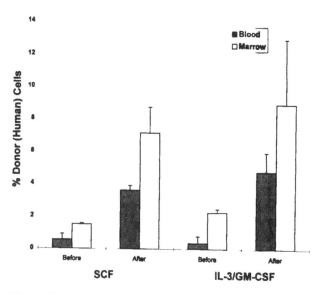

Figure 5 Effect of treatment with recombinant human Interleukin (IL)-3/granulocyte macro-phage-colony stimulating factor (GM-CSF) or stem cell factor (SCF) on the relative expression of donor (human) cells in chimeric sheep. Each value represents mean of results obtained by flow cytometric analysis using a monoclonal antibody against human CD45 in two separate determinations (80).

tors) does not show cross reactivity with human cells. Similarly, human cytokines [interleukin (IL)-3, granulocyte-macrophage colony-stimulating factor (GM-CSF), c-Kit ligand] have little effect on sheep hematopoiesis (77,80). We therefore used several cytokines selectively to investigate the "responsiveness" of the donor (human) cell compartment in chimeric sheep. The administration of human IL-3/GM-CSF or c-Kit ligand to 1- to 2-year-old chimeric sheep with stable levels of human cell engraftment resulted in highly significant increases in human cell multilineage chimerism in bone marrow and blood of these animals (77,80) (Fig. 5). The fact that multilineage preferential stimulation of human cell populations occurs with human cytokine stimulation, even after years of low-level stable engraftment, suggests that a quiescent population of human HSCs remains present (and dormant). It seems likely that although viability and some degree of human hematopoiesis may be maintained by the sheep microenvironment, optimal human cell expression and activity requires the availability of adequate concentrations of human-specific hematopoietins. Recent studies by Almeida-Porada and colleagues (87) suggest that cotransplantation of autologous or allogeneic human stromal elements with human HSCs can significantly improve human HSC engraftment/expression in the sheep, probably by providing the host sheep with some levels of human growth factors. These results suggest that the model may be useful for the in vivo assessment of the role of human hematopoietins.

IV. STUDIES WITH ADULT HUMAN HSCs

In preliminary sheep-to-sheep transplantation studies, we compared different sources of mononuclear cells from fetal liver, cord blood, newborn marrow, and adult bone marrow

Table 2 Role of T Cells in Donor Cell Engraftment and the Development of Graft-Versus-Host Disease in Utero (Sheep to Sheep Transplantation Studies)[a]

Sources of donor cells	No. transplanted/ chimeric	Chimeric animals	
		Donor cells[b]	% GVHD
Fetal liver	32/27	14.6 ± 2.0	0
Cord blood	28/15	11.8 ± 3.3	80
Cord blood-T	24/6	6.3 ± 2.0	0
Newborn marrow	13/6	15.9 ± 4.6	100
Newborn marrow-T	21/7	7.2 ± 2.8	14
Adult marrow	24/12	13.1 ± 8.0	92
Adult marrow-T	31/9	5.3 ± 1.1	0

[a] Equivalent members of viable non–T-mononuclear cells from the different sheep sources were transplanted into preimmune fetal sheep. Donor cells were depleted of T cells as described (89).
[b] Determined by karyotype analysis of cells and progenitor-derived colonies as described (89).

for their engraftment potential. Results summarized in Table 2 indicate that the preimmune fetus engrafts with all four postnatal tissue sources. However, except for the group receiving fetal liver graft (88), all chimeric recipients developed GVHD and died. Table 2 also shows that the development of GVHD in chimeric lambs was directly associated with the presence of donor T lymphocytes in the graft; when cord blood and bone marrow cells were depleted of mature T cells prior to transplantation, there was a significant decrease in GVHD development in chimeric lambs (Table 2) (89). However, the use of T-depleted cells was also associated with failure to engraft in 50–70% of the transplanted fetuses (89). These results clearly indicate that allografting in this model follows the patterns established for postnatal HSC transplantation in animals and humans. This pattern was also seen when we transplanted fetal sheep with preparations of mononuclear cells from human cord blood, adult bone marrow and peripheral blood.

In these xenografts, we found that the preimmune fetal sheep readily permitted the engraftment and multilineage expression of postnatal human HSCs (Table 3) (78,79,81,90). However, as was the case with the allogeneic transplants, animals that were

Table 3 Role of T Cells in Donor Cell Engraftment and the Development of GVHD in Utero (Human to Sheep Transplantation Studies)

Sources of donor cells	No. transplanted/ chimeric	Chimeric animals	
		Donor cells	% GVHD
Fetal liver	47/22	5.2 ± 0.4	0
Cord blood	38/20	6.2 ± 2.5	85
Cord blood-T[a]	15/3	1.7 ± 1.2	0
Newborn marrow	36/17	3.1 ± 0.6	88
Newborn marrow-T[a]	24/5	0.9 ± 0.3	40
Adult marrow	19/11	4.2 ± 1.1	90
Adult marrow-T[a]	9/2	0.7 ± 0.5	0

[a] Bone marrow mononuclear cells depleted of T cells. T cells were removed from human bone marrow or cord blood by rosetting with sheep red cells prior to transplantation.

transplanted with mononuclear cells from postnatal human sources and became chimeric developed severe GVHD and died (Table 3); GVHD was apparently caused by the presence of donor T cells in the graft, since GVHD was not seen in the majority of chimeric sheep transplanted with T-depleted cells. However, T-cell depletion did cause a decrease in the percentage of chimerism (Table 3) (81).

Long-term engraftment/multilineage expression of adult human HSCs without GVHD occurred following the transplantation of highly enriched/purified populations of human HSCs (78,79,90). Adult human CD34$^+$, HLA-DR$^-$ cells have been extensively characterized in vitro and shown to contain a variety of primitive hematopoietic progenitors which possess many functional properties of the HSC (26). We therefore transplanted CD34$^+$, Lin$^-$, HLA-DR$^-$ cells into immune incompetent fetal sheep. Sustained human hematopoietic chimerism and expression of cells belonging to all hematopoietic cell lineages occurred in chimeric sheep for long periods (78,90). The possibility that human HSCs persist in these animals was suggested by the presence of significant numbers of CD34$^+$, HLA-DR$^-$ cells in the marrow of these animals 130 days after the transplant (90). In addition, human high-proliferative potential colony-forming cells (HPP-CFCs), which are primitive hematopoietic progenitor cells capable of multilineage differentiation and self-renewal, properties associated with HSCs (21), were also detected in bone marrow of these chimeric animals (78). Secondary transplant studies in which human CD45$^+$ cells isolated from bone marrow of chimeric sheep more than 2 years posttransplant were transplanted into secondary preimmune fetal sheep (79), with documented multilineage human hematopoietic engraftment in the bone marrow but not in the blood of the secondary recipient for at least 15 months posttransplant (Fig. 6). However, the administration of human hematopoietic growth factors to these human/sheep chimeric animals resulted in the appearance of significant numbers of human cells in circulation (77,80).

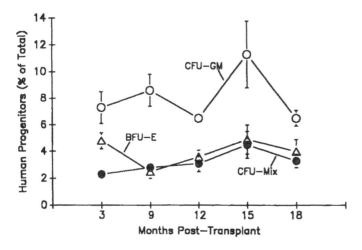

Figure 6   Multilineage human hematopoietic cell engraftment in bone marrow of secondary sheep recipients. CD45$^+$ cells were isolated from bone marrow of primary recipient chimeric sheep more than two years after transplantation and injected into secondary pre-immune fetal sheep. The expression of human cells in secondary recipients was multilineage as also determined by bone marrow flow cytometric cell analysis at 12 months of age with the following antibodies: CD34 0.2%; CD3 1.8%; CD22 0.4%; CD14 0.9% (79).

The demonstration of human cell activity in the secondary sheep recipients strongly suggests that the original graft contained a human HSC with long-term repopulating ability. We also investigated the in vivo engraftment potential of human CD34$^-$, Lin$^-$ cells. In three separate studies transplantation of human CD34$^-$, Lin$^-$ cells into fetal sheep recipients resulted in long-term engraftment and multilineage hematopoietic cell/progenitor expression. Secondary transplantation and limiting dilution studies confirmed the presence of cells with long-term engraftment potential in CD34$^-$ populations (51). The ability to assess long-term function of adult HSCs is unique to the in utero sheep transplantation model and is a consequence of the large size of the chimeric animal which allows repeated sampling of bone marrow and blood at various intervals. Such evaluations over prolonged periods of time permit the type of studies necessary to determine whether a candidate HSC population is capable of long-term hematopoietic engraftment and multilineage differentiation.

V. STUDIES WITH ENRICHED/PURIFIED ADULT HUMAN HSCs

In order to evaluate the relative specificity of the sheep xenograft model to distinguish between different populations of human stem/progenitor cells, we compared different populations containing putative human HSCs for their in vivo long-term engraftment potential. Initially we used the CD34$^+$, Lin$^-$, Thy1$^+$ cells isolated from adult human bone marrow and mobilized peripheral blood, which are felt to be enriched for human HSCs (92,97), provided to us by Ronald Hoffman (University of Illinois, Chicago, IL). When we transplanted blood- or marrow-derived CD34$^+$, Lin$^-$, Thy1$^+$ cells (4 × 10^4 cells/fetus) into preimmune fetal sheep, significant degrees of stable, long-term human cell chimerism were observed postnatally in these animals (93). By contrast, little or no human cell activity was detected in sheep transplanted with Thy1$^-$ cells. This relative specificity of the human/sheep xenograft model was also evident when we evaluated the in vivo potential of a subpopulation of the CD34$^+$, Lin$^-$, Thy1$^+$ cells that is characterized by poor retention of rhodamine 123. Such rhodamine-low cell populations have been shown to be enriched for HSCs. The rhodamine-low but not rhodamine-high population was capable of achieving a remarkable degree of multilineage hematopoietic chimerism in these lambs. For comparative purposes, each of these cell populations were extensively analyzed for their in vitro characteristics, including the frequency of cobblestone area–forming cells (CAFC-). This analysis was also performed on CD34$^+$ cells isolated from bone marrow of a chimeric sheep transplanted with CD34$^+$, Thy1$^+$, Lin$^-$ at 100 days of age (i.e., about 6 months after transplant). These CD34$^+$ rhodamine subpopulations were then assayed for the frequency of CAFCs. The CAFC frequencies in the CD34$^+$ rhodamine-low and rhodamine-mid populations were virtually identical to the frequency of CAFCs in the original graft (92).

Additional evidence that the in utero sheep transplantation approach may serve as a biologically relevant model for the evaluation of the in vivo engraftment/proliferation potential of human stem/progenitor cell populations was obtained in collaboration with Makio Ogawa (Medical University of South Carolina, Charleston, SC) using human bone marrow CD34$^+$ cells further characterized by their expression of c-Kit. In vitro evaluations suggested that the c-Kit^{low} population was enriched for the more primitive HSCs (30). We compared the in vivo activity of three different populations of these cells (c-Kit high, low, and negative) by initially transplanting 3000–4000 cells from each preparation into each preimmune fetal sheep. When the recipients were evaluated at birth, it was found that lambs transplanted with c-Kit[high] cells had no human cells/progenitors in bone marrow or peripheral blood, whereas human cells/progenitors were detected in bone marrow of both remaining groups. However, beginning at about 3 months of age (6 months posttransplant), only lambs who had received c-Kit[low] cells continued to exhibit human cell/progenitor activity (45). Retransplantation studies confirmed the presence of primitive, retransplantable human HSCs in the c-Kit[low] population. This ability of the sheep model to distinguish between the committed and the more primitive human HSC pools may be of value when evaluating the in vivo engraftment/proliferation potential of not only the various human HSC populations, but also of ex vivo expanded human HSCs, especially since the use of growth factors in expansion strategies can potentially alter the long-term engraftment potential of these cells (94).

VI. DISCUSSION

We have developed a xenograft model of human hematopoiesis which has been proven to be extremely useful for the in vivo study of the biology of the human HSC (68,77–79, 90). The human/sheep model has several unique characteristics. Foremost among these are the large size of the sheep, which permits repeated evaluation of human cell activity in the same chimeric sheep over long periods of time, and the fact that this model accomplishes substantial levels of donor HSC engraftment without marrow conditioning by taking advantage of both the immunological naivety of the fetus and the developing "homing" spaces of the fetal bone marrow. The absence of preconditioning regimens such as irradiation and/or chemotherapy ensures that the hematopoietic stroma is still in an intact state at the time of donor cell infusion, enabling donor cells to "home" to a normal bone marrow in direct competition with the recipient's own HSCs. Several other characteristics of the human/sheep xenograft suggest that it represents a biologically relevant model system in which to study the behavior of human HSCs. These include (1) human HSCs colonize the recipient's bone marrow, (2) the engrafted HSCs persist for many years after transplant, (3) these HSCs undergo multilineage differentiation, (4) administration of human-specific hematopoietic growth factors elicits a response from engrafted human HSCs, and (5) the cells that engraft and persist are primitive HSCs, since they are capable of engrafting and differentiating in secondary recipients.

The finding that transplantation of human cells, isolated from bone marrow of human/sheep chimeric animals into secondary recipients results in long-term human cell engraftment and multilineage differentiation suggests that self-renewal/expansion of human HSCs may have occurred in the primary recipients. However, animal models of human hematopoiesis have typically required relatively large numbers of human HSCs for establishing human cell activity in these animals. In these studies, the primary recipients had been transplanted with relatively large numbers of human HSCs, which, although unlikely, raises the possibility that the engraftment in secondary recipients may have resulted from HSCs that had simply persisted in the primary hosts, albeit in some cases for greater than 3 years. Our dose-response studies with CD34$^+$, c-Kit[low] cells demonstrated that significant donor cell engraftment/expression can occur with as few as 700 cells/fetus (95). Of interest was the finding that donor cell expression in animals receiving >700 cells was not appreciably different than in lambs transplanted with the minimal dose of about 700 cells. The absence of a clear dose-response is associated with the relative insensitivity of human cells to sheep hematopoietic growth factors (77). A different dose-response pattern emerged when the lambs were treated with a mixture of human IL-3

(8 μg/kg), GM-CSF (8 μg/kg), and IL-6 (20 μg/kg) daily for 10 days. The administration of human growth factors resulted in a (cell) dose-dependent increase in human cell expression (95).

The ability to detect small numbers of transplanted HSCs is essential for the assay of human HSC–enriched/purified populations, where relatively few cells may be available, and where limiting dilution or competitive repopulation studies may be required for quantitative analysis of HSC frequency within a pool. One concern about a large animal model for the assay of purified human cell populations would be that it may be difficult to assess the proliferation/differentiation of small numbers of cells in the relatively very large bone marrow hematopoietic compartment of the sheep. However, although adult sheep are large, the preimmune fetus at the time of transplantation is quite small, weighing approximately 10 gs. Therefore, in most experiments at the time of transplantation, the donor cell inoculum represents a relatively high cell number relative to the host hematopoietic compartment. This will permit the evaluation of the self-renewal capacity of a given cell type by, among others, quantitating the numbers of cells with the original phenotype in the host chimeric animal and determining whether human cells isolated from such an animal will engraft when transplanted into a secondary recipient. It may, therefore, be possible directly to compare the in vivo engrafting, proliferation, and self-renewal potential of HSCs with different phenotypes from the same source (e.g., bone marrow) or of HSCs with similar phenotypes from different tissue sources.

The biological relevance of this model is also demonstrated by the fact that as in the allogeneic in utero HSC transplantation model, the development of GVHD in the human/sheep xenograft is dependent on the number of infused immunocompetent donor T cells (89). Sheep transplanted with crude preparations of human hematopoietic cells from postnatal sources (marrow, cord blood, peripheral blood) develop GVHD (82). In both allogeneic and xenogeneic transplant settings, we have found that the majority of recipients made chimeric with whole mononuclear cell populations from postnatal sources abort by about 60 days posttransplant; lymphocytic infiltration was seen in all tissues examined (liver, skin, gut) in >90% of the aborted fetuses. By contrast, it is very rare to detect GVHD in chimeric sheep transplanted with T-depleted or enriched/purified human HSC preparations even after many years (77,81,82).

A major drawback to the sheep model has been that on many occasions only a small number of the animals transplanted in utero exhibit significant donor cell engraftment. It is clear, however, that the persistence of human cell activity in chimeric animals and its large size provide unique opportunities for the long-term analysis of human HSC activity not possible in the other models. In addition, it appears that a significant number of transplanted animals acquire tolerance to the source of human HSCs even in the absence of significant human cell activity (96). In 1945, Owen (67) observed that dyzygotic cattle twins which shared cross-placental circulation were hematopoietic chimeras. Subsequent work proved that such chimeric animals were tolerant to skin grafts and kidney transplants from their sibling (70). These findings led to Billingham and Medawar's classic studies on "acquired" immunological tolerance (68,69) showing that preimmune exposure to a foreign antigen resulted in specific tolerance to that antigen. Induction of tolerance has been achieved in a variety of biological models and in our sheep to sheep and human to sheep in utero HSC transplantation studies by prenatal exposure to cells (96). In sheep to sheep transplant experiments, postnatal infusion of donor cells into "tolerized" chimeric lambs resulted in a significant "rise" in donor cell activity (96). Similar increases can occur following the infusion of donor human HSCs to "tolerized" newborn sheep. In three of these lambs, postnatal donor HSC infusion at 3 weeks of age resulted in increasing donor cell activity from 2.1 ± 0.7% to 11.9 ± 6.2% of total bone marrow hematopoietic progenitors [colony-forming units-mix (CFU-Mix), colony-forming units-granulocyte-macrophage (CFU-GM), burst-forming units-erythroid (BFU-E)] determined 6 weeks later.

VII. CONCLUSION

We have developed a large animal model of human hematopoiesis in sheep that permits the engraftment and long-term expression of human hematopoietic stem/progenitor cells. This model has several unique characteristics that distinguish it from other xenograft models. Among these are the large size of the sheep, which permits repeated evaluation of human cell activity in the same chimeric sheep over long periods of time, and the fact that this model allows substantial levels of donor HSC engraftment without marrow conditioning. The absence of preconditioning regimens such as irradiation and/or chemotherapy ensures that the hematopoietic stroma is still in an intact state at the time of donor cell infusion, enabling donor cells to "home" to a normal marrow in direct competition with the recipient's own HSCs. Several other characteristics of the human/sheep xenograft suggest that it represents a biologically relevant model system in which to study the behavior of human HSCs. These include (1) human HSCs colonize the recipient's bone marrow, (2) the engrafted HSCs persist for many years after transplant, (3) these HSCs undergo multilineage differentiation, (4) administration of human-specific hematopoietic growth factors elicits a response from engrafted human HSCs, and (5) the cells that engraft and persist are primitive, retransplantable HSCs, since they are capable of engrafting and differentiating in secondary recipients. Finally, this in utero human/sheep xenograft model appears to distinguish between different populations of human HSCs, exhibiting a sensitivity that suggests it may be useful for the identification, characterization, and study of the in vivo potential and behavior of human HSC from available sources.

ACKNOWLEDGMENT

This work was supported by grants HL40722, HL46566, HL39875, and DK51427 from National Institutes of Health and the Department of Veterans Affairs.

REFERENCES

1. Sullivan KM. Current status of bone marrow transplantation. Transpl Proc 1989; 21(suppl 1): 41–50.
2. Krivit W, Shapiro E, Kennedy W, Lipton M, Lockman L, Smith S, Summers CG, Wenger DA, Tsai MY, Ramsay NK, Kersey JH, Yao JK, Kaye E. Treatment of late infantile metachromatic leukodystrophy by bone marrow transplantation. N Engl J Med 1990; 322:28–32.
3. Krivit W, Shapiro EG. Bone marrow transplantation for storage diseases. In: RJ Desnick, ed. Treatment of Genetic Disease. New York: Churchill-Livingstone, 1991:203–221.
4. Storb R, Champlin RE. Bone marrow transplantation for severe aplastic anemia. Bone Marrow Transplant 1991; 8:69–72.
5. Flowers ME, Doney KC, Storb R, Deeg HJ, Sanders JE, Sullivan KM, Bryant E, Witherspoon RP, Appelbaum FR, Buckner CD, et al. Marrow transplantation for Fanconi anemia with or without leukemic transformation: An update of the Seattle experience. Bone Marrow Transplant 1991; 9:167–173.

6. Clark JG. The challenge of bone marrow transplantation. Mayo Clin Proc 1990; 65:111–114.

7. Bortin MM, Horowitz MM, Rimm AA. Increasing utilization of allogeneic bone marrow transplantation. Results of the 1988–1990 survey. Ann Intern Med 1992; 116:505–512.

8. Harris DT, Schumacher MJ, Locascio J, Besencon FJ, Olson GB, DeLuca D, Shenker L, Bard J, Boyse EA. Phenotypic and functional immaturity of human umbilical cord blood T lymphocytes. Proc Natl. Acad Sci USA 1992; 89:10006–10010.

9. Lowry PA, Tabbara IA. Peripheral hematopoietic stem cell transplantation: current concepts. Exp Hematol 1992; 20:937–942.

10. Cardoso AA, Li MI, Batard P, Hatzfeld A, Brown EL, Levesque JP, Sookdeo H, Panterne B, Sansilvestri P, Clark SC, et al. Release from quiescence of CD34+ CD38-human umbilical cord blood cells reveals their potentiality to engraft adults. Proc Natl Acad Sci USA 1993; 90:8707–8011.

11. Wagner JE, Kerman NA, Broxmeyer HE, Gluckman E. Allogeneic umbilical cord blood transplantation: report of results in 26 patients. Blood 1993; 82:86a.

12. Weaver CH, Buckner CD, Longin K, Appelbaum FR, Rowley S, Lilleby K, Miser J, Storb R, Hansen JA, Bensinger W. Syngeneic transplantation with peripheral blood mononuclear cells collected after the administration of recombinant human granulocyte colony-stimulating factor. Blood 1993; 82:1981–1984.

13. Horowitz MM, Gale RP, Sondel PM, Goldman JM, Kersey J, Kolb HJ, Rimm AA, Ringden O, Rozman C, Speck B, Truitt RL, Zwaan FE, Bortin MM. Graft-versus-leukemia reactions after bone marrow transplantation. Blood 1990; 75:555–562.

14. Sullivan KM. Graft-versus-host disease. In: SJ Forman, KG Blume, ED Thomas, eds. Bone marrow transplantation. Boston: Blackwell, 1994:339.

15. Mitsuyasu RT, Champlin RE, Gale RP, Ho WG, Lenarsky C, Winston D, Selch M, Elashoff R, Giorgi JV, Wells J, et al. Treatment of donor bone marrow with monoclonal anti-T-cell antibody and complement for the prevention of graft-versus-host disease. A prospective, randomized, double-blind trial. Ann Intern Med 1986; 105:20–26.

16. Maraninchi D, Gluckman E, Blaise D, Guyotat D, Rio B, Pico JL, Leblond V, Michallet M, Dreyfus F, Ifrah N, Bordigoni A. Impact of T-cell depletion on outcome of allogeneic bone-marrow transplantation for standard-risk leukaemias. Lancet 1987; 2:175–178.

17. Kernan NA, Bordignon C, Heller G, Cunningham I, Castro-Malaspina H, Shank B, Flomenberg N, Burns J, Yang SY, Black P, Colins NH, O'Reilly RJ. Graft failure after T-cell–depleted human leukocyte antigen identical marrow transplants for leukemia: I. Analysis of risk factors and results of secondary transplants. Blood 1989; 74:2227–2236.

18. Champlin R. T-cell depletion to prevent graft-versus-host disease after bone marrow transplantation. Hematol Oncol Clin North Am 1990; 4:687–698.

19. Civin CI, Stauss LC, Broval C, Fackler MJ, Schwarta JF, Shaper JH. Antigenic analysis of hematopoiesis III. A hematopoietic progenitor cell surface antigen defined by a monoclonal antibody raised against KG1a cells. J Immunol 1984; 133:157–165.

20. Andrews RG, Singer JW, Bernstein ID. Monoclonal antibody 12:8 recognizes a 115-kd molecule present on both unipotent and multipotent hematopoietic colony forming cells and their precursors. Blood 1986; 67:842–845.

21. Brandt J, Baird N, Lu L, Srour EF, Hoffman R. Characterization of human hematopoietic progenitor cell capable of forming blast cell colonies in vitro. J Clin Invest 1988; 82:1017–1027.

22. Sutherland HJ, Eaves AC, Dragowska W, Lansdorp PM. Characterization and partial purification of human marrow cells capable of initiating long-term hematopoiesis in vitro. Blood 1989; 74:1563–1570.

23. Andrews RG, Singer JW, Bernstein I. Human hematopoietic precursors in long-term culture: single CD34+ cells that lack detectable T cell B cell and myeloid cell antigens produce multiple colony-forming cells when cultured with marrow stromal cells. J Exp Med 1990; 172:355–358.

24. Lansdorp PM, Sutherland HJ, Eaves CJ. Selective expression of CD45 isoforms on functional

subpopulations of CD34$^+$ hematopoietic cells from human bone marrow. J Exp Med 1990; 172:363–366.

25. Verfaille C, Blakolmer K, McGlave P. Purified primitive human hematopoietic progenitor cells with long-term in vitro repopulating capacity adhere selectively to irradiated bone marrow stroma. J Exp Med 1990; 172:509–602.

26. Srour EF, Brandt J, Briddell RA, Leemhuis T, van Besien K, Hoffman R. Human CD34$^+$HLA-DR$^-$ bone marrow cells contain progenitor cells capable of self-renewal, multilineage differentiation and long term in vitro hematopoiesis. Blood Cells 1991; 17:287–295.

27. Srour EF, Leemhuis T, Brandt JE, van Besien K, Hoffman R. Simultaneous use of rhodamine 123, phycoerythrin, Texas red and allophycocyanin for the isolation of human hematopoietic progenitor cells. Cytometry 1991; 12:179–183.

28. Terstappen LWMM, Huang S, Safford DM, Lansdorp PM, Loken MR. Sequential generations of hematopoietic colonies derived from single nonlineage-committed CD34$^+$CD38$^-$ progenitor cells. Blood 1991; 77:1218–1227.

29. Baum CM, Weissman IL, Tsukamoto AS, Buckel A-M, Peault B. Isolation of a candidate human hematopoietic stem cell population. Proc Natl Acad Sci USA 1992; 89:2804–2808.

30. Katayama N, Shih JP, Nishikawa S, Kina T, Clark SC, Ogawa M. Stage-specific expression of c-kit protein by murine hematopoietic progenitors. Blood 1993; 82:2353–2360.

31. Orlic D, Bodine DM. What defines a pluripotent hematopoietic stem cell (PHSC): will the real PHSC please stand up. Blood 1994; 84:3991–3994.

32. Ogawa M. Differentiation and proliferation of hematopoietic stem cells. Blood 1993; 81:2844–2853.

33. Spangrude GJ, Heimfeld S, Weissman IL. Purification and characterization of mouse hematopoietic stem cells. Science 1988; 241:58–62.

34. Lemischka IR, Raulet DH, Mulligan RC. Developmental potential and dynamic behavior of hematopoietic stem cells. Cell 1986; 45:917–927.

35. Szilvassy S, Fraser C, Eaves C, Lansdorp P, Eaves A, Humphries R. Retrovirus-mediated gene transfer to purified hemopoietic stem cells with long-term lympho-myelopoietic repopulating ability. Proc Natl Acad Sci USA 1989; 86:8798–8802.

36. Fraser C, Eaves C, Szilvassy S, Humpries K. 1990. Expansion in vitro of retrovirally marked totipotent hematopoietic stem cells. Blood 76:1071–1076.

37. Jordan CT, Lemischka IR. Clonal and systemic analysis of long-term hematopoiesis in the mouse. Genes Dev 1990; 4:220–232.

38. Keller GM, Snodgrass R. Life span of multipotential hematopoietic stem cells in vivo. J Exp Med 1990; 171:1407–1418.

39. Fraser C, Szilvassy S, Eaves C, Humphries K. Proliferation of totipotent hematopoietic stem cells in vitro with retention of long-term competitive in vivo reconstituting ability. Proc Natl Acad Sci USA 1992; 89:1968–1972.

40. Spangrude GJ, Brooks DM, Tumas DB. Long-term repopulation of irradiated mice with limiting numbers of purified hematopoietic stem cells: in vivo expansion of stem cell phenotype but not function. Blood 1995; 85:1006–1016.

41. Udomsakdi C, Eaves CJ, Sutherland HJ, Lansdorp PM. Separation of functionally distinct subpopulations of primitive human hematopoietic cells using rhodamine-123. Exp Hematol 1991; 19:338–342.

42. Berardi AC, Wang A, Levine JD, Lopez P, Scadden DT. Functional isolation and characterization of human hematopoietic stem cells. Science 1995; 267:104–108.

43. Craig W, Kay R, Cutler RL, Lansdorp PM. Expression of Thy-1 on human hematopoietic progenitor cells. J Exp Med 1993; 177:1331–1342.

44. Mayani H, Lansdorp PM. Thy-1 expression is linked to functional properties of primitive hematopoietic progenitor cells from human umbilical cord blood. Blood 1994; 83:2410–2417.

45. Kawashima I, Zanjani ED, Almeida-Porada G, Flake AW, Zeng H, Ogawa M. CD34-positive

human marrow cells that express low levels of Kit protein are enriched for long-term marrow engrafting cells. Blood 1996; 87:4136–4142.

46. Zanjani ED, Almeida-Porada G, Leary AG, Ogawa M. Human bone marrow CD34⁻ cells engraft in vivo and undergo multilineage expression including giving rise to CD34⁺ cells. Blood 1997; 90:252a.

47. Bhatia M, Bonnet D, Dick JE. Identification of a novel CD34⁻ population of primitive human hematopoietic cells capable of repopulating NOD-SCID mice. Blood 1997; 90:258a.

48. Bonnet D, Bhatia M, Dick JE. Development of conditions for the ex vivo culture of a novel CD34⁻ population of primitive human hematopoietic repopulating cells. Blood 1997; 90:160a.

49. Zanjani ED, Almeida-Porada G, Livingston AG, Zeng HO, Ogawa M. Long-term engrafting capabilities of CD34-negative human adult marrow cells. Blood 1998; 92:504a.

50. Almeida-Porada G, Ogawa M, Oh DJ, Palsson B, Zanjani ED. In vivo and in vitro characterization of human bone marrow CD34⁻ cells. Exp Hematol 1998; 26:749a.

51. Zanjani ED, Almeida-Porada G, Livingston AG, Flake AW, Ogawa M. Human bone marrow CD34⁻ cells engraft in vivo and undergo multilineage expression that includes giving rise to CD34+ cells. Exp Hematol 1998; 26:353–360.

52. Osawa M, Hanada K, Hamada H, Nakauchi H. Long-term lymphohematopoietic reconstitution by a single CD34-low/negative hematopoietic stem cell. Science 1996; 273:242–245.

53. Goodell MA, Brose K, Paradis G, Conner AS, Mulligan RC. Isolation and functional properties of murine hematopoietic stem cells that are replicating in vivo. J Exp Med 1996; 183:1797–1806.

54. Morel F, Galy A, Chen B, Svilvassy SJ. Characterization of CD34 negative hematopoietic stem cells in murine bone marrow. Blood 1996; 88:629a.

55. Johnson RP, Rosenzweig M, Goodell MA, Marks DF, Demania M, Mulligan RC. Isolation of a candidate hematopoietic stem cell population that lacks CD34 in rhesus macaques. Blood 1996; 88:629a.

56. Lansdorp PM, Dragowska W, Mayani H. Ontogeny-related changes in proliferative potential of human hematopoietic cells. J Exp Med 1993; 178:787–791.

57. Lansdorp H. Developmental changes in the function of hematopoietic stem cells. Exp Hematol 1995; 23:187–191.

58. Kamal-Reid S, Dick JE. Engraftment of immune-deficient mice with human hematopoietic stem cells. Science 1988; 242:1706–1709.

59. McCune JM, Namikawa R, Kaneshima H, Shultz LD, Leiberman M, Weissman, IL. The SCID-hu mouse: Murine model for the analysis of human hematolymphoid differentiation and function. Science 1988; 241:1632–1639.

60. Namikawa R, Kaneshima H, Lieberman M, Weissman IL, McCune JM. Infection of the SCID-hu mouse by HIV1. Science 1988; 242:1684–1686.

61. Dick JE. Establishment of assays for human hematopoietic cells in immune deficient mice. Curr Top Microbiol Immunol 1989; 152:219–224.

62. Krams SM, Dorshkind K, Gershwin EM. Generation of biliary lesions after transfer of human lymphocytes into severe combined immunodeficient (SCID) mice. J Exp Med 1989; 170:1919–1930.

63. Cannon MJ, Pisa P, Fox RI, Cooper NR. Epstein Barr virus induces aggressive lymphoproliferative disorders of human B-cell origin in SCID/hu chimeric mice. J Clin Invest 1990; 85:1333–1337.

64. Barry TS, Jones DM, Richter CB, Haynes BF. Successful engraftment of human postnatal thymus in severe combined immune deficient (SCID) mice: Differential engraftment of thymic components with irradiation versus anti-asialo GM-1 immunosuppressive regiments. J Exp Med 1991; 173:167–180.

65. Flake AW, Harrison MR, Zanjani ED. In utero stem cell transplantation. Exp Hematol 1991; 19:1061–1064.

66. Zanjani ED, Ascensao JL, Harrison MR, Tavassoli M. Ex vivo incubation with growth factors

enhances the engraftment of fetal hemopoietic stem cells transplanted in sheep fetuses. Blood 1992; 79:3045–3049.

67. Owen RD. Immunogenetic consequences of vascular anastomoses between bovine twins. Science 1945; 1102:400–401.

68. Billingham R, Brent L, Medawar PB. Actively acquired tolerance of foreign cells. Nature 1953; 172:603–607.

69. Billingham R, Brent L, Medawar PB. Quantitative studies on tissue transplantation immunity. III. Actively acquired tolerance. Phil Trans R Soc (Lond) B 1956; 239:357–369.

70. Cragle R, Stone WH. Preliminary results of kidney grafts between cattle chimeric twins. Transplantation 1967; 5:328–335.

71. Binns R. Bone marrow and lymphoid cell injection of the pig fetus resulting in transplantation tolerance or immunity, and immunoglobulin production. Nature 1969; 214:179–181.

72. Barnes RD, Pottinger BE, Marston J, Flecknell P, Ward RH, Kalter S, Heberling RL. Immunological tolerance induced by in utero injection. J Med Genet 1983; 20:41–45.

73. Marrack P, Lo D, Brinster R, Palmiter R, Burkly L, Flavell RH, Kappler J. The effect of the thymic microenvironment on T-cell development and tolerance. Cell 1988; 53:627–634.

74. Schwartz RH. Aquisition of immunologic self-tolerance. Cell 1989; 57:1073–1081.

75. Adams TE. Tolerance of self-antigens in transgenic mice. Mol Biol Med 1990; 7:341–357.

76. Tavassoli M. Embryonic and fetal hemopoiesis: An overview. Blood Cells 1991; 1:269–281.

77. Zanjani ED, Pallavicini MG, Ascensao JL, Flake AW, Langlois RG, Reitsma M, MacKintosh FR, Stutes D, Harrison MR, Tavassoli M. Engraftment and long term expression of human fetal hematopoietic stem cells in sheep following transplantation in utero. J Clin Invest 1992; 89:1178–1188.

78. Srour EF, Zanjani ED, Brandt JE, Leemhuis T, Briddell RA, Heerema NA, Hoffman R. Sustained human hematopoiesis in sheep transplanted in utero during early gestation with fractioned adult human bone marrow cells. Blood 1992; 79:1410–1412.

79. Zanjani ED, Srour EF, Hoffman R. Retention of long-term repopulating ability of xenogeneic transplanted purified adult human bone marrow hematopoietic stem cells in sheep. J Lab Clin Med 1995; 126:24–28.

80. Flake AW, Hendrick MH, Rice HE, Tavassoli M, Zanjani ED. Enhancement of human hematopoiesis by mast cell growth factor in human-sheep chimeras created by the in utero transplantation of human fetal hematopoietic cells. Exp Hematol 1995; 23:252–257.

81. Zanjani ED, Silva MRG, Flake AW. Retention and multilineage expression of human hematopoietic stem cells in human-sheep chimeras. Blood Cells 1994; 20:331–338.

82. Zanjani ED, Almeida-Porada G, Flake AW. Retention and mulitlineage expression of human hematopoietic stem cells in human-sheep chimeras. Stem Cells 1995; 13:101–111.

83. Zanjani ED, MacKintosh FR, Harrison MR. Hematopoietic chimerism in sheep and non-human primates by in utero transplantation of fetal hematopoietic stem cells. Blood Cells 1991; 17:349–363.

84. Zanjani ED, Ascensao JL, Tavassoli M. Liver-derived fetal hemopoietic stem cells selectively and preferentially home to the fetal bone marrow. Blood 1993; 81:399–404.

85. Zanjani ED, Flake AW, Rice HE, Hedrick MH, Tavassoli M. Long term repopulation ability of xenogeneic transplanted human fetal liver hematopoietic stem cells (HSC) in sheep. J Clin Invest 1994; 93:1051–1055.

86. Almeida-Porada G, Ascensao JL, Zanjani ED. The role of sheep stroma in human haemopoiesis in the human/sheep chimaeras. Br J Haematol 1996; 93:795–802.

87. Almeida-Porada GD, Hoffman R, Ascensao JL, Zanjani ED. Co-transplantation of autologous stromal cells with purified adult human hematopoietic stem cells results in increased engraftment and early donor cell expression in sheep. Blood 1994; 84:253a.

88. Flake AW, Harrison MR, Adzick NS, Zanjani ED. Transplantation of fetal hematopoietic cells in utero: the creation of hematopoietic chimeras. Science 1986; 233:776–778.

89. Crombleholme TM, Harrison MR, Zanjani ED. In utero transplantation of hematopoietic cells in sheep: the role of T cells in engraftment and graft-vs-host disease. J Pediatr Surg 1990; 25:885–892.

90. Srour EF, Zanjani ED, Cornetta K, Traycoff CM, Flake AW, Hedrick M, Brandt JE, Leemhuis T, Hoffman R. Persistence of human multilineage, self renewing lymphohematopoietic stem cells in chimeric sheep. Blood 1993; 82:3333–3342.

91. Murray L, Digiusto D, Chen B, Chen S, Combs J, Conti A, Galy A, Negrin R, Tricot G, Tsukamoto A. Analysis of human hematopoietic stem cell populations. Blood Cells 1994; 20: 364–369.

92. Uchida N, Combs J, Murray L, Conti A, Kholodenko T, Almeida-Porada G, Zanjani ED, Hoffman R, Tsukamoto A. Persistence of human hematopoiesis in sheep transplanted in utero with purified human CD34$^+$Thy-1$^+$Lin$^-$ hematopoietic stem cells. Blood 1994; 84:253a.

93. Sutherland DR, Yeo EL, Stewart K, Nayar R, DiGiusto R, Zanjani E, Hoffman R, Murray LJ. Identification of CD34$^+$ subsets following glycoprotease selection: engraftment of CD34$^+$/Thy1$^+$/Lin$^-$ stem cells in fetal sheep. Exp Hematol 1996; 24:795–806.

94. Henschler R, Brugger W, Luft T, Frey T, Mertelsmann R, Kanz L. Maintenance of transplantation potential in ex vivo expanded CD34$^+$-selected human peripheral blood progenitor cells. Blood 1994; 84:2898–2903.

95. Zanjani ED, Kawashima I, Almeida-Porada GD, Zeng HQ, Leary AG, Flake AW, Ogawa M. Human/sheep hematopoietic chimerism: a relatively specific and sensitive model for the in vivo assay of human hematopoietic stem cells (HSC). Blood 1995; 86:487a.

96. Zanjani ED, Ruthven A, Ruthven J, Shaft D, Smith E, Flake AW. In utero hematopoietic stem cell transplantation results in donor specific tolerance and facilitates post-natal "boosting" of donor cell levels. Blood 1994; 84:100a.

97. Zanjani ED, Lim G, McGlave PB, Clapp JF, Mann LI, Norwood TH, Stamatoyannopoulos G. Adult hematopoietic cells transplanted to sheep fetuses continue to produce adult globins. Nature 1982; 295:244–246.

11

Canine Models for Transplantation and Gene Therapy

HANS-PETER KIEM and RAINER STORB

Fred Hutchinson Cancer Research Center and University of Washington, Seattle, Washington

I. HISTORY OF TRANSPLANTATION

In 1902, Alexis Carrel perfected the technique of vascular anastomosis, and beginning in 1905, he reported the experimental transplantation of limbs, kidneys, and other organs. It quickly became apparent that autografts generally succeeded, and allografts almost always failed. He concluded that it was not possible to transplant tissue from one individual to another of different genetic origin without subsequent rejection. He received the Nobel prize for this work in 1912. It was not until after World War II that a group of biologists and immunologists led by Peter Medawar and Macfarlane Burnet provided the scientific base for graft acceptance and rejection. The observation by Owen (1) that nonidentical cattle twins with natural vascular anastomoses in utero were erythrocyte chimeras was the first evidence that rejection of genetically different cells need not always occur. Medawar and colleagues extended these studies and showed that such cattle were unable to reject one another's skin grafts (2). This indicated that tolerance could be induced in utero and initiated a plethora of investigations to understand the phenomenon of immunological tolerance with the goal to overcome the immunological barrier. In 1955, Main and Prehn were the first to recognize the tolerance inducing ability of bone marrow transplants by showing successful skin allografts after the administration of high-dose irradiation and allogeneic marrow from donors that were syngeneic with the skin graft donors (3).

Experiments in mice showed that shielding of the spleen and infusion of marrow conferred radioprotection in lethally irradiated mice (4–7). Most of these studies were aimed at understanding radiation-induced injuries. Further experiments in the mid-50s established the concept that radiation protection was due to the transfer of living cells and that tolerance of the grafted cells to host tissues had been induced (3,8,9). Inbred mice represented a very useful model for studying the basic biology of hematopoiesis and transplantation biology. However, there are limitations to extrapolating data from mice to humans. Mice are much smaller, have a shorter life span, and therefore there is a limited proliferative demand on the hematopoietic stem cell compartment. This is best illustrated by the fact that a mouse makes as many erythrocytes in its lifetime as a human does in 1 day, a dog in 2.5 days, and a cat in 8 days (10); (and H.-P.K., unpublished observations). In fact, early clinical transplantations demonstrated that much of the information obtained in murine models was difficult to transfer to humans, and almost all initial marrow transplants in humans failed (11). Subsequent work has shown large outbred animals to be more predictive for translations to humans, and results from these studies made it feasible to return to marrow grafting in human patients (12–14). The two main large animal models have been the canine and the nonprimate models. Although nonhuman primates are more closely related to humans, the canine model has a number of advantages over nonhuman primates: lower maintenance cost, large litter size, dogs can be kept disease-free in a suitable colony and are easy to work with, and they are large enough to obtain serial blood and marrow samples and organ biopsies (15). Another attraction of the canine model is the availability of spontaneous malignant and nonmalignant hematological diseases resembling those encountered in humans (16–24). Increased understanding of the canine major histocompatibility complex has further facilitated the use of dogs for allogeneic transplantation (15,25–31). In contrast, the nonhuman primate major histocompatibility complex has not been studied as much, and molecular typing is not readily available.

II. CONDITIONING REGIMENS

A. Total Body Irradiation

The purpose of conditioning regimens is to eradicate the recipient's underlying disease and to suppress the recipient's immune system. Given the background of radiation protection studies described above, it is not surprising that total body irradiation (TBI) was the earliest preparative regimen developed for use in the clinic; it has been the most commonly used conditioning regimen for clinical stem cell transplantation and has remained the most effective single agent (21,32–34). Many of the radiation conditions were first worked out in the dog (35,36). Early studies showed that dogs consistently survived lethal irradiation when given autologous marrow, fresh or cryopreserved (37–39). For allogeneic transplants from dog leukocyte antigen (DLA)–identical littermates, at least 9 Gy was required for stable chimerism and doses in excess of 15 Gy for unrelated dogs (40,41).

To take advantage of a dose response in patients with hematological malignancies and to minimize nonhematological toxicities, fractionated TBI with higher total doses and various dose rates were studied first in the dog. Studies by Bodenberger et al. (42) and Deeg et al. (43) showed that up to 23 Gy TBI could be administered when given in fractions and with low dose rates. Long-term complications were significantly less in dogs given fractionated TBI compared with those given a single exposure. In a recent study, we have investigated variations in TBI dose rates and compared single-dose to fractionated TBI. Most DLA-identical grafts failed to engraft with a single dose of 450 cGy TBI delivered at 7 cGy/min; however, all recipients engrafted when the dose rate was increased to 70 cGy/min. These studies have also shown a much higher rate of graft failure when fractionated TBI was used, suggesting that the immunosuppressive effects of fractionated

TBI are inferior to those of single-dose TBI at comparable total doses of radiation (40,44,45).

B. Chemotherapy

Other conditioning regimens included the cytotoxic drugs cyclophosphamide, procarbazine, and busulfan.

1. Cyclophosphamide

Cyclophosphamide (Cy) was one of the first chemotherapeutic agents explored for use in conditioning regimens in dogs. Storb et al. (46) showed that a dose of 100 mg/kg administered as a single 1-h infusion is lethal to dogs. Dogs can be rescued by autologous or allogeneic marrow transplantation; the latter, however, often showed persisting mixtures of host and donor hematopoietic cells (46).

2. Busulfan

Busulfan is a potent stem cell toxin; however, it is less immunosuppressive than radiation at equitoxic doses. The busulfan derivative dimethylbusulfan was studied extensively in the dog (47). When autologous marrow was administered, dogs were able to survive a single intravenous dose of 10 mg/kg. When DLA-identical littermate marrow was transplanted after a single dose of 10 mg/kg, approximately half the animals showed long-term sustained engraftment; however, marrow grafts were not successful when donors were DLA nonidentical. Graft failure could be prevented by the addition of immunosuppression with antithymocyte serum to the dimethylbusulfan preparative regimen (47,48). Many conditioning regimens today contain busulfan. Unfortunately, the most commonly used oral form has highly variable absorption from individual to individual (49). Recent studies have focused on intravenous administration of busulfan dissolved in dimethylsulfoxide. Consistent and highly reproducible blood levels with this agent have been described in both dogs and macaque monkeys (50,51).

C. Other Agents

1. Antithymocyte Serum

Antithymocyte serum (ATS) has been incorporated into conditioning regimens especially in combination with cytotoxic drugs such as procarbazine and dimethylbusulfan, which are potent myeloablative agents. In these combinations, ATS provides powerful immunosuppression as indicated by the successful engraftment of DLA-identical littermate grafts after conditioning with busulfan (48). ATS was found to provide synergistic immunosuppression when given along with alkylating agents, and the combination overcame transfusion-induced sensitization to marrow grafts (52). That finding led to the currently used Cy/antithymocyte globulin (ATG) regimen for patients with aplastic anemia (53). ATS was also found to be useful for the treatment of established graft-versus-host disease (GVHD) but not as a prophylactic agent (54). These studies provided the basis for the use of antihuman ATS in the clinical treatment of GVHD and as an addition to conditioning regimens (55).

2. Monoclonal Antibodies

We and others have developed monoclonal antibodies against dog antigens to study their role in facilitating engraftment in allogeneic transplantation (56). Studies using a monoclonal antibody S5, directed against CD44 antigen, showed that when the antibody was given pretransplant, it resulted in 75% engraftment of DLA-nonidentical marrow grafts compared to 10% engraftment in dogs given an irrelevant antibody or no antibody at all (57,58). In the mouse, monoclonal antibodies directed against T cells have been shown to facilitate hematopoietic engraftment and the establishment of mixed chimerism when sublethal irradiation was used for conditioning (59–63).

III. STEM CELL SOURCE

Traditionally, marrow has been the source of hematopoietic stem cells (HSCs) for autologous and allogeneic transplantation (64). In recent years, alternative sources of HSCs have been receiving increasing attention. Transplants have been carried out in animal models and humans using fetal liver cells (65), umbilical cord and plecenta-derived cells (66), and peripheral blood–derived cells (64). The presence of stem cells in peripheral blood was described very early by Goodman and Hodgson (67) in the mouse. Similar findings were subsequently also reported in guinea pigs, dogs, and baboons (39,68–73). Owing to the low frequency of circulating stem cells in steady state (74), and concern that peripheral blood stem cells (PBSCs) would not include pluripotent stem cells required for long-term hematopoiesis (75), marrow remained the preferred source for stem cell transplantations through the 1980s. In the 1970s, Richman, et al. (76) and Cline and Golde (77) reported the mobilization of hematopoietic progenitor cells in the peripheral blood in humans. Two important observations followed in the dog, and these were crucial for the Introduction of PBSC transplants in humans. First, in the early 1980s, studies in the dog convincingly demonstrated long-term repopulation by allogeneic cells (78,79). Second, Abrams et al. (80) demonstrated that the infusion of cryopreserved PBSCs mobilized after chemotherapy was able to rescue animals after myeloablative TBI, and several years later, Appelbaum et al. (81) reported the successful transplantation of dogs with lymphoma using leukopheresed PBSCs obtained after combination chemotherapy. The first successful PBSC transplant in humans was reported in 1981 by Korbling et al. in a patient with chronic myelogenous leukemia (82). However, it was not until the advent of growth factors that have the ability to mobilize stem cells into the blood (reviewed in Refs. 83 and 84) that prompted the widespread clinical application of chemotherapy-mobilized autologous PBSCs for autologous transplantation for a variety of malignancies, including lymphoma, acute myelogenous leukemia, and breast and ovarian cancers. We have studied the combination of low-dose recombinant canine stem cell factor (rcSCF) (25 µg/kg/day) and recombinant canine granulocyte colony-stimulating factor (rcG-CSF) (10 µg/kg/day) in the dog. rcG-CSF (10 µg/kg/day) alone for 7 days led to a 5.4-fold increase in colony-forming unit-granulocyte-macrophage (CFU-GM)/mL of blood. The combination of rcG-CSF (10 µg/kg/day) and low-dose rcSCF resulted in a 21.6-fold increase in CFU-GM, a significant difference compared to low-dose rcSCF alone ($P = .03$) (85). The basis for using rcSCF at a dose of 25 µg/kg/day were observations in humans suggesting that this may be the approximate maximum tolerated dose. To study the ability of rcG-CSF and rcSCF to mobilize repopulating cells, 1×10^8 mononuclear cells/kg were collected and cryopreserved from dogs after treatment with G-CSF, SCF, or a combination of the two. None of the control animals engrafted. However, all 15 dogs given PBSCs collected after G-CSF, high-dose SCF, or low-dose SCF in combination with G-CSF engrafted. The mean period to obtain an absolute neutrophil count (ANC) >500 µL was 17 days, 18.8 days, and 13.6 days for dogs receiving either G-CSF, high-dose SCF, or the combination of low-dose SCF and G-CSF, respectively. This study demonstrated that both growth factors were able to mobilize PBSCs. Furthermore, G-CSF and SCF act synergistically in mobilizing PBSCs.

For allogeneic transplantation there was still the concern that the higher number of T cells in peripheral blood would be associated with the increased severity of acute GVHD (7). In humans given buffy coat infusions in addition to the marrow graft (resulting in a 1- to 2-log increase in T-cell content compared to marrow alone), there was no increase in the incidence of acute GVHD, but chronic GVHD was seen significantly more frequently in buffy coat cell recipients (86). Although preliminary clinical phase I/II data suggest that there is no increased evidence of acute GVHD in allogeneic human PBSC transplants, randomized controlled studies are ongoing to determine more definitively the incidence of acute and chronic GVHD, relapse, and survival with PBSCs versus marrow. We have transplanted PBSCs mobilized by rcSCF and rcG-CSF into DLA-identical and haploidentical dogs (87). The incidence and severity of acute GVHD was similar to that expected after marrow grafts.

Owing to the concern of increased GVHD in allogeneic transplants using PBSCs, studies have begun in humans to evaluate the role for T-cell depletion by enriching for CD34$^+$ cells. Since many of these manipulations with stem cells in patients with nonmalignant or currently treatable malignant diseases may raise ethical concerns, animal models continue to be necessary for these studies. The recent cloning of the canine CD34 antigen and the development of antibodies to canine CD34 will allow the study of CD34-enriched stem cell transplants in different donor-recipient settings (88).

IV. INFLUENCE OF TRANSFUSIONS ON ENGRAFTMENT OF ALLOGENEIC STEM CELLS

Sensitization of recipients to minor or major histocompatibility antigens present in the marrow donor can lead to graft failure (40). This is usually the case when recipients receive blood transfusions before transplant but can also be mediated through pregnancy. In contrast to kidney transplantations where prior transfusions are thought to enhance the survival of kidney grafts, we have shown in the dog that preceding blood transfusions may jeopardize engraftment of allogeneic marrow. Marrow rejection was 100% when recipients were given three transfusions of whole blood from DLA-identical littermates (21 of 21 instances) (89). Even with only one transfusion, 73% of dogs rejected their marrow grafts. These results suggested sensitization of recipients to polymorphic minor histocompatibility antigens outside the DLA which were not detected with the commonly used in vitro histocompatibility typing techniques available. The fact that 100% of recipients rejected the graft after three transfusions suggested the involvement of at least two polymorphic histocompatibility systems outside the DLA (90–92), which explains why graft rejection is also observed after transfusions from unrelated donors (93). In that situation, rejection of the marrow graft might be expected only when one or more of the blood transfusion donors and the marrow donor share "minor" antigens not present in the recipient. This was, in fact, seen in our studies. Dogs that received nine preceding blood transfusions from randomly chosen unrelated donors had a 40% rejection rate of marrow from DLA-identical littermates. Marrow graft rejection after transfusions prior to transplantation has also been shown for mice (94) and monkeys (95).

Since these findings had considerable implications for transplantation in humans, subsequent studies in the dog were aimed at preventing or suppressing transfusion-induced sensitization. The use of buffy coat–depleted blood products and the combination of cyclosporine (CSP) and procarbazine/antithymocyte serum before transplant successfully reduced the risk of marrow graft rejection due to transfusion-mediated sensitization (52,96,97). Abrogation of transfusion-mediated sensitization was also accomplished by exposing blood products to ultraviolet light irradiation (98) or gamma irradiation (90–92). A strong correlation between pretransplant transfusions and subsequent rejection of human leukocyte antigen (HLA)–identical marrow has also been shown in patients with aplastic anemia (99–101).

V. GRAFT-VERSUS-HOST DISEASE

The era of prophylaxis for acute graft-versus-host disease (GVHD) began with the studies of Uphoff, who demonstrated that aminopterin in mice receiving allogeneic marrow transplantation decreased the incidence of acute GVHD (102). A basic principle of GVHD prevention is that the method used does not interfere with the marrow graft and cause hematopoietic toxicity. This requirement excluded a number of immunosuppressive agents from clinical use as determined by results in canine studies. For example, cyclophosphamide (103), cytosine arabinoside (104), and procarbazine (104) were marrow toxic when given at doses that promised to be immunosuppressive, thereby causing death of the animals from graft failure. Many other drugs were tested in dogs. Some of these drugs, such as 6-mercaptopurine (104), azathioprine (104), CSP (105), tacrolimus (FK506) (106), deoxyspergualin (107), and corticotropin-releasing factor (108), had good immunosuppressive properties in unrelated DLA-nonidentical recipients and resulted in significantly prolonged survival. However, none of the dogs studied became long-term survivors. An exception was methotrexate (MTX), which resulted in a small number of long-term survivors even though the drug was discontinued after 3 months (109). For MTX to be effective it needed to be given for a certain period of time (approximately 3 months), whereas a shorter course of treatment was only partially effective. The early results in dogs led to application of MTX in humans. Despite MTX, acute GVHD occurred in approximately 35–60% of patients transplanted with marrow from HLA-identical sibling donors (110).

CSP became available in the late 1970s. Studies in the dog indicated synergistic immunosuppression between CSP and MTX when they were administered concurrently (111,112). The combination of MTX and CSP was subsequently introduced clinically and compared to either drug alone in two randomized prospective clinical trials. In both trials, the drug combination resulted in significant reduction of acute GVHD (113,114). Although effective in HLA-identical sibling recipients, the combination was less effective in patients with marrow grafts from HLA-haploidentical related donors or from unrelated donors (115,116). More recently, we have investigated the combination of tacrolimus (FK506) with MTX (106) (Fig. 1). Based on the encouraging preclinical results, clinical trials have begun to compare this combination to the standard MTX/CSP combination (117).

A major problem with the MTX/CSP combination is related to the fact that MTX is renally excreted and CSP often produces renal dysfunction. Because of frequent renal dysfunction, MTX generally cannot be administered beyond day 11 after transplant, and 0.25% of transplanted patients do not receive the day 11 dose (118). We, therefore, investigated the MTX-like antimetabolite trimetrexate, which does not depend on renal excretion but rather is metabolized by the liver (119). Encouraging results in the dog have prompted phase I/II studies in HLA-haploidentical and mismatched for no more than one HLA antigen on the nonshared haplotype (120).

Another agent that has recently been explored in the dog is mycophenolate mofetil

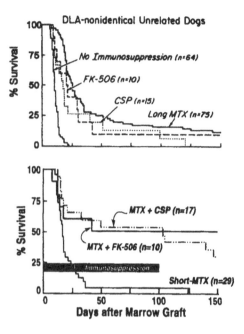

Figure 1 Survival of dogs given 9.2 Gy total body irradiation (TBI) and hematopoietic grafts from dog leukocyte antigen (DLA)–nonidentical unrelated donors. The upper panel shows survival of dogs given no immunosuppression, cyclosporine for the first 100 days, intermittent methotrexate (MTX) for the first 102 days, and FK506 (tacrolimus) for the first 90 days after transplant. The lower panel shows survival of dogs given either a short course of MTX (days 1, 3, 6, and 11), a short course of MTX combined with 100 days of cyclosporine, or a short course of MTX combined with 90 daily doses of FK506 (tacrolimus). (From Ref. 106.)

(MMF). MMF is the 2-(4-morpholino)ethyl ester of mycophenolic acid. It is an immunosuppressive agent that inhibits the production of guanosine nucleotides. We have studied MMF either alone or in combination with CSP for prevention of GVHD in dogs given 9.2 cGy TBI and DLA-nonidentical marrow grafts from unrelated donors. Studies with marrow autografts showed gut toxicity and weight loss to be the limiting side effects of MMF, although hematopoietic engraftment was only slightly delayed. Five dogs received unrelated marrow grafts followed by MMF only given at a dose of 10 mg/kg twice daily (bid) subcutaneously (sc) on days 0–27. These dogs survived significantly better than concurrent and historical control dogs but not significantly different from dogs given CSP alone. Nine dogs were treated with MMF and CSP. All nine dogs engrafted at a rate that was slightly delayed over that of dogs given a standard regimen of MTX/CSP. One dog was euthanized on day 28 because of severe weight loss and two dogs died of infections on days 69 and 97 in the absence of clinical evidence of GVHD. Six dogs were alive between 29 and 92 (median 53) days without evidence of GVHD (121). These results suggested synergism between MMF and CSP with regard to preventing acute GVHD in unrelated DLA-nonidentical marrow graft recipients. Based on these studies in the dog, human studies using MMF for treatment of GVHD have begun.

Studies in the dog showed that there was a quantitative relationship between the number of lymphocytes transplanted and the probability of developing GVHD (34). In our model of DLA-incompatible marrow transplantation from unrelated donors, we gave donor marrow depleted of various lymphocyte subpopulations (122,123); however, most dogs failed to achieve sustained engraftment. Similar results were observed when using L-leucyl-L-leucine methylester (Leu-Leu-OME), a lysosomal tropic agent that selectively kills cytotoxic T cells or other hematopoietic cells. In vitro studies showed that cytotoxic T-lymphocyte responses were completely abrogated with 1000 μM and severe suppression was seen at 250 and 500 μM (124). We then studied whether Leu-Leu-OME would interfere with engraftment of autologous marrow and then in allogeneic transplantation (125). In all donor-recipient settings studied, graft failure was a major problem. Furthermore, all eight dogs that did engraft had fatal GVHD. Overall survival was not improved over controls in DLA-nonidentical recipients and was considerably worse than controls among DLA-identical littermates. SCF did not improve engraftment after Leu-Leu-OME–treated marrow (126). The canine model has been important in developing concepts and approaches for preventing and treating GVHD which have been effective in human marrow transplantation. Many of the drugs that looked promising in inbred murine models were found to be ineffective in dogs and were not introduced clinically (107,108,121,127).

VI. MIXED CHIMERISM STUDIES

In stem cell transplantation, current protocols rely on pretransplant conditioning regimens for suppressing host-versus-graft reactions. Although myeloablative regimens are important for hematological malignancies, this may not be the case for nonmalignant marrow disorders and genetic disorders in which the toxicity of the conditioning regimen is very often responsible for transplant mortality. If engraftment of HSCs could be achieved in these patients without the toxicities of currently applied conditioning regimens, it would be enough to treat many of these disorders. Most preclinical studies involving mixed chimerism have been conducted in inbred mice. The first murine study was reported by Cobbold et al., in 1986, in which pretransplant treatment with anti-CD4 and anti-CD8 monoclonal antibodies were combined with 600 to 850 cGy TBI delivered at 35 cGy/min (59). More recently, investigators have extended these observations and shown mixed chimerism with less TBI and administration of monoclonal antibodies against CD4, CD8, and natural killer (NK) cells before and after transplantation (60,62,128).

We have shown in the dog that postgrafting CSP given for 35 days resulted in the establishment of stable marrow grafts from DLA-identical canine littermates after otherwise suboptimal conditioning with 450 cGy of TBI (129). More recently, we have studied whether sustained allografts could be achieved with a lower dose of TBI. When the TBI dose was lowered to the sublethal range of 200 cGy, CSP alone failed to promote engraftment. All four dogs studied rejected their allografts by 4 weeks but survived with autologous hematopoietic recovery. Next, we combined CSP with the antimetabolite methotrexate given that this drug combination has shown synergism in preventing GVHD in dogs and humans. Three of six dogs became stable mixed chimeras and three rejected their grafts.

We then studied the addition of mycophenolate mofetil, which blocks the de novo purine synthesis pathway by binding to inosine monophosphate dehydrogenase, thereby interfering with lymphocyte proliferation. When MMF was combined with CSP, only 1 of 11 transplanted dogs rejected the allograft at 12 weeks, whereas 10 dogs became stable mixed chimeras for up to 130 weeks after transplant without evidence of GVHD (130,131). These data are summarized in Table 1. Figure 2 illustrates the blood cell changes and the microsatellite marker studies showing mixed chimerism in one of the dogs.

Table 1 Marrow Grafts from DLA-Identical Littermates After Conditioning with Sublethal TBI Delivered at 7 cGy/min or No Conditioning

Group	TBI dose (cGy)	Postgrafting immunosuppression	Recipient no.	Sustained allograft	GVHD		Rejection	Complete autologous recovery	Duration of mixed hematopoietic chimerism by (CA)n dinucleotide repeat marker studies— weeks after marrow graft
					Acute	Chronic			
2	200	MTX[a]/CSP[b]	E126	No	—	—	Yes	Yes	7
			E127	No	—	—	Yes	Yes	2
			E156	No	—	—	Yes	Yes	11
			E157	Yes	No	No	No	No	>8[c]
			E200	Yes	No	No	No	No	>60
			E203	Yes	No	No	No	No	>60
3	200	MMF[d]/CSP[b]	E131	Yes	No	No	No	No	>57[e]
			E219	Yes	No	No	No	No	>54
			E220	Yes	No	No	No	No	>54
			E066	Yes	No	No	No	No	>56
			E069	No	No	No	Yes	Yes	12

DLA, dog leukocyte antigen; TBI, total body irradiation; GVHD, graft-versus-host disease; (CA)n, CA dinucleotide repeats.
[a] MTX, 0.4 mg/kg iv on days 1, 3, 6, and 11.
[b] CSP, 15 mg/kg bid orally on days −1–35.
[c] Dog was euthanized because of massive papillomata on feet related to CSP-induced immunosuppression.
[d] MMF, 10 mg/kg bid sc on days 0–27.
[e] Dog was euthanized at the completion of the study.

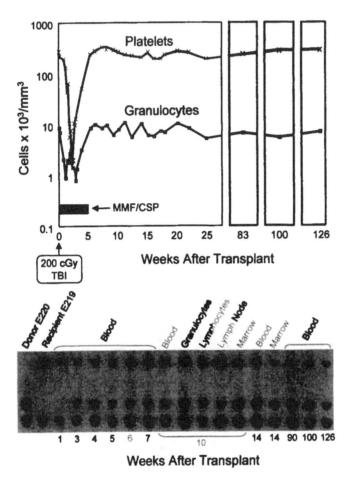

Figure 2 Granulocyte and platelet changes in dog E219 conditioned with 200 cGy TBI, given a marrow graft from a DLA-identical littermate (E220) on day 0, and postgrafting immunosuppression with MMF/CSP for no more than 35 days. The bottom panel shows the results of testing for microsatellite markers of donor and recipient cells before transplantation (lanes 1 and 2) and recipient cells after marrow transplantation (lanes 3–18). (From Ref. 131.)

VII. SECONDARY MALIGNANCIES

There has been great concern about the development of malignant tumors after irradiation in the transplant setting. We have studied the incidence of malignant tumors in marrow grafted dogs. A comparison between radiation chimeras and untreated dogs revealed that dogs receiving TBI as preparation for their transplant had a five times higher incidence of cancer (132). These studies in dogs suggested caution with the use of TBI-based conditioning regimens. A similar correlation between TBI and secondary malignancies has been reported in transplantation in humans, whereas patients with nonmalignant diseases conditioned with cyclophosphamide alone had a significantly lower incidence of secondary cancer (133,134).

VIII. GENE THERAPY

Hematopoietic stem cells are attractive targets for gene therapy, because gene transfer into these cells would presumably lead to the continued presence of the gene in all hematopoietic lineages for the lifetime of the recipient. The accessibility of HSCs in marrow and peripheral blood and the many genetic diseases that could potentially be treated by stem cell gene therapy have provided additional incentives for research in this area.

The use of retroviral vectors is currently the preferred method for gene transfer into HSCs. The ability to integrate genes stably and efficiently into the genome of target cells has not been shown for other gene transfer techniques and is the major advantage of retroviral vectors. Major disadvantages of current retroviral vectors that have mainly derived from murine leukemia viruses include the inability to infect nondividing cells (135) and the requirement for the presence of the appropriate retroviral receptor on the target cell membrane (136). HSCs are, therefore, not ideal targets per se, because they rarely cycle and may express retroviral surface receptors at a low density (137,138). Recently, improved marrow culture conditions and the identification of growth factors that promote the replication of HSCs have increased the gene transfer efficiency into these cells (139,140).

A main obstacle in the development of efficient transduction protocols has been the lack of in vitro assays quantifying transduced stem cells. Although in vitro colony assays have been developed for the quantification of committed and early hematopoietic progenitor cells, none appears directly to assay for the HSC that has self-replication potential. Therefore, the only reliable means of demonstrating stem cell transduction has been proven to be the detection of a vector in mature hematopoietic cells of different lineages after transplantation of stem cells into lethally irradiated recipients. Although much work has been done in inbred strains of mice, we and others chose to work in a large random-bred animal model, the dog, that presents us with problems and issues similar to those encountered in human patients; for example, large size and the limitations imposed by the availability of only a limited number of autologous hematopoietic cells.

A. Retrovirus-Mediated Transduction of Canine Marrow–Derived Stem Cells

Based on observations that gene transduction into canine CFU-GM was increased significantly by combining 24-h cocultivation of marrow on vector-producing cells with 6 days of culture in a vector-containing long-term marrow culture (LTMC) system (141), we tested whether combining cocultivation with LTMC would also lead to the transduction of canine HSCs. In the initial report (142), two different transduction protocols were compared. Retroviral vectors used in both protocols contained the bacterial neomycin phosphotransferase gene (neo) and the human adenosine deaminase gene (*ADA*) gene. In one approach, marrow cells were transduced by 24-h cocultivation on vector-producing cells followed by incubation in a vector-containing LTMC; cells were subsequently infused into dogs after 9.2 Gy TBI. Two of four dogs engrafted, and their marrows showed G418-resistant CFU-GM intermittently after transplant. In a different experimental approach, autologous marrow obtained at the time of peripheral blood neutrophil nadir 7 days after a single dose of Cy (40 mg/kg) was cocultivated for 24 h on vector-producing cells and infused into dogs after 9.2 Gy TBI. One of the three dogs engrafted, showing G418-resistant CFU-GM colonies posttransplant. Culture results were confirmed by polymerase chain reaction (PCR) showing the presence of the *neo* gene in marrow cells, peripheral blood granulocytes, and lymphocytes at low levels (between <0.001 and 0.1%). Both transduction protocols seemed to produce similar results. One dog died 3 years posttransplant of metastatic prostate carcinoma. Two of the dogs were followed for more than 5 years after transplant, and their cells were further analyzed (143). In one of the two dogs, PCR analysis showed the *neo* and *ADA* genes to be present in peripheral blood granulocytes and lymphocytes up to the present time. The estimated percentage of neo-positive cells ranged between <0.001 and 0.1%. Additionally, *ADA* messenger ribonucleic acid (mRNA) expression was detected by reverse transcriptase PCR (RT-PCR) in granulocytes. Studies with cells from the other dog failed to show either persistence or expression of the transduced genes beyond 50 months (Fig. 3). Three additional dogs were transplanted on the same transduction protocols, and persistence of the transduced gene has been documented in peripheral blood myeloid and lymphoid cells along with G418-resistant CFU-GM for more than 2 years. These findings present the longest follow-up of retrovirus-

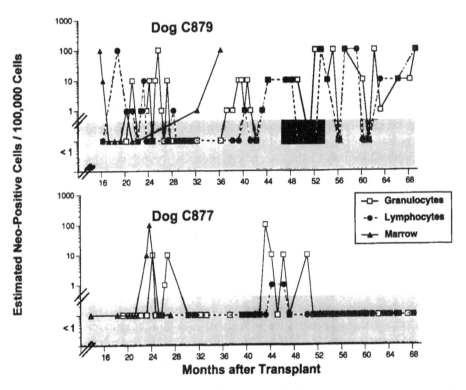

Figure 3 Estimated number of transduced blood and marrow cells present at various timepoints after transplantation of transduced bone marrow cells in two dogs, C877 and C879. Each polymerase chain reaction (PCR) analysis was run with deoxyribonucleic acid (DNA) standards. DNA standards were obtained by making dilutions of DNA from NIH 3T3/LN cells, which contain a single copy of the *neo* gene per cell, with DNA of untransduced dog peripheral blood cells. The intensity of PCR products was compared to the intensity of DNA standards and the number of positive cells was estimated. Assuming that transduced cells contain one copy per cell, the sensitivity of our PCR reaction was 1 copy/cell per 100,000 cells. PCR-negative samples were, therefore, scored <1 cell/copy per 100,000 cells. (From Ref. 143.)

mediated gene transduction in any animal species, although gene transfer rates are very low.

Carter et al. (144) transduced marrow from normal dogs in LTMC by exposing the cells to three supernatant infections with *neo*-containing vector over a 21-day period. No stroma, cocultivation, or growth factors were used. The presence and expression of the *neo* gene was demonstrated in 0.1–1.0% of marrow cells up to 21 months after transplantation. Interestingly, these investigators saw the same degree of engraftment of transduced HSCs regardless of whether transplant recipients were treated with or without myeloablative conditioning. Bienzle et al. (145) updated these results and demonstrated up to 5% G418-resistant hematopoietic progenitors at 24 months after infusion in 2 of 18 dogs receiving transplants without preceding myeloablative conditioning. In most of the animals, however, the percentage of G418-resistant CFU-GM colonies declined to less than 1% by 15 months after infusion of transduced marrow cells. In our experience, myelosuppressive conditioning significantly improved engraftment of genetically marked stem cells.

B. Influence of Different Conditioning Regimens on Engraftment of Genetically Marked Canine Marrow–Derived Stem Cells

Our initial studies using 9.2 Gy TBI were associated with considerable toxicity that would not be acceptable for many clinical applications. We have, therefore, studied the influence of less toxic conditioning regimens on engraftment of transduced stem cells (146). Nineteen dogs received either no conditioning (n = 5), irradiation to both humeri with 10 Gy (n = 4), a sublethal dose of 2 or 3 Gy TBI (n = 3), sublethal dose of Cy (n = 4), or an otherwise lethal dose of 9.2 Gy TBI (n = 3) before administration of transduced autologous hematopoietic cells. Transduction efficiency of hematopoietic cells at the time of infusion into the animals was similar among the different conditioning groups. Dogs were observed for at least 6 months, and peripheral blood granulocytes were examined by PCR for the presence of the transduced gene. Analyzing the percentage of positive PCR results in the different groups showed that engraftment of genetically marked stem cells was significantly improved ($P < .001$) in dogs receiving systemic conditioning with either otherwise lethal TBI, sublethal TBI, or sublethal Cy compared to dogs with local irradiation only or no conditioning. Dogs receiving sublethal Cy, sublethal TBI, or otherwise lethal TBI had comparable engraftment of transduced cells, suggesting that complete myeloablation was not necessary (Fig. 4).

C. Retrovirus-Mediated Transduction of Peripheral Blood–Derived Stem Cells

To study the usefulness of peripheral blood–derived stem cells as target cells for gene transduction and to investigate the contribution of PBSCs to long-term hematopoietic reconstitution after lethal TBI, we transplanted three dogs using genetically marked PBSCs. Dogs were treated with rcSCF for 8 days. Subsequently harvested peripheral blood mononuclear cells were enriched for stem cells with the monoclonal class II antibody 7.2. This antibody has been shown to enrich for hematopoietic repopulating cells in the dog (147,148). The enriched PBSCs were cocultivated for 24 h on irradiated vector-producing packaging cells (PA317/LN, carrying the *neo* gene), followed by an 11-day incubation in a vector-containing LTMC. On the day of transplant, the dogs were irradiated with 9.2 Gy TBI and transduced peripheral blood cells and untransduced cryopreserved marrow cells were infused. Two of three dogs became long-term survivors and were followed for

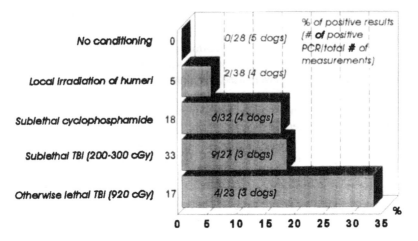

Figure 4 Percentage of polymerase chain reaction (PCR)–positive samples of peripheral blood granulocytes obtained more than 4 weeks after the transplant of transduced hematopoietic cells. Engraftment in dogs that received ''systemic'' conditioning regimens (groups C, D, and E) was significantly better than in dogs receiving ''local'' or no conditioning (groups A and B) ($P < .001$). (From Ref. 146.)

65 and 75 weeks, respectively. Vector-specific sequences were detected by PCR in peripheral blood granulocytes and lymphocytes in both dogs after transplant. Long-term persistence of marked myeloid and lymphoid cells after transplant indicated that the peripheral blood contained repopulating cells that contributed to long-term hematopoietic reconstitution after otherwise lethal TBI.

D. Retrovirus-Mediated Gene Transfer in α-L-Iduronidase–Deficient Dogs

There are many genetic diseases in dogs that resemble diseases in humans. We have chosen canine mucopolysaccharidosis I (MPS I), which has been described in a family of Plott hounds (19) as a model for stem cell gene therapy in genetic diseases. α-L-iduronidase deficiency is a storage disorder affecting the hematopoietic system, and enzyme levels in affected dogs or humans are usually less than 5% of the normal enzyme activity. Affected dogs share many clinical signs with affected humans such as corneal clouding, stunted growth, and joint stiffness. Human MPS I exists as at least three separate syndromes based on clinical severity ranging from Hurler's syndrome (MPS IH), the most severe, to Scheie's syndrome (MPS IS), the mildest. An intermediate form, the Hurler/Scheie form (MPS IHS), appears clinically to be the most analogous to the canine disease. Allogeneic bone marrow transplantation has been reported to improve symptoms in canine MPS I (19). In a collaborative study, six dogs with α-L-iduronidase deficiency were treated with transduced hematopoietic stem cells. Three gene transfer experiments were conducted at the University of Tennessee's College of Veterinary Medicine and one each at the University of Toronto, McMaster University, and the Fred Hutchinson Cancer Research Center. Methods used to treat each of the six dogs were based on experience at each institution with transfer of the *neo* gene into canine marrow (143–145,148). Treatment protocols were well-tolerated by all animals. Leukocyte samples from all six dogs had low (<1%

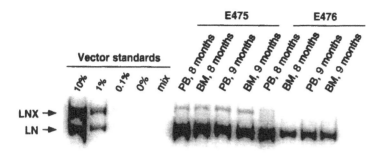

Figure 5 Follow-up of long-term surviving dogs E475 and E476. Detection of vector sequences in PB and BM from dogs transplanted with genetically marked CD34-enriched marrow cells. PCR analysis of amplified vector sequences, LN versus LNX.

of normal) iduronidase activity during the first two months after infusion of transduced cells. Genomic deoxyribonucleic acid (DNA) from leukocytes was generally positive by PCR for the transduced sequences during the period in which enzyme activity was found. By the end of the study, all dogs had been negative by PCR and enzyme assay for between 2 and 9 months. Production of immunoglobulin (IgG) antibody to canine iduronidase was demonstrated in all three dogs tested by enzyme-linked immunosorbent assay (ELISA). These results demonstrated that gene therapy might be further limited by host responses against normal proteins that are introduced to replace the missing proteins that are responsible for the disease state. In this regard, the α-L-iduronidase–deficient dog will be a good model in which to study solutions to this problem.

E. Improved Gene Transfer into Canine Hematopoietic Repopulating Cells

To improve gene transfer efficiency into hematopoietic stem cells, we have used a recently described monoclonal antibody to canine CD34 (149) to enrich for marrow repopulating cells and studied different retroviral pseudotypes for their ability to transduce canine hematopoietic repopulating cells. Cells were divided into two equal fractions that were cocultivated for 72 h with irradiated packaging cells producing vector with different retroviral pseudotypes (GALV, amphotropic, or 10A1). The vectors used contained small sequence differences to allow differentiation of cells genetically marked by the different vectors. Nonadherent and adherent cells from the cultures were infused into four dogs after a myeloablative dose of 920 cGy TBI. PCR analysis of DNA from peripheral blood and marrow posttransplant showed the highest gene transfer rates (up to 10%) were obtained with the GALV–pseudotype vector. Gene transfer levels have remained stable for more than 9 months (Fig. 5). Southern blot analysis confirmed the high gene transfer rate. In summary, our results show that gene transfer into canine hematopoietic repopulating cells is improved using CD34-enriched cells in combination with a GALV–pseudotype vector. Furthermore, these results demonstrate that the monoclonal antibody to canine CD34 used in this study was able to enrich for hematopoietic repopulating cells.

IX. CONCLUSION

A large random-bred animal, the dog, representing an important model for translating preclinical data into clinical trials, strategies for better GVHD prevention, promotion of engraftment across histocompatibility barriers, successful gene transfer, as well as an understanding of the mechanisms of tolerance observed in vivo will be in the center of future research.

ACKNOWLEDGMENTS

The authors thank Harriet Childs and Bonnie Larson for their assistance in preparing the manuscript.

Supported in part by grants CA15704, CA18221, CA78902, CA47748, DK42716, DK47754, DK48265 and HL36444 from the National Institutes of Health, Department of Health and Human Services, Bethesda, MD.

REFERENCES

1. Owen RD. Immunogenetic consequences between vascular anastomoses between bovine twins. Science 1945; 102:400–402.
2. Billingham RE, Brent L, Medawar PB. "Actively acquired tolerance" of foreign cells. Nature 1953; 172:603–606.
3. Main JM, Prehn RT. Successful skin homografts after the administration of high dosage X radiation and homologous bone marrow. J Natl Cancer Inst 1955; 15:1023–1029.
4. Jacobson LO, Marks EK, Robson MJ, Gaston EO, Zirkle RE. Effect of spleen protection on mortality following x-irradiation. J Lab Clin Med 1949; 34:1538–1543.
5. Jacobson LO, Simmons EL, Marks EK, Eldredge JH. Recovery from radiation injury. Science 1951; 113:510–511.
6. Lorenz E, Uphoff D, Reid TR, Shelton E. Modification of irradiation injury in mice and guinea pigs by bone marrow injections. J Natl Cancer Inst 1951; 12:197–201.
7. van Bekkum DW, de Vries MJ. Radiation chimaeras. Radiobiological Institute of the Organisation for Health Research TNO, Rijswijk Z.H. Netherlands, 1967.
8. Ford CE, Hamerton JL, Barnes DWH, Loutit JF. Cytological identification of radiation-chimaeras. Nature 1956; 177:452–454.
9. Nowell PC, Cole LJ, Habermeyer JG, Roan PL. Growth and continued function of rat marrow cells in x-radiated mice. Cancer Res 1956; 16:258–261.
10. Abkowitz JL, Catlin SN, Guttorp P. Evidence that hematopoiesis may be a stochastic process in vivo. Nature Med 1996; 2:190–197.
11. Bortin MM. A compendium of reported human bone marrow transplants. Transplantation 1970; 9:571–587.
12. Crouch BG, van Putten LM, van Bekkum DW, de Vries MJ. Treatment of total-body x-irradiated monkeys with autologous and homologous bone marrow. J Natl Cancer Inst 1961; 27:53–65.
13. Thomas ED, Collins JA, Herman EC Jr., Ferrebee JW. Marrow transplants in lethally irradiated dogs given methotrexate. Blood 1962; 19:217–228.
14. Epstein RB, Thomas ED. Cytogenetic demonstration of permanent tolerance in adult outbred dogs. Transplantation 1967; 5:267–272.
15. Deeg HJ, Storb R. Bone marrow transplantation in dogs. In: Makowka L, Cramer DV, Podesta LG, eds. Handbook of Animal Models in Transplantation Research. Boca Raton, FL: CRC Press, 1994:255–285.
16. Storb R, Marchioro TL, Graham TC, Willemin M, Hougie C, Thomas ED. Canine hemophilia and hemopoietic grafting. Blood 1972; 40:234–238.
17. Weiden PL, Storb R, Deeg HJ, Graham TC, Thomas ED. Prolonged disease-free survival in dogs with lymphoma after total-body irradiation and autologous marrow transplantation

consolidation of combination-chemotherapy-induced remissions. Blood 1979; 54:1039–1049.

18. Appelbaum FR, Deeg HJ, Storb R, Self S, Graham TC, Sale GE, Weiden PL. Marrow transplant studies in dogs with malignant lymphoma. Transplantation 1985; 39:499–504.

19. Shull RM, Hastings NE, Selcer RR, Jones JB, Smith JR, Cullen WC, Constantopoulos G. Bone marrow transplantation in canine mucopolysaccharidosis I: Effects within the central nervous system. J Clin Invest 1987; 79:435–443.

20. Shull RM, Breider MA, Constantopoulos GC. Long-term neurological effects of bone marrow transplantation in a canine lysosomal storage disease. Pediatr Res 1988; 24:347–352.

21. Shull RM, Walker MA. Radiographic findings in a canine model of mucopolysaccharidosis I. Changes associated with bone marrow transplantation. Invest Radiol 1988; 23:124–130.

22. Breider MA, Shull RM, Constantopoulos G. Long-term effects of bone marrow transplantation in dogs with mucopolysaccharidosis I. Am J Pathol 1989; 134:677–692.

23. Storb R, Thomas ED. The scientific foundation of marrow transplantation based on animal studies. In: Forman SJ, Blume KG, Thomas ED, eds. Bone Marrow Transplantation. Boston, MA: Blackwell, 1994:3–11.

24. Whitney KM, Goodman SA, Bailey EM, Lothrop CD Jr. The molecular basis of canine pyruvate kinase deficiency. Exp Hematol 1994; 22:866–874.

25. Raff RF, Deeg HJ, Farewell VT, DeRose S, Storb R. The canine major histocompatibility complex. Population study of DLA-D alleles using a panel of homozygous typing cells. Tissue Antigens 1983; 21:360–373.

26. Bull RW, Vriesendorp HM, Cech R, Grosse-Wilde H, Bijma AM, Ladiges WL, Krumbacher K, Doxiadis I, Ejima H, Templeton J, Albert ED, Storb R, Deeg HJ. Joint Report of the Third International Workshop on Canine Immunogenetics. II. Analysis of the serological typing of cells. Transplantation 1987; 43:154–161.

27. Sarmiento UM, DeRose S, Sarmiento JI, Storb R. Allelic variation in the DQ subregion of the canine major histocompatibility complex: I. DQA. Immunogenetics 1992; 35:416–420.

28. Wagner JL, DeRose SA, Burnett RC, Storb R. Brief communication: nucleotide sequence and polymorphism analysis of canine DRA cDNA clones. Tissue Antigens 1995; 45:284–287.

29. Wagner JL, Burnett RC, DeRose SA, Storb R. Molecular analysis and polymorphism of the DLA-DQA gene. Tissue Antigens 1996; 48:199–204.

30. Wagner JL, Burnett RC, Storb R. Molecular analysis of the DLA DR region. Tissue Antigens 1996; 48:549–553.

31. Wagner JL, Burnett RC, Works JD, Storb R. Molecular analysis of DLA-DRBB1 polymorphism. Tissue Antigens 1996; 48:554–561.

32. Thomas ED, Lochte HL Jr, Lu WC, Ferrebee JW. Intravenous infusion of bone marrow in patients receiving radiation and chemotherapy. N Engl J Med 1957; 257:491–496.

33. Vriesendorp HM, Klapwijk WM, van Kessel AMC, Zurcher C, van Bekkum DW. Lasting engraftment of histoincompatible bone marrow cells in dogs. Transplantation 1981; 31:347–352.

34. Vriesendorp HM, Klapwijk WM, Hogeweg B, Zurcher C, van Bekkum DW. Factors controlling the engraftment of transplanted dog bone marrow cells. Tissue Antigens 1982; 20:63–80.

35. Thomas ED, Ashley CA, Lochte HL Jr, Jaretzki A III, Sahler OD, Ferrebee JW. Homografts of bone marrow in dogs after lethal total-body radiation. Blood 1959; 14:720–736.

36. Thomas ED, LeBlond R, Graham T, Storb R. Marrow infusions in dogs given midlethal or lethal irradiation. Radiat Res 1970; 41:113–124.

37. Mannick JA, Lochte HL Jr., Ashley CA, Thomas ED, Ferrebee JW. Autografts of bone marrow in dogs after lethal total-body radiation. Blood 1960; 15:255–266.

38. Cavins JA, Kasakura S, Thomas ED, Ferrebee JW. Recovery of lethally irradiated dogs following infusion of autologous marrow stored at low temperature in dimethyl-sulphoxide. Blood 1962; 20:730–734.

39. Cavins JA, Scheer SC, Thomas ED, Ferrebee JW. The recovery of lethally irradiated dogs given infusions of autologous leukocytes preserved at −80°C. Blood 1964; 23:38–43.

40. Storb R, Deeg HJ. Failure of allogeneic canine marrow grafts after total body irradiation: allogeneic "resistance" vs transfusion induced sensitization. Transplantation 1986; 42:571–580.

41. Storb R, Raff RF, Appelbaum FR, Schuening FW, Sandmaier BM, Graham TC, Thomas ED. What radiation dose for DLA-identical canine marrow grafts? Blood 1988; 72:1300–1304.

42. Bodenberger U, Kolb HJ, Rieder I, Netzel B, Schäffer E, Kolb H, Thierfelder S. Fractionated total body irradiation and autologous bone marrow transplantation in dogs: hemopoietic recovery after various marrow cell doses. Exp Hematol 1980; 8:384–394.

43. Deeg HJ, Storb R, Longton G, Graham TC, Shulman HM, Appelbaum F, Thomas ED. Single dose or fractionated total body irradiation and autologous marrow transplantation in dogs: effects of exposure rate, fraction size and fractionation interval on acute and delayed toxicity. Int J Radiat Oncol Biol Phys 1988; 15:647–653.

44. Storb R, Raff RF, Appelbaum FR, Graham TC, Schuening FG, Sale G, Pepe M. Comparison of fractionated to single-dose total body irradiation in conditioning canine littermates for DLA-identical marrow grafts. Blood 1989; 74:1139–1143.

45. Storb R, Raff RF, Appelbaum FR, Deeg HJ, Graham TC, Schuening FG, Sale G, Bryant E, Seidel K. Fractionated versus single-dose total body irradiation at low and high dose rates to condition canine littermates for DLA-identical marrow grafts. Blood 1994; 83:3384–3389.

46. Storb R, Epstein RB, Rudolph RH, Thomas ED. Allogeneic canine bone marrow transplantation following cyclophosphamide. Transplantation 1969; 7:378–386.

47. Kolb HJ, Storb R, Weiden PL, Ochs HD, Kolb H, Graham TC, Floersheim GL, Thomas ED. Immunologic, toxicologic and marrow transplantation studies in dogs given dimethyl myleran. Biomedicine 1974; 20:341–351.

48. Storb R, Weiden PL, Graham TC, Lerner KG, Nelson N, Thomas ED. Hemopoietic grafts between DLA-identical canine littermates following dimethyl myleran. Evidence for resistance to grafts not associated with DLA and abrogated by antithymocyte serum. Transplantation 1977; 24:349–357.

49. Grochow LB, Jones RJ, Brundrett RB, Braine HG, Chen T-L, Saral R, Santos GW, Colvin OM. Pharmacokinetics of busulfan: correlation with veno-occlusive disease in patients undergoing bone marrow transplantation. Cancer Chemother Pharmacol 1989; 25:55–61.

50. Dix SP, Bucur SZ, Mullins RE, McCulloch W, Thomas GR, Hillyer CD, McClure HM, Strobert EA, Orkin JL, Winton EF. Studies of the pharmacokinetics and toxicity of once daily bolus intravenous busulfan in non-human primates. Blood 1995; 86(suppl 1):225a.

51. Ehninger G, Schuler U, Renner U, Ehrsam M, Zeller KP, Blanz J, Storb R, Deeg HJ. Use of a water-soluble busulfan formulation—pharmacokinetic studies in a canine model. Blood 1995; 85:3247–3249.

52. Storb R, Floersheim GL, Weiden PL, Graham TC, Kolb H-J, Lerner KG, Schroeder M-L, Thomas ED. Effect of prior blood transfusions on marrow grafts: abrogation of sensitization by procarbazine and antithymocyte serum. J Immunol 1974; 112:1508–1516.

53. Storb R, Etzioni R, Anasetti C, Appelbaum FR, Buckner CD, Bensinger W, Bryant E, Clift R, Deeg HJ, Doney K, Flowers M, Hansen J, Martin P, Pepe M, Sale G, Sanders J, Singer J, Sullivan KM, Thomas ED, Witherspoon RP. Cyclophosphamide combined with antithymocyte globulin in preparation for allogeneic marrow transplants in patients with aplastic anemia. Blood 1994; 84:941–949.

54. Storb R, Kolb HJ, Graham TC, Kolb H, Weiden PL, Thomas ED. Treatment of established graft-versus-host disease in dogs by antithymocyte serum or prednisone. Blood 1973; 42:601–609.

55. Storb R, Gluckman E, Thomas ED, Buckner CD, Clift RA, Fefer A, Glucksberg H, Graham

TC, Johnson FL, Lerner KG, Neiman PE, Ochs H. Treatment of established human graft-versus-host disease by antithymocyte globulin. Blood 1974; 44:57–75.

56. Ladiges W, Deeg HJ, Aprile J, Raff R, Schuening F, Storb R. Differentiation and function of lymphohemopoietic cells in the dog. In: Trnka Z, Miyasaka M, eds. Differentiation Antigens in Lymphohemopoietic Tissues. New York: Marcel Dekker, 1988:307–335.

57. Schuening F, Storb R, Goehle S, Meyer J, Graham TC, Deeg HJ, Appelbaum FR, Sale GE, Graf L, Loughran TP Jr. Facilitation of engraftment of DLA-nonidentical marrow by treatment of recipients with monoclonal antibody directed against marrow cells surviving radiation. Transplantation 1987; 44:607–613.

58. Sandmaier BM, Storb R, Appelbaum FR, Gallatin WM. An antibody that facilitates hematopoietic engraftment recognizes CD44. Blood 1990; 76:630–635.

59. Cobbold SP, Martin G, Qin S, Waldmann H. Monoclonal antibodies to promote marrow engraftment and tissue graft tolerance. Nature 1986; 323:164–166.

60. Sharabi Y, Abraham VS, Sykes M, Sachs DH. Mixed allogeneic chimeras prepared by a non-myeloablative regimen: requirement for chimerism to maintain tolerance. Bone Marrow Transplant 1992; 9:191–197.

61. Colson YL, Wren SM, Schuchert MJ, Patrene KD, Johnson PC, Boggs SS, Ildstad ST. A nonlethal conditioning approach to achieve durable multilineage mixed chimerism and tolerance across major, minor, and hematopoietic histocompatibility barriers. J Immunol 1995; 155:4179–4188.

62. Tomita Y, Khan A, Sykes M. Mechanism by which additional monoclonal antibody (mAB) injections overcome the requirement for thymic irradiation to achieve mixed chimerism in mice receiving bone marrow transplantation after conditioning with anti-T cell mABs and 3-Gy whole body irradiation. Transplantation 1996; 61:477–485.

63. Tomita Y, Sachs DH, Khan A, Sykes M. Additional monoclonal antibody (mAB) injections can replace thymic irradiation to allow induction of mixed chimerism and tolerance in mice receiving bone marrow transplantation after conditioning with anti-T cell mABs and 3-Gy whole body irradiation. Transplantation 1996; 61:469–477.

64. Thomas ED Sr. Stem cell transplantation: past, present and future. Stem Cells 1994; 12:539–544.

65. Ikuta K, Komagata Y. Developmental potential of fetal hematopoietic stem cells. In: Levitt D, Mertelsmann R, eds. Hematopoietic Stem Cells: Biology and Therapeutic Applications. New York: Marcel Dekker, 1995:69–83.

66. Broxmeyer HE, Lu L, Gaddy J, Ruggieri L, Srivastava A, Risdon G. Human umbilical cord blood transplantation: the immunology, expansion, and therapeutic applications of hematopoietic stem and progenitor cells. In: Levitt D, Mertelsmann R, eds. Hematopoietic Stem Cells: Biology and Therapeutic Applications. New York: Marcel Dekker, 1995:297–317.

67. Goodman JW, Hodgson GS. Evidence for stem cells in the peripheral blood of mice. Blood 1962; 19:702–714.

68. Epstein RB, Graham TC, Buckner CD, Bryant J, Thomas ED. Allogeneic marrow engraftment by cross circulation in lethally irradiated dogs. Blood 1966; 28:692–707.

69. Storb R, Epstein RB, Ragde H, Thomas ED. Marrow engraftment by allogeneic leukocytes in lethally irradiated dogs. Blood 1967; 30:805–811.

70. Storb R, Epstein RB, Thomas ED. Marrow repopulating ability of peripheral blood cells compared to thoracic duct cells. Blood 1968; 32:662–667.

71. Storb R, Buckner CD, Epstein RB, Graham T, Thomas ED. Clinical and hematologic effects of cross circulation in baboons. Transfusion 1969; 9:23–31.

72. Storb R, Graham TC, Epstein RB, Sale GE, Thomas ED. Demonstration of hemopoietic stem cells in the peripheral blood of baboons by cross circulation. Blood 1977; 50:537–542.

73. Malnin TI, Perry VP, Kerby CC, Dolan MF. Peripheral leukocyte infusion into lethally irradiated guinea pigs. Blood 1996; 25:693–702.

74. Trobaugh FE Jr, Lewis JP. Repopulating potential of blood and marrow. J Clin Invest 1964; 43:1306.

75. Micklem HS, Anderson N, Ross E. Limited potential of circulating haemopoietic stem cells. Nature 1975; 256:41–43.

76. Richman CM, Weiner RS, Yankee RA. Increase in circulating stem cells following chemotherapy in man. Blood 1976; 47:1031–1039.

77. Cline MJ, Golde DW. Mobilisation of hematopoietic stem cells (CFU-C) into the peripheral blood of man by endotoxin. Exp Hematol 1977; 5:186.

78. Körbling M, Fliedner TM, Calvo W, Ross WM, Nothdurft W, Steinbach I. Albumin density gradient purification of canine hemopoietic blood stem cells (HBSC): long-term allogeneic engraftment without GVH-reaction. Exp Hematol 1979; 7:277–288.

79. Carbonell F, Calvo W, Fliedner TM, Kratt E, Gerhartz H, Körbling M, Nothdurft W, Ross WM. Cytogenetic studies in dogs after total body irradiation and allogeneic transfusion with cryopreserved blood mononuclear cells: observations in long-term chimeras. Int J Cell Cloning 1984; 2:81–88.

80. Abrams RA, McCormack K, Bowles C, Deisseroth AB. Cyclophosphamide treatment expands the circulating hematopoietic stem cell pool in dogs. J Clin Invest 1981; 67:1392–1399.

81. Appelbaum FR, Deeg HJ, Storb R, Graham TC, Charrier K, Bensinger W. Cure of malignant lymphoma in dogs with peripheral blood stem cell transplantation. Transplantation 1986; 42: 19–22.

82. Korbling M, Burke P, Braine H, Elfenbein G, Santos GW, Kaizer H. Successful engraftment of blood-derived normal hemopoietic stem cells in chronic myelogenous leukemia. Exp Hematol 1981; 9:684–690.

83. Demirer T, Buckner CD, Bensinger WI. Optimization of peripheral blood stem cell mobilization (concise review). Stem Cells 1996; 14:106–116.

84. Georges GE, Sandmaier BM, Storb R. Animal models. In: Reiffers J, Goldman J, Armitage J, eds. Blood Stem Cell Transplantation. London: Martin Dunitz, 1998:1–17.

85. de Revel T, Appelbaum FR, Storb R, Schuening F, Nash R, Deeg J, McNiece I, Andrews R, Graham T. Effects of granulocyte colony stimulating factor and stem cell factor, alone and in combination, on the mobilization of peripheral blood cells that engraft lethally irradiated dogs. Blood 1994; 83:3795–3799.

86. Storb R, Prentice RL, Sullivan KM, Shulman HM, Deeg HJ, Doney KC, Buckner CD, Clift RA, Witherspoon RP, Appelbaum FR, Sanders JE, Stewart PS, Thomas ED. Predictive factors in chronic graft-versus-host disease in patients with aplastic anemia treated by marrow transplantation from HLA-identical siblings. Ann Intern Med 1983; 98:461–466.

87. Sandmaier BM, Storb R, Santos EB, Krizanac-Bengez L, Lian T, McSweeney PA, Yu C, Schuening FG, Deeg HJ, Graham T. Allogeneic transplants of canine peripheral blood stem cells mobilized by recombinant canine hematopoietic growth factors. Blood 1996; 87:3508–3513.

88. McSweeney PA, Rouleau KA, Storb R, Bolles L, Wallace PM, Beauchamp M, Krizanac-Bengez L, Moore P, Sale G, Sandmaier B, de Revel T, Appelbaum FR, Nash RA. Canine CD34: Cloning of the cDNA and evaluation of an antiserum to recombinant protein. Blood 1996; 88:1992–2003.

89. Storb R, Weiden PL, Deeg HJ, Graham TC, Atkinson K, Slichter SJ, Thomas ED. Rejection of marrow from DLA-identical canine littermates given transfusions before grafting: antigens involved are expressed on leukocytes and skin epithelial cells but not on platelets and red blood cells. Blood 1979; 54:477–484.

90. Bean MA, Storb R, Graham T, Raff R, Sale GE, Schuening F, Appelbaum FR. Prevention of transfusion-induced sensitization to minor histocompatibility antigens on DLA-identical canine marrow grafts by gamma irradiation of marrow donor blood. Transplantation 1991; 52:956–960.

91. Bean MA, Graham T, Appelbaum FR, Deeg HJ, Schuening F, Sale GE, Storb R. Gamma-

irradiation of pretransplant blood transfusions from unrelated donors prevents sensitization to minor histocompatibility antigens on dog leukocyte antigen-identical canine marrow grafts. Transplantation 1994; 57:423–426.

92. Bean MA, Graham T, Appelbaum FR, Deeg HJ, Schuening F, Sale GE, Leisenring W, Pepe M, Storb R. Gamma radiation of blood products prevents rejection of subsequent DLA-identical marrow grafts: Tolerance vs. abrogation of sensitization to non-DLA antigens. Transplantation 1996; 61:334–335.

93. Storb R, Rudolph RH, Graham TC, Thomas ED. The influence of transfusions from unrelated donors upon marrow grafts between histocompatible canine siblings. J Immunol 1971; 107:409–413.

94. Santos GW, Sensenbrenner LL. A sensitive and quantitative assay for non–H-2 histocompatibility antigens. Exp Hematol 1971; 21:19–20.

95. van Putten LM, van Bekkum DW, de Vries MJ, Balner H. The effect of preceding blood transfusions on the fate of homologous bone marrow grafts in lethally irradiated monkeys. Blood 1967; 30:749–757.

96. Weiden PL, Storb R, Slichter S, Warren RP, Sale GE. Effect of six weekly transfusions on canine marrow grafts: Tests for sensitization and abrogation of sensitization by procarbazine and antithymocyte serum. J Immunol 1976; 117:143–150.

97. Storb R, Deeg HJ, Atkinson K, Weiden PL, Sale G, Colby R, Thomas ED. Cyclosporin-A abrogates transfusion-induced sensitization and prevents marrow graft rejection in DLA-identical canine littermates. Blood 1982; 60:524–526.

98. Deeg HJ, Aprile J, Graham TC, Appelbaum FR, Storb R. Ultraviolet irradiation of blood prevents transfusion-induced sensitization and marrow graft rejection in dogs. Concise Report. Blood 1986; 67:537–539.

99. Storb R, Prentice RL, Thomas ED. Marrow transplantation for treatment of aplastic anemia. An analysis of factors associated with graft rejection. N Engl J Med 1977; 296:61–66.

100. Storb R, Thomas ED, Buckner CD, Clift RA, Deeg HJ, Fefer A, Goodell BW, Sale GE, Sanders JE, Singer J, Stewart P, Weiden PL. Marrow transplantation in thirty "untransfused" patients with severe aplastic anemia. Ann Intern Med 1980; 92:30–36.

101. Storb R, Prentice RL, Thomas ED, Appelbaum FR, Deeg HJ, Doney K, Fefer A, Goodell BW, Mickelson E, Stewart P, Sullivan KM, Witherspoon RP. Factors associated with graft rejection after HLA-identical marrow transplantation for aplastic anaemia. Br J Haematol 1983; 55:573–585.

102. Uphoff DE. Alteration of homograft reaction by A-methopterin in lethally irradiated mice treated with homologous marrow. Proc Soc Exp Biol Med 1958; 99:651–653.

103. Storb R, Graham TC, Shiurba R, Thomas ED. Treatment of canine graft-versus-host disease with methotrexate and cyclophosphamide following bone marrow transplantation from histoincompatible donors. Transplantation 1970; 10:165–172.

104. Storb R, Kolb HJ, Deeg HJ, Weiden PL, Appelbaum F, Graham TC, Thomas ED. Prevention of graft-versus-host disease by immunosuppressive agents after transplantation of DLA-nonidentical canine marrow. Bone Marrow Transplant 1986; 1:167–177.

105. Deeg HJ, Storb R. Experimental marrow transplantation. In: White DJG, ed. Cyclosporin A. Proceedings of an International Conference on Cyclosporin A. Amsterdam: Elsevier, 1982:121–134.

106. Storb R, Raff RF, Appelbaum FR, Deeg HJ, Fitzsimmons W, Graham TC, Pepe M, Pettinger M, Sale G, Van Der Jagt R, Schuening FG. FK506 and methotrexate prevent graft-versus-host disease in dogs given 9.2 Gy total body irradiation and marrow grafts from unrelated DLA-nonidentical donors. Transplantation 1993; 56:800–807.

107. Raff RF, Storb R, Graham T, Deeg HJ, Pepe M, Schaffer R, Sale GE, Schuening F, Appelbaum FR. What role for 15-deoxyspergualin in enhancing engraftment of unrelated, histoincompatible canine marrow grafts and preventing graft-versus-host disease? Transplantation 1993; 55:684–688.

108. Yu C, Storb R, Braude I, Deeg HJ, Schuening FG, Huss R, Graham TC. Corticotropin releasing factor with or without methotrexate for prevention of graft-versus-host disease in DLA-nonidentical unrelated canine marrow grafts. Transplantation 1995; 60:384–404.

109. Storb R, Epstein RB, Graham TC, Thomas ED. Methotrexate regimens for control of graft-versus-host disease in dogs with allogeneic marrow grafts. Transplantation 1970; 9:240–246.

110. Storb R, Prentice RL, Buckner CD, Clift RA, Appelbaum F, Deeg J, Doney K, Hansen JA, Mason M, Sanders JE, Singer J, Sullivan KM, Witherspoon RP, Thomas ED. Graft-versus-host disease and survival in patients with aplastic anemia treated by marrow grafts from HLA-identical siblings. Beneficial effect of a protective environment. N Engl J Med 1983; 308:302–307.

111. Deeg HJ, Storb R, Weiden PL, Raff RF, Sale GE, Atkinson K, Graham TC, Thomas ED. Cyclosporin A and methotrexate in canine marrow transplantation: engraftment, graft-versus-host disease, and induction of tolerance. Transplantation 1982; 34:30–35.

112. Deeg HJ, Storb R, Appelbaum FR, Kennedy MS, Graham TC, Thomas ED. Combined immunosuppression with cyclosporine and methotrexate in dogs given bone marrow grafts from DLA-haploidentical littermates. Transplantation 1984; 37:62–65.

113. Storb R, Deeg HJ, Farewell V, Doney K, Appelbaum F, Beatty P, Bensinger W, Buckner CD, Clift R, Hansen J, Hill R, Longton G, Lum L, Martin P, McGuffin R, Sanders J, Singer J, Stewart P, Sullivan K, Witherspoon R, Thomas ED. Marrow transplantation for severe aplastic anemia: methotrexate alone compared with a combination of methotrexate and cyclosporine for prevention of acute graft-versus-host disease. Blood 1986; 68:119–125.

114. Storb R, Deeg HJ, Whitehead J, Appelbaum F, Beatty P, Bensinger W, Buckner CD, Clift R, Doney K, Farewell V, Hansen J, Hill R, Lum L, Martin P, McGuffin R, Sanders J, Stewart P, Sullivan K, Witherspoon R, Yee G, Thomas ED. Methotrexate and cyclosporine compared with cyclosporine alone for prophylaxis of acute graft versus host disease after marrow transplantation for leukemia. N Engl J Med 1986; 314:729–735.

115. Beatty PG, Anasetti C, Hansen JA, Longton GM, Sanders JE, Martin PJ, Mickelson EM, Choo SY, Petersdorf EW, Pepe MS, Appelbaum FR, Bearman SI, Buckner CD, Clift RA, Petersen FB, Singer J, Stewart PS, Storb RF, Sullivan KM, Tesler MC, Witherspoon RP, Thomas ED. Marrow transplantation from unrelated donors for treatment of hematologic malignancies: effect of mismatching for one HLA locus. Blood 1993; 81:249–253.

116. Anasetti C, Hansen JA, Waldmann TA, Appelbaum FR, Davis J, Deeg HJ, Doney K, Martin PJ, Nash R, Storb R, Sullivan KM, Witherspoon RP, Binger M-H, Chizzonite R, Hakimi J, Mould D, Satoh H, Light SE. Treatment of acute graft-versus-host disease with humanized anti-Tac: an antibody that binds to the interleukin-2 receptor. Blood 1994; 84:1320–1327.

117. Nash RA, Pineiro LA, Storb R, Deeg HJ, Fitzsimmons WE, Furlong T, Hansen JA, Gooley T, Maher RM, Martin P, McSweeney PA, Sullivan KM, Anasetti C, Fay JW. FK506 in combination with methotrexate for the prevention of graft-versus-host disease after marrow transplantation from matched unrelated donors. Blood 1996; 88:3634–3641.

118. Nash RA, Pepe MS, Storb R, Longton G, Pettinger M, Anasetti C, Appelbaum FR, Bowden R, Deeg HJ, Doney K, Martin PJ, Sullivan KM, Sanders J, Witherspoon RP. Acute graft-versus-host disease: analysis of risk factors after allogeneic marrow transplantation and prophylaxis with cyclosporine and methotrexate. Blood 1992; 80:1838–1845.

119. Appelbaum FR, Raff RF, Storb R, Deeg HJ, Graham TC, Sandmaier B, Schuening F. Use of trimetrexate for the prevention of graft-versus-host disease. Bone Marrow Transplant 1989; 4:421–424.

120. Doney KC, Storb R, Beach K, Anasetti C, Deeg HJ, Hansen JA, Martin PJ, Nash RA, Schubert MM, Sullivan KM, Witherspoon RP, Appelbaum FR. A toxicity study of trimetrexate used in combination with cyclosporine as acute graft-versus-host disease prophylaxis in HLA-mismatched, related donor bone marrow transplants. Transplantation 1995; 60:55–58.

121. Yu C, Storb R, Deeg HJ, Schuening FG, Nash RA, Graham T. Synergism between mycophe-

nolate mofetil and cyclosporine in preventing graft-versus-host disease in lethally irradiated dogs given DLA-nonidentical unrelated marrow grafts. Blood 1995; 86(suppl 1):577a.

122. Wulff JC, Deeg H-J, Storb R. A monoclonal antibody (DT-2) recognizing canine T lymphocytes. Transplantation 1982; 33:616–620.

123. Wulff JC, Durkopp N, Aprile J, Tsoi M-S, Springmeyer SC, Deeg HJ, Storb R. Two monoclonal antibodies (DLy-1 and DLy-6) directed against canine lymphocytes. Exp Hematol 1982; 10:609–619.

124. Raff RF, Severns E, Storb R, Martin P, Graham T, Sandmaier B, Schuening F, Sale G, Appelbaum FR. L-Leucyl-L-Leucine methyl ester treatment of canine marrow and peripheral blood cells: inhibition of proliferative responses with maintenance of the capacity for autologous marrow engraftment. Transplantation 1988; 46:655–660.

125. Raff RF, Severns EM, Storb R, Graham TC, Sale G, Schuening FG, Appelbaum FR. Studies of the use of L-leucyl-L-leucine methyl ester in canine allogeneic marrow transplantation. Transplantation 1993; 55:1244–1249.

126. Kiem H-P, Leisenring W, Raff R, Deeg HJ, Schuening FG, Appelbaum FR, Storb R. Failure of recombinant stem cell factor to enhance engraftment of L-leucyl-L-leucine methyl ester treated canine marrow after irradiation (letter to editor). Blood 1996; 88:1896–1897.

127. Yu C, Storb R, Deeg HJ, Fitzsimmons WE, Sale G. Glucocorticoids failed to enhance the effect of FK506 and methotrexate (MTX) on prevention of graft-versus-host disease (GVHD) after DLA-nonidentical unrelated canine marrow transplantation. Blood 1996; 88:232a.

128. Lee LA, Sergio JJ, Sykes M. Natural killer cells weakly resist engraftment of allogeneic, long-term, multilineage-repopulating hematopoietic stem cells. Transplantation 1996; 61: 125–132.

129. Yu C, Storb R, Mathey B, Deeg HJ, Schuening FG, Graham TC, Seidel K, Burnett R, Wagner JL, Shulman H, Sandmaier BM. DLA-identical bone marrow grafts after low-dose total body irradiation: effects of high-dose corticosteroids and cyclosporine on engraftment. Blood 1995; 86:4376–4381.

130. Storb R, Yu C, Wagner JL, Deeg HJ, Nash RA, Kiem H-P, Leisenring W, Shulman H. Stable mixed hematopoietic chimerism in DLA-identical littermate dogs given sublethal total body irradiation before and pharmacological immunosuppression after marrow transplantation. Blood 1997; 89:3048–3054.

131. Storb R, Yu C, McSweeney P, Nash R, Sandmaier B, Wagner J, Woolfrey A. New strategies for hematopoietic stem cell transplantation. In: Proceedings of the Symposium on Transplantation in Hematology and Oncology, May 10–12, 1998, Münster, Germany, Springer-Verlag, 1998.

132. Deeg HJ, Prentice R, Fritz TE, Sale GE, Lombard LS, Thomas ED, Storb R. Increased incidence of malignant tumors in dogs after total body irradiation and marrow transplantation. Int J Radiat Oncol Biol Phys 1983; 9:1505–1511.

133. Witherspoon RP, Deeg HJ, Storb R. Secondary malignancies after marrow transplantation for leukemia or aplastic anemia. Transplant Sci 1994; 4:33–41.

134. Deeg HJ, Socié G, Schoch G, Henry-Amar M, Witherspoon RP, Devergie A, Sullivan KM, Gluckman E, Storb R. Malignancies after marrow transplantation for aplastic anemia and Fanconi anemia: a joint Seattle and Paris analysis of results in 700 patients. Blood 1996; 87:386–392.

135. Miller DG, Adam MA, Miller AD. Gene transfer by retrovirus vectors occurs only in cells that are actively replicating at the time of infection. Mol Cell Biol 1990; 10:4239–4242.

136. Miller DG, Miller AD. A family of retroviruses that utilize related phosphate transporters for cell entry. J Virol 1994; 68:8270–8276.

137. Kavanaugh MP, Miller DG, Zhang W, Law W, Kozak SL, Kabat D, Miller AD. Cell-surface receptors for gibbon ape leukemia virus and amphotropic murine retrovirus are inducible sodium-dependent phosphate symporters. Proc Natl Acad Sci USA 1994; 91:7071–7075.

138. von Kalle C, Kiem H-P, Goehle S, Darovsky B, Heimfeld S, Torok-Storb B, Storb R, Schuen-

ing FG. Increased gene transfer into human hematopoietic progenitor cells by extended in vitro exposure to a pseudotyped retroviral vector. Blood 1994; 84:2890–2897.

139. Crooks GM, Kohn DB. Growth factors increase amphotropic retrovirus binding to human CD34+ bone marrow progenitor cells. Blood 1993; 82:3290–3297.

140. Nolta JA, Smogorzewska EM, Kohn DB. Analysis of optimal conditions for retroviral-mediated transduction of primitive human hematopoietic cells. Blood 1995; 86:101–110.

141. Schuening FG, Storb R, Stead RB, Goehle S, Nash R, Miller AD. Improved retroviral transfer of genes into canine hematopoietic progenitor cells kept in long-term marrow culture. Blood 1989; 74:152–155.

142. Schuening FG, Kawahara K, Miller DA, To R, Goehle S, Stewart D, Mullally K, Fisher L, Graham TC, Appelbaum FR, Hackman R, Osborne WRA, Storb R. Retrovirus-mediated gene transduction into long-term repopulating marrow cells of dogs. Blood 1991; 78:2568–2576.

143. Kiem H-P, Darovsky B, von Kalle C, Goehle S, Graham T, Miller AD, Storb R, Schuening FG. Long-term persistence of canine hematopoietic cells genetically marked by retrovirus vectors. Hum Gene Ther 1996; 7:89–96.

144. Carter RF, Abrams-Ogg AC, Dick JE, Kruth SA, Valli VE, Kamel-Reid S, Dube ID. Autologous transplantation of canine long-term marrow culture cells genetically marked by retroviral vectors. Blood 1992; 79:356–364.

145. Bienzle D, Abrams-Ogg AC, Kruth SA, Ackland-Snow J, Carter RF, Dick JE, Jacobs RM, Kamel-Reid S, Dube ID. Gene transfer into hematopoietic stem cells: long-term maintenance of in vitro activated progenitors without marrow ablation. Proc Natl Acad Sci USA 1994; 91:350–354.

146. Barquinero J, Kiem H-P, von Kalle C, Darovsky B, Goehle S, Graham T, Seidel K, Storb R, Schuening FG. Myelosuppressive conditioning improves autologous engraftment of genetically marked hematopoietic repopulating cells in dogs. Blood 1995; 85:1195–1201.

147. Schuening F, Storb R, Goehle S, Meyer J, Graham T, Deeg HJ, Pesando J. Canine pluripotent hemopoietic stem cells and CFU-GM express Ia-like antigens as recognized by two different class-II specific monoclonal antibodies. Blood 1987; 69:165–172.

148. Kiem H-P, Darovsky B, von Kalle C, Goehle S, Stewart D, Graham T, Hackman R, Appelbaum FR, Deeg HJ, Miller AD, Storb R, Schuening FG. Retrovirus-mediated gene transduction into canine peripheral blood repopulating cells. Blood 1994; 83:1467–1473.

149. McSweeney PA, Rouleau KA, Wallace PM, Bruno B, Andrews RG, Krizanac-Bengez L, Sandmaier BM, Storb R, Wayner E, Nash RA. Characterization of monoclonal antibodies that recognize canine CD34. Blood 1998; 91:1977–1986.

12

Murine Model of In Utero Transplantation

EWA CARRIER

University of California, San Diego, La Jolla, California

I. INTRODUCTION

A. Rationale

To date, 21 in utero transplants have been reported in humans, 4 of which have been successful, all in immunodeficiency disorders (1–3). Despite this limited initial clinical success in humans, the clinical applications of this procedure are likely going to increase. Although many congenital diseases can be cured by postnatal bone marrow transplantation, there are serious limitations associated with its use (4–8). Allogeneic bone marrow transplantation requires ablation and immunosuppression, which may lead to high-risk, frequently life threatening infections. For many congenital disorders, for which damage occurs in utero, postnatal transplants are frequently too late (4–6). Additionally, there is only ~25% chance that a specific patient will have a HLA-matched sibling donor. Even with a matched sibling donor, the risk of graft-versus-host disease (GVHD) is high and is associated with significant mortality and morbidity (9–14). The early gestational fetus is immunologically immature and therefore susceptible to the development of tolerance to specific antigens during its ontogeny. Immunosuppression and myeloablation may not be necessary and therefore alleviate the toxicity and cost of this procedure as compared to the postnatal transplants. If paternal cytokine-stimulated peripheral blood stem cells were to be used, this would provide an unlimited source of donor cells for prenatal transplants and postnatal boosts in tolerant recipients.

B. Clinical Experience

In utero transplantation is becoming an accepted treatment modality in humans. Recent reports demonstrated successful immune reconstitution in patients with severe combined immunodeficiency disease (SCID). To date, 21 in utero transplants have been reported in humans, 4 of which have been successful for immunodeficiency disease (SCID) (1,2) and bare lymphocyte syndrome (3). However, the in utero transplants for β-thalassemia and inborn errors of metabolism were not successful, and no evidence of long-term engraftment nor correction of hemolytic anemia was demonstrated (15–21). This difference in outcome in hosts with defective and normal immune systems suggests the role of immune system in the outcome of in utero transplantation. The up-to-date experience of in utero transplantation in humans is shown in Table 1.

C. Fetal Hematopoiesis

Fetal hematopoiesis starts in the yolk sac, proceeds to fetal liver, and toward the end of pregnancy takes place in the bone marrow (22–26). This migration of the site of hematopoiesis most probably happens due to the upregulation/dowregulation of homing receptors/ligands. In humans, osteoblasts appear at ~10 weeks of gestation and stromal elements at 12 weeks. The first hematopoietic elements from the fetal liver appear at ~15 weeks of gestation, and the process of establishing hematopoiesis in the bone marrow is not finished until 34 weeks of gestation (22,23). Therefore, during the fetal life, there is a "window of opportunity" when bone marrow "niches" are created, but not occupied, by hematopoietic elements. This window of opportunity may allow early engraftment of incoming donor stem cells. The period of fetal development is also associated with the developing, incompetent immune system, which can further increase the chances of allogeneic cells to engraft. Therefore, transplantation of allogeneic donor cells during this time of fetal ontogeny may be performed without immunosuppression or ablation. This is the rationale for in utero transplantation. However, the low degree of engraftment (percentage of donor cells) observed in large and small animal models as well as in humans indicate that there are additional mechanisms that operate during homing and engraftment of allogeneic donor cells. One possible limiting factor may be the difference in the affinity of donor and host cells, allowing preferential engraftment of host cells.

Quesenberry et al. demonstrated engraftment of syngeneic cells achieved by injecting high doses of donor cells over several consecutive days in nonmyeloablated hosts (27,28). The levels of engraftment were higher in mice injected with many doses over consecutive days rather than with one large dose, suggesting that a certain percentage of bone marrow niches are open at any given time. Therefore, when available niches are saturated, any additional injections of cells may not increase engraftment. Further studies are needed to identify the best conditions necessary for high degrees of engraftment after in utero transplantation.

D. Questions for Future Research

The following questions/problems should be addressed in future research:

1. Optimal number and sources of donor cells
2. Precise timing at which donor cells should be injected prenatally for specific congenital disorders
3. Route of prenatal transplants
4. Use of in vivo and in vitro cytokines
5. Tolerance/immunity induced by in utero transplantation

Table 1 Existing Experience of In Utero Transplantation in Humans

Disease	Stem cell source	Gestational age (weeks)	Outcome	Reference
Bare lymphocyte syndrome	FL and thymus	28	Clinically normal requires monthly IVIG.	5
SCID	FL and thymus	26	Alive, engrafted.	6
SCID	Maternal TCD BM	19	Pregnancy terminated at 24 weeks.	7
X-linked SCID	Paternal CD34-enriched BM	16	Alive, with immune function.	1
X-linked SCID	Paternal CD34-enriched BM	20	Alive, mixed chimera.	2
β-Thalassemia major	FL	12	No evidence of engraftment.	7
β-Thalassemia major	FL	19	In utero death following the procedure.	7
β-Thalassemia	Sibling bone marrow (TCD)	25	No evidence of engraftment.	8
β-Thalassemia	Cryopreserved FL	18	No evidence of engraftment.	4
Chédiak-Higashi disease	Maternal TCD bone marrow	26	No evidence of engraftment.	7
GCL	Paternal CD34-enriched BM	13	Extensive donor cell infiltration, death at 20 weeks.	9
α-Thalassemia	Cryopreserved FL	18	No engraftment.	4
α-Thalassemia	Maternal TCD BM		Electively terminated pregnancy at 24 weeks; evidence of donor cells in extramedullary sites.	7

BM, bone marrow; FL, fetal lines; GCL, globoid cell leukodystrophy; TCD, T-cell depleted.

6. Utility and optimal schedule of postnatal boosts with donor cells in tolerant and/or mixed chimeras

In this chapter, we will review existing mouse models of in utero transplantations and discuss directions for future research.

II. ANIMAL MODELS

A. Large Animal Models

1. Monkey Model

To study the feasibility of in utero transplantation in humans, a primate model was developed (29–32). Roodman et al. reported transient low-level chimerism in baboons transplanted in utero with mismatched adult male bone marrow, which was not detectable at birth (29). In contrast, more permanent engraftment was documented with the use of fetal liver as a hematopoietic stem cell (HSC) source, as reported by Harrison et al. (30). Interestingly, transplanted donor cells were fully integrated into the host hematopoiesis, and they responded to hypoxic stress similarly to host cells, as reported by Duncan et al. (32). Generally, only low degrees of engraftment in this model (<0.1%) were demonstrated as well as partial tolerance to donor kidneys (33). Additionally, Rodman et al. showed that the baboon fetuses that engrafted reacted significantly more strongly to their donors than to a pool of unrelated controls in mixed lymphocyte culture (MLC) test postnatally (24). This finding was suggestive of active immunity rather than tolerance and could explain a transient and low degree of engraftment found in this system.

2. Sheep Model

Zanjani et al. showed that human fetal and adult stem cells are capable of engraftment in fetal sheep (34–45). The sheep is particularly tolerant to prenatal manipulations. Owing to its large size and long gestation (145 days), transplants are technically feasible at a relatively early stage of gestational development, as early as 45 days of gestation for intraperitoneal and 60 days for intravenous, which is well within the time of preimmune ontogeny. This model was used to determine the optimal recipient age, route of donor cell administration, and optimal sources of HSCs. Although the sheep is a good model to study human hematopoiesis in vivo, there are few sheep that have manifestations of diseases in humans that can be curable by the in utero transplantation. In contrast, mice are highly useful for studying the effect of in utero transplantation on specific disease models.

A number of mice strains have been identified or developed that have well-defined, naturally occurring identified disorders, including the hematopoietic (46), immune (47), or enzymatic diseases (48). Mice can be altered by recombinant DNA technology and new disease models representing genetic disorders in humans can be established.

III. MURINE MODELS OF IN UTERO TRANSPLANTATION

The following mice models of in utero transplantation have been developed to date:

1. *Anemic*: W^v, W^{41}, β-thalassemic
2. *SCID*:C57BL/6 Sz-scid/scid, NOD/SCID

3. *Xenogeneic*: human–mouse
4. *Metabolic disorders*: MPS VII
5. *Nonanemic mouse model*

A. Anemic Models

1. W^v Mouse Model

The first in utero transplants in this model were performed by Fleischman et al. (49–51). W^v fetal mice were used as recipients, in which macrocytic anemia exists and is most severe in W/W and progressively less severe in W/W^v, W^v/W^v, W/W^f, and W^v/+. The last combination is nonanemic. Genetically anemic recipients were used in order to favor proliferation of nonanemic donor cells. Fetal or adult stem cells from nonanemic donors were injected transplacentally at 13–15 days' gestation (counting the vaginal plug date as day 0). The overall survival was 73%. Engraftment was performed by starch gel electrophoresis separation of strain-specific variants of glucose phosphate isomerase (GPI). Preliminary trails demonstrated that microinjection of normal fetal hematopoietic stem cells into W-series genetically anemic fetuses resulted in rapid and complete substitution of normal erythroid cells and prevention of anemia. The use of the severely anemic W/W recipient was clearly essential to the most rapid and extensive establishment of donor cells colonization and amplification; there were no detectable donor red blood cells (RBCs) in W/+, W^v/+, or +/+ littermates. *This work indicated that fetal hematopoiesis is very active and may prevent successful donor cells engraftment unless conditions for preferential donor cells expression can be established.* It also showed that adult bone marrow contains cells that are capable of proliferating and developing in the fetal environment with a sustained capacity for long-term self-renewal and differentiation into myeloid and lymphoid lineages. The self-renewal capacity of bone marrow cells was decreased as compared to the fetal liver cells.

Howson-Jan et al. investigated the effects of donor strain differences, cell dose, and the number of injections on murine fetal survival and engraftment of congenic marrow into nonanemic and anemic, stem cell–defective W^v/W^v recipients (52). In a series of experiments, 1221 nonanemic C57Bl/6 fetuses were injected transplacentally on day 11 of gestation with 10^6 non–T-cell–depleted adult bone marrow cells from C57Bl/6-CAST (congenic), BALB/c, and DBA/1 (allogeneic) strains without any ablation or immunosuppression. The overall survival rate was 45% and the engraftment rate was 4% in day 5 newborns. Interestingly, a higher incidence of engraftment in allogeneic (5.2%) versus congenic fetal recipients (0.7%) was demonstrated. This engraftment persisted ≥ 6 weeks, increasing in the degree over time. Neither doubling the cell dose nor doubling the number of injections improved engraftment rates in recipients of allogeneic bone marrow. Pretreatment of congenic donors with 5-fluorouracil 4 days prior to harvesting marrow was not effective in increasing engraftment. In contrast, engraftment of congenic marrow into anemic stem cell defective W^v/W^v recipients led to a higher incidence (40%) of engraftment that persisted for ≥ 6 weeks, increasing in the level of engraftment over time. Despite the lack of persisting engraftment of allogeneic cells beyond 6 weeks, 2 of 10 evaluable recipients engrafted with DBA/1 bone marrow cells accepted donor skin grafts with rejection of third party skin grafts. *These studies demonstrated the preferential engraftment and expression of donor cells in hosts with defective hematopoiesis. The low degree of engraftment was correlated with the low rate of tolerance.*

2. W⁴¹ Mouse Model

W⁴¹/W⁴¹ moderately anemic mice were used by Blazar et al. (53), which have different mutation in c-*kit*, than Wᵛ/Wᵛ mice. C57B1/6-W⁴¹/W⁴¹ mice were used as recipients of in utero transplants. These mice have mild anemia, and fertility is not compromised, which is in contrast with nonfertile W/W, W/Wᵛ, or Wᵛ/Wᵛ mice. Two types of C57BL/6 congenic mice were backcloned and intercrossed to obtain homozygous donors expressing both the Ly5 allele and the glucose-phosphate isomerase (GPI) allele. C57B1/6-Ly5.1, GPI-1ᵇ recipients were transplanted with congenic donor bone marrow Ly5.2/GPI-1ᵃ cells and were monitored for erythroid engraftment by the GPI allele as early as day 5. All fetuses were transplanted intraperitoneally. Fifty percent of live-born animals were long-term ($\geq$ 141 days) multilineage chimeras. During the time of injection, extramedullary hematopoiesis (liver/spleen) was present, but transplanted bone marrow cells were found in both extramedullary and intramedullary sites. Adult bone marrow from nondefective recipients was used for intraperitoneal injections in 13–14 fetal recipients. The reported survival rate was 47%. GPI typing and flow cytometry were used for engraftment detection. Multilineage engraftment in T (57–71%), B (10–20%), myeloid cells (27–43%), and erythroid cells (50–70%) was demonstrated. Transplantation of bone marrow from chimeric animals into lethally irradiated secondary recipients resulted in long-term multilineage engraftment, confirming that pluripotent HSCs were engrafted. By secondary transfer studies, the estimation was that the true HSC engraftment level was 10–16%, which is consistent with the proportion of donor cells comprising the B cell (10%) or granulocyte (26%) but not the T cell (42%). This lineage-restricted reconstitution could parallel those typically observed in lymphoid deficiency states such as severe combined immunodeficiency syndrome in children who experience preferential T-cell, but not B-cell, engraftment. *These studies, by serial transfer, showed that true HSCs are engraftable in utero in moderately anemic mice when injected intraperitoneally at midgestation with nonenriched adult bone marrow (BM) progenitor cells.*

3. β-Thalassemic Mouse Model

Postnatal allogeneic cell transplantation is the only curative therapy for homozygous β-thalassemia (54,55), but this procedure is associated with significant morbidity and mortality, which is not acceptable to many physicians and families. The β-thalassemic (C57BL/6-Hbbᵈ³ᵗʰ/H-2kᵇ) mouse was shown to be a good model of human β-thalassemia. Donahue et al. described engraftment in β-thalassemic mice following in utero transplantation with BALB/c (H-2kᵃ) fetal liver cells (56). Increased survival from 10 to 20% after in utero transplantation was observed, demonstrating that correction of anemia in utero increases fetal survival. In 16% of animals, hemoglobin electrophoresis showed 5% of donor cells, which was also detected by mass spectrometry showing α and β major globins of donor type. The improvement of osmotic fragility, reticulocyte count, and hematocrit were observed and indicated that even a low degree of engraftment can improve hematological parameters. Archer et al. demonstrated engraftment of allogeneic purified bone marrow (C.C3/H-2k) cells, which were injected prenatally into C57B1/6 Hbdᵈ³ᵗʰ/th-1 or C57B1/6 Hbbᵗᵐ/ᵘⁿᶜ, th-2/H-2kᵇ) recipients (57). Engraftment was found in the peripheral blood of either moderately (th-2/+) or severely (th-1/th-1) affected mice that persisted for at least 24 weeks. As in the previous experiment, the percentage of donor cells decreased over time. Chimeric animals which received postnatal boosts (transplants without conditioning) of 1 × 10⁶ lineage-depleted donor allogeneic cells at 8-week intervals showed an increase in donor hemoglobin > 40%. This approach indicated the possibility of tolerance induction by prenatal allogeneic cell transplantation with an increase of engraftment with postnatal boosts.

B. SCID Mouse Model

1. C57BL/6 Sz-scid/scid

To determine whether the in utero transplantation could restore the immune system in mice, the SCID model was established (58,59). C57B1/6 Sz-scid/scid fetuses were injected with adult allogeneic bone marrow cells on day 14-15 of gestation and engraftment was tested by GPI and flow cytometry (FACs). Reconstitution of both lymphoid and myeloid lineages was observed and recovery of T-cell function was demonstrated. Pluripotent stem cell engraftment was documented by postnatal transplants with bone marrow of chimeric animals into secondary, lethally irradiated recipients. Twenty-eight percent of recipients (15/54) had evidence of up to 76% of donor cells in peripheral blood (PB) on day 13 postnatally. T- and B-lymphoid cells were entirely of donor origin. *These findings supported the success of in utero transplants in human SCID patients (1–3), in whom T- and/or B-cell reconstitution was documented.*

2. NOD/SCID

Although high levels of donor-derived hematopoiesis have been reported in the SCID model, the majority of chimeric mice exhibited decreasing levels of donor cells over time. To test directly whether the natural killer cells and macrophage activity of the recipients represent a barrier to sustained engraftment, Archer et al. (59) used fetal NOD/SCID mice for injections with an enriched congenic hematopoietic progenitor cell population. The mean number of donor-derived nucleated cells in the peripheral blood was 30%. The majority of circulating donor cells were lymphocytes; up to 15% of cells expressed myelo-monocyte markers. Serial engraftment studies indicated that the percentage of circulating donor cells increased from 17 to 55% between 4 and 24 weeks. Secondary transplants into irradiated congenic recipients demonstrated multilineage donor-derived hematopoiesis up to 6 months posttransplants. This work demonstrated that in utero transplantation of lineage depleted BM cells into fetal NOD/SCID mice results in sustained engraftment of allogeneic cells.

C. Xenogeneic Mouse Model

Xenogeneic mouse models were developed to study in vivo human hematopoiesis. Pallavicini et al. (60) documented a very low (10^{-5}, 10^{-6}) degree of human fetal liver cells engraftment following in utero transplantation in W^v anemic mice. Chimerism was observed in approximately 50% of live-born mice at 5–6 months of age. Human cells were detected in spleen, marrow, thymus, and blood. Engraftment was seen frequently in marrow and spleen and rarely in peripheral blood. Animals carrying human cells in the spleen and marrow also contained human cells in their thymuses. These data were compatible with current theories of tolerance induction, and they suggested that the presence of human cells in the thymic epithelium may be important for both the induction and maintenance of tolerance. Pixley et al. described the rates and the degrees of engraftment in human → mouse xenogeneic model (61). Mixed chimerism with human cells was demonstrated in 29% of 38 live-born mice at 16 weeks of age with the following frequencies: 14% peripheral blood, 8% bone marrow, 8% spleen, 12% thymus. These frequencies were much higher than those previously reported by Pallavicini and could be related to the differences of the techniques used for engraftment detection (PCR vs FACs). *These data demonstrated the utility of xenogeneic transplants in fetal recipients, although further studies are needed to determine the strategies necessary for higher degrees of tolerance and engraftment.*

D. Mucopolysaccharidosis Murine Model of In Utero Transplantation

A stem cell–deficient MPS VII mouse model (W^{41}/W^{41}) MPS VII of in utero transplantation was developed by Soper et al. (62). Mucopolysaccharidosis type VII (MPS VII) belongs to a large family of human heritable lysosomal storage diseases. The MPS VII mouse model for the human disease lacks the enzyme β-glucuronidase (B-GUS), accumulates glycosaminoglycans (GAGs) in the lysosomes, and dies prematurely. The disease in mice and humans is chronic and progressive and is characterized by dwarfism, skeletal abnormalities, and learning disabilities. Purified stem cells of normal congenic recipients were injected prenatally into the W^{41}/W^{41}, gus^{mps}/gus^{mps} recipients. Eighty to 90% donor RBCs population was shown at 30 weeks of age, and multilineage donor cell engraftment was detected (14–30% of donor cells in the liver, 59–100% in the spleen, 2–5% in the kidneys, 8–27% in the lungs). Recipients of 500 enriched cells showed 45–50% donor repopulation at 6 weeks and 80–90% at 30 weeks. Hosts of 35 enriched cells (Sca-1/^{high}/c-kit^{low}) had over 45% donor cell replacement by 14 weeks that subsequently decreased ≤ 25% by 21 weeks. The combinational procedure of greatly enriched population of stem cells showed that they are capable of long-term engraftment of both lymphoid and myeloid lineages and that these cells were therapeutic to MPS VII mice.

1. MPS VII Gene Therapy Murine Model

Sands et al. (63) developed a mouse model for prenatal gene therapy. The MPS VII mouse lacks the enzyme B-GUS and accumulates GAGs in the lysosomes and dies prematurely. The disease is characterized by progressive degenerative syndrome, mucopolysaccharidosis (MPS) type VII (Sly disease), which includes mental retardation. Animal homologues of MPS VII are models for testing somatic gene transfer approaches to treat the central nervous system in this and other lysosomal storage disorders. An in vitro model for cross correction of lysosomal storage disorders from genetically modified cells was developed to approximate the physiological conditions needed for gene therapy in vivo. Gene transfer by retroviral vectors encoding rat or human B-GUS corrected the enzymatic deficiency in cultured MPS VII fibroblasts from humans, dogs, and mice. The vector-transduced cells released β-glucuronidase into the cultured supernatant in an amount proportional to the amounts of cellular enzyme activity. The retrovirus-mediated gene therapy directed to the hematopoietic system or to artificial neo-organs resulted in low levels of enzyme in several tissues and reduced lysosomal storage in the liver and spleen. Partial correction of the disease in the eye was observed following an intra-arterial injection of recombinant adenosines. Neither retrovirus- nor adenovirus-mediated gene transfer resulted in a systemic reduction of lysosomal storage. These attempts to correct murine MPS by gene therapy have successfully treated lesions in some organs but not in the brain. Many diseases affecting the central nervous system are refractory to treatment, because the blood-brain barrier restricts entry of therapeutic molecules. One possible approach is a neural stem cell–based strategy. Multipotent neural progenitors or stem cells are capable of differentiating along multiple central nervous system cell–type lineages. They are capable of engrafting in normal structures throughout the host central nervous system without disturbing neurobiological processes. Therefore, these cells used as vehicles for gene transfer may overcome many of the limitations of nonneural cellular vectors for which the brain-blood barrier exists.

Snyder et al. (64) reported that by transplanting β-glucuronidase–expressing neural progenitors into the cerebral ventricles of newborn donor cells engrafted throughout the entire neuraxis. β-Glucuronidase activity was expressed along the entire neuraxis, resulting in widespread correction of lysosomal storage in neurons and glia in affected mice. This interesting approach of transplanting neural progenitors that intrinsically secrete a missing or therapeutic gene may provide a strategy for the long-term treatment of central nervous system manifestations of a number of neurogenetic diseases.

E. Nondefective Mice Model of In Utero Transplantation

1. Introduction

Kim et al. (65) described chimerism and tolerance in C57B1/6 → BALB/c mouse model. A dose of 10^{10} BM cells/kg was injected intraperitoneally into recipient animals. Peripheral blood of animals which survived beyond 3 weeks of age was analyzed by polymerase chain reaction (PCR) for the presence of donor major histocompatibility (MHC) class I DNA. Tolerance was tested by placement of donor-specific skin grafts after determination of the chimeric status. Of 49 animals injected in utero, 19 (38%) had donor DNA present in the peripheral blood at low levels (<0.1%), whereas only 1 of 18 neonatally injected animals had detectable donor cells. Tolerance to donor-specific skin grafts was found in 6 of 9 animals which were chimeric after in utero HSC transplantation, whereas none of the 18 neonatally injected animals, including the chimeric animals, was tolerant.

Hajdu et al. (66) studied microchimerism in a similar nondefective BALBc → C57B1/6 strain combination. In 9 of 162 surviving recipients (5.6%), cells of donor origin were detected after birth. The highest degree of engraftment was achieved by transplanting of high doses >10^6 cells/fetal gram of fetal liver cells. Only mice with detected chimerism accepted donor skin grafts, whereas rejecting third-party C3H skin grafts.

Carrier et al. (67,68) described engraftment efficiency and tolerance following in utero transplantation with allogeneic fetal liver, bone marrow, and c-kit$^+$ cells in nonanemic BALB/c recipients. The scheme of this model is shown in Figure 1. Previous experiments documented high engraftment rates in defective mice, such as W^v, W^{41}, or SCID, in which the preferential engraftment for stem cells or committed progenitors exists. The nonanemic recipients were chosen to observe the extent of engraftment, kinetics of host/donor cells in chimeric animals, and tolerance to allogeneic donor cells in recipients with a normal immune system. *This model should therefore identify difficulties with engraftment that exist in diseases such as inborn errors of metabolism or β-thalassemia and develop strategies necessary to overcome them.*

The low degree of engraftment in this system was anticipated, and therefore quantitative PCR assay with the sensitivity of 0.0001% was utilized to detect Y chromosomes of male donors in female recipients (69,70). The technique of in utero transplantation was improved, and in utero surgeries could be performed at early gestational ages (11–13 days), when the immunoincompetence of the fetus could potentially permit higher degrees of engraftment. The example of the PCR sample in the engrafted fetal liver recipient showing changes in the percentage of donor cells and the response to a postnatal boost with donor cells is shown in Figure 2.

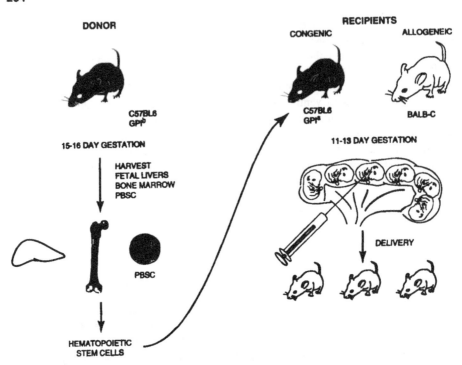

Figure 1 Mouse Model of in utero hematopoietic stem cell transplantation. Donor C57BL/6 fetal liver, bone marrow, and peripheral blood stem cells (PBSCs) are transplanted into 11- to 13-day-old C57BL/6 congenic (GPIa) or allogeneic BALB/c fetuses. Engraftment studies are performed by glucose phosphate isomerase (GPI) assay, polymerase chain reaction (PCR), and FACs analysis. Tolerance is tested postnatally by donor skin graft acceptance, cytotoxicity, mixed lymphocyte culture (MLC), and postnatal boosts with allogeneic cells.

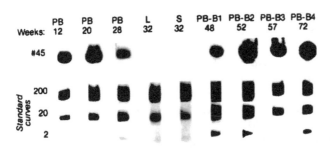

Figure 2 Engraftment in PB/tissues in mouse #45 by PCR, including boosts. Engraftment studies in the blood and tissues were performed by PCR with the sensitivity of 0.00001%. Each sample has a separate standard cure. Postnatal boosts were performed at 44 weeks of age and blood samples were drawn for engraftment studies at 48, 52, 57, and 72 weeks of age. An increasing percentage of donor cells was demonstrated.

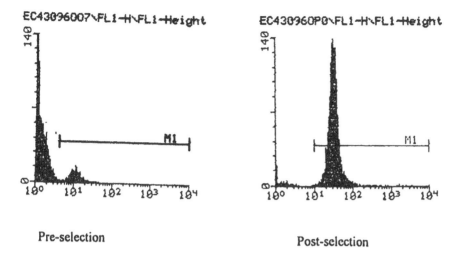

Pre-selection   Post-selection

Figure 3 Purification of c-kit$^+$ cells. Splenectomized donor C57Bl/6 mice were injected subcutaneously (sq) for 7 days with stem cell factor (SCF) and granulocyte colony-stimulating factor (G-CSF). Peripheral blood was RBC depleted and positive selection for c-kit$^+$ cells was performed using Miltenyi microbeads. The purity of c-kit$^+$ cells was 98% ($\pm$1).

The following sources of allogeneic donor cells were used:

Unpurified fetal liver and bone marrow cells
c-kit$^+$ cells from the peripheral blood after cytokine stimulation
Sca-1$^{(+)}$/Lin$^{(-)}$ cells from the spleen after cytokine stimulation

The purity of c-kit$^+$ cells and Sca-1$^{(+)}$/Lin$^{(-)}$ cells after microbeads positive selection (Miltenyi, Auburn, CA) is shown in Figures 3 and 4, respectively.

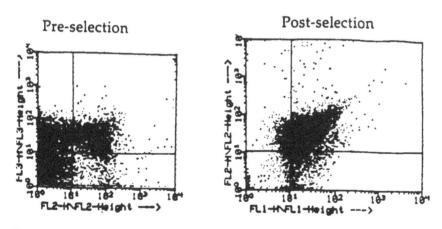

Pre-selection   Post-selection

Figure 4 Purification of Sca-$^+$/Lin$^-$ mice stem cells. Murine bone marrow and peripheral blood stem cells from BALB/c and C57Bl/6 donors were lineage depleted and positively selected for Sca-1$^+$ cells using magnetic Miltenyi microbeads. These microbeads are 0.5 μm in size and do not need to be detached prior to in utero transplantation. The purity of Sca-$^+$/Lin$^-$ cells was ~98% ($\pm$1).

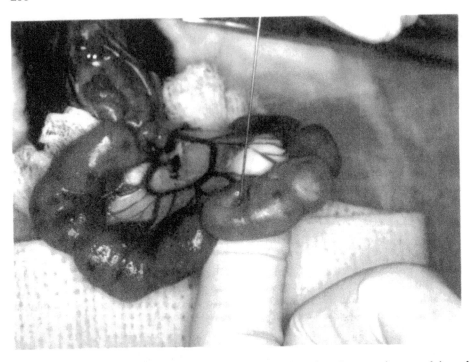

Figure 5 In utero surgery scheme. For the in utero transplantation, the uterus is exposed through a vertical laparotomy incision. Micropipettes are prepared from the glass microcapillaries using a Brown and Flaming micropipette automated puller (T-87). The sharpened micropipette with 30 μm OD (outer diameter) tip is inserted onto the Hamilton syringe containing cell suspension to be injected. The tip of micropipette is inserted through the uterine wall into each fetus intraperitoneally (ip) in 12- to 13-day-old fetuses and transplacentally into 11-day-old fetuses. Owing to the active fetal hematopoiesis present at this gestational age (landmark for ip injection), ip injection can be easily achieved.

2. The In Utero Transplantation Technique

Micropipettes are prepared from the glass microcapillaries using a Brown and Flaming micropipette puller (T-87) as described (67). The end of the pulled needle is cut under a microscope with jeweler's forceps and the tip sharpened on a micro-grinding wheel. Eleven- to 13-day pregnant recipient mice are anesthetized with isoflurane inhalation anesthesia. The uterus is exposed through a vertical laparotomy incision. The tip of the micropipette is inserted through the uterine wall into each fetus intraperitoneally in 12–13 days old fetuses and transplacentally in 11-day-old fetuses. Owing to the fetal hematopoiesis, the liver is visible and provides an excellent landmark for microinjection. Preliminary experiments with India ink demonstrated the appearance of the dye in the peritoneal cavity as well as general circulation (see under inverted microscope). The scheme of the in utero surgery is shown in Figure 5, and the photograph of the India ink–injected fetus is shown in Figure 6.

3. Engraftment with Unpurified Fetal Liver and Bone Marrow Cells

Female mice were evaluated by PCR at 2- to 4-month intervals starting at 1–2 weeks of age. Tissues (livers and spleens) were tested at 6 months of age and bone marrows post-

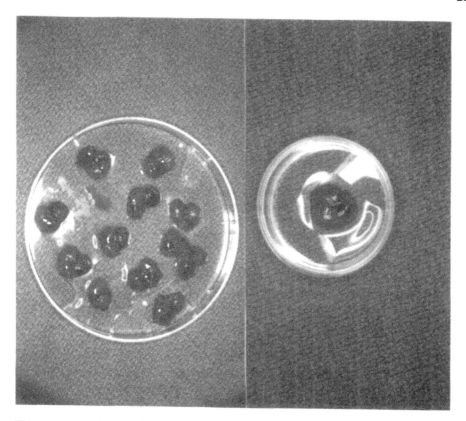

Figure 6   India ink injections. Twelve-day-old fetuses from C57B1/6 mice were injected intraperitoneally with India ink. India ink could be demonstrated in the heart and blood vessels under the inverted microscope immediately after the injection.

mortem. Durable engraftment was defined as donor cells present beyond 20 weeks of age in any tissue or blood. No difference in the overall engraftment rate between allogeneic and congenic recipients was observed and results were combined ($P > .3$) (Table 2). There was no statistical difference between engraftment in the blood, bone marrow, or spleen ($P > .3$), but a two-fold higher engraftment rate in the liver was observed in the group transplanted with the fetal liver cells ($P < .01$).

4.   Degree of Engraftment

The PCR assay was used to estimate the percentage of donor cells in the blood, liver, spleen, and bone marrow. There was no significant difference in the percentage of donor

Table 2   Engraftment Rate by PCR Following In Utero Transplantation with Fetal Liver and Bone Marrow Cells

Recipients	Liver	Spleen	Bone marrow	Blood	Overall
Fetal liver	14/39 (36)[a]	8/40 (20)	7/8 (88)	6/49 (12)	23/49 (47)
Bone marrow	4/41 (19)	9/41 (22)	2/3 (67)	2/3 (13)	20/45 (44)

[a] Number engrafted/number tested (% engrafted).

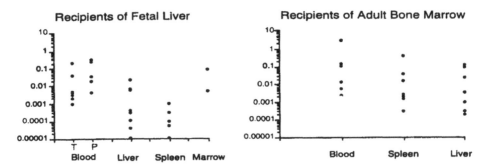

Figure 7 Percentage of donor cells in the blood and tissues of engrafted recipients transplanted with fetal liver and bone marrow cells. Each point represents the average (when more than one time point was evaluated) degree of engraftment in the blood or tissues of individual mice. T, donor cells transiently detected in the blood; P, donor cells permanently detected in the blood.

cells between allogeneic and congenic recipients ($P > .3$) and results were combined. *All mice were engrafted at a very low level (usually below 1%).* The median degree of engraftment in the peripheral blood was 0.01% in both groups with the range of 0.0004–0.6% and 0.002–2.4% in mice transplanted with fetal liver and bone marrow, respectively (Fig. 7). Similarly, a very low degree of engraftment was observed in the tissues with the median of 0.0001% in the fetal liver group and 0.01% in the bone marrow group. The degree of engraftment in tested bone marrow samples were in the range seen for peripheral blood. Similar degrees of engraftment were seen in mice transplanted with c-kit$^+$ cells.

5. Kinetics of Engraftment

When peripheral blood was evaluated in the recipients of fetal liver and bone marrow cells, as many as half the congenic recipients had donor cells present during the first 20 weeks of age. The presence of these short-lived circulating cells probably did not represent permanent engraftment, as only a small number of recipients had detectable circulating donor cells beyond 20 weeks of age. Some animals never showed evidence of engraftment in the blood, spleen, or liver, whereas others showed early engraftment with subsequent loss of donor cells, and some had donor cells present in the peripheral blood during each test. In the animals transplanted with c-kit$^+$ cells, there was no evidence of circulating donor cells beyond 6 months of age (Fig. 8).

6. Recruitment of Donor Cells into the Peripheral Circulation by Postnatal Cytokine Injection

A very high (~80%) engraftment rate in the bone marrow of mice transplanted in utero with fetal liver cells but at a very low degree (<0.01%) was observed. This high engraftment rate of bone marrow did not correlate with the presence of donor cells in the peripheral blood (8% engraftment rate). The hypothesis was that the low degree of engraftment in the bone marrow did not permit the expression of donor cells in the peripheral blood. If these engrafted bone marrow cells were indeed hematopoietic cells, they should respond to the in vivo administration of cytokines. Allogeneic and congenic mice transplanted in utero were injected with fetal liver or bone marrow with 25 µg/kg of pegylated recombinant rat stem cell factor (rrSCF-PEG) and 200 µg/kg of recombinant human granulocyte-colony stimulating factor (rhG-CSF) at 1 year postnatally. On day 8 after cytokine

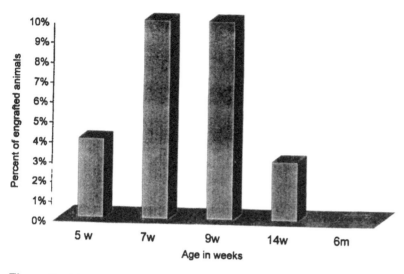

Figure 8 Kinetics of engraftment with c-kit+ cells. Blood was obtained for engraftment studies at 5, 7, 9, and 14 weeks and 6 months. At 1 month of age, only 4% of tested mice showed circulating donor cells, whereas by 2 months of age, this number increased to 10%. No animal had evidence of engraftment by 6 months of age.

injection, a significant number of mice expressed circulating donor cells in the blood. The number of recipients expressing donor cells in the blood return to preinjection levels 2 months postinjection (Table 3). Although there were significant increases in the total white cell counts, the percentage of donor cells remained the same, indicating that the engrafted donor cells were capable of responding to exogenous cytokines, although there was no selective advantage for donor cells. The engraftment in congenic and allogeneic recipients was similar and results were combined.

7. Characteristics of Injected Cells

c-kit+ cells from peripheral blood were characterized for Sca-1+ and CD3+ cells, as shown in Figure 9. Seventy-five thousand to 500,000 cells/fetus were injected with 1–5% CD3+ cells and 5–20% Sca-1+ cells. Therefore, 750–250,000 of CD3+ cells were injected/fetus, but no graft-versus-host disease (GVHD) was observed in any of these mice. All recipient mice were observed for 2 years and no runting, hunched posture, weight loss, or skin changes were observed in any of the transplanted animals. Histological examination con-

Table 3 Kinetics of Donor Cell Appearance in the Peripheral Blood Following Postnatal Injection with Cytokines

Day postinjection	Day 8	2 Weeks	1 Month	2 Months
Fetal liver	7/13 (54)[a]	2/13 (15)	4/13 (30)	0/13 (13)
Bone marrow	9/15 (60)	1/15 (6)	5/15 (33)	0/15 (0)
Combined	16/28 (57)	3/28 (9)	9/28 (32)	0/28 (0)

[a] Number of mice with new expression of donor cells in the peripheral blood at this time point/ number of mice responsive to exogenous cytokines at any time point tested (%).

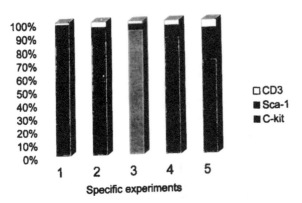

Figure 9   Characteristics of injected cells. Five purification experiments were performed to obtain c-kit⁺ cells for the in utero transplantation using MiniMACS microbeads positive selection. The purity of c-kit⁺ cells was 98%. Depending on the experiment, there were 1–5% CD3⁺ cells and 5–20% Sca-1⁺ cells in the injected population.

firmed no evidence of GVHD. These findings are similar to those observed in humans, in which no active GVHD has been observed thus far after in utero transplantation with allogeneic cells.

8. Tolerance

Donor skin graft acceptance was used to test for tolerance induction following in utero transplantation. In the fetal liver recipients, 13 nonengrafted (i.e., no donor cells detected in the blood or tissues at any time point evaluated) mice rejected skin grafts within 2 weeks. Three mice, all with engraftment in the blood and/or tissues, accepted donor skin grafts permanently, and six mice, with donor cells in the tissues only (liver, spleen, and/ or bone marrow), showed prolonged skin graft acceptance. In none of the bone marrow or c-kit⁺ cells recipients was durable skin graft acceptance achieved. *This difference in tolerance between fetal liver, bone marrow, and c-kit⁺ cells could be related to the difference in the degree of engraftment, possibly the intrinsic differences between various stem cell sources, or the presence of dendritic cells (DCs) in the injected populations.* The correlation of engraftment in the blood and tissues with tolerance by skin graft acceptance in fetal liver recipients are shown in Figure 10. Tolerant mice showed evidence of donor cells in CD3⁺ population (Fig. 11).

    Less than 0.1% donor cells in recipient blood or tissues was sufficient for tolerance induction, and even smaller numbers of donor cells could maintain permanent tolerance. In one mouse, the skin graft was permanently accepted even after donor cells disappeared from the blood shortly after the graft placement (Fig. 10).

9. Postnatal Boosts

The main limitation of in utero transplantation is the low degree at which HSCs engraft. This may be insufficient for the correction of a majority of the diseases unless proliferative advantage for donor progenitor cells exists, such as in β-thalassemia and SCID. *It was observed that the percentage of circulating donor cells may significantly increase after a postnatal boost in tolerant mice with even a small number of donor cells.* One mouse which was durably engrafted in the peripheral blood and the liver and tolerant by skin

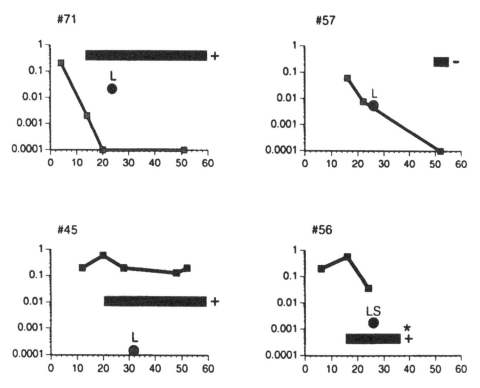

Figure 10 Correlation of degree of engraftment in the blood and tissues with tolerance induction. (X), percentage of donor cells in the peripheral blood tested at specific time points; (•), engraftment in the liver (L) and/or spleen (S) tested at one time point. Hatched bar represents duration of skin graft acceptance: (+), permanent; (−), prolonged.

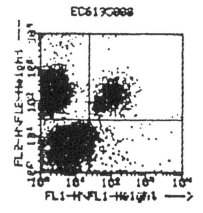

Figure 11 Detection of donor T cells in tolerant mice. Peripheral blood from tolerant mice (accepted donor skin graft) was obtained and stained with 1 µg/10⁶ cells phycoerythria (PE)–anti-CD3 monoclonal antibody (mAb) and 1 µg/10⁶ cells fluorescent isothiocyanate (FITC)–anti–H-2K^{b}D^b mAb. The cells were subsequently stained with propidium iodide (0.5 mg/100 mL) and analyzed by three-color flow cytometry; dead cells were excluded. The data for CD3$^+$ T cells of donor (i.e., H-2K^b) origin, gated for PE/FITC–positive events are presented in two-color immunofluorescence probability dot plot with quadrant markers set relative to negative controls. Total of 9712 live events were analyzed. Of these cells, 34.8% were stained with CD3 and 1.43% with H-2K^b alone and 5.3% were double stained with PE/FITC indicating T lymphocytes of donor origin.

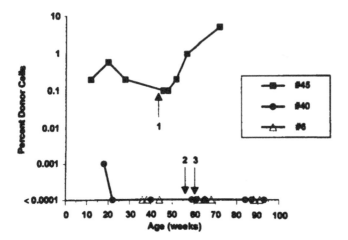

Figure 12 Postnatal boosts in tolerant and nontolerant mice. Mouse #45 was transplanted in utero with fetal liver cells, showed ~1% of circulating donor cells in the blood and accepted permanently donor skin grafts. When boosted with allogeneic donor cells at 44 weeks of gestation, it showed 25-fold increase in circulating donor cells at 72 weeks of age. Mouse #40 had transiently circulating donor cells at 15 weeks of age of 0.001%, which subsequently disappeared at 20 weeks of age. It rejected donor skin grafts and did not respond to postnatal boosts similar to the nonengrafted, nontolerant mouse #6.

graft acceptance showed a 5- and 25-fold increase of donor cells in the peripheral blood 3 and 6 months after boost, respectively (Fig. 12). Similar response was seen in another fetal liver (FL) recipient, who accepted a donor skin graft and showed five-fold increase in donor cells 3 weeks postboost (Fig. 13). A mouse with a transient presence of donor cells in the peripheral blood and a nongrafted mouse who rejected skin grafts and had no

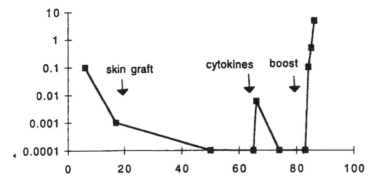

Figure 13 Response to postnatal boosts in tolerant fetal recipient. BALB/c fetal mouse was transplanted with unpurified fetal liver cells at 12 days of gestation. It showed circulating donor cells of 0.1% at 1 month of age with subsequent disappearance to 0.001% at 20 weeks of age and no evidence of engraftment at 50 weeks of age. Donor skin graft was placed at 20 weeks of gestation and was accepted throughout life. Postnatal cytokines (stem cell factor/granulocyte colony-stimulating factor, SCF/G-CSF) recruited donor cells from other sites of engraftment into the blood (0.01%) at 65 weeks of gestation. Postnatal boost with allogeneic donor cells and no conditioning was performed at 85 weeks of age with allogeneic donor cells and showed a significant increase in circulating donor cells at 3 weeks postboost. No signs of GVHD were detected.

evidence of circulating donor cells at various times following a postnatal boost. High-dose boosts of 40 million bone marrow cells for 5 days were performed in syngeneic (δ BALB/c $\rightarrow$ $\female$ BALB/c) and allogeneic (δ C57B1/6 $\rightarrow$ $\female$ BALB/c) combinations in age-matched mice not transplanted in utero. The percentage of donor cells in the recipients of syngeneic cells ranged from 25 to 45% and allogeneic cells from 0.1 to 3.5%. The in utero transplanted mice received 1M–4.9M of purified c-kit$^+$ cells at 1 year of age and showed circulating donor cells up to 6 months post boost, but of a very low degree (<0.1%), suggesting possible immune rejection of these cells. The percentage of donor cells in control syngeneic and allogeneic recipients as well as in mice transplanted in utero is shown in Figure 14.

a.   Immunity

All c-kit$^+$ recipients were evaluated for tolerance/immunity by mixed lymphocyte culture (MLC), cytotoxicity, and natural killer (NK) cell assay at 2 years of age. The results suggested active immunity against allogeneic donor cells in 30% of mice at 2 years of age. The work of Brent and Billingham demonstrated that tolerance to allogeneic cells can be induced after in utero transplantation. However, the low degree of engraftment and tolerance observed in recipients with a full immune system suggests the possibility of active rejection of allogeneic cells after in utero transplantation. The following figures show evidence of alloreactivity to donor cells at 2 years of age after in utero transplanta-

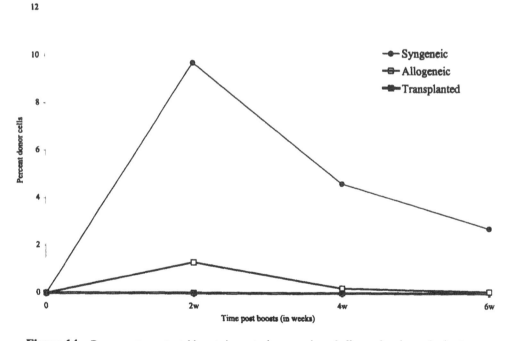

Figure 14   Response to postnatal boosts in control syngeneic and allogeneic mice and mice trans-planted in utero. Age-matched control syngeneic and allogeneic mice nontransplanted in utero re-ceived 40 M × 5 days of allogeneic donor cells without any conditioning. The percentage of donor cells detected in syngeneic controls was ~10%, allogeneic controls 1%, and in utero transplanted mice 0.1%, suggesting the possibility of active immune rejection of donor cells in mice exposed in utero to these cells.

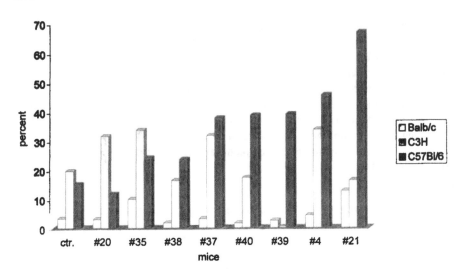

Figure 15 Cytotoxicity indicating immune response in mice transplanted in utero with allogeneic donor cells. All mice transplanted in utero with c-kit⁺ cells had cytotoxicity assay performed at 2 years of age. Control mice nontransplanted in utero showed <15% lysis of allogeneic C57B1/6 target cells. Mice #40, #39, #4, and #21 showed >40% lysis of donor cells, which was much higher than that of third-party (C3H) or syngeneic (BALB/c) cells, indicating active immunity against these cells.

tion: Figure 15 Cytotoxicity; Figure 16 MLC; Figure 17 NK number and function. Of interest is a high number of NK cells in the majority of tested animals, suggesting nonspecific immune activation. Additionally, all these recipients survived up to 25 months of age and were active and robust, as shown in Figure 18, which is uncharacteristic for old BALB/c mice.

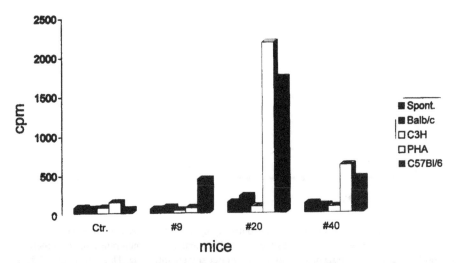

Figure 16 Mixed lymphocyte culture (MLC) assay of BALB/c cells transplanted in utero against syngeneic (BALB/c), third-party (C3H), phytohemagglutinin (PHA), and allogeneic donor cells (C57B1/6) showed active proliferation against donor cells in mice #9, #20, and #40.

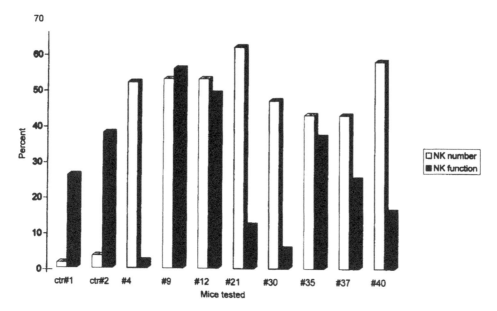

Figure 17 Natural killer (NK) number and function in mice transplanted in utero with c-kit⁺ cells. All mice transplanted in utero with c-kit⁺ cells were phenotyped and functional assay for NK cells was performed. Most of these mice had a very high number of NK cells (>40%) when compared to the controls (~5%). About 30% of mice showed increased NK function (>40%) when compared to controls, suggesting no specific immune activation in response to in utero transplantation with c-kit⁺ cells.

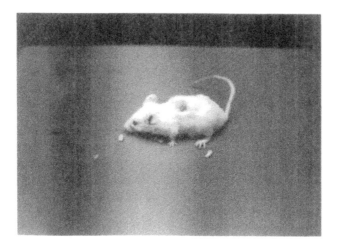

Figure 18 Photograph of mice transplanted in utero with c-kit⁺ cells at 25 months of age. All surviving mice transplanted in utero with c-kit⁺ cells had no evidence of GVHD throughout life. They appeared active, robust, and well nourished, which is uncharacteristic of old BALB/c mice. The pink patch on the skin represents accepted syngeneic graft placed at 6 months of age. Allogeneic (C57Bl/6) and third-party (C3H) skin grafts were rejected and the surgery site was completely healed.

IV. TOLERANCE/IMMUNITY

In 1945, Owen observed that dizygotic cattle twins which showed cross-placental circulation developed hematopoietic chimerism. Postnatally, they were tolerant to skin or kidney grafts from their siblings (71,72). This naturally occurring tolerance was observed in humans and primates as well (73,74). This initial experiment of nature led Billingham and Medawar to the development of a classic "tolerance experiment" of actively acquired immunological tolerance, which showed that preimmune exposure to foreign antigen will result in specific tolerance to this antigen (75,76). The self–nonself theory indicates that a fetus will develop tolerance to alloantigens when exposed to them during a specific "window of opportunity." The "danger" model proposed by Matzinger et al. develops this theory further and indicates that the immune system will reject a foreign antigen only if it presents a danger (77–90). Therefore, the outcome of in utero transplantation may depend on the conditions at which it is performed, such as timing, number and ratio of injected cells, T-/B-cell ratio, and the presence of DCs in the injected population. Further studies are needed to address this and define the best conditions required for the development of a high degree of tolerance. Experimental evidence indicates that the fetal thymic environment plays a major role in the determination of self-recognition (91). Recent studies, however, challenge the self–nonself theory and demonstrated the possibility that, depending on the condition of the transplant, immunity or tolerance may develop in a newborn system (77). When conditions of the classic tolerance experiment are changed, immunity rather than tolerance follows (78).

The in utero transplantation provides an excellent opportunity to induce tolerance to allogeneic cells with the possibility of postnatal high-dose transplants in diseases such as inborn errors of metabolism or congenital hemoglobinopathies in which full myeloablation may not be necessary. However, the low degree of chimerism and tolerance induced in recipients with a full immune system and unsuccessful transplants in humans with β-thalassemia suggests the possibility of active immunity. We have developed a model of tolerance/immunity in which either one may develop, depending on the conditions of transplants, as shown in Figure 19. The classic "tolerance" experiment of Brent and Billingham has been challenged by the Matzinger group and others (77–90), who showed

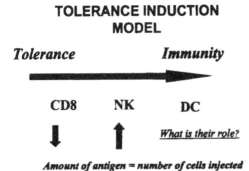

Figure 19 The development of tolerance/immunity following in utero transplantation. This diagram represents the hypothesis that, depending on the conditions of in utero transplantation, such as number of injected cells, T/B ratio, number of dendritic cells injected, tolerance or immunity may develop.

that under specific conditions, active immunity will develop following allogeneic cell exposure in newborn life. Specifically, it was speculated that in the classic "tolerance" experiment in which spleen and kidneys were injected prenatally, there was a large number of B cells in relation to T cells and DCs. B cells could therefore disarm T cells and tolerance followed. However, when the conditions were reversed, immunity followed (78). This possibility of the development of active immunity after in utero transplantation is intriguing and may explain the low and transient engraftment in hosts with an intact immune system. It needs to be further investigated to define better the conditions for induction of a high degree of tolerance as well as to explore the possibility of fetal immunization against infectious diseases.

The following questions must therefore be addressed in the upcoming experiments:

1. What are the strategies for increasing the degree of engraftment? The possible approaches to this problem include:

    a. Purified sources of stem cells
    b. Optimal number of cells injected
    c. Optimal time for transplant
    d. In vitro and in vivo cytokines
    e. Strategies leading to upregulation of homing receptors
    f. Suppression of endogenous (host) hematopoiesis

2. How to increase the number of animals with higher degree tolerance?

    a. Exploring mechanisms of tolerance/immunity induction
    b. Role of NK cells
    c. Role of DCs
    d. Role of the specific T/B-cell ratio

3. The role of postnatal boosts in maintaining a high percentage of donor cells in the blood.

    a. Identifying the optimal boost protocols
    b. Using high-dose boosts
    c. Using sublethal irradiation or low-dose chemotherapy for ablation
    d. Creating successful miniablative regimens in tolerant recipients for the treatment of metabolic disorders and hemoglobinopathies

ACKNOWLEDGMENT

This work was supported, in part, by grant K08HL03603-01 from the National Institutes of Health, DHHS RMHC medical grant, and March of Dimes grant (95-0954).

REFERENCES

1. Flake AW, Roncarolo MG, Puck JM, Alameida-Porada G, Evans MI, Johnson MP, Abella EM, Harrison DD, Zanjani ED. Treatment of X-linked severe combined immunodeficiency by in utero transplantation of paternal bone marrow. N Engl J Med 1996; 335:1806–1810.
2. Wengler GS, Lanfranchi A, Frusca T, Verardi R, Neva A, Brugnoni D, Giliani S, Fiorini M, Mella P, Guandalini F, Mazzolari E, Pecorelli S, Notarangello LD, Porta F, Ugazio AG. In-utero transplantation of parental CD34 haematopoietic progenitor cells in a patient with X-linked severe combined immunodeficiency (SCIDXI). Lancet 1996; 348:1484–1487.

3. Touraine JL, Raudrant D, Royo C, Rebaud A, Roncarolo MG, Sovillet G, Phillipe N, Touraine F, Betuel H. The in utero transplantation of stem cells in bare lymphocyte syndrome. Lancet 1989; 1:1382.

4. Krivit W, Shapiro E, Kennedy W, Lipton M, Lockman L, Smith S, Summers CG, Wenger DA, Tsai MY, Ramsay NK, et al. Treatment of late infantile metachromatic leukodystrophy by bone marrow transplantation. N Engl J Med 1990; 322:28–32.

5. Krivit W, Pierpont ME, Ayaz K, Tsai M, Ramsay NK, Kersey JH, Weisdorf S, Sibley R, Snover D, McGovern MM, et al. Bone-marrow transplantation in the Maroteaux-Lamy syndrome (mucopolysaccharidosis VI). Biochemical and clinical status 24 months after transplantation. N Engl J Med 1984; 311:1606–1611.

6. Parkman R. The application of bone marrow transplantation to the treatment of genetic diseases. Science 1986; 232:1373–1378.

7. Sullivan KM. Current status of bone marrow transplantation. Transplant Proc 1989; 21(Suppl 1):41–50.

8. Clark J. The challenge of bone marrow transplantation. Mayo Clin Proc 1990; 65:111–114.

9. Sasazuki T, Juji T, Morishima Y, Kinukawa N, Kashiwabara H, Inoko H, Yoshida T, Kimura A, Akaza T, Kamikasji N, Kodera Y, Takaku F. Effect of matching of class I HLA alleles on clinical outcome after transplantation of hematopoietic stem cells from an unrelated donor. Japan Marrow Donor Program. N Engl J Med 1998; 339:1177–1185.

10. Exner BG, Acholonu I, Ildstad ST. Hematopoietic chimerism, tolerance induction and graft-versus-host disease: considerations for composite tissue transfer. Transplant Proc 1998; 30:2718–2720.

11. Ellison C, Gartner J. Acute, lethal graft-versus-host disease in a F1-hybrid model using grafts from parental-strain, T-cell receptor-delta gene knockout donors. Scand J Immunol 1998; 48:272–276.

12. Asplund S, Gramlich TL. Chronic mucosal changes of the colon in graft-versus-host disease. Mod Pathol 1998; 11:513–515.

13. Nagler A, Condiotti R, Nabet C, Naparstek E, Or R, Samuel S, Slavin S. Selective CD34$^+$–T cell depletion does not prevent graft-versus-host disease. Transplantation 1998; 66:138–141.

14. Klingebiel T, Schlegel PG. GVHD: overview on pathophysiology, incidence, clinical and biological features. Bone Marrow Transplant 1998; 21(suppl 2):S45–S49.

15. Touraine JL. In utero transplantation of fetal liver cells into human fetuses. Hum Reprod 1992; 7:44–48.

16. Westgren M, Ringden O, Eik-Nes S, Ek S, Anvret M, Brubakk AM, Bui TH, Giambona A, Kiserud T, Kjaeldgaard A, Maggio A, Markling L, Seiger A, Orlandi F. Lack of evidence of permanent engraftment after in utero fetal stem cell transplantation in congenital hemoglobinopathies. Transplantation 1996; 61:1176–1179.

17. Flake AW, Zanjani ED. In utero transplantation for thalassemia. Ann NY Acad Sci 1998; 850:300–311.

18. Flake AW, Zanjani ED. In utero hematopoietic stem cell transplantation. A status report. JAMA 1997; 278:932–937.

19. Hayward A, Ambruso D, Battaglia F, Donlon T, Eddelman K, Giller R, Hobbins J, Hsia YE, Quinones R, Shpall E, Trachtenberg E, Giardina P. Microchimerism and tolerance following intrauterine transplantation and transfusion for alpha-thalassemia-1. Fetal Diagn Ther 1998; 13:8–14.

20. Slavin S, Naparstek E, Ziegler M, Lewin A. Clinical application of intrauterine bone marrow transplantation for treatment of genetic diseases—feasibility studies. Bone Marrow Transplant 1992; 9(Suppl 1):189–190.

21. Diukman R, Golbus MS. In utero stem cell therapy. J Reprod Med 1992; 37:515–520.

22. Tavassoli M. Embryonic and fetal hemopoiesis: an overview. Blood Cells 1991; 17:269.

23. Bessler H, Djaldetti M. Ultrastructural studies on bone marrow development in embryonic mice. Biol Neonate 1992; 61:243–252.

24. Djaldetti M, Ovadia J, Bessler O, Fishman P, Halbrefht I. Ultrastructural study of the erythropoietic events in human embryonic livers. Biol Neonate 1975; 28:367–374.

25. Sminia T, Djkstra CD. The origin of osteoclasts: an immunohistochemical study on macrophages and osteoclasts in embryonic rat bone. Calcif Tissue Int 1986; 39:263–266.

26. Hann IM, Bodger MP, Hoffbrand AV. Development of pluripotent hematopoietic progenitor cells in the human fetus. Blood 1983; 62:118–123.

27. Stewart FM, Crittenden RB, Lowery PA, Pearson-White S, Quesenberry PJ. Long-term engraftment of normal and post–5-fluorouracil murine bone marrow into normal nonmyeloablated mice. Blood 1993; 81:2566–2571.

28. Quesenberry PJ, Ramshaw H, Crittenden RB, Stewart FM, Rao S, Peters S, Becker P, Lowry P, Blomberg M, Reilly J, et al. Engraftment of normal murine marrow into nonmyeloablated host mice. Blood Cells 1994; 20:348–350.

29. Roodman GD, Kuehl TJ, Vandeberg JL, Muirhead DY. In utero transplantation of fetal baboons with mismatched adult baboon marrow. Blood Cells 1991; 17:367–375.

30. Harrison MR, Slotnik RN, Crombleholme TM, Golbus MS, Tarantal AF, Zanjani ED. In utero transplantation of fetal liver haematopoietic stem cells in monkeys. Lancet 1989; 2:1425–1427.

31. Cowan MJ, Tarantal AF, Capper J, Harrison M, Garovoy M. Long term engraftment following in utero T-cell depleted parental marrow transplantation into fetal rhesus monkeys. Bone Marrow Transplant 1996; 17:1157–1165.

32. Duncan BW, Harrison MR, Crombleholme TM, Clemons G, Tavassoli M, Zanjani ED. Effect of erythropoietic stress on donor hematopoietic cell expression in chimeric rhesus monkeys transplanted in utero. Exp Hematol 1992; 20:350–353.

33. Mychaliska GB, Rice HE, Tarantal AF, Stock PG, Capper J, Garovoy MR, Olson JL, Cowan MJ, Harrison MR. In utero hematopoietic stem cell transplants prolong survival of postnatal kidney transplantation in monkeys. J Pediatr Surg 1997; 32:976–981.

34. Zanjani ED, Flake AW, Rice H, Hedrick M, Tavassoli M. Long-term repopulating ability of xenogeneic transplanted human fetal liver hematopoietic stem cells in sheep. J Clin Invest 1994; 93:1051–1055.

35. Zanjani ED, Almeida-Porada G, Flake AW. The human/sheep xenograft: a large animal model of human hematopoiesis. Int J Hematol 1996; 63:179–192.

36. Almeida-Porada GD, Hoffman R, Manolo P, Gianni AM, Zanjani ED. Detection of human cells in human/sheep chimeric lambs with in vitro human stroma-forming potential. Exp Hematol 1996; 24:482–487.

37. Shimizu Y, Ogawa M, Kobayashi M, Almeida-Porada G, Zanjani ED. Engraftment of cultured human hematopoietic cells in sheep. Blood 1998; 91:3688–3692.

38. Zanjani ED, Almeida-Parada G, Livingston AG, Flake AW, Ogawa M. Human bone marrow CD34$^-$ cells engraft in vivo and undergo multilineage expression that includes giving rise to CD34$^+$ cells. Exp Hematol 1998; 26:353–360.

39. Zanjani ED. The human/sheep xenograft model for assay of human HSC (discussion). Stem Cells 1997; 15:209.

40. Almeida-Porada G, Ascensao JL, Zanjani ED. The role of sheep stroma in human haemopoiesis in the human/sheep chimaeras. Br J Haematol 1996; 93:795–802.

41. Zanjani ED, Srour EF, Hoffman R. Retention of long-term repopulating ability of xenogeneic transplanted purified adult human bone marrow hematopoietic stem cells in sheep. J Lab Clin Med 1995; 126:24–28.

42. Flake AW, Hedrick MH, Rice HE, Tavassoli H, Zanjani ED. Enhancement of human hematopoiesis by mast cell growth factor in human-sheep chimeras created by the in utero transplantation of human fetal hematopoietic cells. Exp Hematol 1995; 23:252–257.

43. Zanjani ED, Almeida-Porada G, Flake AW. Retention and multilineage expression of human hematopoietic stem cells in human-sheep chimeras. Stem Cells 1995; 13:101–111.

44. Zanjani ED, Flake AW, Rice HE, Hedrick M, Tavassoli M. Long-term repopulating ability of xenogeneic transplanted human fetal liver hematopoietic stem cells in sheep. J Clin Invest 1994; 93:1051–1055.

45. Zanjani ED, Silva MR, Flake AW. Retention and multilineage expression of human hematopoietic stem cells in human-sheep chimeras. Blood Cells 1994; 20:338–340.

46. Shehee WR, Oliver P, Smithies O. Lethal thalassemia after insertional disruption of the mouse major adult beta-globin gene. Proc Natl Acad Sci USA 1993; 90:1777–1781.

47. Bosma GC, Custer RP, Bosma MJ. A severe combined immunodeficiency mutation in the mouse. Nature 1983; 301:527–530.

48. Wolfe JM, Sands MS, Barker JE, Gwynn B, Rowe LB, Vogler CA, Birkenmeier EH. Reversal of pathology in murine mucopolysaccharidosis type VII by somatic cell gene transfer. Nature 1992; 360:749–753.

49. Fleischman RA, Mintz B. Prevention of genetic anemias in mice by microinjection of normal hematopoietic stem cells into the fetal placenta. Proc Natl Acad Sci USA 1979; 76:5736–5740.

50. Fleischman RA, Mintz B. Development of adult bone marrow stem cells in H-2–compatible and –incompatible mouse fetuses. J Exp Med 1984; 159:731–745.

51. Blanchet JP, Fleischman RA, Mintz B. Murine adult hematopoietic cells produce adult erythrocytes in fetal recipients. Dev Genet 1982; 3:197.

52. Howson-Jan K, Matloub YH, Vallera DA, Blazar BR. In utero engraftment of fully H-2 incompatible versus congenic adult bone marrow transferred into nonanemic or anemic murine fetal recipients. Transplantation 1993; 56:709–716.

53. Blazar BR, Taylor PA, Vallera DA. Adult bone marrow–derived pluripotent hematopoietic stem cells are engraftable when transferred in utero into moderately anemic fetal recipients. Blood 1995; 853:833–841.

54. Lucarelli G, Galinberti M, Polchi P, Angelucci E, Baronciani D, Giardini C, Politi P, Durazzi SM, Muretto P, Albertini F. Bone marrow transplantation in patients with thalassemia. N Engl J Med 1990; 322:417–421.

55. Lucarelli G, Clift RA, Galinberti M, Polchi P, Angelucci E, Baronciani D, Giardini C, Andreani M, Manna M, Nesci S, Agostinelli F, Rapa S, Ripalti M, Albertini F. Marrow transplantation for patients with thalassemia: results in class 3 patients. Blood 1996; 87:2082–2088.

56. Donahue J, Kuypers F, Witkowska E, Carrier E et al. Engraftment and tolerance following in utero transplantation in β-thalassemic mice. Blood 1998; 92:286b.

57. Archer DR, Hester LE, Gu Y et al. Successful in utero engraftment of allogeneic hematopoietic cells in murine β-thalassemia. Blood 1998; 92:267a.

58. Blazar BR, Taylor PA, Vallera DA. In utero transfer of adult bone marrow cells into recipients with severe combined immunodeficiency disorder yields lymphoid progeny with T- and B-cell functional capabilities. Blood 1995; 86:4353–4366.

59. Archer DR, Turner CW, Yeager AM, Fleming WH. Sustained multilineage engraftment of allogeneic hematopoietic stem cells in NOD/SCID mice after in utero transplantation. Blood 1997; 90:3222–3229.

60. Pallavicini MG, Flake AW, Madden D, Bethel C, Duncan B, Gonzalgo ML, Haendel S, Montoya T, Roberts L. Hemopoietic chimerism in rodents transplanted in utero with fetal human hematopoietic cells. Transplant Proc 1992; 24:542–543.

61. Pixley JS, Tavassoli M, Zanjani ED, Shaft MD, Futamachi KJ, Sauter T, Tavassoli A, MacKintosh FR. Transplantation in utero of fetal human hematopoietic stem cells into mice results in hematopoietic chimerism. Pathobiology 1994; 62:238–244.

62. Soper BW, Duffy T, Barker JE. Corrective therapy for mucopolysaccharidosis type VII by transplantation of syngeneic lineage[low], SCA-1[high], hoechst 33342[low] marrow into W[41]/W[41]/gus[mps]/gus[mps] recipients. Blood 1997; 90:364a.

63. Sands MS, Wolfe JH, Birkenmeier EH, Barker JE, Vogler C, Sly WS, Okuyama T, Freeman

B, Nicholes A, Muzyczka N, Chang PL, Axelrod HR. Gene therapy for murine mucopolysaccharidosis type VII. Neuromuscul Disord 1997; 7:352–360.

64. Snyder EY, Taylor RM, Wolfe JH. Neural progenitor cell engraftment corrects lysosomal storage throughout the MPS VII mouse brain. Nature 1995; 374:367–370.

65. Kim HB, Shaaban AF, Yang EY, Milner R, Flake AW. Donor specific tolerance in a murine model of in utero stem cell transplantation requires hematopoietic microchimerism and is dependent on donor cell source. Blood 1997; 1618:95a.

66. Hajdu K, Tanigawara S, Mclean LK, Cowan MJ, Golbus MS. In utero allogeneic hematopoietic stem cell transplantation to induce tolerance. Fetal Diag Ther 1996; 11:241–248.

67. Carrier E, Lee TH, Busch MP, Cowan MJ. Induction of tolerance in non defective mice after in utero transplantation of major histocompatibility complex mismatched fetal hematopoietic stem cells. Blood 1995; 86:4681–4690.

68. Carrier E, Lee TH, Busch MP, Cowan MJ. Recruitment of engrafted donor cells potentially into the blood with cytokines after in utero transplantation in mice. Transplantation 1997; 64: 627–633.

69. Lee TH, Stromberg RR, Heitman J, Tran K, Busch MP. Quantification of residual white cells in filtered blood components by polymerase chain reaction amplification of HLA DQ-A DNA. Transfusion 1994; 34:986–994.

70. Goodarzi MO, Lee TH, Pallvicini MG, Donegan EA, Busch MP. Unusual kinetics of white cell clearance in transfused mice. Transfusion 1995; 35:145–149.

71. Owen RD. Immunogenetic consequences of vascular anastomoses between bovine cattle twins. Science 1945; 10:400.

72. Cragle RG, Stone WH. Preliminary results of kidney grafts between cattle chimeric twins. Transplantation 1967; 5:328.

73. van Dijk BA, Boomsma DI, de Man AJ. Blood group chimerism in human multiple births is not rare. Am J Med Genet 1996; 61:264–268.

74. Picus J, Aldrich WR, Letvin NL. A naturally occurring bone-marrow–chimeric primate. I. Integrity of its immune system. Transplantation 1985; 39:297–303.

75. Billingham RE, Brent L, Madawar PB. Actively acquired tolerance of foreign cells. Nature 1953; 4379:603.

76. Billingham R, Brent L, Madawar PB. Quantitative studies on tissue transplantation immunity. Actively acquired tolerance. Phil Trans R Soc(Lond) B 1956; 239:357.

77. Sarzotti M, Robbins DS, Hoffman PM. Induction of protective CTL responses in newborn mice by a murine retrovirus. Science 1996; 271:1726–1728.

78. Fuchs EJ, Matzinger P. B cells turn off virgin but not memory T cells. Science 1992; 258: 1156–1159.

79. Matzinger P. Tolerance, danger, and the extended family. Annu Rev Immunol 1994; 12:991–1045.

80. Sarzotti M, Dean TA, Remington MP, Ly CD, Furth PA, Robbins DS. Induction of cytotoxic T cell responses in newborn mice by DNA immunization. Vaccine 1997; 15:795–797.

81. Matzinger P. The immune system's role in graft loss: theoretical considerations. Transplant Proc 1997; 29:11S–12S.

82. Goodnow CC. Balancing immunity and tolerance: deleting and tuning lymphocyte repertoires. Proc Natl Acad Sci USA 1996; 93:2264–2271.

83. Matzinger P. Immunology. Memories are made of this? Nature 1994; 369:605–606.

84. Di Rosa F, Matzinger P. Long-lasting CD8 T memory in the absence of CD4 T cells or B cells. J Exp Med 1996; 183:2153–2163.

85. Sarzotti M, Robbins DS, Hoffman PM. Induction of protective CTL responses in newborn mice by a murine retrovirus. Science 1996; 271:1726–1728.

86. Bonney EA, Matzinger P. The maternal immune system's interaction with circulating fetal cells. J Immunol 1997; 158:40–47.

87. Ridge JP, Fuchs EJ, Matzinger P. Neonatal tolerance revisited: turning on newborn T cells with dendritic cells. Science 1996; 271:1723–1726.

88. Ridge JP, Di Rosa F, Matzinger P. A conditioned dendritic cell can be a temporal bridge between a CD4$^+$ T-helper and a T-killer cell. Nature 1998; 393:474–478.

89. Epstein MM, Di Rosa F, Jankovic D, Sher A, Matzinger P. Successful T cell priming in B-cell deficient mice. J Exp Med 1995; 182:915–922.

90. Lehmann PV, Forsthuber T, Miller A, Sercarz EE. Spreading of T-cell autoimmunity to cryptic determinants of an autoantigen. Nature 1992; 358:155–157.

91. Guidos CJ, Danska JS, Fathman CG, Weissman IL: T cell receptor-mediated negative selection of autoreactive T lymphocyte precursors occurs after commitment to the CD4 or CD8 lineages. J Exp Med 1990; 172:835.

13

CD34 Selection Using Immunomagnetic Beads

ROBERT A. PRETI

Progenitor Cell Therapy, L.L.C., Hackensack, New Jersey

ANDREW L. PECORA

Hackensack University Medical Center, Hackensack, New Jersey

TAUSEEF AHMED

New York Medical College, Valhalla, New York

TIMOTHY J. FARLEY

New York Blood Center, Valhalla, New York

I. INTRODUCTION

In consideration of the recent advances in the field of hematopoietic stem cell transplantation, it is important to recognize the critical contributions that certain technologies have made to the significant progress of the field. To this end, CD34 selection culminates a line of graft engineering strategies designed to prepare the hematopoietic stem cell product for transplantation. In effect, the evolution from technologies based on the exploitation of broad differences in cell size (centrifugation and elutriation) and surface characteristics (soybean agglutination and E rosetting) to specific surface antigens [monoclonal antibody (mAb)–based approaches] has represented a progressive refinement in cell processing expectations. Such development makes possible a nontoxic, passive removal of cells considered to act as contaminants of the hematopoietic stem cell product, has opened the doors to cellular therapeutics through gene therapy and immunotherapy, and has advanced these experimental technologies to within the realm of possibility.

The idea of specific targeting of cells based on cell characteristics is not new (Kemshead, 1991). However, its progression from negative selection of cells for tumor cell removal in the autograft or T-lymphocyte depletion from the allograft has made more routine positive selection for cells bearing the CD34 antigen (Civin, 1984). Current advantages including volume reduction of the hematopoietic graft, T-cell depletion for allogeneic transplantation, and tumor cell depletion in the autologous setting can be ascribed to this technology. Refinements to these processes have thus accomplished direct benefit to patient care, whereas limiting the nonspecific loss of progenitor and stem cell populations, reducing the posttransplant mortality and morbidity historically associated with earlier attempts to purify the hematopoietic progenitor cell product.

Through the isolation of these cells in the posttransplant setting, CD34 selection affords the opportunity to gain greater understanding of the role that CD34$^+$ cells play in hematopoiesis and hematopoietic reconstitution. Additionally, although it remains a distant goal, we are also beneficiaries of a setting in which it is possible to evaluate the relative contribution of micrometastases to relapse of disease following transplantation. And, finally, as clinical researchers continue to tease apart graft-versus-host disease and graft-versus-leukemia in order to strike the perfect balance between the two phenomena, selection technologies make possible the production of tailored allografts containing mixed populations of variously represented T lymphocytes to reach this end.

Beyond these immediate and more obvious benefits lie possibilities yet to be uncovered as purer cell populations lend themselves to more sophisticated manipulations such as ex vivo expansion, immunotherapy, and gene therapy. It is the intent of this chapter to focus on the immunomagnetic bead–based approaches to CD34 selection, variations on the methods using the Isolex300i Automated Cell Separator (Baxter Immunotherapy, Irvine, CA), and provide an initial glimpse into the clinical and laboratory data which will ultimately determine the fate of this technology.

II. ISSUES FROM THE LABORATORY

Immunomagnetic bead (MagB) (Chang, 1985; Ugelstad, 1986) selection includes preparation of the cell sample, labeling of target cells with an antibody raised specifically against them, capture of the labeled cells with an immunomagnetic bead, passage of the cell suspension over a magnetic field to attract the labeled cells, and release of the captured cells from the immunomagnetic bead if this population represents the cells required for further manipulation or transplantation. Alternatively, magnetic beads that have been presensitized with monoclonal antibody may be incubated with the cell population in a single step prior to passage over the magnetic field.

Regardless of whether peripheral blood, cord blood, bone marrow, or a peripheral blood apheresis collection is used, there are several considerations that are required for each of the elements to be performed with maximum efficiency.

A. Sample Preparation

The quality of the starting material is an important consideration for any immunomagnetic bead selection. Owing to a lack of vast experience using these technologies, most laboratories initiate specimen processing as soon as possible after arrival of the product. However, in an attempt to optimize utilization of resources, it is often desirable to combine two products from a single patient in preparation for the selection procedure. In these cases, the first apheresis product may be stored overnight and added to the second apheresis product from the same individual on the following day. Consequently, the age of the specimen and the storage conditions are considerations in this setting. The key factors that affect product quality appear to be storage temperature, cellular concentration, the gas permeability characteristics of the storage bag, and the requirement for agitation. Although the clinical findings are somewhat incomplete, storage at either 20 or 4°C appears to have no effect on the subsequent selection procedure. However, although our data are mixed, it does appear to be beneficial to dilute highly concentrated cell suspensions with a buffer solution or autologous plasma for overnight storage. This is particularly important for apheresis products generated using the CS3000 Apheresis System (Fenwal, Deerfield, IL), which produces a relatively small, highly concentrated mononuclear cell preparation. Further, the use of gas-permeable plastic containers to allow for adequate gas exchange is recommended as well.

The purity of the target cell population has a direct impact on the efficiency of selection of that population. Collected over a number of years, our early data were in agreement with those of many other groups in that a marked decrease in postselection recovery is observed when the starting purity falls below 0.5% target cells (Fig. 1A), given a fixed selection procedure, since the efficiency of target cell capture by the immunomagnetic beads is directly proportional to the relative purity of the target cell population in the fresh product (Farley, 1997). Further, although the yield of target cells increased as a function of the starting target cell concentration, the purity of the final product decreased proportionately. Enrichment of the target population prior to selection can be achieved through density-gradient centrifugation, elutriation, and automated cell processing (Preti, 1994). However, these methods are often time consuming and may result in some toxicity to and losses of target cells prior to selection. In addition, if the purity rather than the yield of the final product is of prime importance to the investigator, then preenrichment may not be desirable. Thus, consideration of the intended characteristics and requirements of the final product must balance the use of any enrichment procedure prior to selection.

Even in the event that no additional target cell enrichment is required or desirable, platelet reduction is recommended prior to selection (Kvalheim et al., 1988). The presence of high numbers of platelets in the specimen may ultimately result in decreased yields of target cells postselection. Interference by platelets can be reduced by performing two rounds of centrifugation (250 × g for 10 min with the brake in the off position) followed by removal of supernatant (Fig. 2). Alternatively, the Isolex300i automated selection device reduces platelets via a spinning membrane module containing a 2.5-μm filter that enables the platelets to be drawn off, in process, with no loss of cells from the specimen and precluding the need for separate, preparative "platelet-wash" step.

Finally, as is customary with all antibody-based selections and assays, nonspecific binding (of predominantly mature myeloid cells) with labeling antibody and immunomagnetic beads is reduced through the use of a wash/incubation solution containing human serum albumin (1%) or autologous plasma and/or human immunoglobulin (IvIg). Generally, this may be accomplished during the overnight storage, if it is required, and/or during the incubation of the mAb with the target cells.

B. Antibody Labeling of Target Cells and Target Cell Capture with Immunomagnetic Beads

Murine mAbs with a high degree of specificity for the target populations are generally employed for the selection procedure. This process entails selection of an antibody specific

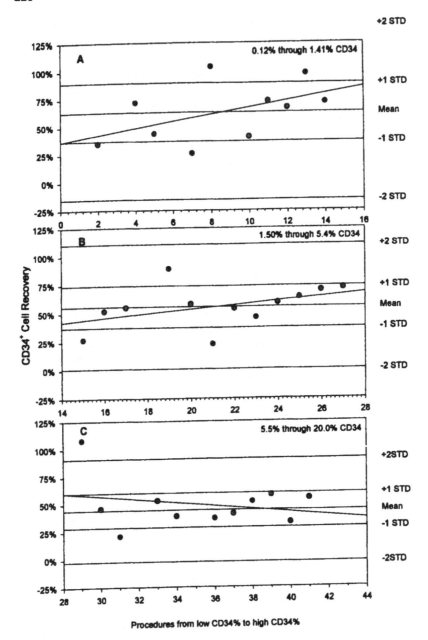

Figure 1 (A) At a median starting purity of 0.5%, recovery of CD34 cells following selection increases proportionately with starting purity. (B) This relationship is dampened (decreased slope) as the starting purity of the product increases and ultimately, (C) is associated with a reduction in recovery of target cells. Note the mean recovery decreases from 62.0% in 1A to 55.2% (B) and 43% above a starting purity of 5.5% (C).

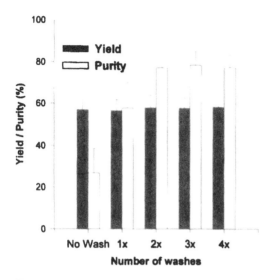

Figure 2   Platelet washes prior to selection. Although the yield is not effected by the wash procedure, significant ($P < .004$) increases in CD34 purity following selection were associated with two washes prior to incubation of the cell suspension with anti-CD34 mAb.

for an antigen that exhibits minimal expression outside of the target cell population. In the case of the CD34 antigen, capture of nonprogenitor cells is rarely a problem, since the CD34 antigen is normally expressed only by cells in the early stages of hematopoietic development. Class I antigens are recommended owing to the lack of universal expression on leukemic cells bearing the CD34 surface antigen (Sutherland and Keating, 1992).

In the "indirect method," the cells are incubated with the mAb for a minimum of 15 mins. Although extending the incubation period for longer periods (≥ 30 mins) did not increase the efficiency of the selection process, no decrease in yield or purity was observed. Additionally, at 4 and 22°C, no effect was seen as a function of cell concentration for the range tested. Following a wash step to remove unbound mAb, the cell suspension is mixed with immunomagnetic beads coated with an antimouse immunoglobulin (IgG), generally obtained from immunized sheep. In many protocols, the bead is coated with antibodies specific for mouse IgG, since the majority of labeling antibodies available for use in a selection procedure are of the IgG class [Sheep–anti-Mouse (SAM)–IgG Magnetic Beads, Dynal, Oslo, Norway].

Alternatively, the immunomagnetic beads may be sensitized with the mAb prior to incubation with the cell product. This "direct method" requires that, during or prior to the initial processing of the specimen on the Isolex instrument, the mAb be incubated with the magnetic beads and prepared for inoculation into the product.

The procedure using the Isolex300i automated cell selection system combines the antibody and magnetic bead incubations using a presensitization step. The protocol combines the wash, platelet filtration, and sensitized-bead incubation steps into one seamless procedure, which is controlled by the instrument software. This modification to the previous protocol using the Isolex semiautomated device (SA), an earlier version of the Isolex300i) has resulted in a reduction in total processing time from approximately 6 h to roughly 3.5 h. The process requires minimal operator intervention, providing a relatively "hands-off" 2.5-h device operation time.

The key factor that influences the recovery and purity of CD34 cells after selection is the interaction of the mAb and the CD34 surface antigen. By optimizing this interaction, significant efficiencies can be achieved ultimately resulting in improvements in the quality of the product. As an alternative to a fixed selection procedure, given that apheresis products may contain variable percentages of target cells, we attempted to design a selection algorithm specifically tailored to each product. In this manner, we hoped to optimize the selection of cells and the use of reagents as well. Using this protocol, the target cell population must be enumerated by flow cytometry prior to the selection procedure. In this scenario, the number of target cells in the starting product determines the amount of reagents required to perform the procedure. In preceding experiments, we determined the optimal per target cell amounts of mAb and magnetic beads required to result in the most effective and most efficient utilization of reagents (Fig. 3). Through these experiments, we determined that optimal yields and recoveries were obtained using 25 pg/target cell antibody with 100 magnetic beads for each target cell present in the starting material.

Although not prohibitively difficult for a well-equipped laboratory, this protocol does require additional coordination with the flow cytometry staff, additional flow analyses, and calculation and dispensing of the amounts of reagents required. In addition, this approach limits the use of the cell-selection technologies to laboratories with greater resources and more specialized staff. In part to avoid these cumbersome and potentially error-prone complications, the manufacturer has optimized the protocol through the design of the Isolex300i and the provision of single-use kits with reagents dispensed in saturating amounts for a standard apheresis products. Although this approach may slightly increase the costs of reagents used for each procedure, it provides a more streamlined and less labor-intensive approach to accomplish the same goal.

Peripheral blood stem cell apheresis following chemotherapy and growth factor mobilization generally provides a sufficient product for CD34 cell selection, generating consistently high yields and purities after selection (Table 1). However, more effective mobilization strategies have been developed in recent years. Our data now indicate that some apheresis products contain greater than saturating amounts of CD34$^+$ cells (Pecora, 1998), reaching as many as 110×10^6 CD34$^+$ cells/kg patient body weight. Such numbers are orders of magnitude beyond those for which many of today's selection technologies were originally designed. Selection of these products, therefore, has resulted in a reduction in overall percentage yield for CD34 cells; presumably by overloading either the available reagent base and/or magnetic strength of the instrument. Greater cell numbers with an ever-increasing CD34 content have begun to erode the yield of CD34$^+$ cells in a dose-dependent manner (Fig. 4); reducing the mean yield to 50% in our last series of 39 selections. Currently, we are investigating the use of additional reagents and/or setting limits to the number of CD34$^+$ cells for each selection procedure in order to increase the mean yield of target cells.

C. Removal of Nontarget Cells

Once the immunomagnetic beads (MagBs) have formed rosettes with the target cells, a magnetic field is applied to the specimen in order to initiate the selection process. In practice, the MagB/target cell rosettes move through the cell suspension to the point in the chamber where the magnetic field strength is at its greatest. With the magnetic field still in place, the unattached cell suspension is removed and wash buffer is added to replace the lost fluid. At least two washes are required to ensure that nontarget cells that may

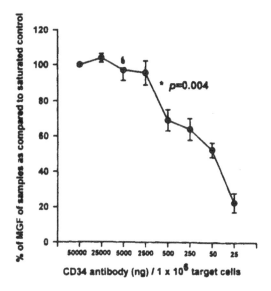

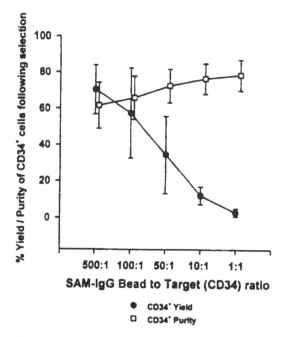

Figure 3   (Top) Significant decrease in saturation of antibody binding sites as determined by the strength of the mean green fluorescence signal (MGF) were seen at 500 ng/1 million target cells. (Bottom) A MagB target cell ratio of 100:1 gave the optimal combination of yield and recovery.

Table 1 High Yields and Purities Derived from CD34
Selection of Products with Historically Standard CD34
Starting Purities

	Preselection	Postselection	Recovery (%)
N = 12		Median (range)	
Purity (%)	0.9 (0.4–7.4)	92.4 (78.8–99.3)	
Dose ($\times 10^6$)	2.0 (0.55–11.0)	1.4 (0.25–7.4)	54 (39–68)

These data were derived from a series of patients whose mobilization regimen included cytoxan and G-CSF.

have adhered to the chamber or become entrapped by the rosettes are removed from the selected product.

Two different strength magnets are employed during this step. For negative selection procedures, where the viability of the selected cells is not of concern, a rare earth magnet possessing an intensely strong field strength is used. Such a magnet ensures the least degree of escape of MagBs during the wash steps. For procedures where high cell viability of the captured population is critical, such as the case for CD34 selection, magnets of considerably less strength which provide for more gentle collection of the cells are employed. In either case, secondary magnets are employed to capture MagBs that escape the primary magnet before they enter the final product container.

D. Release of Captured Target Cells from the Immunomagnetic Beads

Several different strategies have been employed to effect target cell release from the magnetic beads where such an endpoint is required. This may be accomplished by incubating the MagB/target cell rosettes at 37°C for a period of approximately 8–12 h. During the incubation, the antigen-antibody complex "caps" on the cells and is ultimately shed in to the medium. Although relatively simple, concerns of poor viability and cell maturation discourage the use of this approach. In addition, the released cells will require further incubation in suitable conditions to promote regeneration of the shed cell membrane antigens.

Alternatively, enzymatic treatment of the MagB/target cell complex is an effective and rapid method by which cells may be removed from the MagBs. Typically, following incubation with the proteolytic enzyme, chymopapain, a magnetic field is reapplied and the detached cells are washed from the beads. Using this approach, however, a portion of the cell surface antigens is cleaved and regeneration of the cell membrane proteins is required (Rubbi, 1993).

The safest and most specific method for release of MagB-bound target cells is through competitive binding with the antigen-binding site of the labeling monoclonal antibody. In order to use this technique, the compound needs to be epitope specific and has been developed for release of CD34$^+$ cells. The reagent is supplied with the kits used in the Isolex300i processing protocol [Peptide (PR34$^+$) Releasing Agent (Baxter Immuno-

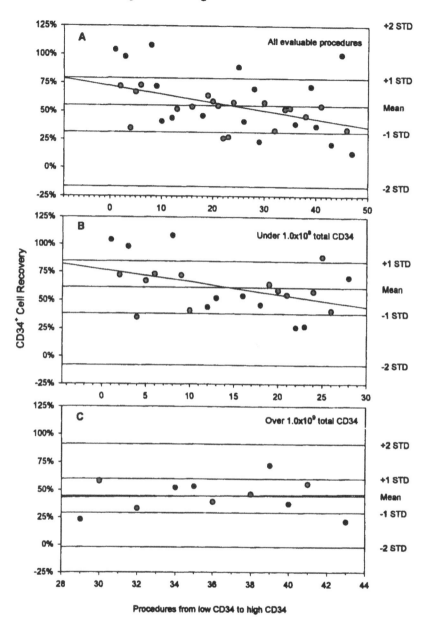

Figure 4 Relationship between CD34 dose loading and recovery. Loading the Isolex300i with over 1×10^9 CD34+ cells may saturate the selection system and reduce overall yield. Multivariate analysis of these data need to be performed in order to isolate the variables most responsible for this observation, primarily to include the effect of overall cell count on recovery of CD34 cells.

therapy, Irvine, CA; Hansen 1996)]. This engineered oligopeptide is incubated with the MagB/target cell rosettes for 30 min at ambient temperature. Passing the product through the magnetic field once more and collecting the MagB-free cell suspension results in the collection of the released cells in high purity. The selected cells retain their normal surface antigen phenotype and may advance immediately cryopreserved, transfused, cultured, or used for antibody-based diagnostic testing without further manipulation (Silvestri, 1993).

III. CLINICAL ISSUES

Although there may be many potential uses for enriched cell products, ideally CD34[+] cells enriched in the manner described above must provide a suitable product for transplantation. Successful CD34 selection produces the highest recovery of CD34[+] cells with the least amount of nontarget cell contamination, since the number of CD34[+] cells has a direct impact on the kinetics of engraftment. This phenomenon is most easily demonstrated by the observation that, to a point, the greater the per kilogram dose of CD34[+] cells derived from the peripheral blood or bone marrow, the least dependence on transfusion support and the shortest period of bone marrow aplasia are observed (Fig. 5) (Pecora, 1997). The quantity of CD34 cells in a graft is an acceptable surrogate measure for graft quality.

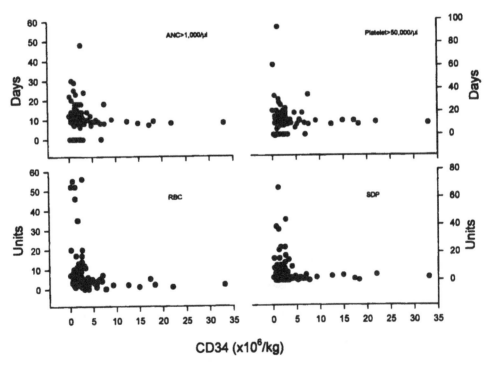

Figure 5 Relationship between CD34 dose and engraftment. Transplantation of between 2–5 × 10[6] CD34[+] cells begins to reduce the range of recovery indices including ANC > 1000/μL, platelets (Plt) > 50,000μL, and units of red blood cells (RBC) and single donor platelet (SDP) equivalents required until hematopoietic recovery posttransplant. Doses of 5 × 10[6] CD34[+] cells consistently produce rapid recovery for each parameter. Transplantation of more than 5 × 10[6] does not appear to bestow any advantage in the autologous transplant setting.

Table 2 Comparison of Recovery Following Transplant of Similar Doses of CD34 Cells, CD34-Selected vs CD34-Unselected PBSCs

Engraftment index	Unselected	Selected
Area under the curve > 1000/μL (days)	10	11
	(9–13)	(9–13)
Platelets > 20,000/μL (days)	13	15
	(10–16)	(10–19)

No significant differences in engraftment kinetics have been reported following transplantation of CD34-selected peripheral blood aphereses.

Many issues surround the accuracy of CD34 enumeration in different stem cell sources and at different stages of processing. We are, therefore, left with inadequate laboratory techniques to assess precisely the effectiveness of the transplant product and must continue to rely on the posttransplant engraftment kinetics to evaluate the quality of the graft. It is well accepted that transplantation of between 2 and 5×10^6 CD34$^+$ cells derived from the peripheral blood results in prompt and durable engraftment. In a trial involving autologous transplantation in 12 patients, transplantation of a median of 1.4×10^6 selected CD34$^+$ cells/kg (ranging from 0.25 to 7.4) resulted in no decrease in engraftment kinetics or increase in transfusion requirements following transplantation (Table 2). Although the precise minimal dose of CD34 cells required to effect prompt and durable engraftment is not known, it has been documented that transplantation of greater than 5×10^6 of these cells to a myelosuppressed or myeloablated patient confers no additional advantage to the patient in terms of engraftment kinetics. However, it has also been demonstrated that the greater the number of CD34$^+$ cells transplanted, the greater the chance that the graft will overcome the barriers imposed by HLA disparity in the allogeneic setting (Yabe, 1996) and that increased numbers of aphereses are associated with an increased rate of tumor cell contamination (Kahn, 1997). In either case, therefore, it is critical to recover as great a number of these crucial cells following any laboratory graft manipulation procedure. However, methods that recover great numbers of target cells are also sometimes prone to return nontarget cells as well. Particularly for T-lymphocyte depletion where T-cell dose is clearly associated with the occurrence and severity of graft-versus-host, these impure cell populations defeat the purpose of CD34 selection and may only serve to add time, expense, and hematopoietic cell losses to transplantation procedures.

IV. TUMOR CELL DEPLETION OF THE AUTOGRAFT

Much attention has been paid to the relevance of tumor cell contamination in the autograft. It has been most difficult to correlate outcome prognosis and tumor cell purging the graft. Is the resistance to purging responsible for the poor outcome or that residual cells were left behind? Perhaps outcome is dependent on a combination of both. To a degree, the answers to these questions will be based on a more clear understanding of the degree of contamination of the autograft and the impact of this degree (Moss, 1997). With the development of polymerase chain reaction (PCR) techniques, some micrometastatic detection can occur in as discrete a population as 1 in 1 million normal cells. It remains to be determined whether this level of detection is of the appropriate sensitivity; that is, does the tumor burden at one point not reflect the probability of relapse, or is the reinfusion of one tumor cell too many? Therefore, it is clear that any study undertaken to address the issue of the relevance of purging must necessarily consider that the extent to which the degree of contamination may influence the rate and frequency of relapse.

Although the significance of tumor cell contamination remains to be definitively determined, there is evidence that occult tumor cells in the graft contribute in some measure to relapse (Brenner, 1993; Deisseroth, 1994). It has also been well documented that tumor cell contamination is found in hematopoietic progenitor cell products intended for adjunct therapy for all types of cancer. Immunocytochemical analysis of peripheral blood progenitor cells in our laboratory and others has revealed that the overall frequency of breast cancer cell contamination increases as the disease progresses from adjuvant to stage IV disease (Table 3). The same has been found true particularly for metastatic disease or other oncological disorders and is particularly manifest in examination of bone marrow samples from these patients (Pecora, 1997). In these cases, where the degree of tumor cell contamination is sufficiently high that detection patterns become obvious and where tumor cell antigen expression does not include the CD34 antigen, the use of CD34 selection is well suited to prepare the product for transplantation. As previously discussed, however, selection of class I antibodies for the selection process may discourage the collection of CD34$^+$ leukemia cells, whose antigen glycoform is poorly detected by this class of antibody.

Although a clinically relevant degree of tumor cell depletion has yet to be defined, the ideal purging technique is capable of complete eradication of the contaminating cancer cells. Although this goal is likely to be unachievable, it is constructive to set a goal for purging techniques. Peripheral blood progenitor cell products generally contain total cell numbers on the order of $1-2 \times 10^{10}$ cells. Although the range is quite great, quantitative analysis of many of these products reveals a contamination of one to two tumor cells per 100,000 hematopoietic cells. It follows that a typical contaminated graft may contain as many as $1-4 \times 10^5$ tumor cells. Therefore, an effective purging technique must remove 5 $\log_{10}$ of contaminating cells. Depletion of tumor cells using immunomagnetic beads and mAb directed against tumor cells is capable of reducing the tumor burden by 2–3 $\log_{10}$, whereas CD34 selection passively removes a mean 3.67 $\log_{10}$ of these cells (Fruehauf, 1994) (Table 4). Data such as these have prompted investigators to seek dual purging strategies (positive/negative) that combine different methods of purging to approach the theoretical purging goal of removing 5 $\log_{10}$ of tumor cells. Data using Isolex300i CD34

Table 3 Immunocytochemical Analysis of Peripheral Blood Stem Cells in Breast Cancer

No. of contaminated aphereses	Stage II	Stage III	Stage IV	Total
	No. (%) of patients in each group			
	13 (34)	4 (11)	21 (55)	38 (100)
0	8 (61)	3 (75)	10 (48)	23 (61)
1	4 (31)	1 (25)	2 (10)	8 (21)
>1	1 (8)	0	9 (43)	7 (18)

As the stage of disease progresses, so does the likelihood that at least one peripheral blood progenitor cell apheresis for a single patient contains breast cancer cells detectable by immunocytochemistry (ICC). ICC performed by BIS Laboratories (Reseda, CA).

Table 4 Passive Depletion of Spiked CAMA-1 Cells Following CD34 Selection

Preselection	Mean ± std
CD34 purity (%)	7.9 ± 4.8
CAMA-1 (%)	1.02 ± 0.16

Postselection	Mean ± std
CD34 purity (%)	93.8 ± 4.7
CAMA-1 (%)	0.0092 ± 0.0075
CD34 Recovery (%)	49.9 ± 3.8
Depletion of CAMA-1 ($\log_{10}$)	3.67 ± 0.25

CAMA-1 cells (an established breast cancer cell line) were spiked at 1.0% into peripheral blood apheresis products. CD34 selection was performed using the Isolex300i. Tumor cell detection was performed by immunocytochemistry at Baxter Biotech, Chicago, IL.

selection followed by negative depletion using immunomagnetic beads sensitized with monoclonal antibodies against CD8 and CD4 cells has shown marked improvement in T-lymphocyte depletion and progress toward achieving 5 $\log_{10}$ reduction (Loudavaris, 1997). Similar positive/negative strategies using immunomagnetic beads and a cocktail of mAbs raised against epithelial cell cytokeratin antibodies have been used in laboratory investigation on products spiked with breast cancer cells and have shown similar results (our own preliminary data).

V. CD34 SELECTION OF CRYOPRESERVED PRODUCTS

For a variety of operational reasons, it may be desirable to select CD34$^+$ cells from cryopreserved samples. We evaluated the procedures for CD34 selection on samples of peripheral blood progenitor cells (PBPCs) cryopreserved in hydroxyethyl starch and 5% dimethyl sulfoxide (DMSO) (Stiff, 1987) for over 18 months and stored at $-95°C$. Cryopreserved PBPCs were thawed at 37°C and immediately diluted with a Ca^{2+}/Mg^{2+}–free solution of buffered saline containing 1% human serum albumin. The cells were centrifuged and the supernatant decanted. Cells thawed in this manner were CD34 selected as previously described and the recovery of viable CD34 and colony-forming units granulocyte macrophage (CFU-GM) was assessed. In our series of 10 selections perform in this manner, although mean nucleated cell recovery was only 67.7 ± 9.3% after wash and CD34 selection, we recovered 79.6 ± 11.0% of the CD34$^+$ cells present in the starting product. Of particular interest was the viability of the CD34$^+$ cells isolated from the thawed PBSC collections. Using a propidium iodide exclusion to measure membrane integrity revealed an average viability for the CD34 population postthaw of 100% (Table 5). The cells maintained this complete viability throughout the selection procedure. In contrast, there was a mean reduction of 20.2% (±13.3%) viability in the remaining nucleated cell populations. Remarkably, cryopreservation of the thawed, CD34 selected cells resulted in a mean CD34 viability of 85.6% (±4.7% after a subsequent second thaw in contrast to 1.1% (±0.8%) for the other nucleated cells. The refrozen/thawed cells recovered 72.3% (±10.9%) of the CFU-GM, indicating that these cells were functionally viable as well.

Table 5 Postthaw Viability of CD34$^+$ Cells

	Post 1st thaw	Post 2nd thaw
All nucleated cells	83.4 ± 12.9	70.9 ± 16.7
CD34$^+$ cells	100	85.6 ± 4.7
CD45$^+$/34$^-$ fraction	98.2 ± 0.9	1.1 ± 0.8

Whole aphereses thawed and subjected to CD34 selection yield high CD34$^+$ cell viability as assessed by dual staining with anti-CD34 mAb and propidium iodide. High viability was achieved following thaw of the refrozen, selected CD34$^+$ cells, in contrast to a drastic reduction in viability for CD45$^+$/CD34$^-$ cells.

VI. CONCLUSION

CD34 selection is shaping up to be an excellent tool for passive depletion of the nontarget cell types, although a combined positive/negative depletion may be advantageous to approach more closely the theoretical limits of depletion. Simple modification of the CD34 selection procedure, adding no additional processing time, is likely to accomplish this goal. Issues relating to additional apheresis due to cell loss through purging have been managed by the consistently high percentage of recovery of CD34$^+$ cells and better mobilization regimens. It will be some time before the impact of tumor cell contamination in the transplant setting can be evaluated, but a reduction in transplant-related morbidity due to DMSO-related toxicity through transplantation of selected products has been well documented. Cost and operational concerns will likely be addressed by the ability to store products and combine them prior to selection. Moreover, as the CD34 selection technology seeks its level, we are only at the threshold of defining its possibilities and liabilities. At the present time, the data indicate that the liabilities of such a procedure are few and the full benefits are yet to be realized.

REFERENCES

Brenner MK, Rill DR, Moen RC. Gene marking to trace origin of relapse after autologous bone marrow transplantation. Lancet 1993; 341:85.

Chang M, Richards G, Rembaum A. Polyacrolein microspheres: preparation and characteristics. Methods Enzymol 1985; 112:150.

Civin CI, Strauss LC, Brovall C. Antigenic analysis of hematopoiesis III. A hematopoietic progenitor cell surface antigen defined by a monoclonal antibody raised against KG-1a cells. J Immunol 1984; 133:157.

Deisseroth AB, Zu Z, Claxton D. Genetic marking shows that Ph+ cells present in autologous transplants of chronic myelogenous leukemia (CML) contribute to relapse after autologous bone marrow in CML. Blood 1994; 83:3068.

Farley TJ, Ahmed A, Fitzgerald M, Preti RA. Optimization of CD34+ cell selection using immunomagnetic beads: implications for use in cryopreserved peripheral blood stem cell collections. J Hematother 1997; 6:53–60.

Fruehauf S, Haas R, Zeller WJ, Hunstein W. CD34 selection for purging in multiple myeloma and analysis of CD34+ B cell precursors. Stem Cells (Dayt) 1994; 12:95–102.

Hansen M, Mansour V, Yacob D, Schaeffer A, Karandish S, Schilling M, Guillermo R, Burgess J, Deans R. Performance of a novel peptide CD34+ releasing agent for the Isolex system. Bone Marrow Transplant 1996; 17(Suppl 1):S29.

Hardwick RA, Kulchinski D, Mansour V. Design of large-scale separation systems for positive and negative immunomagnetic selection of cells using superparamagnetic microspheres. J Hematother 1992; 1:386.

Kahn DG, Prilutskaya M, Cooper B, Kennedy MJ, Meagher R, Pecora AL, Preti RA, Moreb J, Wingard J, Rosenfeld C, Herzig RM, Glassco JE, Umeil T, Copelan E, Lazarus HM, Moss TJ. The relationship between the incidence of tumor cell contamination and number of phereses for stage IV breast cancer (abstr). Blood 1997; 90(Suppl 1):2514.

Kemshead JT. The immunomagnetic manipulation of bone marrow. In: Gee AP, ed. Bone Marrow Processing and Purging: A Practical Guide. Boca Raton, FL, CRC Press, 1991:293–305.

Kvalheim G, Sorenssen O, Fodstad O, Finderud S, Kiesel S, Dorken B, Nustad K, Jakobsen E, Ugelstad J, Pihl A. Immunomagnetic removal of B-lymphoma cells from human bone marrow: a procedure for clinical use. Bone Marrow Transplant 1988; 3:31.

Loudavaris M, Unverzagt K, Martinson J, Jarmillo J, Bender J, Deans R. Simultaneous positive/negative selection for t cell depletion with the Isolex 300i magnetic cell separator, Blood 1997; 90(Suppl 1):1874.

Moss TJ, Umiel T, Herzig RM, Meagher R, Cooper B, Kennedy MJ, Preti RA, Pecora AL, Lazarus HM, Rosenfeld C. The presence of clonogenic breast cancer cells in peripheral blood stem cell products correlates with an extremely poor prognosis for patients with stage IV disease (abstr). Blood 1997; 90(Suppl 1):4570.

Pecora AL, Lazarus H, Cooper B, Kennedy MJ, Umiel T, Meagher R, Herzig RM, Copelan M, Prilutskaya M, Glasco J, Kahn DG, Moss TJ. Breast cancer contamination in peripheral blood stem cell collections associates with bone marrow disease and type of mobilization (abstr). Blood 1997; 90(Suppl 1):434.

Pecora AL, Gleim GW, Preti RA, Jennis A, Zahos K, Cantwell S, Doria L, Isaacs R, Gillio AP, Michelis MA, Brochstein JA. Cd34$^+$ cd33$^-$ cells influence days to engraftment and transfusion requirements in autologous blood stem cell recipients. J Clin Oncol 1998; 16:2093–2104.

Preti RA, Farley TJ, Fan Y, Ahmed T, Rose M, Ciavarella D. The combined use of soybean agglutinin and immunomagnetic beads for t lymphocyte subset depletion of bone marrow allografts: a laboratory analysis. J Hematother 1994; 3:111–120.

Preti RA, Nadasi S, Murawski J, McMannis J, Karandish S, Pecora AL. Single step positive/negative purging for breast cancer using the Isolex 300i magnetic cell separator, Blood 1997; 90(Suppl 1):4306.

Rubbi CP, Patel D, Rickwood D. Evidence of surface antigen detachment during incubation of cells with immunomagnetic beads. J Immunol Methods 1993; 166:233–341.

Silvestri F, Banavali S, Savignano C, Presiler HD, Baccarin M. CD34 cell selection: focus on immunomagnetic beads and chymopapain. Int J Artif Organs 1993; 16(Suppl 5):96–101.

Stiff PJ, Koester AR, Weidner MK. Autologous bone marrow transplantation using unfractionated cells cryopreserved in dimethylsulfoxide and hydroxyethyl starch without controlled-rate freezing. Blood 1987; 70:974–980.

Sutherland DR, Keating A. The CD34 Antigen: structure, biology, and potential clinical applications. J Hematother 1992; 1:131–142.

Treleaven JG, Gibson FM, Ugelstad J, Rembaum J, Philip T, Caine GD, Kemshead JT. Removal of neuroblastoma cells from bone marrow with monoclonal antibodies conjugated to polymer particles. Lancet 1984; 1:70.

Ugelstad J, Berge A, Schmidt R. New developments in production and application of monosized polymer particles. In: Reichert KH, Geiselar W, eds. Polymer Reaction Kinetics. Huthig & Wepf, 1986:219.

Yabe H, Yabe M, Hattori K, Hinohara T, Morimoto T, Nakmura Y, Noma M, Takei M, Kobayashi N, Tsuji KM, Kato S. Successful engraftment of allogeneic CD34-enriched marrow cell transplantation from HLA-matched parental donors. Bone Marrow Transplant 1996; 17:985–991.

14

Autologous and Allogeneic Transplantation with Blood CD34$^+$ Cells
A Pediatric Experience

YOSHIFUMI KAWANO, TSUTOMU WATANABE, YASUHIRO OKAMOTO, TAKANORI ABE, and YASUHIRO KURODA

University of Tokushima, Tokushima, Japan

YOICHI TAKAUE

National Cancer Center Hospital, Tokyo, Japan

ARATA WATANABE

University of Akita and Naka-dori Hospital, Akita, Japan

I. ADVANTAGES OF BLOOD STEM CELLS OVER BONE MARROW FOR PURIFICATION AND TRANSPLANT

In bone marrow transplantation (BMT), only hematopoietic stem cells (HSCs) that exist in the iliac bone can be collected by aspiration under general anesthesia. However, hematopoietic activity in this area decreases with age, which very often makes the procedure inefficient. On the other hand, collection of peripheral blood stem cells (PBSCs) does not require anesthesia or multiple marrow aspirations and, hence, is far less invasive than bone marrow collection. Most importantly, PBSCs can be collected from the body's entire pool of HSCs to provide more stem cells than bone marrow aspiration performed at localized iliac bones; this leads to the faster recovery of hematopoiesis after PBSC transplantation (PBSCT) than after BMT and makes "cell component therapy" far more effective with PBSCs. Accordingly, insurance reimbursement policy has been cleared for PBSCT

239

since 1994, and this has become an accepted treatment modality for a variety of malignant disorders in Japan.

Currently, an effective procedure for allogeneic transplantation with PBSCs is also being developed. Since a PBSC graft contains approximately 10-fold more T lymphocytes (T cells) than bone marrow, the establishment of a carefully constructed bulk purging procedure that may reduce the number of T cells below the critical threshold for developing graft-versus-host disease (GVHD), whereas still retaining engraftment potential, becomes critical, particularly for matched-unrelated or mismatched-related pairs at a high risk of developing severe GVHD. To support this effort, recent techniques which enable the positive selection/enrichment of CD34$^+$ cells from PBSCs provide a convenient method for concentrating HSCs and depleting T cells ("indirect purging"). This should also make autografts more effective by depleting contaminating cancer cells. At the same time, a decrease in the graft volume and dimethyl sulfoxide (DMSO), which is ultimately administered, enables the elimination of toxicities at graft infusion and saves cryopreservation space (1).

In the mouse and human, the use of CD34 antigen as a marker for HSCs has been questioned (2–4). Nevertheless, through extensive clinical studies, it has now become quite obvious that CD34$^+$ cells contain "true" stem cells that are required in the transplantation procedure. Again, to overcome the inevitable loss of HSCs during purification procedures, leaving an adequate number of cells for safe transplant, expansion of the initial inoculum by the use of PBSCs rather than bone marrow has become mandatory. This chapter will present our pediatric experience of transplants with CD34$^+$ cells, which were purified from granulocyte colony-stimulating factor (G-CSF)–mobilized blood cells.

II. MOBILIZATION AND PURIFICATION OF BLOOD CELLS FROM PEDIATRIC DONORS

A. Mobilization by G-CSF

Identification of the optimal cytokines and a protocol for use in the PBSC collection procedure, with which the fewest number of apheresis procedures are required, has emerged as the major subject of intense research in hemato-oncology. Although ethical problems related to giving G-CSF to young sibling donors still need to be resolved, this should be balanced against the existing risk of multiple marrow aspiration under general anesthesia. Studies on the kinetics of circulating progenitor cell mobilization are critical to the development of successful G-CSF mobilization protocols. At the University of Tokushima, realizing the rapidly increasing demand for allogeneic PBSCT, G-CSF (10 µg/kg/day) was given to normal donors subcutaneously for 5 days and two consecutive aphereses are performed on days 5 and 6 using a CS 3000 plus cell separator (Baxter Healthcare Corporation, Deerfield, IL) with a maximum processed volume the higher of twice the donor blood volume or 10 L, as previously reported (5,6). Commonly reported side effects related to G-CSF treatment were observed in essentially all of the 25 adult healthy donors (median age 37 years; range 18–49 years), whereas no complaints were made by 16 pediatric donors (median age, 6 years; range, 2–16 years), who all maintained their usual activity. All toxicities, if any, were acceptable and negligible in related transplant settings.

The results of simultaneous pharmacokinetics study disclosed that serum trough levels of G-CSF determined by enzyme-linked immunosorbent assay (ELISA) varied widely among donors, but they were significantly lower in the pediatric donors evaluated than in adults on days 3 and 4 ($P < .05$) even though the same dose of G-CSF was used. Serum trough levels of G-CSF became maximal on the second day of treatment in most of the donors and declined on continuing G-CSF treatment. Subsequent aphereses were uneventful and the number of blood CD34+ cells collected per unit of blood processed was identical in both donor populations. Thus, we confirmed that PBSCs could be safely mobilized and collected in small children so that they could be donors for adult patients. It might be indicated that higher doses of G-CSF are recommended in pediatric donors for more effective mobilization.

We also observed wide interdonor variations in the kinetics of circulating CD34+ cells and in the subsequent final cell yield by apheresis (Fig. 1), which could not be predicted by an evaluation before G-CSF therapy. Hence, we feel that real-time evaluation of CD34+ cells should become part of a routine examination during G-CSF treatment. These results also suggest that collected cells should be cryopreserved to prevent the possibility that an adequate amount of graft may not be available after the preparative regimen has started in allogeneic settings, although cryopreservation of cells may result in some degree of stem cell loss on freezing and thawing. This approach allows for the time to perform a thorough analysis of harvested graft for engraftment potential and T-cell contamination and, thus, has become mandatory in our transplant program. The results of our previous study indicate that, in terms of preserving engraftment potential, a simplified cryopreservation method that incorporates 6% hydroxyethyl starch and 5% DMSO without a programmed freezer (PF) is at least as effective as the traditional controlled-rate freezing procedure with PF (7).

B.   Other Mobilization Mechanisms

Following initiation of G-CSF administration, a substantial increase in circulating CD34+ cells does not occur until day 4 or 5 of G-CSF treatment. We then hypothesized that endogenous cytokine-mediated regulation of hematopoiesis is involved in this delayed appearance of circulating progenitor cells, and one of the most logical cytokines to have such a mechanism is interleukin-8 (IL-8). To investigate the role of endogenous cytokine expression in G-CSF–induced progenitor cell mobilization, we examined the serum levels of these cytokines in healthy normal donors who received G-CSF for the harvest of PBSCs.

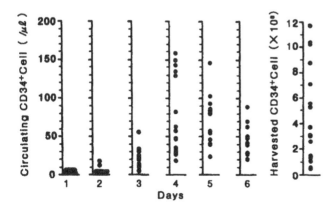

Figure 1   Circulating level of CD34+ cells during G-CSF treatment (left) and the absolute numbers of CD34+ cells collected by apheresis in pediatric donors.

The results suggested that IL-8 production may be critical to G-CSF–induced stem cell mobilization (8). In addition, serum IL-8 measurement appear to be a useful tool to define the time for apheresis and identify donors with poor mobilization potential.

C. Purification

There has been increasing development in the technology for cell processing ("graft engineering") moving from the experimental to the clinical settings. The effective depletion of cancer cells or T cells may be possible through the use of purified CD34$^+$ cells. To make the procedure clinically effective, the purity of CD34$^+$ cells needs to be high enough to ensure satisfactory depletion of target cells. To develop a cost-effective and clinically applicable procedure for the bulk purification of CD34$^+$ cells with anti-CD34 monoclonal antibody (mAb) and magnetic microspheres, we modified the manufacturer's original protocol (9). Briefly, platelet-rich plasma was removed by low-speed centrifugation and cells were diluted to a concentration of 2–5 × 10^7/mL. The same volume of 10 mM l-phenylalanine methyl ester hydrochloride (PME) (Terumo Medical Corp., Elkton, MD) supplemented with 40 U/mL of deoxyribonuclease and 2 mM ethylenediaminetetraacidic acid (EDTA) was then added to the cell suspension. The mixture was incubated for 30 min at room temperature and placed on double-layered Percoll (diameter = 1.046/1.077). After centrifugation for 25 min at 400 g, the cells in the interface were harvested. In this step, 95% of the contaminating granulocytes and monocytes, which nonspecifically bind to antibody or immunomagnetic beads, were removed from the mononuclear cell fraction. At the same time, red blood cells and cell debris which induce cell clumping on thawing were removed and the number of cells which were to undergo a costly isolation procedure with mAb can be reduced to about 40% of the initial inoculum (9).

III. ENGRAFTMENT WITH CD34$^+$ CELLS

A. Autologous Transplantation

In a subsequent study, 22 children were autografted with purified CD34$^+$ cells. In a previous study with 54 infusions of unmanipulated PBSC graft in 52 children, we made a toxicity assessment in which the volume of PBSCs infused varied from 46 to 500 mL (219.6 ± 118.4 mL) (1). In this cohort without a postthaw washing maneuver, we found that transient toxicity was rather common at graft infusion. On the other hand, in the current study with purified CD34$^+$ cells, the mean volume of the grafts the patients received was 8.8 mL (range 3–30 mL), and no adverse effects directly related to graft infusion were observed (Table 1). Hence, the cell isolation procedure resulted in the complete elimination of infusion toxicities.

After the infusion of cells, the median number of days to achieve an absolute granulocyte count (AGC) of >0.5 × 10^9/L and a platelet count of >50 × 10^9/L was, respectively, 11 (range 9–18) and 26 (range 13–90). Although the potential disadvantage of CD34$^+$ cell selection is that the reconstitution of hematological functions may be delayed, these engraftment data were identical to our historical data of 74 transplants that were performed with unmanipulated PBSCs containing an equivalent number of CD34$^+$ cells (Fig. 2).

Then we performed a randomized trial in children to determine whether engraftment after PBSCT is improved by the addition of exogenous G-CSF (10). The patients were prospectively randomized at diagnosis to evaluate the effectiveness of exogenous G-CSF

Table 1 Engraftment Data After Autografts with Purified CD34+ Cells

Case	Age/sex	Diagnosis	Reinfused volume (mL)	Infused CD34+ cells (×10⁶/kg)	No. of Days to	
					AGC (0.5 × 10⁹/L)	Platelets (50 × 10⁹/L)
1	5/F	NB	70	3.4	10	18
2	6/F	PNET	58	7.0	10	15
3	2/M	NB	30	2.3	9	18
4	8/M	T-ALL	13	5.7	13	22
5	3/F	T-ALL	7.5	1.1	14	23
6	11/F	OC	11	4.3	13	17
7	15/M	GCT	15	1.5	14	18
8	8/F	RB	7	3.9	13	20
9	1/M	RBS	7.0	0.6	11	32
10	5/M	GCT	3.0	3.3	16	35
11	9/M	WT	5.0	5.9	18	51
12	7/M	NHL	3.8	2.1	11	55
13	1/F	WT	3.8	2.0	11	45
14	4/M	NB	9.1	1.2	11	36
15	18/M	NHL	8	2.0	N.E.	N.E.
16	40/F	OC	22	2.4	11	15
17	30/F	UC	8	2.3	11	32
18	56/F	BC	18	0.53	13	17
19	60/F	BC	20	2.1	10	13
20	10/M	AML	5	1.9	12	26
21	31/F	OC	8.8	0.74	16	26
22	56/F	BC	7.8	0.43	18	44
Median			8.8	2.1	12	23
(range)			(3–30)	(0.43–5.9)	(9–18)	(13–55)
		Median	8.4	2.1	12	23
		Min	3	0.43	9	13
		Max	30	5.9	18	55

NB, neuroblastoma; PNET, peripheral neuroectodermal tumor; T-ALL, acute lymphoblastic leukemia (T-cell type); RB, retinoblastoma; RBS, rhabdomyosarcoma; GCT, germ cell tumor; WT, Wilms' tumor; NHL, non-Hodgkin's lymphoma.

treatment in accelerating hematopoietic recovery after PBSCT. We demonstrated that the use of G-CSF does not provide a marked clinical benefit in patients undergoing PBSCT with more than a threshold level of PBSCs, although this expensive strategy appears to be associated with a tendency for the delayed recovery of platelets. We recommend that the routine application of costly G-CSF therapy in children undergoing PBSCT should be seriously reconsidered.

B. Tandem Transplants with CD34-Selected Cells

Dose intensification and the sequential use of agents to overcome drug resistance may benefit some patients, and interest in the concept of tandem transplants has been growing. The principal objective of this procedure is to reduce the size of the cancer cell mass by repeated, closely timed courses of high-dose chemotherapy, each given with HSC rescue. To ensure the safety of repeated intense therapy, the risks and hazards of prolonged cytope-

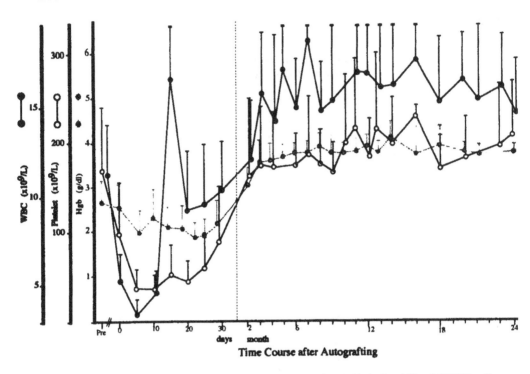

Figure 2   Hematopoietic recovery after autologous transplant with isolated blood CD34⁺ cells.

nia should be minimized by infusion of an adequate amount of stem cells. To improve the therapeutic efficacy under these conditions by depleting contaminating tumor cells in the grafts, positively selected CD34⁺ cells have been used. Although the number of stem cells can be increased when PBSCs are used, purification procedures have been associated with inevitable cell loss, and approximately half of the CD34⁺ cells in the initial inoculum are discarded with the purged cancer cells. Thus, a substantial proportion of patients could not have a purified graft sufficient for the support of multiple courses of transplant.

To maximize the intensity of therapy at an acceptable cost in toxicity, we developed a new tandem transplant strategy in which cells recovered in the CD34⁻ fraction, which still contains a large amount of clonogenic progenitor cells identified as colony-forming unit granulocyte-macrophage (CFU-GM), are used in the initial transplant. This was followed by two to three courses of regular-dose chemotherapy without rescue for further in vivo purging before the final transplant with purified CD34⁺ cells, which enables the ultimate eradication of reinfused cancer cells. The results of a feasibility study with six patients was previously published, and we speculate that this approach makes multiple-course combination high-dose therapy more feasible by ameliorating cytopenia with an improved cost/benefit ratio (11). To further prove the safety and efficacy of this procedure, a follow-up study has been performed with 10 patients, as summarized in Table 2.

Although tumor cells contaminating the CD34⁻ fraction might be of clinical concern, the presence of these cells in the graft is not necessarily capable of producing a relapse of the disease on reinfusion. This risk associated with our procedure must be weighed against the likelihood of a significant benefit. We believe that the number of cancer cells in the first graft is far smaller than the tumor burden remaining in the entire body at the

Table 2 Comparison of Engraftment Days Between Transplants with Cells in CD34⁻ (First Transplant) and CD34⁺ Fractions (Second Transplant)

	1ˢᵗ/CD34⁻ n = 10		2ⁿᵈ/CD34⁺ n = 10	
Infused CFU-GM (×10⁵/kg)	2.5	(0.3–5.0)	1.0	(0.2–4.6)
AGC > 0.5 × 10⁹/L	13	(11–16)	12	(10–16)
Platelet > 2 × 10⁹/L	12	(11–50)	16	(13–23)
Platelet > 5 × 10⁹/L	15	(11–40)	25	(15–51)

AGC, absolute granulocyte count.

first transplant and that infused cancer cells can be purged by the subsequent transplant. Nevertheless, recognizing that cancer cells might be enriched in the CD34⁻ fraction, the use of an additional purification of this fraction for negative depletion of cancer cells will be evaluated.

C. Intramedullar Injection of CD34⁺ Cells

When bone marrow transplantation was first developed, the direct injection of graft into the bone marrow space was considered to be a very appropriate maneuver. However, the large amount of cell suspension required eventually prevented the widespread use of this procedure, and intravenous infusion is currently the preferred approach. Nevertheless, it is likely that in this case only a limited portion of cells enter into the marrow space, since many cells are "trapped" in the microcirculation including the reticuloendothelial system, pulmonary vessels, and other capillary bed during the first pass through the systemic circulation. Therefore, we speculate that direct puncture of the marrow cavity to implant the graft might provide a more stable engraftment only when cells are purified with a recently developed technique (12).

IV. ALLOGRAFTS WITH CD34⁺ CELLS

A. Transplants with Unmanipulated PBSCs in Matched Sibling Pairs

Although PBSCs may be an acceptable alternative source of stem cells for future allogeneic donors who hesitate to undergo bone marrow harvest under anesthesia, the advantages/disadvantages of the use of PBSCT still need to be clarified, particularly in children. At the University of Tokushima, 12 children have thus far received a cytoreductive regimen followed by the infusion of unmanipulated PBSCs obtained from an HLA-identical sibling donor. After the infusion of graft containing a mean of 8.1 (1.7–11.5) × 10⁶/kg CD34⁺ cells, the number of days to achieve an AGC of >0.5 × 10⁹/L and a platelet count of >50 × 10⁹/L was, respectively, 10 (8–19) and 22 (12–36). Thus, the rapid recovery of hematopoiesis inherent to autologous PBSCT is also found after allogeneic transplant.

B. Transplants in HLA-Mismatched Related Pairs

The major limitation of allogeneic BMT is the lack of possible donors, in that only one third of the potential recipients have an HLA-identical sibling donor. Extension of the donor pool to a partially matched family member or matched unrelated donor, or the use of PBSCs, will indeed be associated with an increased risk of GVHD with respect to both incidence and severity and graft rejection. In this regard, routine application of T-cell depletion will become mandatory. On the other hand, major risks of T-cell depletion include increased graft rejection, loss of graft-versus-leukemia (GVL) effect, and development of lymphoproliferative disorders and serious viral infection due to delayed recovery of immune function (13). Various methods for isolating CD34$^+$ cells from harvested PBSCs have been tested to achieve indirect T-cell purging, but the optimal composition of the graft remains to be determined. With these results in mind, our current clinical research regarding allogeneic PBSCT is focussed on adapting our findings in HLA-matched sibling pairs to develop a finely tuned transplant procedure for HLA-nonidentical related pairs. Successful development of this procedure would avoid the need for lengthy matching procedures and would provide donors for >90% of patients who can benefit from an allogeneic transplantation procedure.

In our feasibility phase I study in patients who lacked an HLA-matched donor, 13 children were enrolled and PBSCs were collected from healthy mismatched family donors (14). Subsequent bulk depletion of T cells from PBSCs was accomplished with an Isolex300. (Baxter Immunotherapy, Irvine, CA). The median yield of CD34$^+$ cells was 32% (range 6–112%) with a median purity of 78% (range 19–98%), as summarized in Table 3. Preliminary result may suggest that this approach may become a universal therapeutic approach in a substantial fraction of patients who will be candidates for allogeneic transplant by providing a readily available donor.

C. Periodic Donor Leukocyte Infusion (DLI) after Transplant in Mismatched Pairs

In our program, patients who attained a stable engraftment and did not develop GVHD by day 28 were scheduled to receive a weekly infusion of a graded incremental add-back of cryopreserved mononuclear cells in the CD34$^-$ fraction, which is mostly composed of lymphocytes, over the 2 months posttransplant, with the development of grade II GVHD or clearance of viremia used as a cutoff for subsequent infusion. In our initial study, the starting dose of cells was 1×10^5/kg and patients received cyclosporine at least during this period (14). Although DLI has been effective not only for the treatment of relapsed chronic myelocytic leukemia (CML) but also for allogenic BMT patients who developed virus-induced complications (15), the GVL effect and GVHD are intimately associated, and separation of the two has been difficult (16).

Table 3 Allogeneic Cell Purification Data Using Isolex300

	Cells in the bags			CD34$^+$ cell fraction		
	MNC ($\times 10^{10}$)	Purity of CD34$^+$ cells (%)	No. of CD34$^+$ cells ($\times 10^8$)	Purity of CD34$^+$ cells (%)	Yield (%)	No. of CD34$^+$ cells ($\times 10^6$)
Median	4.20	0.69	2.40	78.1	32.3	85
(range)	(1.2–10.4)	(0.10–1.78)	(0.17–18.5)	(19–98)	(6.4–112)	(13–365)
Mean	4.35	0.70	3.19	73.7	30.0	113
(SD)	2.2	0.35	3.0	21.3	20.4	87

MNC, mononuclear cells.

The release of inflammatory cytokines, such as IL-1 and tumor necrosis factor-α from host tissues as a result of conditioning regimen-related toxicity is limited and resolves within 7–10 days when allogeneic T cells are not present. On the other hand, in the early presence of allogeneic T cells, this leads to the augmentation of their alloactivation and further cytokine release to induce a cytokine storm (17). In a mouse system, it has been reported that multiple weekly infusions of donor lymphocytes could be given to transplanted chimeras starting on day 21 after BMT without increasing the risk of developing GVHD in both major histocompatibility complex (MHC)–matched and MHC-haplomismatched combinations (18).

Based on these considerations, we postulated that by delaying the infusion of donor cells until 28 days after transplantation with purified CD34⁺ cells, posttransplant events, including a cytokine storm, conditioning regimen-related tissue damage and profound cytopenia with resultant infection to induce macrophage activation, could be resolved. Therefore, instead of the use of freshly prepared lymphocytes obtained by apheresis from the same donor, we use cryopreserved/thawed cells in the CD34⁻ fraction which were cryopreserved the same as CD34⁺ cells, thereby decreasing the burden to the donor. Thus, with the use of PBSCs rather marrow cells, one-step preparation for comprehensive cell therapy can be possible. The optimal timing and dose of DLI have not yet been determined. Although the threshold dose of lymphocytes to induce GVHD is likely to be far lower in mismatched than matched sibling settings, whether any dose-response effect exists with DLI remains unclear. In mismatched pairs, we feel that the starting dose of mononuclear cells needs to be adjusted to below 5×10^4/kg. The ultimate clinical benefit of this approach remains to be determined by a prospective randomized study.

D. Solid Organ Transplantation

Recipients of solid organs must receive life-long immune-suppressive therapy. When donated organs are from related donors, simultaneous harvest and infusion of hematopoietic stem cells from the same donor may induce allograft acceptance with a limited period of immune suppression. The expertise developed in PBSCT, as noted above, could be modified and applied to this strategy. Although there are many obstacles to be overcome, we predict that this procedure will play a major role in organ transplantation.

V. APPLICATION TO GENE TRANSDUCTION THERAPY

Recent developments in gene manipulation have led to the clinical application of gene therapy in patients with congenital metabolic diseases. An additional advantage of PBSCs is that multiple collection procedures can be performed without invasive surgery; which may be an important consideration in gene therapy, since the target patients could be very small children. It has been reported that the purification of CD34⁺ cells is necessary to improve the transduction and/or long-term expression of marker genes by reducing both the amount of retrovirus supernatant and the risk of insertion mutagenesis. To establish an effective gene therapy protocol for patients with congenital metabolic diseases, we evaluated retrovirus-mediated transduction and long-term expression of the *NeoR* gene in cryopreserved and thawed CD34⁺ cells purified from G-CSF–mobilized peripheral blood of infants and found that these cells are suitable and realistic targets for clinical gene therapy (19). Tandem transduction procedures can be achieved by combining cord blood and PBSCs.

REFERENCES

1. Okamoto Y, Takaue Y, Saito S, Hirao A, Shimizu T, Suzue T, Abe T, Sato J, Watanabe T, Kawano Y, Kuroda Y. Toxicities associated with infusion of cryopreserved and thawed peripheral blood stem cell autografts in children with active cancer. Transfusion 1993; 33:578–581.

2. Osawa M, Hanada K, Hamada H, Nakauchi H. Long-term lymphohematopoietic reconstitution by a single CD34-low/negative hematopoietic stem cell. Science 1996; 273:242–245.

3. Zanjani ED, Almeida-Porada G, Livingston AG, Flake AW, Ogawa M. Human bone marrow CD34− cells engraft in vivo and undergo multilineage expression that includes giving rise to CD34+ cells. Exp Hematol 1998; 26:353–360.

4. Bhatia M, Bonnet D, Murdoch B, Gan OI, Dick JE. A newly discovered class of human hematopoietic cells with SCID-repopulating activity. Nature Med 1998; 4:1038–1045.

5. Takaue Y, Kawano Y, Abe T, Okamoto Y, Suzue T, Saito S, Sato J, Watanabe T, Ito M, Kuroda Y. Collection and transplant of peripheral blood stem cells in very small children weighing 20 kg or less. Blood 1995; 86:372–380.

6. Takaue Y, Kawano Y, Kuroda Y. Application of recombinant granulocyte colony-stimulating factor in peripheral blood stem cell transplantation: a pediatric experience. In: Levit DJ, Mertelsmann R, eds. Hematopoietic Stem Cells: Biology and Therapeutic Applications. New York: Marcel Dekker, 1995: 611–630.

7. Takaue Y, Abe T, Kawano Y, Suzue T, Saito S, Hirao A, Sato J, Makimoto A, Kawahito M, Watanabe T, Shimokawa T, Kuroda Y. Comparative analysis of engraftment after peripheral blood stem cell autografts cryopreserved by controlled vs uncontrolled-rate method. Bone Marrow Transplant 1994; 13:801–804.

8. Watanabe T, Kawano Y, Kanamaru S, Onishi T, Kaneko S, Wakata Y, Nakagawa R, Makimoto A, Kuroda Y, Takaue Y, Talmadge JE. Endogenous interleukin (IL)-8 surge in granulocyte-colony stimulating factor induced peripheral blood stem cell mobilization. Blood 1999; 93:1157–1163.

9. Kawano Y, Takaue Y, Law P, Abe T, Okamoto Y, Makimoto A, Sato J, Suzue T, Nakagawa R, Kajiume T, Watanabe T, Ikeda K, Watanabe A, Ito M, Kuroda Y. Clinically applicable bulk isolation of blood CD34+ cells for autografting in children. Bone Marrow Transplant 1998; 22:1011–1017.

10. Kawano Y, Takaue Y, Mimaya J, Horikoshi Y, Watanabe T, Abe T, Katsuura T, Matsushita T, Kikuta A, Watanabe A, Iwai A, Ito E, Endo M, Kotani N, Ohta S, Gushi K, Azuma H, Etoh T, Hattori H, Okamoto Y, Kuroda Y (for the Japanese Cooperative Study Group of PBSCT). Marginal benefit/disadvantage of granulocyte colony-stimulating factor (G-CSF) therapy after autologous blood stem cell transplantation in children: A result of prospective randomized trial. Blood 1998; 92:4040–4046.

11. Kajiume T, Kawano Y, Takaue Y, Abe T, Watanabe T, Okamoto Y, Makimoto A, Suenaga K, Suzuya H, Sato J, Yokobayashi A, Hashimoto Y, Yoshida K, Ishibashi H, Takehara H, Tashiro S, Kuroda Y. New consecutive high-dose chemotherapy modality with fractionated blood stem cell support in the treatment of high-risk pediatric solid tumors: a feasibility study. Bone Marrow Transplant 1998; 21:147–151.

12. Yano M, Watanabe A, Kawano Y, Watanabe T, Takaue Y. Facilitated engraftment by intramedullary administered enriched allogeneic CD34+ cells? Bone Marrow Transplant 1999; 23:847–848.

13. Bacigalupo A, Mordini N, Pitto A, Piaggio G, Podesta M, Benvenuto F, van Lint MT, Valbonesi M, Lercari G, Carlier P, Lamparelli T, Gualandi F, Occhini D, Bregante S, Figari O, Soracco M, Vassallo F, De Stefano G. Transplantation of HLA-mismatched CD34+ selected cells in patients with advanced malignancies: severe immunodeficiency and related complications. Br J Haematol 1997; 98:760–766.

14. Kawano Y, Takaue Y, Watanabe A, Takeda O, Arai K, Itoh E, Ohno Y, Teshima T, Harada M,

Watanabe T, Okamoto Y, Abe T, Kajiume T, Matsushita T, Kuroda Y, Asano S, Yamaguchi K, Law P, McMannis JD. Partially mismatched pediatric transplants with allogeneic CD34+ blood cells from a related donor. Blood 1998; 92:3123–3130.

15. O'Reilly RJ, Small TN, Papadopoulos E, Lucas K, Lacerda J, Koulova L. Biology and adoptive cell therapy of Epstein-Barr virus–associated lymphoproliferative disorders in recipients of marrow allografts. Immunol Rev 1997; 157:195–216.

16. Porter DL, Antin JH. Graft-versus-leukemia effect of allogeneic bone marrow transplantation and donor mononuclear cell infusions. In: Winter JN, ed. Blood Stem Cell Transplantation. Boston: Kluwer, 1997:57–85.

17. Krenger W, Hill GR, Ferrara JL. Cytokine cascades in acute graft-versus-host disease. Transplantation 1997; 64:553–558.

18. Johnson BD, Truitt RL. Delayed infusion of immunocompetent donor cells after bone marrow transplantation breaks graft-host tolerance and allows for persistent antileukemic reactivity without severe graft-versus-host disease. Blood 1995; 85:3302–3312.

19. Abe T, Ito M, Okamoto Y, Kim HJ, Takaue Y, Yasutomo K, Makimoto A, Yamaue T, Kawano Y, Watanabe T, Shimada T, Kuroda Y. Transduction of retrovirus-mediated NeoR gene into CD34+ cells purified from granulocyte-colony stimulating factor (G-CSF)–mobilized infant and cord blood. Exp Hematol 1997; 25:696–701.

has been increasing emphasis placed on an improved quality of life following transplantation. If the beneficial properties of allogeneic BMT are to be exploited in this new era, the 40–50% up-front mortality must be significantly reduced and the quality of life must be improved for the survivors.

T-cell depletion (TCD) of donor marrow was initially viewed as a major advance toward conquering the above problems, since both animal and human studies implicated T cells as the primary mediators of GVHD (Noga and Hess, 1993). Indeed, early clinical studies demonstrated that radical (3–4 $\log_{10}$) TCD successfully reduced the incidence of acute GVHD (Filipovich et al., 1984; Antin et al., 1991). Surprisingly, the few randomized TCD trials did not show improved overall disease-free survival (DFS) over those patients receiving an unmanipulated graft (Mitsuyasu et al., 1986; Ash et al., 1990). Although the latter showed high death rates from GVHD, TCD marrow recipients were dying from graft failure, leukemic relapse, and B-cell lymphoproliferative disease: all previously low-incidence complications (Martin et al., 1988; Champlin, 1993). These studies persuaded many transplant centers to curtail TCD and other methods of allogeneic marrow manipulation.

Subsequent studies have confirmed that ancillary marrow (other than pluripotent stem) cell populations do mediate GVHD, but that they and/or other cells also facilitate engraftment and possess antileukemic properties (Vogelsang et al., 1988; Noga and Hess, 1993). Animal studies also suggested that the ancillary immunocompetent donor lymphocyte component could facilitate engraftment by overcoming host-vs-graft resistance: a host immune response that is not extinguished by myeloablative therapy (Martin and Kernan, 1997; Truitt et al., 1997). Many of the TCD techniques radically deplete ancillary cell populations (including committed progenitor cells) via nonspecific loss (Reisner et al., 1981; Martin et al., 1987; Hale et al., 1988). The use of pan–T-cell monoclonal antibodies (well characterized only against peripheral blood T cells), variability in complement lots, and numerous washing steps all contributed to low cell doses for infusion. A systematic approach was needed to investigate carefully whether ancillary cells are required for optimal survival following an allogeneic transplant. The complexities that were emerging in the donor/host relationship also suggested that future trials utilize a multidisciplinary approach toward engineering the hematopoietic graft. The approach we developed was termed "graft engineering," and it relied on a series of interdependent phase I and I/II clinical trials used in succession to alter systematically the lymphohematopoietic characteristics of the graft and/or the host to improve long-term survival (Noga, 1992). Where possible, animal models were utilized to guide the preclinical development of new approaches. This design also facilitated the incorporation of new technology (investigational devices) whose performance characteristics could be easily evaluated and compared to the previous study that did not include this step. Each graft manipulation step had to be thoroughly characterized to allow comparison to further or new manipulations that would be added in subsequent trials. This also allowed a direct comparison of various graft characteristics [(e.g., stem cell content, lymphocyte subsets, natural killer (NK) activity] to "performance" characteristics which are represented in patient outcomes such as acute and chronic GVHD, engraftment, inpatient hospitalization stay, infections, blood product utilization, relapse, performance status, and overall quality of life. This approach would allow total flexibility, including the eventual incorporation of genetic engineering strategies. At present, however, the bulk manipulation of cell populations combined with immunological/pharmacological modulation of the donor/host or graft comprises the currently available tools for graft engineering. This chapter summarizes our decade of experience in allogeneic graft engineering. The results and outcomes of several clinical trials will emphasize the many achievements made in this field as well as cover several of the unsuccessful approaches, which have now been modified. We will conclude with a discussion of the current status of graft engineering and outline the future directions and clinical trials that could further improve patient outcome.

II. USING ELUTRIATION FOR PRIMARY GRAFT MODIFICATION

A. Lymphocyte-Modified Grafts

Although the long-term complications of TCD outweighed its beneficial effects, it was extraordinarily successful in abrogating the early post-BMT morbidity associated with acute GVHD (Mitsuyasu et al., 1986; Martin and Kernan, 1997). Rather than abandon TCD altogether, we hypothesized that long-term complications could be minimized by "dosing back" a predetermined number of lymphocytes into the TCD graft. Preclinical studies suggested that the physical separation technology of elutriation was well suited for this approach. Elutriation can rapidly and reliably separate bulk cell populations differing in sedimentation coefficient (size and density) into distinct cellular fractions with virtually no loss in either recovery or viability (Noga et al. 1986; Noga, 1988; Kauffman et al., 1990). A consistent 2.0–2.5 $\log_{10}$ TCD of an entire marrow graft could be achieved in 40 mins. The only surrogate marker that was available to assess engraftment during these initial studies was the colony-forming unit (CFU). Over 90% of the CFU–granulocyte-macrophage (CFU-GM) or granulocyte/erythroid/macrophage/megakaryocyte (CFU-GEMM or Mix) were recovered in this large-sized TCD fraction (Noga et al., 1986). Not knowing which of the ancillary cells comprising the lymphoid-rich elutriation fractions were beneficial, the initial trials utilized morphology to determine lymphocyte dose. Patients received the TCD graft fraction and, if necessary, a second product derived from the lymphoid-rich fractions to construct a graft containing either 1×10^6 or 5×0^5 lymphocytes/kg recipient ideal body weight (Wagner et al., 1988, 1990). Limiting dilution analysis demonstrated that this correlated with a functional T-cell dose of 4×10^5 or 2×10^5 cells/kg, respectively (Noga et al., 1990). Cyclosporine A (CSA) was administered for 180 days for GVHD prophylaxis because of the intentional inclusion of T cells. Using elutriation combined with lymphocyte dose modification, clinically significant (stage $\geq$ 2) acute GVHD was reduced from 46 and 38% (historical matched controls, 1×10^6 lymphocytes/kg, respectively) to 11% at a lymphocyte dose of 5×10^5/kg (Wagner et al., 1990). The 5-year probability of developing chronic GVHD was also decreased from 56 to 6% (Noga et al., 1991). Although considered only a minor complication with this approach, 10% of the patients still demonstrated early graft failure (Table 1). Perhaps more worrisome, a considerable number of elutriated graft recipients showed delayed engraftment kinetics with the median day to an ANC > 500/µL of 22 days and the median day to an untransfused platelet count of $\geq$50,000/µL of 44 days (Wagner et al., 1990) (Fig. 1). An additional 4% of patients eventually showed complete loss of the donor graft, whereas mixed hematopoietic chimerism could be documented in an additional 32% (Noga et al., 1992). In contrast to patients with acute leukemia, 79% of patients transplanted with TCD grafts for chronic myelogenous leukemia (CML) relapsed within 2 years (Wagner et al., 1992). These patients had nearly a 100% probability of relapse by 30 months as compared to <10% for non-TCD patients transplanted for CML.

     Over a 6-year period (1986–1992), 106 patients received lymphocyte-modified, elutriated grafts. Patients with CML were excluded from elutriation protocols after 1988.

Table 1 Summary of TCD Using Elutriation
for HLA-Matched BMT

N[a]	106
Acute leukemia (CR1,CR2)	44
CML/Other	40/16
Failure to engraft/chimerism[b]	10/19
Acute GVHD	12 (11%)
Chronic GVHD	6 (6%)
DFS/survival: acute leukemia[c]	52%/52%
DFS/survival: CML[c]	3%/32%

CML, chronic myelogenous leukemia; TCD, T-cell
depletion; HLA, histocompatibility antigen; BMT, bone
marrow transplant; CR, complete remission; GVHD,
graft-versus-host disease; DFS, disease-free survival.
[a]Combined phase I and II studies from 1985 to 1992.
[b]Excludes patients with CML (97% of which demonstrated mixed chimerism).
[c]10-year follow-up.

Benefits derived from this procedure included decreased morbidity from acute and chronic
GVHD and the inclusion of patients up to age 45 for allogeneic BMT without increased
peritransplant morbidity. Sufficient patient numbers were transplanted for the acute leukemias to assess DFS (Fig. 2). For combined first complete remission (CR1) and second
complete remission (CR2) acute myeloid leukemia (AML) patients, DFS now at 10 years
is 45% and, surprisingly, combined CR1 and CR2 acute lymphocytic leukemia (ALL)

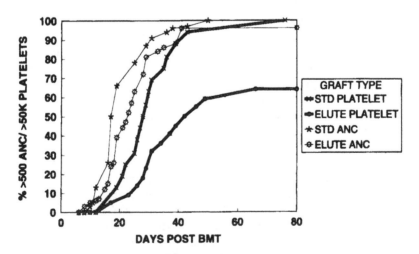

Figure 1 Engraftment kinetics of elutriated allogeneic marrow recipients. Engraftment curves
display the second day of achieving a granulocyte count ≥ 500/μL or a platelet count ≥ 50,000/
μL for 43 patients who received only elutriated marrow/cyclosporine A (CSA) prophylaxis along
with the respective curves for a similar patient cohort who received unmanipulated marrow and
CSA/methotrexate prophylaxis. A small proportion of patients receiving elutriated grafts required
> 6 months to achieve platelet independence.

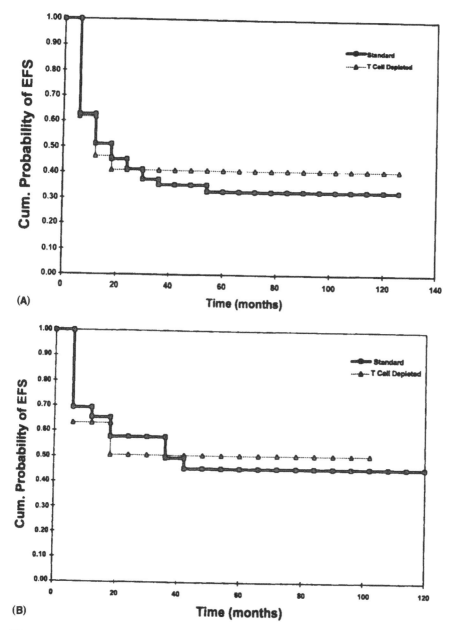

Figure 2 Disease-free survival following elutriation for patients with acute leukemia. (A). Acute myeloid leukemia (AML): CR1 and CR2 (10-year followup). (B). Acute lymphocytic leukemia (ALL): CR1 and CR2 (10-year followup). CR1, first complete remission; CR2, second complete remission.

recipients have a 10-year DFS of 62% (Noga et al., 1992). Therefore, the GVL effect of allogeneic BMT is not compromised by this graft modification technique. There was also no secondary B-cell malignancies documented for any elutriation study and the risk of infection was not increased (Flinn et al., 1995). Several drawbacks were also discovered during this time period. Despite having less engraftment problems than with radical TCD, elutriation still demonstrated a 10% graft failure rate and showed delayed engraftment kinetics, especially for platelets, when compared to unmanipulated marrow. The presence of mixed hematopoietic chimerism was also troublesome, although the Nijmegen group had also reported similar findings with elutriation. Similar to our cohort, it was not associated long term with relapse (Schattenberg et al., 1989). Obviously, this approach was not acceptable for CML, thus excluding a fairly large transplant population of older age. Lastly, one phase I study utilized elutriation without CSA prophylaxis. This study was terminated after enrolling four patients owing to a 100% incidence of initial failure to engraft (FTE) or subsequent graft failure (Wagner et al., 1988). Apparently this form of TCD had an absolute CSA requirement to ensure durable engraftment in addition to CSA's role in suppressing GVHD. All subsequent elutriation protocols maintained CSA prophylaxis for 6 months post-BMT. Laboratory investigation was then directed toward improving engraftment kinetics and in determining what conditions, if any, would allow elutriation to be used again in CML.

III. CD34⁺ STEM CELL AUGMENTATION

A. Preclinical Development

Using an animal elutriation model, it had become apparent that a small-sized lineage undefined cell residing in the lymphoid-rich elutriation fraction was responsible for long-term durable engraftment (Jones et al., 1990). This cell population was distinct from the larger-sized lineage-defined cell population found in the TCD fraction which generated 14-day hematopoietic colonies. In humans, the development of the anti-CD34 monoclonal antibody which defined early hematopoietic progenitor cell populations and more sophisticated flow cytometric systems, which could easily discern rare events, permitted a detailed reevaluation of the currently generated elutriation fractions. This data indicated that two thirds of the CD34⁺ cells were small in size and coeluted with the lymphocytes that were not included in the graft (Noga et al., 1994).

If these smaller-sized CD34⁺ cells (which did not give rise to appreciable 14-day colonies) were similar to the phenotype^{neg} long-term repopulating cells in the mouse, then their loss from the graft could account for the delayed engraftment kinetics seen with elutriated marrow. Furthermore, animal data also suggested that higher stem cell doses may also out compete malignant stem cells during repopulation, thus reducing the probability of relapse (Reisner et al., 1994). This could be particularly important in CML where most patients are transplanted in chronic phase and have a significant tumor burden at the time of transplant. DeWitte et al. (1996) used incremental flow rates to separate these smaller-sized stem cells away from their lymphoid counterparts. Unfortunately, this resulted in variable CD34⁺ cell recoveries and lymphocyte contamination.

Soon after the human stem cell (or at least its earliest identifiable progenitor) epitopes were characterized, several biotechnology companies developed methods of capturing and isolating these CD34⁺ cells from marrow (Berenson et al., 1996; Civin et al., 1996). Although high purity (>90%) could be achieved using marrow aspirate-sized samples, the use of whole marrows with clinical scale devices yielded purities between 50 and 70% (Noga and Civin, 1996). This was acceptable for autologous stem cell concentration but unsatisfactory for allogeneic TCD. A typical marrow harvest of $2-4 \times 10^8$ nucleated cells/kg has an average lymphocyte contamination of 20% ($4-8 \times 10^7$/kg); this would result in a lymphocyte contamination of $1.5-3.0 \times 10^7$/kg if an entire allograft was processed via CD34$^+$ selection. This degree of lymphocyte contamination would result in significant GVHD. Alternatively, elutriating the marrow first results in a well-defined TCD fraction containing almost all the committed progenitor cells and also provides defined smaller-sized fractions which contain cells of uniform size with significantly less platelets and mature erythrocytes than whole marrow. Since the lymphoid-rich small cell fractions were previously discarded, they were available for large-scale CD34$^+$ cell selection procedures. These fractions were pooled, incubated with biotinylated anti-CD34, and washed. Passing them over an avidin gel column (Fig. 3) could then capture the labeled cells. Using the CellPro CEPRATE SC Stem Cell Concentrator system (CellPro, Inc., Bothell, WA), only 2% of the cells loaded onto the column were recovered in the adsorbed fraction, but the median CD34$^+$ purity and yield was 80 and 60%, respectively. The T cells comprised only 5% of the positively selected cells; $<1 \times 105$ T cells/kg would be derived from this fraction if it were infused. The total graft CD34$^+$ cell dose could be effectively doubled if this product were to be given along with the elutriated TCD fraction (Noga et al., 1994).

B. Clinical Trials of CD34$^+$ Augmentation/Elutriation

If engraftment kinetics are affected by stem (CD34$^+$) cell dose, especially in the TCD setting, then the ability to recover twice as many CD34$^+$ cells should impact on this outcome. The initial phase I trial (N = 10) utilized an elutriated, TCD graft as used in the preceding elutriation trials. Instead of discarding the small-sized lymphocyte-rich frac-

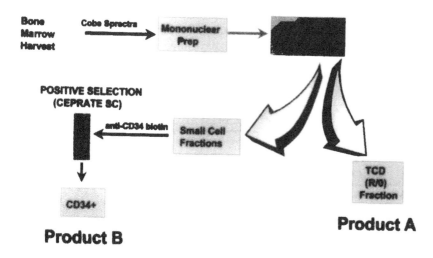

Figure 3 Schema for elutriation combined with CD34$^+$ augmentation. The donor marrow harvest is processed using the Cobe Spectra to obtain a mononuclear cell preparation for elutriation. The large-sized T-cell–depleted (TCD) elutriated fraction (R/O) is infused immediately. The lymphocyte-rich small-sized fractions are pooled, washed, incubated with anti CD34-biotin, and the stem cells concentrated over an avidin (CEPRATE SC) column (CellPro, Inc., Bothell, WA). The CD34$^+$ fraction is then infused.

tions, they were concentrated, incubated with biotinylated anti-CD34 monoclonal antibody, and then positively selected over the CellPro CEPRATE avidin column. Post-BMT CSA prophylaxis was maintained for 180 days. The use of the CD34$^+$ selected product effectively doubled the graft's CD34$^+$ cell dose to 3.2 × 10^6/kg, whereas the total T-cell content averaged 5 × 10^5/kg (S.J. Noga, personal communication). As with elutriation alone, the CD34$^+$ fraction contributed very few committed progenitor cells (only 10% of the CFU-GMs), but the majority of the cells capable of initiating long-term hematopoiesis on marrow stromal layers resided in this fraction. Granulocyte and platelet engraftment was rapid and durable with a median of 18 and 22 days, post-BMT, respectively. No patient had stage 3 or 4 acute GVHD; one patient had stage 2 which resolved and no patient developed chronic GVHD. Several phase II trials were then conducted to explore the durability and characteristics of engraftment using this approach. Since CSA was an absolute requirement with elutriation alone, different posttransplant intervals were investigated. CSA has several deleterious side effects such as hypertension, nephrotoxicity/neurotoxicity, immune suppression, and increased relapse risk which significantly affect posttransplant morbidity. The long-term outcome may be improved by CSA reduction post-BMT. The ability to reproducibly engineer the hematopoietic graft combined with the use of standardized preparative and supportive care regimens permits the investigation of single variables such as the duration of CSA administration. In this way, their effect on transplant outcome (e.g., engraftment, GVHD, morbidity, costs) can be determined. The following sections demonstrate the effect of CSA duration on several outcome parameters. Later sections discuss other active or planned phase II protocols aimed at addressing other factors (e.g., CML, relapse, HLA disparity) that affect outcome.

C. Effect of CSA Duration on Engraftment

Animal data suggested that 30–60 days of CSA were required to ensure durable TCD allogeneic engraftment (A.D. Hess, unpublished data). Three consecutive phase II graft engineering studies examined post-BMT CSA duration (Noga et al., 1997). The daily dosing schedule was constant while CSA was administered for 180 (CSA180, N = 28), 30 (CSA30, N = 30), and 80 (CSA80, N = 52) days. In terms of graft composition, the results for all three studies were pooled, since there were no statistical differences detected in the engineered graft product (Table 2). The majority of the T cells (86%) and CFU-

Table 2   Composition of Elutriated/CD34$^+$-Augmented Allogeneic Grafts

	Nucleated cells/kg (×10^6)	CD3$^+$ cells/kg (×10^5)	CFU-GM/kg (×10^4)	CD34$^+$ cells/kg (×10^6)	%CD34+	%CD3+
Large (R/O) cell fraction	41 (37–45)	4.2 (2.9–5.5)	11.6 (9.4–13.8)	1.8 (1.4–2.2)	4.4	1.0
Small (CD34$^+$) selected fraction	2.0 (1.6–2.4)	1.3 (1.0–1.6)	3.5 (2.7–4.3)	1.5 (1.3–2.7)	79 (64–94)	6.5
Engineered graft	43 (40–46)	5.5 (4.1–6.9)	15.1 (13.5–16.7)	3.3 (3.1–3.5)	7.7	1.3

CFU-GM, colony-forming units, granulocyte-macrophage; R/O, rotor off; TCD, T-cell depletion.
Values represent the mean (95% confidence intervals) for 110 consecutive allogeneic donor marrow harvests processed using elutriation for TCD and CD34$^+$ selection of the pooled, elutriated small cell fraction (CellPro CEPRATE SC).

GMs (76%) were contributed by the TCD fraction obtained when the elutriator rotor is turned off [(R/O) fraction]. The enriched CD34$^+$ small cell fraction represented 0.4% of the initially harvested cells but contained 49% of the combined graft CD34$^+$ cells. The average engineered graft had a CD34$^+$ cell dose of 3.3 × 10^6/kg. The majority (96.5%) of patients demonstrated prompt granulocyte and platelet engraftment: The median days to reach an ANC > 500/μL and platelet count >50,000/uL were 16 and 24 days on the CSA30 study and 17 and 26 days for the CSA80/180 trials (P.V. O'Donnell, personal communication). It should also be noted that no hematopoietic growth factors were given to these patients during the immediate transplant period. These results are significantly improved over the kinetics of granulocyte and platelet engraftment seen with elutriated marrow only (20 and 41 days, respectively) and compare favorably with historical controls that received unmanipulated marrow [17 and 22 days, respectively (Mitsuyasu et al., 1986; Martin et al., 1987; Noga et al., 1991)]. Four patients (3.6%) failed to engraft (two in CSA80, two in CSA180 cohort). One patient experienced late graft failure at 6 months (CSA80) but had complete hematopoietic recovery following a boost from his donor. This is less than the incidence of FTE seen with elutriation alone (10% incidence) or with other forms of TCD. However, it is still higher than the ≤1% incidence reported for unmanipulated marrow grafts (Martin and Kernan, 1997). Two of the four patients (AML CR2, CR3) were highly alloimmunized and had received platelet products from their donor during induction therapy (prior to BMT). The third patient had AML arising out of myelo-dysplastic syndrome (MDS) and the fourth had MDS presenting after aplastic anemia. It is now evident that the cohort of patients transplanted for MDS stand apart from those transplanted for acute leukemia, lymphoma, or multiple myeloma (MM) in having some-what delayed engraftment kinetics (Fig. 4). The disease status of these four patients sug-gests the possibility of an underlying microenvironmental marrow disorder predisposing to graft failure. All patients received an optimal engineered graft product. The total num-bers of mononuclear cells, CD34$^+$ cells, and CFU-GM per graft were all within the 95% confidence intervals for these graft parameters.

As discussed previously, the use of elutriated grafts has been associated with high rates of mixed hematopoietic chimerism. Although apparently not influencing the relapse rate in acute leukemia or lymphoma, it is conceivable that diseases that have strong marrow microenvironmental components, such as CML or MDS, may require higher CD34$^+$ cell doses to establish normal hematopoiesis. Southern blot analysis of restriction fragment length polymorphisms (RFLPs) was used to evaluate hematopoietic chimerism in the 78 patients who survived beyond the peritransplant period. There was no evidence of persis-tent, mixed chimerism (>20% host BM cells >60 days post-BMT). A shift to mixed chimerism from 100% donor engraftment was seen in 16 patients (20%), but 14 of these patients had documented relapse (P.V. O'Donnell, personal communication). The duration of CSA had no impact on mixed hematopoietic chimerism. Therefore, CD34$^+$ augmen-tation of elutriated grafts resulted in rapid and durable engraftment and the disappearance of mixed hematopoietic chimerism when compared to elutriation alone. Similarly, it ap-peared that the absolute requirement for post-BMT CSA had been abrogated. Either dou-bling the CD34$^+$ cell dose or the inclusion of previously discarded stem cell populations had eliminated this complication of elutriation/TCD.

D. Effect of CSA Duration on GVHD

CSA duration was not expected to have an impact on the incidence of GVHD, since this had not been a problem in the phase I trial. The incidence of stage I (grade 2 skin biopsy;

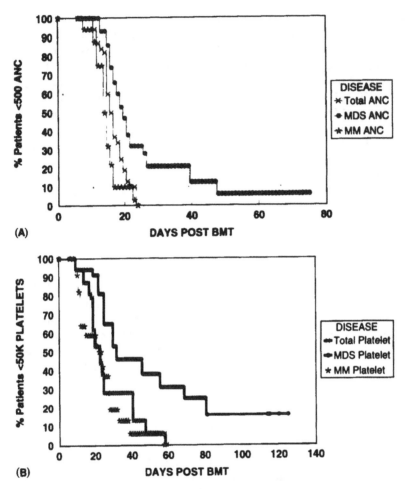

Figure 4 Disease-specific differences in engraftment kinetics in recipients of elutriated/CD34+-augmented allografts. The mean curve for granulocyte (A) and platelet (B) engraftment for patients transplanted for acute myelogenous leukemia (AML), acute lymphocytic leukemia (ALL), non-Hodgkin's and Hodgkin's lymphoma, multiple myeloma (MM), chronic lymphocytic leukemia (CLL) (all diagnoses except MDS) versus those transplanted for MDS or MM.

clinically insignificant) acute GVHD approached but did not achieve statistical significance between the CSA groups indicating that CD34+ augmentation/elutriation has minimal effects on mild GVHD even with differing CSA duration regimens. With all groups combined, the overall incidence of clinically significant acute GVHD (>stage I) for all CSA dosing schedules combined (N = 104 evaluable patients) was 11% (Fig. 5). This was similar to the previous elutriation studies using elutriation alone combined with 180 days of CSA (Noga et al., 1990; Wagner et al., 1990). However, the overall incidence of >stage I acute GVHD differed significantly between 30 and 80 days of CSA (P = .002) and between 30 and 180 days of CSA (P = .02), but there was no difference observed between 80 and 180 days (P = .67). For this discussion, the results of CSA prophylaxis can be discussed in terms of 30 versus >30 days' duration. The incidence was 23% for

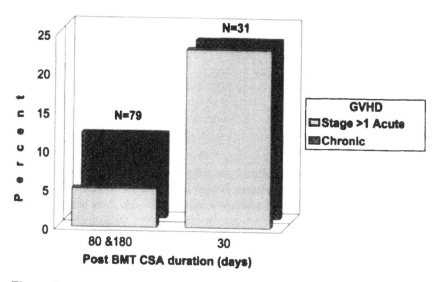

Figure 5 Incidence of acute and chronic chronic graft-versus-host disease (GVHD). Results of 110 patients who received elutriated/CD34$^+$-augmented grafts but with different durations of cyclosporine A (CSA) prophylaxis. Patients receiving either 80 or 180 days of posttransplant CSA were similar and combined for statistical purposes. Stage >1 acute GVHD represents grade ≥ 2 skin biopsy, ≥25% surface area involvement, and a requirement for corticosteroids. Chronic GVHD includes both limited and extensive disease.

the CSA30 group versus 5% ($P = .012$) for those receiving >30 days of CSA. The incidence of chronic GVHD also approached, but did not achieve, statistical significance between the CSA groups. The overall incidence of chronic GVHD was higher than that observed with elutriation/CSA180 (15 vs 6%, respectively). However, there was a 23% incidence in the CSA30 group compared to an 11% incidence in the >CSA30 group ($P = .10$). More importantly, there was a significant difference between the groups in the number of patients with chronic GVHD who had prior acute GVHD (80% in the CSA30 group vs 25% in the >CSA30 group, $P = .019$). The latter observation gives support to the hypothesis that acute and chronic GVHD may be independent immune phenomena which are separable only in settings where the incidence of acute GVHD is minimal, such as the >CSA30 cohort (Hakim and Mackall, 1997).

E. Effect of CSA Duration on Early Posttransplant Morbidity

Again the two groups (CSA30 and >CSA30) can be compared. Overall post-BMT infectious complications accounted for a 5% mortality for both studies combined. Peritransplant mortality was significantly higher in the group of patients receiving 30 days of CSA prophylaxis (10 vs 2%, $P = .013$) with the excess mortality due to infection and acute GVHD. The two deaths from acute GVHD and one death from chronic GVHD also were restricted to the CSA30 group; patients succumbing to infectious complications all had antecedent GVHD requiring corticosteroid therapy. The majority of these deaths were complicated by opportunistic infections [cytomegalovirus (CMV), pneumocystitis, aspergillosis pneumocystis carinii pneumonia (PCP)]. There did not appear to be any disease-specific effect on mortality, which was distributed approximately equally among the various diagnoses

[AML, ALL, MDS/AML, non-Hodgkin's lymphoma (NHL), Hodgkin's disease (HD), MM]. The causes of mortality differed between the peritransplant and late-transplant (>100 days post-BMT) periods. The incidence of infectious deaths was about equal. In the peritransplant period, 64% of mortality was due to FTE, acute GVHD, veno-occlusive disease, and organ failure, whereas in the late-transplant period, 67% of mortality was due to relapse-related causes. As with standard elutriation, there have been no primary B-cell malignancies developing in the CD34$^+$-augmented patients post-BMT.

F. Effect of Age at Transplant

A significant effect of age on peritransplant mortality was observed. The mortality of patients <50 years of age was 16% compared to 36% for patients >50 years of age ($P =$ .027). When the patient population was stratified at 40 years of age, there was no significant difference between mortality in the two groups (15 and 24%, respectively; $P = .25$). These data are important, since only a few patients aged 40 years or over were transplanted prior to elutriation owing to high post-BMT mortality. Mortality in the late-transplant period in the <50-year and ≥50-year age groups approached but did not achieve statistical significance at a median follow-up period of 296 days (range 3–1284 days).

G. Overall Assessment of CD34$^+$ Augmentation/Elutriation

An unexpected benefit of these phase II studies was that the rapid engraftment, lack of significant GVHD, decreased febrile episodes, decreased blood product and antibiotic utilization, reduced gastrointestinal complications, and improved oral intake led to shorter inpatient hospitalization stays (median 12-day reduction) and a concomitant 40% reduction in patient charges (Noga et al., 1994a, 1994b). This provided the impetus for performing allogeneic BMT (using engineered grafts) in an intensive outpatient setting in carefully selected individuals, 40% of whom never have a febrile episode or have an inpatient admission during their aplastic period.

To summarize, one variable (i.e., CSA duration) can significantly impact on transplant outcome when using TCD engineered grafts. Reducing CSA duration in patients receiving a CD34$^+$-augmented/elutriated graft did not effect hematopoietic engraftment. However, there was a substantial increase in both acute and chronic GVHD. This was accompanied by increased mortality related to GVHD and its associated complications (immunosuppression, infection). It appears that hematopoietic allografts containing even low numbers of intentionally included T cells require a moderate period of posttransplant CSA administration to control GVHD. Durable engraftment, however, is no longer dependent on long-term CSA usage. The minimal period for CSA therapy has not been established. These studies would indicate that at least 2–3 months of CSA are required to prevent excess morbidity in the posttransplant period. If additional cell populations are to be administered (i.e., CD56$^+$ NK cells, donor leukocytes) at intervals post-BMT to augment antitumor activity, it may be necessary to extend immunosuppressive coverage to beyond the last treatment cycle to minimize complications.

IV. ENGINEERING GRAFTS TO REDUCE RELAPSE

The major goals of our previous marrow manipulation protocols centered on decreasing short-term morbidity (GVHD, engraftment) associated with allogeneic BMT without affecting the GVL effect, especially in the older patient cohort. As we enter the next decade of graft engineering, our focus has shifted toward modulation of the antitumor properties of the graft (or host). Attention has been focused on patients who are especially at high risk of relapse, since their long-term survival is significantly impaired. Radical TCD and other methods which nonspecifically remove other cell populations (including stem cells) demonstrated the importance of ancillary graft cells. However, it is still unclear which cell population(s) is important in combating relapse. Are different ancillary cell populations more effective for specific diseases? Can specific donor graft ancillary cell populations be stimulated/augmented in the peritransplant period via cytokines to decrease the incidence of relapse? For the most part, these questions have not been fully answered.

Over the last 5 years, several investigators have successfully used donor leukocyte infusions to induce durable remissions in patients who have relapsed after TCD BMT (Kolb et al., 1990; Bar et al., 1993; Drobyski et al., 1993; Hertenstein et al., 1993; Kolb et al., 1993; Collins et al., 1994; Porter et al., 1994; van Rhee et al., 1994; MacKinnon et al., 1995; Raffoux et al., 1995). As expected, the majority of patients were treated for relapsed CML, but responses have also been seen in AML, MM, MDS, and lymphoma. Complications of this therapy include aplasia (graft failure, infection) and acute and chronic GVHD. Very few groups have looked at the effect of specific donor leukocyte populations for reducing these complications while maintaining antitumor activity. Champlin and colleagues (Champlin et al., 1992; Giralt et al., 1995) have demonstrated that CD8 depletion of donor lymphocyte grafts can achieve molecular remissions in CML patients who have relapsed following TCD BMT. The use of CD8-depleted donor leukocyte infusion (DLI) products is associated with a lower incidence of GVHD and aplastic complications (Giralt et al., 1995). It is unclear as to which cells are responsible for achieving remission in this setting since CD4$^+$ T cells, CD56$^+$ NK cells, and other rarer cell populations are still all present in the donor graft. These data support previous trials showing that specific CD8 depletion of the initial donor graft can be equally effective in reducing relapse in CML (Champlin et al., 1992). Animal data suggest that CD56$^+$ NK cells may also provide effective antitumor activity in AML and other diseases (Truitt et al., 1997). Together, these clinical trials suggest that modulation or enhancement of specific ancillary cell populations following TCD may reduce the incidence of relapse in high relapse–risk patients.

More benefit may be derived from administering specific ancillary cell populations prophylactically (Johnson and Truitt, 1995; Dimitrios et al., 1996). While one approach may be to infuse unmanipulated donor leukocytes at various time points following a TCD transplant, another possibility may be to utilize the ancillary cells from graft manipulation for this purpose. These graft-derived ancillary cells may include beneficial antitumor subpopulations in higher frequency than those available via donor leukopheresis. New developments in positive selection technology now permit sequential selection of ancillary cell populations from the graft (Berenson et al., 1996; Risdon et al., 1996). One can envision the complete dissection of the hematopoietic graft into specific fractions that can be used either immediately to construct the engineered graft or stored for later use (Fig. 6). Preliminary large-scale experiments using the ''CD34$^-$'' cells that are not infused following CD34$^+$ augmentation/elutriation show that CD4$^+$, CD8$^+$, and CD56$^+$ cells can be sequentially obtained in high purity and yield (Fig. 7) using the respective biotinylated monoclonal antibodies and the CellPro CEPRATE avidin column (Turner et al., 1995; Eby et al., 1997). In vitro functional (cytolytic) activity (Fig. 8) can be demonstrated against appropriate targets using the purified CD4$^+$ and CD56$^+$ cells even after control rate freezing, cryopreservation and thawing (Turner et al., 1995; Eby et al., 1997). There is some

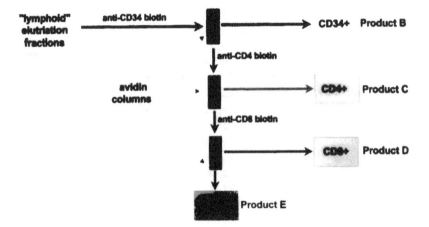

Figure 6   Schema for sequential positive selection. Initial graft processing is identical to Figure 3. Following CD34+ selection, the CD34- fraction is concentrated and washed using a Cobe 2991, incubated with the designated biotin-conjugated antibody, and selected over the CEPRATE avidin column. This process is repeated for each cell population desired.

concern that "uncaptured" antibody-coated cells from the first selection will be carried over into the subsequent sequentially selected product. We have shown that this does occur with the avidin-biotin selection, but this "contamination" can be quite beneficial depending on the initial positive selection performed (Eby et al., 1997). If the cells were first selected for CD34, which is the most likely process, the contaminating population comprises CD34+ stem cells. Although representing only a small percentage of the total selected product, they would still equal as much as 20–40% of the initial CD34+ cell population (Fig. 9). The use of both selected products results in near total recovery of all

	pre-sep fraction →	CD34+ →	CD4+ →	CD8+ →	CD4neg CD8neg
Total Nuc cells	4.4x10E9	7.0x10E7	4.9x10E8	4.2x10E8	1.6x10E9
Target purity	N/A	83%	91%	86%	N/A
Yield	N/A	48%	45%	46%	N/A
CD3+ purity	46%	8%	93%	96%	20%

Figure 7   Purity and yield of cells obtained by sequential positive selection. The values are the mean of four preclinical large-scale experiments using actual donor grafts. The CD34+ cells are infused, but the CD34- fraction is available for further manipulation. In a separate series, CD56+ natural killer (NK) cells were selected from the CD4-CD8- fraction.

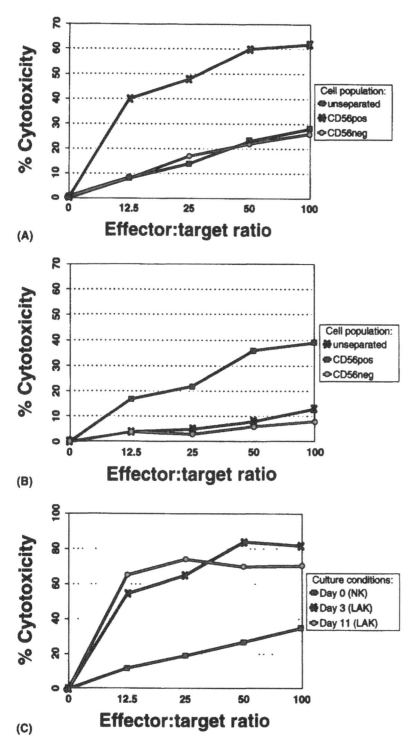

Figure 8 Natural killer (NK) activity of CD56⁺ selected cells following sequential selec-
tion. Results are the mean of seven experiments using a ^{51}Cr 4-h release assay. (A). Using K562
(NK-sensitive) cell line as targets. (B). Using Raji (NK-resistant) cell line as targets. (C). Using
K562 cell line on cells that have been frozen, thawed, and cultured in the presence of interleukin
(IL)–2 (200 U/mL) at various time points to determine lymphokine-activated killer (LAK) activity.

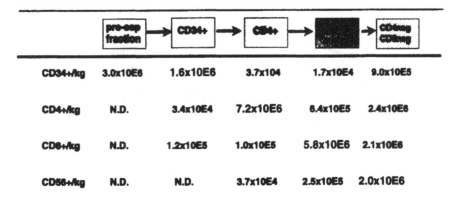

CD34+/kg	3.0x10E6	1.6x10E6	3.7x104	1.7x10E4	9.0x10E5
CD4+/kg	N.D.	3.4x10E4	7.2x10E6	6.4x10E5	2.4x10E6
CD8+/kg	N.D.	1.2x10E5	1.0x10E5	5.8x10E6	2.1x10E6
CD56+/kg	N.D.	N.D.	3.7x10E4	2.5x10E5	2.0x10E6

Figure 9 Cell yield following sequential positive selection of allogeneic marrow. Values are the mean of four consecutive experiments using actual donor grafts. The CD34+ cells are infused, but the CD34− fraction is available for further manipulation.

the CD34+ cells contained in the unmanipulated graft. Few would argue that this type of contamination is detrimental to clinical outcome.

The use of specific biological response modifiers or cytokines could increase GVL activity in the posttransplant period and lead to higher remission rates (Truitt et al., 1997). Current experimental data suggest that interleukin (IL)–2 used at a low dose will be sufficient to stimulate NK/lymphokine–actived killer (LAK) cells but would not trigger the abundant low-affinity receptors found on T cells, thus preventing their participation in a GVHD reaction (Sykes et al., 1990). The use of a TCD or "cytotoxic effector modulated graft" also reduces the life-threatening side effects that would otherwise occur from protean T-cell stimulation. Several recent studies have demonstrated that the use of post-BMT IL-2 can increase NK function and absolute peripheral blood CD56+ cell counts (Leever et al., 1987; Soiffer, 1994; Soiffer et al., 1995). Soiffer et al. (1995) were able to increase CD56+ cell numbers from a baseline of 16–54% in 8 weeks using low-dose IL-2 starting on day 80 (mean) post-BMT. No patient developed GVHD; fevers were the most common side effect. An earlier study by Soiffer (1994) also showed that low-dose continuous infusion (CI) IL-2 could be safely started 60 days post-BMT (mean) with compliance to 12 weeks of therapy. Follow-up was sufficient in the latter study to show a significant decrease in relapse rates in patients who completed the course of posttransplant IL-2 therapy. We have currently opened an optimal dose–finding trial of post-BMT IL-2 in patients at high risk of relapse to determine if NK function and CD56+ cell numbers can be increased without incurring increased morbidity. All patients first receive a CD34+–augmented/elutriated graft to minimize post-BMT complications. We are also accruing patients with high-risk CML to receive CD34+–augmented/elutriated grafts and post-BMT granulocyte macrophage colony-stimulating factor (GM-CSF). As previously discussed, patients receiving elutriated grafts alone have unacceptably high relapse rates. Increased stem cell dose (CD34+ augmentation) and the antiapoptotic effect (on BCR/ABL+ stem cells) of high-dose myeloid growth factors are expected significantly to decrease this risk (Bedi et al., 1993). The seven patients currently enrolled (median follow up 18 months) remain both cytogenetically and molecularly free of disease (R. J. Jones, personal communication).

A. Future Trials

If toxicity remains acceptable on trials such as these, but sufficient cytolytic activity has not been achieved, future studies may incorporate positively selected ancillary cell populations (i.e., CD56$^+$ NK cells, CD4$^+$ T cells) along with cytokines (e.g., IL-2, IL-12, IL-15) to augment activity further. Specific ancillary cell populations can also be expanded ex vivo using various cytokine combinations. These effectors can be (1) used fresh, and/or (2) cryopreserved for use at relapse, or (3) given back at defined times post-BMT. Currently, we and other investigators are expanding Epstein-Barr virus (EBV)–specific donor lymphocyte clones for use against B-cell lymphoproliferative disorders (Davis et al., 1996, Hestop et al., 1997). Although this has not been a complication of elutriation, it has a high incidence after solid organ transplantation, human immunodeficiency virus (HIV) infection, and also with other forms of TCD. It is likely that different disease states will require different ancillary effectors and cytokine combinations. Current DLI trials (especially those employing selected subpopulations) may help define a disease hierarchy for future up-front graft engineering studies.

V. CONCLUSION

A systematic approach to hematopoietic graft manipulation will minimize several of the variables inherent to BMT. Through this approach, we have been able to impact significantly on morbidity and quality of life following allogeneic transplantation. Acute and chronic GVHD, blood product and antibiotic usage, inpatient hospitalization, acuity, costs, and survival (especially in patients older than age 40 years) have been improved. The HLA barrier still presents a formidable obstacle to achieving a more widespread use of this therapy. The complications encountered in HLA-matched/TCD grafts occur with even greater magnitude in the HLA-mismatched or unrelated donor setting. Several centers are now engaged in studies using TCD grafts which are augmented with high doses of PBSCs derived CD34$^+$ cells to ensure engraftment while reducing the incidence of GVHD (Reisner et al., 1994; Bacigalupo et al., 1995; Friedrich et al., 1995; Yeager et al., 1995). Similar groups of phase II graft engineering trials are now active at our center for patients receiving mismatched and unrelated graft products.

The continued use of animal and in vitro models to assess new graft engineering approaches must be encouraged in the future. Several biomedical devices geared toward hematopoietic cell manipulation will be entering the field over the next decade. Patient outcome must be continually assessed with respect to changes in graft manipulation or stem cell source. A newly emerging example is the manipulation of allogeneic PBSC grafts. Mobilized allogeneic PBSCs appear to be an excellent source of stem cells for BMT (Korbling et al., 1994; Lane et al., 1995; Link et al., 1995). Earlier reports showed decreased rates of GVHD despite having T-cell burdens 10 times higher than those found in unmanipulated bone marrow (Korbling et al., 1995; Schmitz et al., 1995). However, several of these centers now report a high incidence of chronic GVHD (along with its attendant morbidity) following allogeneic PBSC transplantation (Korbling et al., 1995; Bensinger et al., 1996). Initial results of TCD in these PBSC grafts using CD34$^+$ selection are disappointing in those recipients developed unexpectantly high incidences of both acute and chronic GVHD (Bensinger et al., 1996). There are certainly significant differences between ancillary marrow and PBSC populations. For example, two laboratories

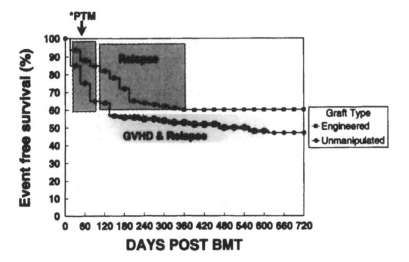

Figure 10 Characteristics of survival curves contrasting recipients of elutriated/CD34⁺ augmented and unmanipulated grafts. Idealized curves emphasizing the differences in Kaplan-Meyer event-free survival plots for these two patient cohorts. Essentially all relapse events occur within the first year of receiving an engineered graft. *PTM, peritransplant mortality.

now report the presence of natural suppressor cells in these allogeneic PBSC products in both an animal model (B. Storb, unpublished data) and a human model (R. Negrin, unpublished data). Thus, the same, stepwise model approach would be expected to improve graft performance when using PBSCs, cord blood, fetal tissue, xenografts, or genetically engineered products as a stem cell source.

Allogeneic BMT survival curves characteristically fall precipitously during the first 100 days owing to peritransplant mortality. The slope of the curve then falls gradually over the next few years. This has been attributed to deaths from late complications (chronic GVHD, infection) or relapse. Survival curves generated from patients who have received engineered grafts do not have an initial steep slope but rather fall gradually during the first year of transplant. The downward curve, in this case, represents a large percentage of patients who have relapsed (Fig. 10). For acute leukemia in CR1 and CR2, no patient receiving an elutriated graft (median follow up 6.5 years, range 4.5–11.0 years) has relapsed past 13 months posttransplant. This suggests that any further graft manipulation aimed at decreasing relapse must be initiated soon after transplant to be successful. An unexpected, but encouraging, finding is the present difficulty encountered in plotting DFS for engineered graft recipients. Several patients who had relapsed are now in long-lasting remission following DLI and are maintaining a good quality of life. It is hoped that future graft engineering approaches will be as successful as previous studies and will extend this form of therapy to an even larger patient population.

ACKNOWLEDGMENTS

I wish to thank the members of the Graft Engineering Laboratory and the BMT physicians and nurses for their dedication and devotion to the patients enrolled in these studies. This work was supported through funding from the National Institutes of Health (grants CA15396, CA67787 and HL46533).

REFERENCES

Antin J, Bierer B, Smith B, et al. Selective depletion of bone marrow T lymphocytes with anti-CD5 monoclonal antibodies: effective prophylaxis for graft-versus-host disease in patients with hematologic malignancies. Blood 1991; 78:2139–2149.

Ash RC, Casper JT, Chitambar CR, et al. Successful allogeneic transplantation of T cell depleted bone marrow from closely HLA matched unrelated donors. N Engl J Med 1990; 322:485–494.

Bacigalupo A, Mordini N, Pitto A, Piaggio G, Podesta M. CD34+ selected stem cell transplants in patients with advanced leukemia from 3 loci mismatched family donors. Blood 1995; 86:937a.

Bar BMAM, Schattenberg A, Mensink EJBM, et al. Donor leukocyte infusions for chronic myeloid leukemia relapsed after allogeneic bone marrow transplantation. J Clin Oncology 1993; 11:513–519.

Bedi A, Zehnbauer BA, Collector MI, et al. BCR-ABL gene rearrangement and expression of primitive hematopoietic progenitors in chronic myeloid leukemia. Blood 1993; 81:2898–2902.

Bensinger WI, Buckner CD, Shannon-Dorcy K, Rowley S, Appelbaum FR, Benyunes M, Clift R, Martin P, Demirer T, Storb R, Lee M, Schiller G. Transplantation of allogeneic CD34$^+$ peripheral blood stem cells in patients with advanced hematologic malignancy. Blood 1996a; 88:4132–4138.

Bensinger WI, Clift R, Martin P, Appelbaum FR, Demirer T, Gooley T, Lilleby K, Rowley S, Sanders J, Storb R, Buckner CD. Allogeneic peripheral blood stem cell transplantation in patients with advanced hematologic malignancies: a retrospective comparison with marrow transplantation. Blood 1996b; 88:2794–2800.

Berenson RJ, Shpall EJ, Auditore-Hargreaves K, Heimfeld S, Jacobs C, Krieger MS. Transplantation of CD34+ hematopoietic progenitor cells. Cancer Inves 1996; 14:589–596.

Champlin R. T-cell depletion for allogeneic bone marrow transplantation: impact on graft-versus host disease, engraftment, and graft-versus-leukemia. J Hematother 1993; 2:27–42.

Champlin R, Giralt S, Przepiorka D, et al. Selective depletion of CD8-positive T-lymphocytes for allogeneic bone marrow transplantation: engraftment, graft-versus-host disease, and graft-versus-leukemia. Prog Clin Biol Res 1992; 377:385–398.

Civin CI, Trishmann T, Kadan NS, Davis J, Noga S, Cohen K, Duffy B, Groenewegen I, Wiley J, Law P, Hardwick A, Oldham F, Gee A. Highly purified CD34-positive cells reconstitute hematopoiesis. J Clin Oncol 1996; 14:2224–2233.

Collins R, Wolff S, List A, et al. Prospective multi center trial of donor buffy coat infusion for relapsed hematologic malignancy post-allogeneic bone marrow transplantation (BMT). Blood 1994; 84:333a.

Davis JM, Orentas R, Eby LL, Flinn I, Lemas MV, Noga SJ, Ambinder R. Generation/expansion of Epstein-Barr Virus (EBV)–specific cytotoxic T cells (CTLs) in gas permeable cell culture bags. Blood 1996; 88:111a.

DeWitte T, Hoogenhout J, De Pauw B, Joldrinet R, Janssen J, Wessels J, Van Daal W, Justinx T, Haanen C. Depletion of donor lymphocytes by counterflow centrifugation successfully prevents acute graft-vs-host disease in matched allogeneic marrow transplantation. Blood 1986; 67:1302–1308.

Dimitrios M, Read E, Cottler-Fox M, et al. CD34$^+$ cell dose predicts survival, post transplant morbidity, and rate of hematologic recovery after allogeneic marrow transplant for hematologic malignancies. Blood 1996; 88:3223–3229.

Drobyski WR, Keever CA, Roth MS, et al. Salvage immunotherapy using donor leukocyte infusions as treatment for relapsed chronic myelogenous leukemia after allogeneic bone marrow transplantation: Efficacy and toxicity of a defined T cell dose. Blood 1993; 82:2310–2318.

Eby L, Davis-Sproul JM, Harris DP, Thoburn CJ, Hess AD, Risdon G, Noga SJ. Sequential positive selection of CD34$^+$ stem cells and CD4$^+$ and CD8$^+$ lymphocytes for allogeneic bone marrow transplant (BMT). J. Hematother 1997; 6:372a.

Filipovich AH, McGlave PB, Ramsay NK. Ex-vivo treatment of donor bone marrow with monoclonal antibody okt3 for prevention of acute graft-vs-host disease in allogeneic histocompatible bone marrow transplantation. Lancet 1984; 1:469–471.

Flinn I, Orentas R, Noga SJ, Marcellus D, Vogelsang GB, Jones RJ, Ambinder RF. Low risk of Epstein-Barr virus (EBV)–associated post-transplant lymphoproliferative disease (PTLD) in patients receiving elutriated allogeneic marrow transplants may reflect depletion of EBV infected lymphocytes from the graft. Blood 1995; 86:626a.

Friedrich W, Muller S, Schreiner T, et al. The combined use of positively selected, T-cell depleted blood and bone marrow stem cells in HLA non-identical bone marrow transplantation in childhood leukemia. Exp Hemat 1995; 23:854a.

Giral S, Hester J, Huh Y, Hirsch-Ginsberg C, Rondon G, Seong S, Lee M, Gajewski J, Van Besien K, Khouri I, Mehra R, Przepiorka D, Korbling M, Talpaz M, Katarjian H, Fischer H, Deisseroth A, Champlin R. CD8-depleted donor lymphocyte infusion as treatment for relapsed chronic myelogenous leukemia after allogeneic bone marrow transplantation. Blood 1995; 86:4337–4343.

Hakim FT, Mackall CL. The Immune system: Effector and target of graft-versus-host disease. In: Ferrara J, Deeg H, Burakoff S, eds. Graft-vs-Host Disease. 2nd ed. New York: Marcel Dekker, 1997:257–289.

Hale G, Cobbold S, Waldmann H. T cell depletion with CAMPATH-1 in allogeneic bone marrow transplantation. Transplantation 1988; 45:753–759.

Hertenstein B, Wiesneth M, Novotny J, et al. Interferon-a and donor buffy coat transfusions for treatment of relapsed chronic myeloid leukemia after allogeneic bone marrow transplantation. Transplantation 1993; 56:1114–1118.

Heslop HE, Cunningham JM, Jane SM. Gene Therapy. In: Ferrara J, Deeg H, Burakoff S, eds. Graft-vs-Host Disease. 2nd ed. New York: Marcel Dekker, 1997:755–773.

Horowitz MM, Gale RP, Sondel PM, Goldman JM, Kersey J, Kolb HJ, Rimm AA, Ringden O, Rozman C, Speck B, Truitt RL, Zwaan FE, Bortin MM. Graft-versus-leukemia reactions after bone marrow transplantation. Blood 1990; 75:555–562.

Johnson BD, Truitt RL. Delayed infusion of immunocompetent donor cells after bone marrow transplantation breaks graft-host tolerance and allows for persistent anti-leukemia reactivity without severe graft-versus-host disease. Blood 1995; 85:3302–3312.

Jones RJ, Wagner JE, Celano P, Zicha MS, Sharkis SJ. Separation of pluripotent hematopoietic stem cells from spleen colony-forming cells (CFU-S). Nature 1990; 347:188–189.

Kauffman MG, Noga SJ, Kelly TJ, Donnenberg AD. Isolation of cell cycle fractions by counterflow centrifugal elutriation. Analyt Biochem 1990; 191:41–46.

Keever CA, Welte K, Small T, et al. Interluekin 2-activated killer cells in patients following transplants of soybean lectin-separated and E rosette-depleted bone marrow. Blood 1987; 70:1893–1903.

Kolb HJ, Mittermuller J, Clemm J, Holler E, Ledderose G, Brehm G, Heim M, Wilmanns W. Donor leukocyte transfusions for treatment of recurrent chronic myelogenous leukemia in marrow transplant patients. Blood 1990; 76:2462–2465.

Kolb HJ, deWitte T, Mittermuller J, Hertenstein B, Goldman JM, Ljungman P, Verdonck L, Holler E, Thalmaer K, Bartram C. Graft-versus-leukemia effect of donor buffy coat transfusions on recurrent leukemia after marrow transplantation. Blood 1993; 82:214a.

Korbling M, Przepiorka D, Engel H, et al. Allogeneic blood stem cell transplantation (Allo-PBSCT) in 9 patients with refractory leukemia and lymphoma: Potential advantage of blood over marrow allografts. Blood 1994; 84:396.

Korbling M, Przepiorka D, Hug Y, Engel H, van Besien K, Giralt S, Andersson B, Kleine HD, Seong D, Deisseroth AB, Andreeff M, Champlin R. Allogeneic blood stem cell transplantation for refractory leukemia and lymphoma: Potential advantage of blood over marrow allografts. Blood 1995; 85:1659–1665.

Lane TA, Law P, Maruyama M, Young D, Burgess J, Mullen M, Mealiffe M, Terstappen LWMM, Hardwick A, Moubayed M, Oldham F, Corringham RET, Ho AD. Harvesting and enrichment of hematopoietic progenitor cells mobilized into the peripheral blood of normal donors by granulocyte-macrophage colony-stimulating factor (GM-CSF) or G-CSF: potential role in allogeneic marrow transplantation. Blood 1995; 85:275–282.

Link H, Arseniev L, Bahre O, et al. Transplantation of allogeneic peripheral blood and bone marrow CD34+ cells after immunoselection. Exp Hematol 1995; 23:855a.

Mackinnon S, Papadapoulos EB, Carabasi MH, et al. Adoptive immunotherapy evaluating escalating doses of donor leukocytes for relapse of chronic myeloid leukemia after bone marrow transplantation; separation of graft-versus-leukemia responses from graft-versus-host disease. Blood 1995; 86:1261–1268.

Martin PJ, Hansen JA, Storb R, Thomas ED. Human marrow transplantation: an immunological perspective. Advan Immunol 1987; 40:379–438.

Martin PJ, Hansen JA, Torok-Storb B, Durnam D, Przepiorka D, O'Quigley J, Sanders J, Sullivan KM, Witherspoon RP, Deeg HJ, et al. Graft failure in patients receiving T-cell depleted HLA-identical allogeneic marrow transplants. Bone Marrow Transplant 1988; 3:445–456.

Martin PJ, Kernan NA. T-cell depletion for GVHD prevention in humans. In: Ferrara I, Deeg H, Burakoff S, eds. Graft-vs-host disease. 2nd ed. New York: Marcel Dekker, 1997:615–637.

Mitsuyasu RT, Champlin RE, Gale RP. Treatment of donor bone marrow with monoclonal anti-T-cell antibody and complement for the prevention of graft-versus-host disease. A prospective, randomized, double-blind trial. Ann Int Med 1986; 105:20–26.

Noga SJ. Elutriation: new technology for separation of blood and bone marrow. Lab Med 1988; 19:234–239.

Noga SJ. Graft Engineering: the evolution of hematopoietic transplantation. J Hematother 1992; 1:3–17.

Noga SJ, Civin CI. Positive stem cell selection of hematopoietic grafts for transplantation. In: Ferrara J, Deeg H, Burakoff S, eds. Graft-vs-Host Disease. 2nd ed. New York: Marcel Dekker, 1997:717–731.

Noga SJ, Hess AD. Lymphocyte depletion in bone marrow transplantation: will modulation of graft-versus-host disease prove to be superior to prevention? Semin Oncol 1993; 20:28–33.

Noga SJ, Vogelsang GB, Seber A, Davis JM, Schepers K, Hess AD, Jones RJ. CD34+ stem cell augmentation of allogeneic, elutriated marrow grafts improves engraftment but cyclosporine A (CSA) is still required to reduce GVHD and morbidity. Transplant Proc 1997; 29:1–5.

Noga SJ, Berenson RJ, Davis JM, Hess AD, Braine HG, Vogelsang GB, Miller CA, Jones RJ. CD34+ stem cell augmentation of T-cell depleted allografts reduces engraftment time, GVHD, and length of hospitalization. Br J Hematol 1994a; 87:41a.

Noga SJ, Davis JM, Schepers K, Eby L, Berenson RJ. The clinical use of elutriation and positive stem cell selection columns to engineer the lymphocyte and stem cell composition of the allograft. Prog Clin Biol Res 1994b; 392:317–324.

Noga S, Miller C, Berenson R. Braine H, Sproul J, Jones R. Combined use of CD34+ stem cell augmentation and elutriation reduces the morbidity and cost of allogeneic bone marrow transplantation. Proc Am Soc Clin Oncol 1994c; 13:309a.

Noga SJ, Vogelsang GB, Santos GW. Allograft lymphocyte dose modification (LDM) prevents GVHD without compromising GVL following BMT for acute leukemia. Blood 1992; 78:136a.

Noga SJ, Wagner JE, Santos GW, Donnenberg AD. Allograft lymphocyte-dose modification with counterflow centrifugal elutriation (CCE): Effects on chronic GVHD and survival in a case/control study. Blood 1991; 78:227a.

Noga SJ, Wagner JE, Rowley SD, Davis JM, Vogelsang GB, Hess AD, Saral R, Santos GW, Donnenberg AD. Using elutriation to engineer bone marrow allografts. Prog Clin Biol Res 1990; 333:345–361.

Noga SJ, Donnenberg AD, Schwartz CL, Strauss LC, Civin CI, Santos GW. Development of a simplified counterflow centrifugation-elutriation procedure for depletion of lymphocytes from human bone marrow. Transplantation 1986; 41:220–229.

Porter DL, Roth MS, McGarigle C, et al. Induction of graft-versus-host disease as immunotherapy for relapsed chronic myeloid leukemia. N Engl J Med 1994; 330:100–106.

Raffoux E, de Revel T, Pignon JM, et al. Adult Philadelphia positive acute lymphoblastic leukemia (Ph+ ALL) in relapse after allogeneic bone marrow transplantation (BMT): successful treatment with donor leukocyte infusions. Exp Hematol 1995; 23:858a.

Reisner Y, Kapoor N, Kirkpatrick D, Pollack MS, Dupont B, Good RA, O'Reilly RJ. Transplantation for acute leukaemia with HLA-A and B nonidentical parental marrow cells fractionated with soybean agglutinin and sheep red blood cells. Lancet 1981; 2:327–331.

Ringden O, Horowitz M. Graft-versus-leukemia reactions in humans. Transplant Proc 1989; 21: 2989–2992.

Risdon G, Read EJ, Potter M, Kanz L, Auditore-Hargreaves K. Pan T-cell depletion of PBSC: allograft engineering with the CEPRATE TCD system. Blood 1996; 88:254a.

Santos GW. Bone marrow transplantation in hematologic malignancies. Cancer 1990; 65:786–791.

Schattenberg A, De Witte T, Salden M, et al. Mixed hematopoietic chimerism after allogeneic transplantation with lymphocyte-depleted bone marrow is not associated with a higher incidence of relapse. Blood 1989; 73:1367–1372.

Schmitz N, Dreger P, Suttorp M, Rohwedder EB, Haferlach T, Loffler H, Hunter A, Russell NH. Primary transplantation of allogeneic peripheral blood progenitor cells mobilized by filgrastim (granulocyte colony-stimulating factor). Blood 1995; 85:1666–1672.

Soiffer RJ. Effect of low-dose interleukin-2 on disease relapse after T cell depleted allogeneic bone marrow transplantation. Blood 1994; 84:964–971.

Soiffer R, Murray C, Richardson P, Ayash L, Elias A, Ritz J. Prolonged subcutaneous administration of low dose IL-2 following bone marrow (BMT) and peripheral blood stem cell (PBSCT) transplantation. Blood 1995; 86:567a.

Sykes M, Romick ML, Sachs DH. Interleukin 2 prevents graft-versus-host disease while preserving the graft-versus-leukemia effect of allogeneic T-cells. Proc Natl Acad Sci USA 1990; 87:5633–5637.

Truitt RL, Johnson BD, McCabe CM, Weiler MB. Graft. Graft versus leukemia. In: Ferrara J, Deeg H, Burakoff S, eds. Graft-vs-Host Disease. 2nd ed. New York: Marcel Dekker, 1997:385–424.

Turner CE, Davis JM, Harris DP, Schepers KG, Eby LL, Noga SJ. Graft engineering V: isolation, cryopreservation, and activation of CD56+ cells recovered after CD34+ selection of elutriated bone marrow. Blood 1995a; 86:117a.

Turner CE, Davis JM, Harris DP, Schepers KG, Eby LL, Berenson RJ, Noga SJ. Graft engineering IV: CD56+ selection following elutriation and CD34+ selection. J Hematother 1995b; 4: 75a.

van Rhee F, Lin F, Cullis JO, et al. Relapse of chronic myeloid leukemia after allogeneic bone marrow transplant: the case for giving donor leukocyte transfusions before the onset of hematologic relapse. Blood 1994; 83:3377–3383.

Vogelsang GB. Acute and chronic graft-vs-host disease. Curr Opin Oncol 1993; 5:276–281.

Vogelsang GB, Hess AD, Santos, GW. Acute graft-versus-host disease: clinical characteristics in the cyclosporine era. Medicine 1988; 67:163–174.

Wagner JE, Donnenberg AD, Noga SJ, Cremo CA, Gao IK, Yin HJ, Vogelsang GB, Rowley SD, Saral R, Santos GW. Lymphocyte depletion of donor bone marrow by counterflow centrifugal elutriation: Results of a phase I clinical trial. Blood 1988a; 72:1168–1176.

Wagner JE, Donnenberg AD, Noga SJ, Rowley SD, Santos GW. The role of post-transplant cyclosporine A (CsA) immunosuppressive therapy on engraftment of lymphocyte depleted bone marrow. Blood 1988b; 72:412a.

Wagner JE, Santos GW, Noga SJ, Rowley SD, Davis J, Vogelsang GB, Farmer ER, Zehnbauer BA, Saral R, Donnenberg AD. Bone marrow graft engineering by counterflow centrifugal elutriation: results of a phase I–II clinical trial. Blood 1990; 75:1370–1377.

Wagner JE, Zahurak M, Piantadosi S, et al. Bone marrow transplantation of chronic myelogenous leukemia in chronic phase: Evaluation of risks and benefits. J Clin Oncol 1992; 10:779–789.

Yeager AM, Holland HK, Mogul MJ, Forte K, Lauer M, Boyer MW, Turner CW, Vega RA, Beatty PG, Jacobs CA, Benyunes MC, Wingard JR. Transplantation of positively selected CD34[+] cells from haploidentical parental donors for relapsed acute leukemia in children. Blood 1995; 86:291a.

16

Detection and Significance of Minimal Residual Disease from Solid Tumor Malignancies in Stem Cell Autografts

AMY A. ROSS

Nexell Therapeutics Inc., Irvine, California

I. INTRODUCTION

The increasing use of autologous stem cell transplantation (ASCT) as a means of hematopoietic reconstitution following high-dose chemotherapy (HDC) has heightened the concern about tumor contamination of autologous grafts. Post-ASCT relapse may be due to persistence of disease, the infusion of clonogenic tumor cells, or a combination of the two. Although no study to date has demonstrated that infused tumor cells in contaminated ASCT grafts are solely responsible for posttransplant relapse, the presence of gene-marked, infused tumor cells at sites of disease relapse has been documented in three malignancies (1–3). The presence of tumor cells in autologous grafts is also correlated with poor post-ASCT clinical outcome in a variety of solid-tumor malignancies (4–8). Thus, the sensitive and specific identification of minimal residual disease (MRD) in ASCT grafts is of great concern.

This chapter will discuss the various methodologies that are used for MRD detection, the benefits and pitfalls of each, and how MRD detection assays are crucial for tracking the clinical significance of infused tumor cells. An overview of what is known to date about the clinical consequences of infused tumor cells in HDC/ASCT therapy of solid tumor malignancies will also be discussed.

II. DETECTION OF MRD

The earliest attempt to detect epithelium-derived tumor cells in peripheral blood by routine microscopy was over 125 years ago (9). Since then, the possible clinical significance of circulating tumor cells has been hotly debated. Attempts to improve detection methods were spotty, as vocal skeptics viewed the information as clinically irrelevant. However, the past 20 years has witnessed vast improvements in the methodologies used to detect MRD. The emphasis has been to develop detection assays that are both sensitive and specific for any given tumor type. Table 1 outlines MRD assays currently in use and their respective limits of detection sensitivity.

Several important caveats of MRD assays cannot be overemphasized. First, the sensitivity and, most importantly, the specificity of the assay are influenced by the source of tissue analyzed. For example, certain anticarcinoma monoclonal antibodies (mAbs) that react strongly with breast cancer cells show no false-positive immunostaining of venous peripheral blood or bone marrow cells. However, cross-reactive immunostaining of myeloid progenitor cells with certain antibodies can be observed in hematopoietic tissues that are stimulated to differentiate by the administration of chemotherapeutic agents or recombinant growth factors (10). Similarly, the use of anticytokeratin antibodies can result in the false-positive staining of epidermal cells or weak cytoplasmic staining of phagocytic cells that contain cytokeratin debris. In these cases, definitive confirmation of the malignant cytology of the immunostained cells is crucial.

Molecular-based MRD assays can be influenced by the same phenomena discussed above. False-positive reactions for epithelial cell–specific cytokeratins using the reverse-transcriptase polymerase chain reaction (RT-PCR) have been reported in peripheral blood, peripheral blood stem cell (PBSC) collections, and bone marrow (11–14). This suggests that growth factors used in the mobilization of hematopoietic progenitor cells may upregulate pseudogenes in myeloid cells that are detected as cytokeratin transcripts, or that cytokeratin debris-containing phagocytic cells register as RT-PCR positive.

Second, one must consider the number of cells analyzed in MRD assays. If the frequency of occult tumor cells in ASCT samples is as few as one tumor cell in 10^6–10^7 hematopoietic cells, then it is necessary to examine an adequate number of cells to assure that infrequently occurring tumor cells can be detected with reasonable certainty. For example, assuming a detection sensitivity of 1 tumor cell in 10^6 hematopoietic cells, a mathematical model of tumor contamination of ASCT products concludes that the probability of detecting at least one tumor cell in a single apheresis sample is 0.08. If five apheresis specimens from the same patient are tested, the detection probability rises to 0.32 (15). This model highlights the point that finding a single tumor cell in a single apheresis collection is a "needle in a haystack" endeavor. Thus, the best sensitivity for MRD assays is achieved when a substantial number of hematopoietic cells ($>2 \times 10^6$) from multiple samples are analyzed. Using such assay parameters in a model system, it has been demonstrated that immunology-based assays can detect between 2 and 4 tumor cells seeded at a concentration of 10 tumor cells in 10^6 marrow cells, and, by mathematical

Table 1 Minimal Residual Disease (MRD) Assays

MRD assay	Detection sensitivity
Conventional cytology	1–$5:10^3$
Immunocytochemistry	$1:10^5$–$1:10^6$
Flow cytometry	$1:10^4$–$1:10^7$
In vitro culture	Variable
Polymerase chain reaction	$1:10^5$–$1:10^7$

extrapolation, a 95% confidence interval of detecting a single tumor cell at a concentration of 2 tumor cells in 10^6 hematopoietic cells (16).

Third, MRD assays are hampered by the lack of tumor-specific markers for detecting rare tumor cells. As outlined above, epithelial cell–associated cytokeratin components may be detected in hematopoietic cells as a function of phagocytosis, aberrant gene expression, or epidermal cell contamination. To complicate matters even further, so-called "tumor-specific" markers can be present in nontumor cells. Prostate-specific antigen (PSA) expression has been documented in normal and malignant breast and endometrial tissues. The (t14;18) translocation associated with low-grade non-Hodgkin's lymphoma and other hematological malignancies is observed with increasing frequency in normal lymphocytes as a function of age (13).

To help circumvent these problems, it may be possible to increase both the sensitivity and the specificity of tumor cell detection by incorporating additional tumor-specific markers (e.g., oncogenes, hormonal receptors, chromosomal aberrations) into MRD assays (17–19). Although extremely useful in the experimental setting, application of multiple-marker assays in the routine performance of clinical laboratory analysis of MRD is problematic, extremely time and labor consuming, and costly.

III. MRD ASSAYS

A. Immunocytochemistry

Immunocytochemical (ICC) assays rely on the specific binding affinity of antibodies to cellular antigens. Antibodies can be derived from polyclonal antisera or from monoclonal immunoglobulin fractions. Most current ICC assays rely on the use of mAbs for improved specificity.

Following incubation with the mAb, a series of secondary antibody-bridging steps are performed to link the mAb to a color-based detection system. The number and complexity of these secondary bridging steps determine how strong the color-based reaction will be. The most commonly used color-based detection chemistries utilize fluorescein, phycoerythrin (both are birefringent under polarized light), alkaline phosphatase, and immunoperoxidase. The color-reacted cells are then visible against a sea of unstained or counterstained hematopoietic cells.

The advantages of ICC assays are: (1) they allow the use of multiple mAbs for tumor cell detection; (2) they can amplify the detection signal to increase the detection sensitivity of weakly reacting antigens, and (3) of primary importance, they allow for the morphological verification of immunostained tumor cells. The disadvantages of ICC assays are: (1) they are extremely labor intensive; (2) results are often not reproducible; (3) endogenous levels of alkaline phosphatase and peroxidase in hematopoietic cells can result in unacceptable background staining that obscures true tumor staining; (4) cross reactivity with nontumor antigens on hematopoietic cells can cause false-positive results; and (5) a pathologist skilled in ICC of hematopoietic tissues is needed for diagnostic interpretation.

B. Flow Cytometry

Flow cytometry relies on the automated analysis of cells labeled with mAb-fluorochrome complexes that are passed single-file in a continuous fluid stream through a laser beam. Emitted fluorescence and scattered light from each cell are captured by light detectors, amplified, and sent to a computer where information from millions of cells can be accumulated and analyzed. Flow cytometry measures both the immunofluorescent signal of stained cells as well as the light-scattering properties of cells. Most currently used MRD flow cytometric assays rely on the use of multiparameter analysis. These assays detect tumor cells with antitumor or anti–epithelial cell mAbs and differentiate their staining with the use of fluorescent antihematopoietic mAbs (e.g., anti-CD45). The unique size and light-scattering properties of the various cells are analyzed using sophisticated software gating techniques. By examining the staining and morphological properties of hematopoietic samples, it is possible to profile the normal cells versus the tumor cells.

The advantages of flow cytometry are: (1) assay reproducibility is high, as millions of cells can be analyzed in a few minutes; and (2) owing to the fact that multiple mAbs and two light-scatter parameters can be measured simultaneously, instantaneous multiparameter and statistical analyses can be performed on companion software programs. The disadvantages of flow cytometric assays are: (1) it is very difficult to detect accurately low numbers ($<10^{-4}$) of tumor cells; (2) nontumor cells may stain nonspecifically; and (3) tumor cell morphology cannot be verified.

C. Culture Methods

Although capricious in nature, culture methods for MRD detection are the only assays that provide information as to the viability and clonogenicity of tumor cells. Sharp and colleagues pioneered the use of Dexter-type culture methods for the in vitro growth of breast and non-Hodgkin's lymphoma MRD (5). Emerman and colleagues (20) have developed a similar culture assay for the successful growth of breast cancer cells from marrow and effusion fluids. These assays use either serum-supplemented or serum-free culture media and standard culture vessels. Over a period of weeks, the normal hematopoietic cells will differentiate and die out, whereas the malignant cells proliferate. Thus, it is possible to obtain an expanded population of tumor cells for postculture analyses.

Ross and colleagues (21–24) developed a soft agar-based clonogenic assay for the in vitro growth of breast cancer micrometastases from marrow and PBSCs. In contrast to the Sharp method, this assay uses culture medium, fetal bovine serum, and recombinant growth factor–supplemented soft agar in small culture dishes. Tumor colonies, along with a limited number of hematopoietic colonies, grow in 2 weeks' time in this assay.

Advantages of culture methods are: (1) they are the only assays that can measure tumor cell viability and clonogenicity; (2) the population of tumor cells can be expanded for subsequent analyses; (3) effects of ex vivo purging of MRD can be measured; and (4) a greater volume of cells can be analyzed, as most culture methods plate considerably more cells than are analyzed by immunological or molecular methods. The disadvantages of culture methods are: (1) they are prone to problems with contamination; (2) the lack of tumor growth may reflect poor culture conditions rather than lack of tumor cell viability; and (3) they are technically demanding and can be time consuming (up to 8 weeks).

D. Molecular Methods

The most commonly used molecular method for the detection of MRD is the polymerase chain reaction (PCR). Although more frequently used for hematological malignancies, PCR assays are being used for MRD detection in certain solid tumor malignancies. PCR-based assays amplify specific sequences of deoxyribonucleic acid (DNA) or messenger ribonucleic acid (mRNA). By greatly amplifying sequences that are unique to tumor cells,

PCR assays are theoretically capable of unparalleled sensitivity (up to 1 tumor cell in 10^7–10^8 cells).

PCR assays that detect DNA rearrangements are routinely used to detect MRD in leukemias and lymphomas. For example, (t14;18) occurs in up to 80% of follicular non-Hodgkin's lymphomas, and 20–30% of diffuse large cell lymphomas. Likewise, the (t9; 22) translocation occurs in the majority of chronic myelogenous leukemia (CML) tumor cells. By amplifying these DNA rearrangements, it is possible to detect rare tumor cells in marrow and PBSC specimens. However, PCR assays for the detection of MRD in hematological malignancies that have no common DNA translocation are considerably more complex. For diseases such as multiple myeloma and (t14;18)-negative lymphomas, where DNA rearrangements are patient unique, it is necessary to make patient-specific primers using DNA sequencing technology.

PCR assays for the detection of solid tumor MRD are a bit more complicated. These assays rely on the amplification of transcripts of proteins that are expressed in tumor cells but, presumably, not in hematopoietic cells. RT-PCR assays involve the initial synthesis of complementary DNA (cDNA) from cellular RNA using the enzyme reverse transcriptase. Once this process is accomplished, the target-specific RT-PCR primers are used to amplify the target cDNA. For example, the most widely used RT-PCR assay for the detection of solid tumor MRD is for PSA in prostate cancer. In this circumstance, RT-PCR is capable of detecting rare tumor cells in histologically normal marrow and peripheral blood (13).

RT-PCR technology has recently been applied to the detection of MRD in breast cancer (8,11,14,25,26) and other epithelium-derived tumors (27,28). These assays target cellular expression of epithelial cell–associated cytokeratins (usually cytokeratins 18 or 19) or cellular enzymes that are presumably lacking in hematopoietic and lymphoid tissues. However, several studies have reported the expression of cytokeratin "pseudogenes" (closely related DNA sequences that react as positives in PCR assays) in hematopoietic cells that result in an unacceptable rate of RT-PCR false-positives in certain instances (11,12,29).

The advantages of PCR assays are: (1) they are relatively easy and straightforward to perform; (2) they are capable of achieving the highest reported detection sensitivity levels; (3) primers for various DNA and mRNA sequences are readily available through commercial sources; and (4) PCR assays can analyze large numbers of cells.

Uniform acceptance of PCR assays for MRD detection in solid tumor malignancies has been hampered by some significant disadvantages. They include (1) all PCR assays are exquisitely sensitive to contamination either from cells shed from the operator, ambient DNA, or contamination of the PCR equipment; (2) the results are only semiquantitative, with additional dilution experiments being required to approximate the number of tumor cells present in a sample; (3) the expression of "pseudogenes" can yield false-positive results; and (4) true expression of tumor-associated DNA rearrangements occur in normal populations (e.g., PSA expression in some women and the increasing frequency of *bcl-2* rearrangements in normal hematopoietic cells as a function of patient age). Nonetheless, PCR technologies offer exciting potential applications to the field of MRD detection.

IV. CLINICAL APPLICATIONS OF MRD TESTING

Because the presence of MRD in solid tumor malignancies is of clinical concern at various stages of HDC/ASCT therapy, MRD assays are currently used at several clinical points in time to document and monitor tumor micrometastases. As will be discussed below, MRD assays are useful for monitoring (1) the response of tumor micrometastases to induction chemotherapy or HDC; (2) the mobilization of tumor cells as a consequence of growth factor administration and apheresis; (3) the presence of tumor cells in the autograft; and (4) the tumor-purging effects of graft manipulation. Table 2 outlines the results of several MRD studies on tumor contamination of ASCT grafts.

A. MRD Response to Chemotherapy

Most patients with solid tumor malignancies are treated with successive cycles of induction chemotherapy prior to HDC/ASCT. This regimen is capable of reducing tumor burden in chemosensitive patients. However, it has been documented that patients with histologically normal marrow may still have low levels of MRD present. Researchers from Johns Hopkins University (22) used sensitive ICC assays to track marrow MRD clearance in breast cancer patients following successive cycles of combination chemotherapy. ICC analysis was able to document tumor cell reduction or ablation in marrow and PBSC collections from cycle two to cycle five of induction therapy. Further, 15 of 20 patients had no ICC-detectable MRD in the marrow harvests following five cycles of induction chemotherapy. Similar data have been reported in chemosensitive neuroblastoma patients (30).

Table 2 Minimal Residual Disease (MRD) in Autologous Stem Cell Transplantation (ASCT) Grafts

Disease	% Tumor-positive grafts	MRD assay method	Reference
Neuroblastoma	26% (marrow/PBSC)	ICC/TCA	Moss et al., 1994 (36)
Neuroblastoma	57% (CR marrow)	RT-PCR	Miyajima et al., 1996 (27)
	14% (CR PBSCs)		
	100% (pre-CR marrow)		
	82% (pre-CR PBSCs)		
Breast cancer (stage IV)	50% marrow	Long-term culture	Sharp et al., 1992 (5)
Breast Cancer (stage III-IV)	62% marrow	ICC/TCA	Ross et al., 1993 (21)
	10% PBSCs		
Breast cancer (stage IV)	83% marrow	RT-PCR	Datta et al., 1994 (11)
	0% PBSCs		
Breast cancer (stage II-III)	36% marrow	ICC	Vredenburgh et al., 1997 (6)
	4% PBSCs		
Breast cancer (stage II-III)	38% marrow	Short-term culture	Greer et al., 1996 (34)
Breast cancer (stage II-IV)	52% stage II marrow	RT-PCR	Fields et al., 1996 (8)
	57% stage III marrow		
	82% stage IV marrow		
Breast cancer (stage II-IV)	30% marrow	ICC	Franklin et al., 1996 (35)
	11% PBSCs		
Breast cancer (stage II-IV)	14% stage II-III PBSCs	ICC	Weaver, et al., 1998 (47)
	24% stage IV PBSCs		
Breast cancer (stage IV)	27% marrow	ICC	Cooper et al., 1998 (44)
	14% PBSCs		

PBSC, peripheral blood stem cell; CR, complete remission; RT-PCR, reverse transcriptase-polymerase chain; ICC, immunocytochemical; TCA, tumor cell clonogenic assay.

B. MRD in Stem Cell–Mobilization Procedures

Because the majority of ASCT procedures are performed with mobilized peripheral blood, there is justifiable concern about the concomitant mobilization of tumor cells. Brugger et al. (31) reported the mobilization of breast cancer and lung cancer cells into the peripheral blood following priming with chemotherapy followed by granulocyte colony-stimulating factor (G-CSF). Although this study examined mobilization of tumor cells into venous peripheral blood in previously untreated patients, the implication was that the same phenomenon might be observed in the HDC/ASCT setting.

To examine this issue, several studies have monitored the mobilization of tumor cells into PBSC collections using ICC and cell culture techniques. Passos-Coelho and colleagues (23,24) reported no increase in tumor cell contamination in a single, large-volume apheresis collection in chemosensitive advanced-stage breast cancer patients who were mobilized with either G-CSF alone or with cyclophosphamide followed by granulocyte-macrophage colony-stimulating factor (GM-CSF). Of particular interest, the in vitro tumor clonogenic assay (TCA) technique showed that inclusion of cyclophosphamide in the mobilization protocol may have the additional benefit of rendering the tumor cells incapable of subsequent clonogenic growth (24). The results of these two studies are summarized in Table 3.

Three retrospective studies of PBSC collections from advanced-stage breast cancer patients also demonstrated no significant increase in tumor cell mobilization in sequential apheresis collections (32). However, in a cohort of patients who had a median of 10 aphereses collected, a statistically significant ($P = .0064$) association was observed in the trend for the first three PBSC collections to be tumor contaminated (33).

Table 3 Effects of Stem Cell–Mobilization Protocols on Minimal Residual Disease (MRD) in Autologous Stem Cell Transplantation (ASCT) Grafts from Advanced-Stage Breast Cancer Patients

Patients/mobilization protocol G-CSF-(5 µg/kg/5–7 days)	Nonmobilized peripheral blood		Nonmobilized bone marrow		Peripheral blood stem cell apheresis collection	
	ICC[a]	TCA[b]	ICC	TCA	ICC	TCA
Patient 1	0	ND[c]	0	Negative	3	Positive
Patient 2	0	Negative	0	Negative	2	Positive
Patient 3	1	Negative	1	Positive	0	Negative
Cy/GM-CSF (4 g/m²/5 µg/kg/14 days)	ICC	TCA	ICC	TCA	ICC	TCA
Patient 1	0	Negative	18	Incl.[d]	0	Negative
Patient 2	0	Negative	2	Incl.	0	Negative
Patient 3	0	ND	8	Incl.	0	Negative
Patient 4	2	Positive	4	Positive	1	Negative

G-CSF, granulocyte colony-stimulating factor; Cy = cyclophosphamide.
[a] Number of tumor cells detected by immunocytochemical staining per 100,000 hematopoietic cells.
[b] Tumor colony growth in vitro in tumor cell clonogenic assay.
[c] Not done.
[d] Inconclusive.

C. MRD in ASCT grafts

Numerous investigators have documented the presence of MRD in marrow or PBSC auto-grafts from patients with solid tumors whose marrow was histologically normal. Sharp et al. (5) used a long-term culture assay to document the presence of contaminating breast cancer cells in marrow harvests. Approximately 50% of marrow cultures from 35 patients with histologically normal marrow were positive for culture growth. In intriguing follow-up studies, this group recently reported that the number of hematopoietic progenitor cells was greater in cultures that were tumor contaminated than those that were tumor free (from cancer patients and normal donors) (5). They postulated that the production of cytokines by the tumor cells, and/or direct tumor cell/hematopoietic cell contact, may explain this hematopoietic phenomenon. Further, a symbiotic relationship between tumor cells and hematopoietic cells may explain the affinity of epithelium-derived tumor cells for bone marrow.

Greer et al. (34) used a similar culture assay to document tumor cell growth in 10 of 26 (38%) marrow harvests from stage II-III breast cancer patients. Only 7 of the 10 culture-positive specimens were ICC positive prior to culture.

In a multicenter prospective study of 48 advanced-stage breast cancer patients, Ross et al. (21) used ICC and TCA analyses to document that 32 of 48 (67%) patients had marrow contamination, whereas only 9 of 48 (19%) patients had PBSC contamination. Results of this study are detailed in Table 4. Immunostained tumor cells were detected in 13 of 133 PBSC collections (10%) versus 38 of 61 (62%) marrow harvest specimens. The decreased tumor contamination frequency between PBSCs and marrow, as well as the number of patients with tumor-contaminated autografts, was significant ($P < .005$). Further, the geometric mean concentration of tumor cells was $0.8/10^5$ in PBSC specimens versus $22.9/10^5$ in marrow specimens ($P < .0001$). However, it must be appreciated that, owing to the large number of PBSC cells that comprise the ASCT graft, the actual number of infused tumor cells may equal or even surpass those in a marrow harvest. Similar to the culture results described above, this study also documented the in vitro clonogenic capacity of contaminating tumor cells in both marrow and PBSC specimens.

Franklin and colleagues (35) also used an ICC assay to document the presence of contaminating tumor cells in marrow and PBSC autografts from poor-prognosis breast

Table 4 Minimal Residual Disease (MRD) in Autologous Stem Cell Transplantation (ASCT) Grafts from Stage III-IV Breast Cancer Patients: Immunocytochemical (ICC) and Tumor Cell Clonogenic Assay Results

Autologous stem cell source	Immunostaining for tumor cells	In vitro growth of tumor colonies
Bone marrow (n = 31)	Positive = 21[a]	Growth = 17
		No growth = 4
	Negative = 10	Growth = 2
		No growth = 8
Peripheral blood stem cells (n = 27)	Positive = 5[a]	Growth = 4
		No growth = 1
	Negative = 22	Growth = 0
		No growth = 22

[a] ICC detection of tumor cells correlated significantly with clonogenicity ($P < .0001$, χ^2 test).

cancer patients. Overall, 30% of 240 patients had ICC-detectable MRD in marrow harvests. This included 70 of 190 (37%) patients with stage IV disease, 0 of 7 patients with stage III disease, and 3 of 43 (7%) patients with stage II disease. With respect to tumor contamination of PBSC collections, 73 of 657 (11%) from 26 of 155 (17%) patients were ICC positive. Stage IV patients were more likely to have tumor-contaminated PBSC [21 of 107 (20%)] versus 5 of 44 (11%) stage II patients.

In a retrospective study of 83 high-risk stage II-III breast cancer patients, Vredenburgh and colleagues (6) used an ICC assay to measure MRD in marrow and PBSC products. They found that 30 of 83 (36%) marrow specimens had tumor contamination versus only 2 of 57 (4%) PBSC specimens.

Using molecular-based assays, several groups have compared marrow versus peripheral blood or PBSC contamination in breast cancer patients. Datta and colleagues (11) used RT-PCR for cytokeratin 19 (CK19) to examine blood and marrow specimens from stage IV breast cancer patients. Four of 19 (12%) patients had RT-PCR–positive peripheral blood specimens, whereas 5 of 6 (83%) had RT-PCR–positive marrow following induction chemotherapy. Interestingly, all four PBSC collections from this cohort were RT-PCR negative. Of 39 non–breast cancer patients analyzed, one had RT-PCR–positive marrow (a patient with CML).

Of like note, Fields and colleagues (8) used RT-PCR for CK19 in a retrospective study to detect breast cancer micrometastases at transplant from stage II, III, and IV patients whose marrows were histologically normal. Fifty-two percent of 19 stage II, 57% of 14 stage III, and 82% of 50 stage IV patients had RT-PCR–positive marrow specimens. The increase in number of patients with RT-PCR–positive marrow as a function of clinical stage was significant ($P = .0075$).

In pediatric neuroblastoma, recent studies have documented the presence of tumor cells in autologous grafts. Using ICC and in vitro clonogenic assay methods, Moss et al. (36) documented tumor contamination of marrow harvests and peripheral blood collections. Overall, ICC showed 19/74 (26%) specimens to be tumor contaminated. Thirteen of the specimens grew tumor colonies in vitro with 6% of samples that were ICC negative showing tumor growth in vitro. Of additional interest, this group demonstrated that, although circulating neuroblastoma cells could be detected in 75% of blood specimens at diagnosis and in 36% of blood specimens during induction therapy, only 14% of PBSC collections were tumor positive (30). Thus, the incidence of neuroblastoma-contaminated PBSC collections, even in patients with MRD in marrow, is remarkably similar to that reported in breast cancer.

In a prospective study of 15 stage IV neuroblastoma patients, Miyajima and colleagues (27) used RT-PCR for tyrosine hydroxylase mRNA to detect MRD in paired marrow and PBSC collections. They compared tumor contamination rates in specimens obtained during complete remission (CR) or before CR was achieved. They found that 16 of 28 (57%) marrow and 4 of 28 (14%) PBSC samples taken during CR were RT-PCR positive versus 17 of 17 (100%) marrow and 14 of 17 (82%) PBSC samples taken prior to CR that were RT-PCR positive. These results were highly significant ($P < .0001$ for PBSC and $P < .01$ for marrow). Thus, although marrow and PBSC tumor contamination are apparently lower during CR than prior to CR, the risk of tumor contamination of autografts from chemoresponsive neuroblastoma patients is still considerable.

Although in the minority of HDC/ASCT cases select patients with ovarian cancer are being treated with this therapy. Because ovarian cancer metastasizes primarily by direct extension into body cavities, it was assumed that tumor contamination of marrow was nonexistent. However, two studies have used sensitive ICC techniques to document the presence of MRD in marrow harvests from patients with ovarian cancer. Cain et al. (37) reported that 23% of patients with histologically normal marrow had ICC-documented MRD.

Using similar ICC techniques, Ross et al. (38) compared the incidence of tumor contamination in marrow and PBSC collections from ovarian cancer patients in the HDC/ASCT setting. They found that 10 of 23 (43%) marrow specimens from 9 of 19 (47%) patients were ICC positive. Only 1 of the 10 ICC-positive marrows contained tumor by routine histopathological analysis. Further, ICC-detectable tumor cells were cleared from the marrows of two patients during induction chemotherapy. None of seven PBSC collections was ICC positive for tumor cells.

D. MRD and Tumor Purging

In an attempt to minimize tumor contamination of autologous grafts, a number of investigators have pursued methods of eradicating or "purging" tumor cells from marrow (7,39). Briefly, tumor cells can be removed by so-called "negative selection," which involves the specific depletion of tumor cells, or by so-called "positive selection," which involves the passive removal of tumor cells via the specific capture of hematopoietic cells.

Negative purging can be accomplished by pharmacological means (e.g., in vitro treatment with 4-hydroperoxycyclophosphamide) or by immunomagnetic depletion. In both instances, MRD assays are required to document tumor removal. Although somewhat laborious, limiting dilution assays of pharmacologically purged marrow can document tumor purging (40). It is also possible to use both ICC and TCA assays to document ex vivo purging effects (22). The advantage of using combined assays is that, although tumor cells may be detectable by ICC assays, only functional in vitro assays can measure the cytocidal effect of the pharmacological treatment. Results of combined ICC and TCA assays in breast cancer are summarized in Table 5.

Positive-selection purging involves the passive removal of tumor cells by the selective adsorption of selected hematopoietic cell populations (41–43). Because most epithelium-derived tumor cells are $CD34^-$, this results in the depletion of tumor cells in $CD34^+$-selected grafts. Preclinical and clinical studies have used culture methods and ICC to

Table 5 Detection of Minimal Residual Disease (MRD) by Immunocytochemical (ICC) and Tumor Cell Clonogenic Assay (TCA) in 4-Hydroperoxycyclophosphamide (4-HC)–Purged Marrow from Breast Cancer Patients

Pre–4-HC		Post–4-HC	
ICC[a]	TCA	ICC[a]	TCA
10	Positive	4	Negative
10	Positive	0	Negative
10	Positive	0	Negative
2	Negative	1	Negative
Not done	Negative	4	Negative

[a] Number of stained tumor cells per 10^5 marrow cells.

document between 2–4 logs of tumor cell depletion in neuroblastoma and breast cancer ASCT grafts (41). Of particular interest, Rill and colleagues (3) used in vitro culture techniques to demonstrate that residual gene-marked neuroblastoma cells in pharmacologically purged autologous grafts were not only present at sites of posttransplant disease relapse, but the tumor cells were capable of in vitro clonogenic growth as well.

To summarize, MRD assays are valuable tools in determining (1) the optimum time to obtain ASCT grafts; (2) whether induction therapy has been effective in clearing or reducing disease; (3) if MRD is present in ASCT grafts; and (4) if ex vivo graft manipulation has resulted in tumor purging. Certainly, the routine inclusion of MRD assays in the HDC/ASCT setting should be considered as a means of identifying and, ultimately, documenting the reduction of tumor contamination of autologous grafts.

V. CLINICAL SIGNIFICANCE OF MRD IN SOLID TUMOR MALIGNANCIES

Although the clinical significance of MRD in hematological malignancies is considerably more characterized, several recent studies have examined the posttransplant clinical consequences of MRD in solid tumor malignancies. The studies discussed below are the first attempts to define the possible role that infusion of tumor cells plays in the HDC/ASCT setting.

A. Breast Cancer

Although a number of studies have provided definitive evidence of the prognostic significance of marrow micrometastases in primary breast cancer, the first study to document the clinical significance of tumor contamination of ASCT grafts was published by Sharp et al. in 1992 (5). They used their long-term culture assay to detect MRD in marrow and PBSC collections from breast cancer and non-Hodgkin's lymphoma patients. Thirteen of 31 (42%) marrows from breast cancer patients were culture positive, whereas 4 of 25 (16%) of the PBSC collections were culture positive. Follow-up data demonstrated that the patients who had culture-positive PBSC collections had a poor prognosis. Overall, four of six (67%) PBSC-positive patients died shortly before or after transplant. Conversely, 7 of 18 (39%) of the culture-negative PBSC patients were alive at 1-year follow-up. Owing to low sample size, statistical analysis of the data is not available.

In follow-up studies of a cohort of the advanced-stage breast cancer patients reported initially by Ross et al. (21), subsequent analysis at greater than 36 months posttransplant indicates that no correlation was found with tumor contamination of the PBSC collection and time to disease progression, sites of relapse, or overall survival (44). Another retrospective study of a small cohort (n = 26) of advanced-stage breast cancer patients with tumor-contaminated marrow found a trend toward decreased overall survival ($P = .11$) at the 84-month follow-up (45). Insufficient power due to low sample size precluded any subset analyses in this cohort. Similar trends toward decreased progression-free and overall survival in advanced-stage breast cancer patients who received tumor-contaminated PBSC collections have also been reported by Gluck et al. (33).

By contrast, the retrospective study of MRD in marrow by Fields et al. (8) concluded that the probability of relapse at 36 months posttransplant was 32% for stage II-III and 94% for stage IV CK19 RT-PCR–positive patients. Conversely, the probability of relapse was 10% for stage II-III and 14% for Stage IV CK19 RT-PCR–negative patients. The difference was significant ($P = .0002$) for stage IV patients.

In a similar retrospective study, Duke University found that stage II-III breast cancers patients with ICC-positive marrow harvests had significantly shorter disease-free and overall survival (6). Unfortunately, too few patients had tumor-contaminated PBSCs for comparable statistical analysis. Moss et al. (46) reported that tumor contamination of autologous marrow grafts in 246 stage IV breast cancer patients was significantly associated with reduced disease-free survival ($P = .0001$). Patients who had both marrow and PBSCs contaminated with tumor had a worse posttransplant clinical course than did all other patients ($P = .015$). However, this study was a retrospective analysis of patients from a number of transplant centers who were treated with a variety of HDC/ASCT protocols.

In a prospective study (47) of 223 stage II-IV breast cancer patients analyzed with the same immunocytochemical assay used by Moss et al. (46), the investigators detected tumor cells in 17 of 122 (14%) stage II-III patients and in 24 of 101 (24%) stage IV patients ($P = .06$). Eleven percent of all patients who had one to two aphereses tested were tumor positive versus 32% of nine patients who had at three or greater aphereses tested. This difference was statistically significant ($P < .001$). However, similar to the results reported by Cooper et al. in stage IV patients, the presence of tumor cells in the ASCT graft was not associated with a significant decrease in early relapse or tumor progression. The discordant conclusions of the above-mentioned studies in breast cancer highlight the need for additional prospective analyses in expanded patient populations to more completely understand the role of tumor infusion in the HDC/ASCT setting.

B. Neuroblastoma

As is the case with breast cancer, several studies have documented the poor prognostic significance of tumor-contaminated marrow and peripheral blood in neuroblastoma (4,27,36). These studies concluded that the presence of MRD in ASCT grafts is associated with poor prognosis. However, it was the unique and elegant study of Rill and colleagues at St. Jude's Hospital (3) which conclusively demonstrated that infused neuroblastoma cells directly contribute to disease relapse. They transfected ASCT grafts with a neomycin-resistant gene to mark the cells in the graft prior to infusion. At relapse, the tumor cells were removed and plated into a clonogenic assay. The resulting tumor colonies were analyzed for the presence of the neomycin-resistant gene. The presence of gene-marked tumor cells at existing and new sites of relapse directly demonstrated that infusion of tumor cells from a solid tumor malignancy do contribute to posttransplant relapse.

VI. CONCLUSION

One issue in HDC/ASCT therapy is clear. Until chemotherapy regimens are more effective in eradicating systemic disease, HDC/ASCT therapy will likely result in increased survival, but the "cure" remains elusive. The advent of sensitive assays for the detection of MRD has shown us that, although bulk tumor may be greatly reduced by therapy, stubborn, occult tumor cells may still reside in hematopoietic tissue compartments. In fact, as the gene-marking studies have illustrated, it may be that these occult remaining tumor cells are the therapy-resistant progeny that have the capacity to give rise to disease recurrence posttransplant.

It is unclear at this point whether the presence of MRD in solid-tumor malignancies is merely a marker of aggressive, treatment-resistant disease, if MRD cells are singularly capable of reseeding systemic disease posttransplant, or if a combination of these factors are at play. It may be, short of complete disease eradication, that the infusion of tumor-free or tumor-reduced ASCT grafts results in prolonged treatment and disease-free survival but has a limited impact on overall survival. Residual tumor cells likely possess tremendous heterogeneity with respect to genetic characteristics, metastatic potential, and chemoresistance. It is safe to say that their lingering presence despite the arsenals of cancer therapy is indicative of some survival advantage.

The challenge for those of us who study MRD is to uncover the secrets of these elusive cells. To do so will require the development of more sophisticated, sensitive, and specific assays. Further, it will also require that prospective clinical trials incorporate carefully designed, empirically tested and validated MRD assays into their protocols. In conclusion, these tumor cells have something very important to tell us; it behooves us to listen.

ACKNOWLEDGMENTS

The author gratefully acknowledges Dr. Karen Auditore-Hargreaves, Tamara Layton, Anita Ostrander, and Mark Rehse for helpful manuscript review and Tina Loucks and Anne O'Connell for expert manuscript preparation assistance.

REFERENCES

1. Brenner MK, Rill DR, Moen RC, Krance RA, Mirro J, Anderson WF, Ihle JN. Gene-marking to trace origin of relapse after autologous bone-marrow transplantation. Lancet 1993; 341:85–86.
2. Deisseroth AB, Zu Z, Claxton D, Hanania EG, Fu S, Ellerson D, Goldberg L, Thomas M, Janicek K, Anderson WF, Hester J, Korbling M, Durett A, Moen R, Berenson R, Heimfeld S, Hamer J, Calvert L, Tibbits P, Talpaz M, Kantarjian H, Champlin R, Reading C. Genetic marking shows that Ph⁺ cells present in autologous transplants of chronic myelogenous leukemia (CML) contribute to relapse after autologous bone marrow in CML. Blood 1994; 83: 3068–3076.
3. Rill DR, Santana VM, Roberts WM, Nilson T, Bowman LC, Krance RA, Heslop HE, Moen RC, Ihle JN, Brenner MK. Direct demonstration that autologous bone marrow transplantation for solid tumors can return a multiplicity of tumorigenic cells. Blood 1994; 84:380–383.
4. Moss TJ, Reynolds CP, Sather HN, Romansky SG, Hammond GD, Seeger RC. Prognostic value of immunocytologic detection of bone marrow metastases in neuroblastoma. N Engl J Med 1991; 324:219–226.
5. Sharp JG, Kessinger A, Vaughan WP, Mann S, Crouse DA, Dicke K, Masih A, Weisenburger DD. Detection and clinical significance of minimal tumor cell contamination of peripheral stem cell harvests. Int J Cell Cloning 1992; 10:92–94.
6. Vredenburgh JJ, Silva O, Broadwater G, Berry D, DeSombre K, Tyer C, Petros WP, Peters WP, Bast Jr RC. The significance of tumor contamination in the bone marrow from high-risk primary breast cancer patients treated with high-dose chemotherapy and hematopoietic support. Biol Blood Marrow Transplant 1997; 3:91–97.
7. Shpall EJ, Gee AP, Hogan C, Cagnoni P, Gehling U, Hami L, Franklin W, Bearman SI, Ross M, Jones RB. Bone marrow metastases. Hematol/Oncol Clin North Am 1996; 10:321–343.
8. Fields KK, Elfenbein GJ, Trudeau WL, Perkins JB, Janssen WE, Moscinski LC. Clinical significance of bone marrow metastases as detected using the polymerase chain reaction in pa-

tients with breast cancer undergoing high-dose chemotherapy and autologous bone marrow transplantation. J Clin Oncol 1996; 14:1868–1876.

9. Salsbury AJ. The significance of the circulating cancer cell. Cancer Treat Rev 1975; 2:55–72.

10. Moss TJ, Ross AA. Detection of tumor cells in the peripheral blood of patients with solid tumor malignancies. J Hematother 1992; 1:225–232.

11. Datta YH, Adams PT, Drobyski WR, Ethier SP, Terry VH, Roth MS. Sensitive detection of occult breast cancer by the reverse-transcriptase polymerase chain reaction. J Clin Oncol 1994; 12:475–482.

12. Neumaier M, Gerhard M, Wagener C. Diagnosis of micrometastases by the amplification of tissue-specific genes. Gene 1995; 159:43–47.

13. Pelkey TJ, Frierson Jr HF, Bruns DE. Molecular and immunological detection of circulating tumor cells and micrometastases from solid tumors. Clin Chem 1996; 42:1369–1381.

14. Schoenfeld A, Kruger KH, Gomm J, Sinnett HD, Gazet JC, Sacks N, Bender HG, Luqmani Y, Coombes RC. The detection of micrometastases in the peripheral blood and bone marrow of patients with breast cancer using immunohistochemistry and reverse transcriptase polymerase chain reaction for keratin 19. Eur J Cancer 1997; 33A:854–867.

15. Wolin MJ, Ross AA, Rigor RL, Gale RP, Klein J. Are single apheresis collections of blood stem cells less likely to contain cancer cells than multiple collections? (abstr). Blood 1995; 86:235a.

16. Chaiwun B, Saad AD, Groshen S, Chen SC, Mazumder A, Imam A, Taylor CR, Cote RJ. Immunohistochemical detection of occult carcinoma in bone marrow and blood. Diagn Oncol 1992; 2:267–276.

17. Pantel K, Felber E, Schlimok G. Detection and characterization of residual disease in breast cancer. J Hematother 1994; 3:315–322.

18. Pantel K, Riethmüller G. Methods for detection of micrometastatic carcinoma cells in bone marrow, blood and lymph nodes. Onkologie 1995; 18:394–401.

19. Müller P, Weckermann D, Riethmüller G, Schlimok G. Detection of genetic alterations in micrometastatic cells in bone marrow of cancer patients by fluorescence in situ hybridization. Cancer Genet Cytogenet 1996; 88:8–16.

20. Emerman JT, Stingl J, Petersen A, Shpall EJ, Eaves CJ. Selective growth of freshly isolated human breast epithelial cells cultured at low concentrations in the presence or absence of bone marrow cells. Breast Cancer Res Treat 1996; 41:147–159.

21. Ross AA, Cooper BW, Lazarus HM, Mackay W, Moss TJ, Ciobanu N, Tallman MS, Kennedy MJ, Davidson NE, Sweet D, Winter C, Akard L, Jansen J, Copelan E, Meagher RC, Herzig RH, Klumpp TR, Kahn DG, Warner NE. Detection and viability of tumor cells in peripheral blood stem cell collections from breast cancer patients using immunocytochemical and clonogenic assay techniques. Blood 1993; 9:2605–2610.

22. Passos-Coelho J, Ross AA, Davis JM, Huelskamp A-M, Clarke B, Noga SJ, Davidson NE, Kennedy MJ. Bone marrow micrometastases in chemotherapy-responsive advanced breast cancer: Effect of ex vivo purging with 4-hydroperoxycyclophosphamide. Cancer Res 1994; 54:2366–2371.

23. Passos-Coelho JL, Ross AA, Moss TJ, Davis JM, Huelskamp A-M, Noga SJ, Davidson NJ, Kennedy MJ. Absence of breast cancer cells in a single-day peripheral blood progenitor cell collection after priming with cyclophosphamide and granulocyte-macrophage colony-stimulating factor. Blood 1995; 85:1138–1143.

24. Passos-Coelho JL, Ross AA, Kahn DJ, Moss TJ, Davis JM, Huelskamp A-M, Noga SJ, Davidson NE, Kennedy MJ. Similar breast cancer cell contamination of single-day peripheral-blood progenitor-cell collections obtained after priming with hematopoietic growth factor alone or after cyclophosphamide followed by growth factor. J Clin Oncol 1996; 14:2569–2575.

25. Berois N, Varangot M, Osinaga E, Babino A, Caignault L, Musé I, Roseto A. Detection of

rare human breast cancer cells. Comparison of an immunomagnetic separation method with immunocytochemistry and RT-PCR. Anticancer Res 1997; 17:2639–2646.

26. Mapara MY, Körner IJ, Hildebrandt M, Bargou R, Krahl D, Reichardt P, Dörken B. Monitoring of tumor cell purging after highly efficient immunomagnetic selection of CD34 cells from leukapheresis products in breast cancer patients: comparison of immunocytochemical tumor cell staining and reverse transcriptase-polymerase chain reaction. Blood 1997; 89:337–344.

27. Miyajima Y, Horibe K, Fukuda M, Matsumoto K, Numata S-I, Mori H, Kato K. Sequential detection of tumor cells in the peripheral blood and bone marrow of patients with stage IV neuroblastoma by the reverse transcription-polymerase chain reaction for tyrosine hydroxylase mRNA. Cancer 1996; 77:1214–1219.

28. Zippelius A, Kufer P, Honold G, Köllermann MW, Oberneder R, Schlimok G, Riethmüller G, Pantel K. Limitations of reverse-transcriptase polymerase chain reaction analyses for detection of micrometastatic epithelial cancer cells in bone marrow. J Clin Oncol 1997; 15:2701–2708.

29. Noguchi S, Motomura K, Inaji H, Imaoka S, Koyama H. Clonal analysis of human breast cancer by means of the polymerase chain reaction. Cancer Res 1992; 52:6594–6597.

30. Moss TJ, Sanders DG, Lasky LC, Bostrom B. Contamination of peripheral blood stem cell harvests by circulating neuroblastoma cells. Blood 1990; 76:1879–1883.

31. Brugger W, Bross KJ, Glatt M, Weber F, Mertelsmann R, Kanz L. Mobilization of tumor cells and hematopoietic progenitor cells into peripheral blood of patients with solid tumors. Blood 1994; 83:636–640.

32. Ross AA, Layton TJ, Ostrander AB, Passos-Coelho JL, Davis JM, Huelskamp AM, Noga SJ, Davidson NE, Kennedy MJ, Cooper BW, Gerson SL, Lazarus HM, Holland K, Gluck S, Moss TJ, Kaubish A, Vahdat L, Antman K. Comparative analysis of breast cancer contamination in mobilized and nonmobilized hematopoietic grafts. J Hematother 1996; 5:549–552.

33. Gluck S, Ross AA, Layton TJ, Ostrander AB, Goldstein L, Porter K, Ho AD. Decrease in tumor cell contamination and progenitor cell yield in the leukapheresis products after consecutive cycles of chemotherapy for breast cancer. Biol Blood Marrow Transplant 1997; 3:316–323.

34. Greer G, Franklin W, Hami L, Williams S, Jones K, Stoltz J, Emmerman J, Shpall EJ. A clonogenic culture method for the identification of breast cancer cells in marrow aspirates of patients receiving high-dose chemotherapy (abstr). Blood 1996; 88:252a.

35. Franklin WA, Shpall EJ, Archer P, Johnston CS, Garza-Williams S, Hami L, Bitter MA, Bast Jr RC, Jones RB. Immunocytochemical detection of breast cancer cells in marrow and peripheral blood of patients undergoing high dose chemotherapy with autologous stem cell support. Breast Cancer Res Treat 1996; 41:1–13.

36. Moss TJ, Cairo M, Santana VM, Weinthal J, Hurvitz C, Bostrom B. Clonogenicity of circulating neuroblastoma cells: Implications regarding peripheral blood stem cell transplantation. Blood 1994; 83:3085–3089.

37. Cain JM, Ellis GK, Collins C, Greer BE, Tamimi HK, Figge DC, Gown AM, Livingston RB. Bone marrow involvement in epithelial ovarian cancer by immunocytochemical assessment. Gynecol Oncol 1990; 38:442–445.

38. Ross AA, Miller GW, Moss TJ, Kahn DG, Warner NE, Sweet DL, Louie KG, Schneidermann E, Pecora AL, Meagher RC, Herzig RH, Collins RH, Fay JW. Immunocytochemical detection of tumor cells in bone marrow and peripheral blood stem cell collections from patients with ovarian cancer. Bone Marrow Transplant 1995; 15:929–933.

39. Kvalheim G. Purging of autografts: Methods and clinical significance. Ann Med 1996; 28:167–173.

40. Shpall EJ, Jones RB, Bast Jr RC, Rosner GL, Vandermark R, Ross M, Affronti ML, Johnston C, Eggleston S, Tepperburg M, Coniglio D, Peters WP. 4-Hydroperoxycyclophosphamide purging of breast cancer from the mononuclear cell fraction of bone marrow in patients receiv-

ing high-dose chemotherapy and autologous marrow support: a phase I trial. J Clin Oncol 1991; 9:85–93.

41. Shpall EJ, Jones RB, Bearman SI, Franklin WA, Archer PG, Curiel T, Bitter M, Claman HN, Stremmer SM, Purdy M, Myers SE, Hami L, Taffs S, Heimfeld S, Hallagan J, Berenson RJ. Transplantation of enriched CD34-positive autologous marrow into breast cancer patients following high-dose chemotherapy: Influence of CD34-positive peripheral-blood progenitors and growth factors on engraftment. J Clin Oncol 1994; 12:28–36.

42. Handgretinger R, Greil J, Schurmann U, Lang P, Gonzalez-Ramella O, Schmidt I, Fuhrer R, Neithammer D, Klingbiel T. Positive selection and transplantation of peripheral CD34$^+$ progenitor cells: feasibility and purging efficacy in pediatric patients with neuroblastoma. J Hematother 1997; 6:235–242.

43. Hohaus S, Pförsich M, Murea S, Abdallah A, Lin YS, Funk L, Voso MT, Kaul S, Schmid H, Wallwiener D, Haas R. Immunomagnetic selection of CD34$^+$ peripheral blood stem cells for autografting in patients with breast cancer. Br J Haematol 1997; 97:881–888.

44. Cooper BW, Moss TJ, Ross AA, Ybanez J, Lazarus HM. Occult tumor contamination of hematopoietic stem-cell products does not affect clinical outcome of autologous transplantation in patients with metastatic breast cancer. J Clin Oncol 1998; 16:3509–3517.

45. Brockstein BE, Ross AA, Moss TJ, Kahn DG, Hollingsworth K, Williams SF. Tumor cell contamination of bone marrow harvests products: Clinical consequences in a cohort of advanced-stage breast cancer patients undergoing high-dose chemotherapy. J Hematother 1996; 5:605–616.

46. Moss TJ, Cooper B, Kennedy MJ, Meagher R, Pecora AL, Rosenfeld C, Herzig RM, Umiel T, Copelan E, Lazarus HM. The prognostic value of immunocytochemical (ICC) analysis on bone marrow (BM) and stem cell products (PBSC) taken from patients with stage IV breast cancer undergoing autologous transplant (ABMT) therapy (abstr). Proc Am Soc Clin Oncol 1997; 16:90a.

47. Weaver CH, Moss T, Schwartzberg LS, Zhen B, West J, Rhinehart S, Campos L, Beeker T, Lautersztain L, Messino M, Buckner CD. High-dose chemotherapy in patients with breast cancer: evaluation of infusing peripheral blood stem cells containing occult tumor cells. Bone Marrow Transplant. 1998; 21:1117–1124.

17

Stem Cell Isolation with Immunomagnetic Beads and Tumor Cell Contamination

GUNNAR KVALHEIM, ANNE PHARO, HARALD HOLTE, ELISABETH LENSCHOW, MENGYU WANG, BJORN ERIKSTEIN, STEIN KVALØY, JOHN MAGNE NESLAND, and ERLEND SMELAND

The Norwegian Radium Hospital, Oslo, Norway

I. INTRODUCTION

High-dose chemoradiotherapy (HDCRT) with autologous stem cell support is increasingly being used to treat selected patients with hematological cancer as well as other malignancies (1). The use of hematopoietic growth factors can significantly increase the number of peripheral blood progenitor cells (PBPCs) when administered in the recovery phase after cytotoxic treatment (2). Collection and reinfusion of such cells following high-dose treatment gives several advantages compared to the use of bone marrow (BM). In particular, PBPCs can be collected without general anesthesia, and the use of PBPCs reduces the number of days until neutrophils and platelets have reached pretransplant levels (3–5).

In spite of these advantages, the disease-free survival of patients treated with high-dose therapy has not improved significantly. Relapse of the underlying disease still represents the major cause of death. The possible contribution of tumor cell purging to the efficacy of HDCRT with autologous stem cell transplantation is unknown, as prospective clinical studies have not been performed. However, gene-marking studies of autografted cells to trace the origin of relapse after autologous bone marrow transplantation (ABMT) have indicated that tumor cells remaining in the reinfused stem cell product contribute to recurrence of the disease at least in myeloid leukemias and neuroblastomas (6,7). This conclusion is further supported by results in patients with follicular lymphomas, which indicate that efficient BM purging improves disease-free survival (8).

A variety of techniques have been developed for the purpose of removing tumor cells from BM grafts (9). Monoclonal antibodies (mAbs) directed against tumor-associated antigens can be used for specific removal of the malignant cells. The mAbs can either be used together with complement (10), coupled to toxins as immunotoxins (11,12), or in combination with iron-containing polymer beads coated with a secondary antibody (13–17). Previously we have reported our experiences with purging of lymphoma cells from BM employing anti–B-cell or anti–T-cell mABs and magnetizable bead, Dynabeads M-450 (Dynal A/S, Oslo, Norway) (18). Based on this, a purging procedure to deplete PBPCs of lymphoma cells has been developed. Moreover, we have obtained data showing that the use of anti–breast cancer mAbs in combination with immunobeads efficiently removes breast cancer cells from leukapheresis products.

Most solid tumor cells such as breast cancer and lymphoma cells do not express CD34 antigens. Positive enrichment of CD34 cells from leukapheresis products obtained from breast cancer patients has resulted in a tumor cell depletion of only 2 log (19,20). As will be discussed in this chapter, our own experiences with CD34 cell enrichment employing Isolex300 (Baxter Immunotherapy, Irvine, CA) and immunobeads has shown a similar purging efficacy in patients with breast cancer. However, a 2–4–log depletion is often not sufficient to eradicate all tumor cells from the enriched CD34$^+$ cell population. Therefore, a positive enrichment of CD34 cells followed by the purging procedure for the tumor cells might by warranted.

II. MINIMAL RESIDUAL DISEASE IN BM AND PERIPHERAL BLOOD

Sensitive immunocytochemical methods using tumor-associated mABs and alkaline phosphatase anti-alkaline phosphatase (APAAP) staining techniques to detect occult micrometastatic tumor cells in blood and BM have been developed (21,22). In patients with breast cancer, neuroblastoma and lymphomas, tumor cells can be found in 30–60% of the BM autografts and in 10–30% of the PBPC products (23–26). Available data indicate that patients with tumor cells in the BM and PBPC collections detected by immunohistochemistry have an unfavorable prognosis (26). A possible explanation for the relatively frequent presence of tumor cells in PBPC harvests is the recent observation that stem cell mobilization with hematopoietic growth factors can induce the release of tumor cells into the bloodstream (27).

In Scandinavia, high-risk stage II breast cancer patients with a life expectancy of <30% disease-free survival after 5 years are randomized to be given adjuvant treatment with tamoxifen for 5 years and either dose-escalating chemotherapy plus granulocyte colony-stimulating factor (G-CSF) or high-dose therapy with PBPC support. Among 124 breast cancer patients entering this study in Norway, detection of micrometastases has been evaluated in BM and peripheral blood (PB) at diagnosis, and in PBPCs, BM and PB after treatment. Immunocytochemistry using anticytokeratin antibodies (AE-1/AE-3, Sanbio Laboratories Inc., Uden, The Netherlands) and APAAP staining technique was applied (28). One to 2 × 10^6 cells were examined from each individual patient sample. At diagnosis, 29% had tumor cells present in the BM, whereas only 8% had tumor cells in the blood. Figure 1 shows that, among 60 patients randomized to have high-dose therapy, 24 (36%) presented with tumor cells in BM and 6 (10%) in PB at diagnosis. In spite of tumor reductive therapy with three cycles of chemotherapy, 14 of 60 (23%) PBPC products were contaminated. Among these patients, only two of six presented with tumor cells in PB at diagnosis. This shows that tumor cells are mobilized together with CD34$^+$

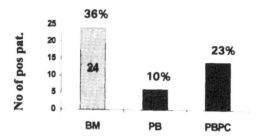

Figure 1   Monitoring micrometastatic cells in 60 high-risk breast cancer patients in bone marrow (BM) and peripheral blood (PB) at diagnosis and in peripheral blood progenitor cells (PBPC) mobilized with chemotherapy and granulocyte-colony stimulating factor (G-CSF). All patients were treated with two cycles of chemotherapy prior to mobilization of PBPCs.

cells into the blood and that tumor cell depletion of the PBPC products might be important even in patients with limited disease treated with high-dose therapy. The mean number of tumor cells found in each patient sample was 6 (1–100) per $1-2 \times 10^6$ cells. To further improve the reproducibility and sensitivity of tumor cell detection and further characterize the tumor cells, methods for tumor cell enrichment employing immunomagnetic beads are currently being tested (29).

Polymerase chain reaction (PCR) is based on an in vitro enzymatic amplification of a specific target deoxyribonucleic acid (DNA) segment resulting in a highly specific, 10^5- to 10^6-fold enrichment of the sequence of interest. Cloning the breakpoints of specific translocations makes it possible to use amplification by PCR to detect lymphoma cells containing the translocation. The t(14;18) translocation appears in approximately 85% of patients with follicular lymphomas and in 30% of high-grade diffuse non-Hodgkin's lymphomas (NHLs). This translocation results in the juxtaposition of the proto-oncogene *bcl-2* with the immunoglobulin heavy-chain locus on chromosome 14. The PCR technique permits the detection of as little as one lymphoma cell among 10^5 normal cells. In low-grade lymphomas, BM infiltration is common at diagnosis, and in spite of successful tumor reduction with the disappearance of enlarged lymph nodes, residual BM infiltration can be frequently demonstrated by BM biopsies. In addition, the use of PCR has shown that patients with advanced lymphomas with a *bcl-2* translocation invariably have BM infiltration even when in complete remission after conventional chemotherapy. Although tumor cells can be detected in 100% of the BM harvests, 50–80% of the PBPC harvests also contain tumor cells (25). As in the case of breast cancer, low-grade lymphoma cells are also mobilized into the PB with growth factors (G. Sharp, personal communication). Similar findings have been found in other types of cancers (30). Based on these observations, and if purging of tumor cells is of clinical benefit in autotransplants employing BM, it will also be important in high-dose therapy employing PBPC products.

III.   IMMUNOMAGNETIC PURGING OF B- AND T-MALIGNANT CELLS FROM AUTOGRAFTS

At The Norwegian Radium Hospital, we developed an efficient indirect immunomagnetic purging procedure to deplete lymphoma cells from BM anti–B-cell or anti–T-cell monoclonal antibodies and magnetizable beads [Dynabeads M-450 sheep-antimouse (14,15)].

Before initiation of the purging procedure, the total number of antibody-binding cells in the BM is determined by immunocytochemistry or by flow cytometry. A mononuclear cell preparation of harvested marrow is incubated at 4°C for 30 min with saturated amounts of a mixture of mABs reactive with the B-cell antigens CD19, CD20, CD22, CD23, and CD37, or the T-cell antigens CD2, CD3, CD4, CD5, CD7, and CD8. Excess antibody is removed by washing BM cells twice with cold medium. Desired amounts of beads are added and incubated at 4°C for 30 min. The bead/cell rosettes are formed and excess beads are removed using our own purging device or the MAX-SEP Cell Separator (Baxter Biotech, Deerfield, IL). After a second cycle of purging, for which the same amount of beads is added, the cell suspension is concentrated and frozen.

As previously reported (18), 83 lymphoma patients have been transplanted with immunomagnetic purged BM. Ten Burkitt's lymphomas, 6 B-cell lymphoblastic lymphomas, and 21 T-cell lymphoblastic lymphomas were transplanted in first complete remission (CR). Twenty-seven high-grade lymphomas and 19 low-grade lymphomas were transplanted in second or later CR. High-dose therapy consisted of fractionated total body irradiation (1.3 Gy twice daily for 5 days) followed by 2 days of cyclophosphamide 60 mg/kg. After high-dose therapy, the median number of days to recover granulocytes ($>0.5 \times 10^9$/L) was 24 (range 11–117 days) and platelets ($>20 \times 10^9$/L) 24 (range 8–566 days). Patients who experienced late engraftment had all been treated before high-dose therapy with multiple cycles of chemotherapy.

Sixty percent of 21 T-cell lymphoma patients treated with high-dose therapy and purged BM are in CR with a median observation time of 25 (10–79) months. Of the B-cell lymphomas, 10 of 10 Burkitt lymphomas and 4 of 6 B-cell lymphoblastic lymphomas are in CR with a median observation time of 28 (12–82) months. Forty-three percent of the 27 relapsed high-grade lymphomas are in CR with an observation time of 18 (9–100) months. Thirty-seven percent of the 19 low-grade lymphomas transplanted are in CR with an observation time of 35 (12–76) months. The overall survival was 75%, indicating that many low-grade lymphomas remain alive with disease after transplantation.

Previously we have shown that purging lymphoma cells with immunomagnetic beads is 10–100 times more efficient than targeted cell lysis with complement-activating antibodies and rabbit complement (31). In agreement with these experimental findings, it has been demonstrated that full-scale immunomagnetic purging of BM from low-grade NHL patients gave up to 5 log depletion of tumor cells when PCR was used to detect residual lymphoma cells after purging (32).

Based on our work with purging of lymphoma cells from BM, a purging procedure to deplete leukapheresis products of lymphoma cells has been developed (33). Six relapsed lymphoma patients in clinical remission were treated with MIME [mitoguazon, 500 mg/m² (body weight), day 1; ifosfamide, 1000 mg/m², daily from days 1–4; metothrexate, 30 mg/m², day 3; and etoposide, 100 mg/m², daily days 1–3 Uromitexan, 400 mg, was given daily every 4–8 h on days 1–5]. Two days after the end of chemotherapy, the patients were given daily subcutaneous (sc) G-CSF injection (Filgrastim, 5 µg/kg; Amgen/Roche, Basel, Switzerland). When peak levels of CD34⁺ cells appeared in the blood leukapheresis was performed with a CS 3000 Fenwall Cell Separator (Baxter, Deerfield, IL) with a flow rate of 70 mL/min. Each day, 10 L of blood was processed. The first day, the leukapheresis product was washed and stored overnight. After finishing the second day's leukapheresis, both products were pooled together, washed in a COBE 2991 Cell Separator (COBE Laboratories, Inc., Lakewood, CO), and resuspended in medium to give a cell concentration of $1-2 \times 10^8$ cells/mL. The cells were then incubated at 4°C for 30 min with a total amount of 1 mg of each of the clinical grade B-cell antibodies, as previously described. Excess antibody was removed by washing the cells twice with cold medium in the COBE 2991 Cell Separator. The cells were resuspended in medium to give a cell concentration of $1-2 \times 10^8$ cells/mL. Based on a previous estimation of the number of B cells or T cells present in the leukapheresis product, the desired amount of sheep-antimouse IgG Dynabeads M-450 was added. Since in B-cell lymphomas the number of B cells in all cases was less than 5%, the ratio of beads to total nucleated cells was 1 to 1. In contrast, the T-cell lymphomas contained >10% T cells in the PBPC product and the ratio of beads to total cells was 2 to 1. After incubation at 4°C for 30 min, the bead/cell rosettes and excess beads were removed by the use of the MAX-SEP Cell Separator. After a second cycle of purging, in which the same amount of beads was added, the cell suspension was concentrated and frozen.

The immunomagnetic purging procedure always gives some unspecific cell loss. Among the five lymphoma patients, the mean PBPC loss was 25% (12–40%), and all patients given high-dose therapy had a rapid reconstitution of hematopoiesis without post-transplant administration of G-CSF, reaching >0.5 × 10^9/L granulocytes at days 8–10 and >20 × 10^9/L platelets at days 9–27. The purging efficacy is demonstrated in Figure 2, which shows data from a T-cell lymphoma patient in remission but with a previous history of a T-cell lymphoma expressing of CD4 and CD8 analysis. After mobilization

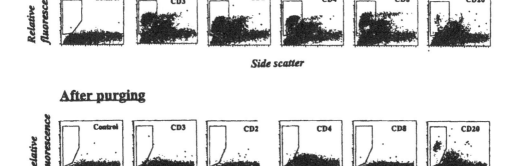

Figure 2 The leukapheresis product from a patient with T-cell lymphoma was purged (×2) with CD2, CD3, CD5, CD7, CD4, and CD8 monoclonal antibodies and sheep-antimouse IgG Dynabeads M-450. Immunophenotyping was performed before and after purging by use of fluorescein isothiocyanate (FITC)–labeled monoclonal antibodies against CD3, CD2, CD4, CD8, and CD20 antigens. Control cells received an isotope-matched irrelevant monoclonal antibody. Flow cytometry was performed on a Beckton Dickinson FACscan flow cytometer using the CellQuest software (Becton Dickinson Immunotherapy Systems, San Jose, CA). Before purging, approximately 40% of the cells expressed T-lineage antigens. After purging, less than 1% (range 0.05–0.7%) of the cells expressed weakly various T-lineage antigens. The number of B cells was relatively unchanged by the purging procedure (2.5% CD20 cells before purging and 2.7% CD20$^+$ cells after purging).

with MIME and G-CSF, the apheresis product contained 40% T cells. After immunomagnetic purging employing the antibodies anti-CD2, -CD3, -CD5, -CD7, -CD8, and -CD4, only a minor fraction (<1%) of low T-cell antigen-expressing cells could be detected. Although efficient, the immunomagnetic bead purging procedure is expensive, especially when used to purge leukapheresis products, since 10 times more beads are required as when BM is used. To achieve a purging efficacy in the lymphoma patients as described here, 6.4×10^{10} beads (16 vials) were used for each purging cycle.

IV. PURGING OF BREAST CANCER CELLS FROM AUTOGRAFTS

Previously it has been shown that mixtures of anti–breast cancer antibodies attached to beads efficiently deplete breast cancer cells from autografts (34). Since some of the antibodies originally used were not for clinical use, we tested a new protocol employing purified and clinical grade antibreast antibodies 9189.9187 and 9184 of IgG1 subtype (Baxter, Munich, Germany) (33). A mixture of individual antibodies attached to sheep-antimouse IgG Dynabeads M-450 particles was experimentally used to purify PBPC products from lymphoma patients admixed with 1% breast cancer cells. When a ratio of beads and total nucleated cells of 1 to 1 was used, a 4-log tumor cell depletion could be obtained with a total cell loss of less than 20%. To further deplete breast cancer cells from the graft, one additional cycle of immunomagnetic purging was required. Therefore, like in lymphoma patients, purging of breast cancer cells from PBPCs is costly.

V. IMMUNOMAGNETIC ENRICHMENT OF CD34+ CELLS FROM LEUKAPHERESIS PRODUCTS

Autografts consisting of isolated CD34+ progenitor cells from PBPCs appear to give similar reconstitution of hematopoiesis after high-dose therapy as unmanipulated PBPC (19,35). Since most solid tumor cells do not express the CD34 antigen, isolation of CD34+ cells should not contain malignant cells. However, previous results show only a 2–3–log depletion of tumor cells (19). Since the purity of CD34 cells in this study varies from 50 to 85%, one explanation for the modest purging effect could be that the malignant cells are contaminating the CD34⁻ fraction of the selected cells.

Previously we reported our clinical experience with enrichment of CD34+ cells from leukapheresis products from breast cancer and lymphoma patients employing immunobeads and the Isolex300 Cell Separator (36). This experience has been further extended. Briefly, pooled leukapheresis products were prepared from breast cancer and lymphoma patients in the same manner as when immunomagnetic purging was performed. The PBPCs were incubated with saturated amounts of anti-CD34 mABs for 30 min at 4°C and excess antibodies were removed by washing twice in the COBE 2991 Cell Separator. Then 1×10^8 cells/mL were introduced into the Isolex300 and the desired amount of immunobeads coated with sheep-antimouse IgG was added. At room temperature, the incubation of beads and detachment of CD34 immunobead/cell complexes was done in the Isolex300 device. To release beads from CD34+ cells, Chymo-Cell in appropriate amounts was used in samples from 24 patients (17 breast cancers and 7 lymphomas). In 25 patients (18 breast cancers plus 7 lymphomas) the recently developed PR34+[TM3] Stem Cell–releasing agent was used. Chymo-Cell releases beads from CD34+ cells by an unspecific removal of membrane antigens. In contrast, the new system conserves all antigens on the CD34$^+$ cell after the release of the beads. The reason for the latter is that this product consists of a genetically engineered peptide that mimics the CD34 antigen–binding cite and thus competes with the CD34 antibody. The yield of CD34$^+$ cells was slightly better with Chymo-Cell than with PR34^{+TM3} Stem Cell–releasing agent (62 vs 54%). No significant differences were observed with regard to purity.

VI. ISOLEX300 CD34$^+$ CELL ENRICHMENT IN PATIENTS

Fifty-four patients (35 breast cancers plus 19 lymphomas) have been treated with high-dose therapy and isolated CD34$^+$ cells as stem cell support. Four high-grade NHLs and 15 Hodgkin's patients in clinical remission were treated with MIME and G-CSF. The first day, leukapheresis product was washed and stored overnight. After finishing the second day leukapheresis, both products were resuspended in medium to give a cell concentration of 1–2 × 10^8 cells/mL. After CD34$^+$ enrichment, CD34 cell numbers and purity were calculated, and the cells were frozen until use.

Thirty-five high-risk breast cancer patients were treated with FEC (5-fluorouracil, 600 mg/m^2; epiadriamycin, 90 mg/m^2; and cyklophosphamide, 1200 mg/m^2 body weight). Three days after the end of chemotherapy, the patients were given daily G-CSF subcutaneously (Filgrastim 5 μg/kg). When a peak of CD34$^+$ cells appeared in the blood, usually at days 11–12 after initiating the chemotherapy, leukapheresis was performed as described previously. After CD34$^+$ cell enrichment, cells were frozen and stored until use.

Of the 35 patients, the mean number of PBPCs processed in the Isolex was 3.0 × 10^{10} (0.6–7.2 × 10^{10}). The mean percentage of CD34$^+$ cells in the PBPC products before enrichment was 2.2% (0.6–6.1). Mean purity of CD34$^+$ cells after positive selection was 98% (91.5–99.7) with a mean yield of 51% (19–81). The purity of CD34$^+$ cells was independent of the percentage of CD34$^+$ cells in the PBPC product. In contrast, we observed a lower yield of CD34$^+$ cells among patients with a high percentage of CD34$^+$ cells in the starting material.

VII. RECOVERY OF HEMATOPOIESIS AFTER HIGH-DOSE THERAPY BY THE USE OF CD34$^+$ CELLS AS STEM CELL SUPPORT

High-dose therapy for breast cancer patients consisted of a daily administration for 4 days with cyclophosphamide, 1.5 g/m^2; carboplatin, 200 mg/m^2; thiotepa, 125 mg/m^2; and Uromitexan, 15 mg/kg every 4 hs. Three days after finalizing the chemotherapy, the cells were reinfused.

For two high-grade lymphoma patients, high-dose therapy consisted of total body irradiation in doses of 1.3 Gy twice daily for 5 days. A lung shield was used for 2 of the 10 fractions, limiting the total lung dose to 10.4 Gy. For two consecutive days, the patients received cyclophosphamide, 60 mg/kg, and 2 days later the purged leukapheresis product was reinfused. The remaining lymphoma patients were given high-dose therapy with carmustine, 300 mg/m^2 at day 1; Vepeside 150, mg/m^2 daily from days 1–4; Cytosar, 200 mg/m^2 twice a day daily from days 1–4; and melfalan, 140 mg/m^2 on day 5. Three days after finalizing chemotherapy, the cells were reinfused. Only the breast cancers and the non-Hodgkin's lymphoma patients were given G-CSF subcutaneously (Filgatrim 5 μg/kg) from day 2 after reinfusion of CD34$^+$ cells daily until reconstitution. Except for one breast cancer patient and one Hodgkin's lymphoma patient, all patients had reinfused >4 × 10^6 CD34$^+$ cells/kg body weight after high-dose therapy. This resulted in a fast

Table 1   High-Dose Therapy in 52 Breast Cancer Patients Autotransplanted with PBPCs (n = 16) or Enriched CD34$^+$ Cells (n = 35)

Type of cells	CD34$^+$ cells infused ($\times 10^6$/kg)	CFUs infused ($\times 10^5$/kg)	Leukocytes >0.5 × 10^9/L (n = days)	Platelets >20 × 10^9/L (n = days)	Platelet infusions (n = units)	In hospital (n = days)
PBPC (n = 16)	11.1 (2.6–24)	25 (9–76)	9.0	10.0	5	16.5
CD34$^+$ cells (n = 35)	5.6 (2.3–17)	10 (4–22)	10.0	11.0	6	17

Mean number of CD34 cells and CFUs reinfused and time to hematopoietic recovery, mean number of platelet transfusions needed, and mean number of days in the hospital are shown.
PBPC, peripheral blood progenitor cells; CFU, colony-forming units.

recovery of granulocytes and platelets (Tables 1 and 2). Time to recovery of hematopoiesis, number of platelet transfusions required, and number of days in the hospital were calculated among breast cancer patients given CD34$^+$ cells or nonmanipulated PBPCs. No significant differences could be observed among patients reconstituted with PBPCs or CD34$^+$ cells (Table 1). These data, like others, suggest that immunomagnetic CD34$^+$-enriched cells can be used safely as stem cell products.

VIII.   PURGING EFFICACY OF CD34$^+$ CELL ENRICHMENT

In patients with Hodgkin's disease, atypical CD30$^+$ cells were found in all PBPC products. After CD34$^+$ cell enrichment, no such cells were detected. Among the breast cancer patients, immunocytochemical examination of isolated CD34$^+$ cells showed that one to five breast cancer cells per 10^6 CD34$^+$ cells were present in two of six positive PBPC products. Furthermore, in lymphoma patients, 1% B cells, including malignant B cells, were present among the isolated cells even when a purity of 99.7% CD34$^+$ cells was achieved.

Table 2   High-Dose Therapy in 15 Hodgkin's and 4 Non-Hodgkin's Lymphoma Patients Autotransplanted with CD34$^+$ cells. Dose of CD34$^+$ Cells Infused and Time to Hematopoietic Recovery

Patient group	CD34$^+$ cells ($\times 10^6$/kg) infused	Leukocytes >0.5 × 10^9/L (n = days)	Leukocytes >1.0 × 10^9/L (n = days)	Platelets >20 × 10^9/L (n = days)	Platelets >50 × 10^9/L (n = days)
Hodgkin's lymphoma (n = 15)	4.6 (2.5–16.0)	12 (11–17)	13 (12–19)	11 (7–15)	13 (8–17)
Non-Hodgkin's lymphoma (B-cell)	5.3	14	15	11	16
Non-Hodgkin's lymphoma (B-cell)	5.0	11	12	9	13
Non-Hodgkin's lymphoma (T-cell)	5.2	12	14	13	18
Non-Hodgkin's lymphoma (T-cell)	20.6	7	8	9	12

Because of these clinical findings, we are exploring the use of a negative purging following CD34$^+$ isolations. For breast cancer, the direct immunobead method, as discussed previously, is currently being tested. Preliminary experiments indicate that the combination of CD34$^+$ enrichment followed by purging eradicates all detectable tumor cells with a modest loss of CD34$^+$ cells. Similar data have been observed by employing a semiquantitative PCR for detection of lymphoma cells and where a mixture of B-cell antibodies in conjunction with beads used after CD34$^+$ cell enrichment give a negative PCR (G. Kvalheim et al., unpublished data).

IX.   FUTURE DIRECTIONS

Recently, a new device, Isolex300i, has been developed by Baxter. When this device was tested and compared with the previous Isolex300 using PBPCs from breast cancer patients, we found the Isolex300i gave similar purity of CD34$^+$ cells (Fig. 3) and a comparative yield of CD34$^+$ cells. The new device is completely closed and automatic. A program for

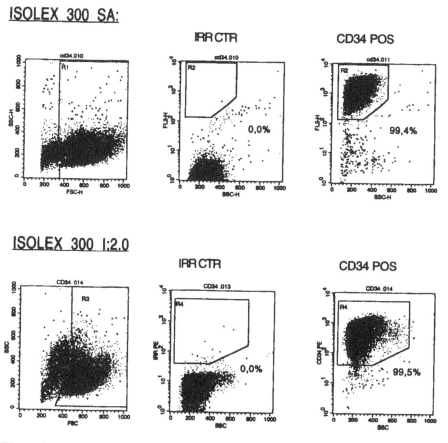

Figure 3   Clinical scale immunomagnetic enrichment of CD34$^+$ cells from peripheral blood progenitor cells obtained from breast cancer patients. Comparison between the automated Isolex300i 2,0 device and the previous Isolex300SA. Data show flow cytometric measurements of CD34$^+$ cells purity employing the different devices.

CD34$^+$ cell enrichment followed by purging by lymphoma or breast cancer cells is currently being made in Isolex300i. If this turns out to be efficient and safe, the use of purified CD34$^+$ cells as stem cell products might be the best choice for future high-dose protocols. Still, the type of patients that should be offered such highly purified and costly CD34 cells remains to be defined. Owing to health and economical reasons, and unless it can be proven that a patient group such as metastatic breast cancer patients will have a clinical benefit of being autotransplanted with purified CD34$^+$ cells, such a program will most likely be turned down by our authorities. Therefore, studies addressing the clinical relevance of purging must be performed.

REFERENCES

1. Coiffer B, Philip T, Burnett AK, Symann ML. Concensus on intensive chemotherapy plus hematopoietic stem cell transplantation in malignancies. 1993; Ann Oncol (Lyon) 5:19–23.
2. Gianni AM, Bregni M, Siena S, Tarella C. Use of recombinant growth factors after chemotherapy and high-dose chemo-radiotherapy. Haematology 1989; 74(suppl 5):511–526.
3. Eaves CJ. Peripheral blood stem cells reach new heights. Blood 1993; 82:1957–1959.
4. Haas R, Mohle R, Fruehauf S, Goldschmidt H, Witt B, Flentje M, Wannenmacher M, Hunstein W. Patient characteristics associated with successful mobilizing and autografting of peripheral blood progenitor cells (PBPC) in malignant lymphoma. Blood 1994; 83:3787–3794.
5. Bensinger W, Appelbaum F, Rowley S, Storb R, Sanders J, Lilleby K, Gooley T, Demirer T, Schiffman K, Weaver C. Factors that influence collection and engraftment of autologous peripheral-blood stem cells. Blood 1995; 13:2547–2555.
6. Brenner MK, Rill DR, Moen RC, Krance RA, Mirro J Jr, Anderson WF, Ihle JN. Gene-marking to trace origin of relapse after autologous bone-marrow transplantation. Lancet 1993; 341:85–86.
7. Deisseroth A, Zu Z, Claxton D, Hanania EG, Fu S, Ellerson D, Goldberg L, Thomas M, Janicek K, Anderson WF. Genetic marking shows that Ph+ cells present in autologous transplants of chronic myelogenous leukemia (CML) contribute to relapse after autologous BM in CML. Blood 1994; 83:3068–3076.
8. Gribben JG, Freedman AS, Neuberg D, Roy DC, Blake KW, Woo SD, Grossbard ML, Rainbowe SN, Coral F, Freeman GJ. Immunologic purging of marrow assessed by PCR before autologous BM assessed by PCR before autologous BM transplantation for B-cell lymphoma. N Engl J Med 1991; 28:1525–1533.
9. Kvalheim G. Purging of autografts. Methods and clinical significance. Ann Med 1996; 28:167–173.
10. Gee AP, Boyle MD. Purging tumor cells from BM by use of antibody and complement: a critical appraisal. J Natl Cancer Inst 1988; 80:154–159.
11. Vitetta ES, Uhr JW. Immunotoxins: redirecting nature's poisons. Cell 1985; 41:653–654.
12. Fodstad Ø, Kvalheim G, Pihl A, Godal A, Funderud S. New indirect approach to the therapeutic use of immunotoxins. J Natl Cancer Inst. 1988; 80:439–443.
13. Kvalheim G, Fodstad Ø, Pihl A, Nustad K, Pharo A, Ugelstad J, Funderud S. Elimination of B-lymphoma cells from human BM: Model experiments using monodisperse magnetic particles coated with primary monoclonal antibodies. Cancer Res 1987; 47:846–851.
14. Kvalheim G, Sørensen O, Fodstad Ø, Funderud S, Kiesel S, Dorken B, Nustad K, Jakobsen E, Ugelstad J, Pihl A. Immunomagnetic removal of B-lymphoma cells from human BM: a procedure for clinical use. Bone Marrow Transplant 1988; 3:31–41.
15. Wang MY, Kvalheim G, Kvaløy S, Beiske K, Jakobsen E, Wijdenes J, Pihl A, Fodstad Ø. An effective immunomagnetic method for BM purging in T-cell malignancies. Bone Marrow 1992; 9:319–323.

16. Ogniben E, Hohaus S, Holhaus S, Kvalheim G, Dorken H, Haas R. Successful autologous transplantation of immunogenic bead purged BM in non-Hodgkin's lymphoma. Prog Clin Res 1992; 377:189–195.

17. Atta J, Martin H, Bruecher J, Elsner S, Wassman B, Rode C, Russ A, Kvalheim G, Hoelzer D. Residual leukemia and immunomagnetic bead purging in patients with BCR-ABL-positive acute lymphoblastic leukemia. Bone Marrow Transplant 1996; 18:541–548.

18. Kvalheim G, Holte H, Jakobsen E, Kvaløy S. Immunomagnetic purging of lymphoma cells from autografts. J Hematother 1996; 5:561–562.

19. Shpall EJ, Jones RB, Bearman SI, Franklin WA, Archer PG, Curiel T, Bitter M, Claman HN, Stemmer SM, Purdy M. Transplantation of enriched CD34 positive autologous marrow into breast cancer patients following high-dose chemotherapy: influence of CD34-positive peripheral-blood progenitors and growth factors on engraftment. J Clin Oncol 1994; 12:28–36.

20. Mapara MY, Korner LJ, Hildebrandt M, Bargou R, Krahl D, Reichardt P, Dorken B. Monitoring of tumor cell purging after highly efficient immunomagnetic selection of CD34 cells from leukapheresis products in breast cancer patients: comparison of immunocytochemical tumor cell staining and reverse transcriptase-polymerase chain reaction. Blood 1997; 89:337–344.

21. Pantel K, Felber E, Schlimok G. Detection and characterization of residual disease in breast cancer. J Hematother 1994; 3:315–322.

22. Diehl LJ, Kaufmann M, Goerner R, Costa SD, Kaul S, Bastert G. Detection of tumor cells in BM of patients with primary breast cancer: a prognostic factor for distant metastasis. J Clin Oncol 1992; 10:1534–1539.

23. Moss TJ, Ross AA. The risk of tumor cell contamination in peripheral bloodstem cell collections. J Hematother 1992; 1:225–232.

24. Ross AA, Cooper BW, Lazarus HM, Mackay W, Moss TJ, Ciobanu N, Tallman MS, Kennedy MJ, Davison NE, Sweet D. Detection and viability of tumor cells in peripheral blood stem cell collections from breast cancer patients using immunocytochemical and clonogenic assay techniques. Blood 1993; 82:2605–2610.

25. Negrin RS, Pesando, J. Detection of tumor cells in purged BM and peripheral-blood mononuclear cells by polymerase chain reaction amplification of bcl-2 translocations. J Clin Oncol 1994; 12:1021–1027.

26. Brockstein BE, Ross AA, Moss TJ, Kahn DG, Hollingsworth K, Williams SF. Tumor cell contamination of BM harvest products: consequences in a cohort of advanced-stage breast cancer patients undergoing high-dose chemotherapy. J Hematother 1996; 5:617–624.

27. Brugger W, Bross, KJ., Glatt M, Wever F, Mertelmann R, Kantz L. Mobilization of tumor cells and hematopoietic progenitor cells into peripheral blood of patients with solid tumors. Blood 1994; 83:636–640.

28. Kvalheim G. Detection of occult tumor cells in BM and blood in breast cancer patients—methods and clinical significance. Acta Oncol 1996; 35(Suppl 8):13–18.

29. Naume B, Borgen E, Beiske K, Herstad TK, Ranås G, Renolen A, Trachsel S, Thrane-Steen K, Funderud S, Kvalheim G. Immunomagnetic techniques for enrichment and detection of isolated breast carcinoma cells in BM and peripheral blood. J Hematother 1997; 6:103–114.

30. Corradini P, Voena C, Astolfi M, Ladetto M, Tarella C, Boccadoro M, Pileri A. High-dose sequential chemotherapy in multiple myeloma: residual tumor cells are detectable in bone marrow and peripheral blood harvest after autografting. Blood 1995; 85:1596–1602.

31. Kiesel S, Haas R, Moldenhauer G, Kvalheim G, Pezzutto A, Dorken B. Removal of cells from malignant B-cell line from BM with immunomagnetic beads and with complement and immunoglobulin switch variant mediated cytolysis. Leukemia Res 1987; 11:1119–1125.

32. Straka C, Kroner C, Dorken B, Kvalheim G. Polymerase chain reaction monitoring shows a high efficacy of clinical immunomagnetic purging in patients with centroblastic-centrocytic non-Hodgkin's lymphoma. Blood 1992; 15:2688–2690.

33. Kvalheim G, Wang M-Y, Pharo A, Holte H, Jakobsen E, Beiske K, Kvaløy S, Smeland EB,

Funderud S, Fodstad Ø. Purging of tumor cells from leukapheresis products: experimental and clinical aspects. J Hematother 1996; 5:427–436.

34. Myklebust AT, Godal A, Juell S, Pharo A, Fodstad Ø. Comparison of two antibody-based methods for elimination of breast cancer cells from human BM. Cancer Res 1994; 54:209–214.

35. Dunbar CE, Cottler-Fox M, O'Shaugnessy JA, Doren S, Carter C, Berneson R, Borwn S, Moen RC, Greenblatt J, Stewart FM. Retrovirally marked CD34-enriched peripheral blood and BM. Blood 1995; 85:3048–3057.

36. Kvalheim G, Pharo A, Holte H, Jakobsen E, Ugland K, Nesland J, Kvaløy S, Smeland EB. The use of immunomagnetic beads and ISOLEX 300 gives high purity and yield of CD34$^+$ cells from peripheral blood progenitor cell products. Bone Marrow Transplant 1996; 17(Suppl 1):57.

18

CD34 Cell Culture
Clinical Needs and Applications

DENNIS E. VAN EPPS

Nexell Therapeutics Inc., Irvine, California

I. INTRODUCTION

Stem cell transplantation has undergone a dramatic change over the past few years both in the numbers of transplants and in the way that these transplants are being done. Stem cell transplants are increasing at a rate of more than 20% per year with current estimates showing that more than 40,000 transplants were done in 1997. The drivers of this increase include the effectiveness of high-dose chemotherapy in lymphoma and some early studies suggesting a similar remission and/or survival advantage in patients with breast cancer and myeloma (1–3). In addition, the discovery and use of hematopoietic growth factors both to treat patients posttransplant and to mobilize CD34 cells to the peripheral blood where they can be harvested by apheresis has also affected the increase in stem cell transplants. Peripheral blood stem cell (PBSC) transplants have been used primarily in the autologous setting and eliminate the need for general anesthesia to harvest stem cells as is required for bone marrow transplants. In the United States, the cost of a transplant has decreased from the $150,000 range to $60,000–$70,000 because of the use of autologous PBSCs. Although decreased cost has been a factor in the increase in stem cell transplants, the primary reason for this trend is the observed decrease in engraftment time. Neutrophil recovery time has been reduced to approximately 10 days and platelet recovery time to approximately 15 days (4–6). This is a dramatic decrease from prolonged engraftment times with bone marrow where platelet recovery could take 4–6 weeks. Although most stem cell transplants have been autologous to date, allogeneic PBSC transplants are now being evaluated in many centers. Most of these use stem cells from matched related donors where CD34 cells have been mobilized with growth factors. Currently, the emphasis of stem cell transplantation is to support high-dose chemotherapy, although its application is potentially much broader. Other therapeutic applications include both the use of allogeneic CD34 cells to treat patients with congenital and acquired blood cell deficiencies or autologous CD34 cells as target cells for gene therapy.

As stem cell transplantation evolves, so does technology to produce a standardized purified stem cell preparation. Selection of CD34 cells to produce a clinical scale, purified cell product has now been accomplished using specific monoclonal antibody and magnetic particles (7,8), flow cytometry (9), or avidin columns and biotinylated antibody (10,11). CD34 selection addresses the need to reduce contaminating cell populations such as tumor cells in autologous transplants (12–16) or T cells responsible for graft-versus-host disease in allogeneic transplants (17). In addition, the selection of CD34 cells offers an opportunity to more efficiently transfer genes into stem and progenitor cells for correction of defects or for conveying resistance to chemotherapy (18,19) or viral infection (20,21). CD34 selection also provides a starting cell population for CD34 cell expansion and differentiation (22–25).

The availability of recombinant growth factors capable of stimulating progenitor cell expansion and differentiation along with the ability to isolate CD34 cells from blood, cord blood, and marrow have made it possible to consider the culture expansion of these cells or their progeny for clinical use. Table 1 summarizes some of these potential applications of cultured CD34 cells.

Over the past several years there have been many studies on the culture of human CD34 cells. Many of these efforts have focused on the expansion of primitive stem cells which represent only a small portion of the CD34 cell population. One of the major technical hurdles with this approach is that there is not a simple assay truly to identify functional

Table 1 Clinical Applications of Cultured CD34 Cells

Cell population generated and/ or expanded	Growth factors needed	Clinical application
Multi potential primitive CD34 cell	Exact mix unknown, although may contain FLT3, stem cell factor, IL-3, Tpo, and/or unknown factor with stem cell activity. Stromal cell factor(s) may contribute.	Patients with deficient stem cell numbers Multiple transplants Gene therapy Cord blood Large-scale production of blood cells
Neutrophil progenitors	IL-3 + GM-CSF or G-CSF (amplified by SCF or FLT3)	Neutropenia Neutrophil dysfunction
Megakaryocyte progenitors	IL-11 or Tpo, MDGF + IL-3, PIXY321; SCF and MDGF and G-CSF	Thrombocytopenia
Dendritic cells	GM-CSF, TNF-α	In vitro generation of antigen specific T cells Treatment of chronic myelogenous leukemia Vaccines

FLT3, fetal liver tyrosine kinase 3; G-CSF, granulocyte-colony stimulating factor; GM-CSF, granulocyte-macrophage colony-stimulating factor; IL, interleukin; MDGF, megakaryocyte development and growth factor; SCF, stem cell factor; TNF, tumor necrosis factor; Tpo, thrombopoietin.

pluripotential human stem cells. Animal model systems for human cells have been developed in severe combined immunodeficient (SCID) mice (26) and neonatal sheep (27–29), but even these models are fraught with difficulties. Some of these include the complexity of the assay, a lack of quantitation, a failure to produce the entire repertoire of mature cells, or a failure of these cells to circulate in sufficient numbers in the peripheral blood. Some phenotypic assays using flow cytometry have subdivided CD34 cells into subsets enriched for primitive cells based on Thy1, DR antigen, CD38, or rhodamine 123 staining (26,30–36). These assays, however, do vary between laboratories, and often analysis is reduced to determining the intensity of staining rather than a positive or negative cell population.

In vitro assays for primitive human cells have been described, although these are complex assays and it is still unproven whether they truly represent a measure of the "multipotential stem cell." One of the most widely used assays is the long-term culture-initiating cell (LTCIC) assay (34,37,38). Using this assay, several investigators have reported the expansion or maintenance of LTCICs (22,39). The primary technical issue with achieving primitive stem cell expansion is obtaining stem cell expansion without differentiation. It is clearly possible to culture CD34 cells and increase by manyfold the total cell number in vitro. Most studies show only limited increases in the absolute number of CD34 cells, and for the most part the final cell preparation is predominantly negative for the CD34 antigen (7). It has been shown by many investigators that there is a synergy between growth factors when culturing CD34 cells and measuring the increase in total cell number and the number of colony-forming cells (7,23,40–44). For example, in previous studies (40,45), a mixture of interleukin-1 (IL-1), IL-3, IL-6, granulocyte colony-stimulating factor (G-CSF), granulocyte-macrophage colony-stimulating factor (GM-CSF), and stem cell factor (SCF) stimulated nearly double the number of colony-forming unit granulocyte-macrophage (CFU-GM) as compared to a mixture of IL-3, IL-6, G-CSF, and SCF. More than a 10-fold greater number of CFU-GM was observed when compared to SCF, GM-CSF, G-CSF, IL-6, or IL-3 alone. Obviously the mix and type of growth factors make a difference in the phenotype of the final cell population. Figure 1 summa-

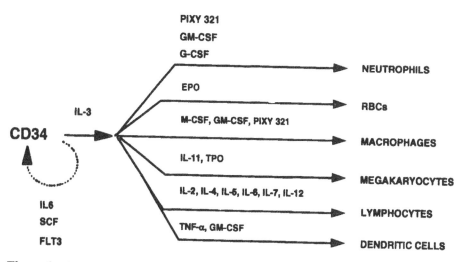

Figure 1 Schematic of primary growth factors involved in generating potentially therapeutic cell populations from CD34 stem cells.

rizes the cell populations that may be generated using various mixtures of growth factors. The pathways shown in Figure 1 do not represent all of the possible progeny of CD34 cells, but they do define some primary differentiation pathways leading to cell populations with clinical application.

II. CLINICAL APPLICATIONS FOR PRIMITIVE CD34 CELL (STEM CELL) CULTURE

As shown in Table 1, there are a variety of clinical applications for culture and/or expansion of primitive CD34 cells (stem cells). These include increasing the number of stem cells where a therapeutic dose of these cells cannot be obtained by conventional harvesting of marrow or blood. This may be applicable to many patients where CD34 mobilization is insufficient or where marrow has become fibrotic or damaged by chemotherapy or radiation. Similarly, expansion of stem cells for use as a transplant product would be beneficial in patients who require multiple transplants where graft failure has occurred or where multiple chemotherapeutic doses are required. The ability to expand true multipotential stem cells in these patients would allow for the harvesting of such cells when only a limited amount of chemotherapy has been given. Thus, stem cells will have had least exposure to potentially toxic drugs or radiation. Such cells theoretically may be more responsive to stimulation with growth factors. Expanded cells may also be useful in dose-intensification regimens where apheresis products are given to reduce the toxicity of chemotherapy (46). Finally, stem cell expansion would also be most beneficial in the evolving field of cord blood transplantation. Clear evidence of human stem cell expansion has not been achieved. However, there are data supporting the fact that cultured CD34 cells can at least be used as a transplant product with engraftment times similar to uncultured cells. Previous studies (22) suggest that "stem/progenitor cells" capable of short-term autologous engraftment can be maintained in vitro and upon transplantation can result in hematopoietic reconstitution in time frames similar to uncultured cells. Whether long-term engraftment attributable to the cultured cells can be maintained under these conditions remains to be seen. This may only be determined when allogeneic transplants or gene therapy trials show successful long-term engraftment of the transplanted cells. In these cases, the progeny of the transplant cells bear the markers of the donor cells and can be easily tracked over time.

Another application of stem cell expansion is its use in cord blood transplantation. Cord blood transplants are rapidly on the rise and will continue to increase with the establishment of cord blood banks and evidence for successful engraftment. This is a particularly important source of stem cells for patient ethnic groups that are poorly represented in current bone marrow transplant registries. One primary issue in cord blood banking is that there is only one opportunity to obtain the sample and overall it is limited in volume and cell number. Therefore, efficient transplantation may be limited to children or by weight, since the therapeutic dose of stem cells to obtain rapid engraftment in adults may not be reached in a cord blood sample. This may in part be why cord blood transplants usually have a slower engraftment time than PBSC transplants (47–49). The ability to expand this population of stem cells to reach a therapeutic dose even for adults would be a major advantage and could potentially augment the use of cord blood transplantation.

Another area where stem cell culture and expansion would be of clinical benefit is in the field of stem cell gene therapy. First, for retroviral gene transfer, there is a requirement for cells to be in cycle to attain efficient integration of the vector. This may not be accomplished without stem cell culture, since many "true" stem cells are believed to be in a quiescent G_0 state. Second, the efficiency of transduction with viral vectors is low where only a small percentage of the cells exposed to vector actually incorporate and express the gene. One option for increasing the percentage of cells containing and expressing the gene is to use a growth-selection gene. For example, a neomycin resistance gene inserted in the vector allows for the selective survival in culture of only those cells that can grow in the presence of neomycin. This gene has also been used as a marker gene for tracking cells in clinical trials (50). A parallel approach is also being tested in vivo where the multidrug resistance gene has been inserted into stem cells to reduce their sensitivity to chemotherapy (18). Finally, effective culture expansion of stem cells would allow for the expansion of a genetically modified cell so that a therapeutic dose of modified stem cells may be more easily attained. There are many clinical diseases where genetic defects have been identified or where genetic modifications have been proposed which would benefit from the ability to isolate and culture CD34 cells. Table 2 summarizes some of these potential therapeutic targets which are being tested or may potentially be in trials in the future.

The examples in Table 2 are just some potential applications of gene therapy which are dependent on or may benefit from the culture of CD34 cells. Besides the proposed and current therapeutic clinical trials with CD34 cells, there are about an equal number of gene-marking studies underway using CD34 cells. These studies are focused primarily on evaluating hematopoietic reconstitution following transplantation or for determining the fate of tumor cell contamination in stem cell grafts following a transplant. The optimal mix of growth factors to stimulate CD34 proliferation has not been established. A variety

Table 2 Disease or Therapies Utilizing CD34 Cells as Targets for Gene Transfer

Disease	Genetic defect
Chronic granulomatous disease[a]	NADH oxidase deficiency (p47-phox, p22-phox, gp91-phox)
Adenosine deaminase (ADA) severe combined immune deficiency (SCID)[a]	Adenosine deaminase deficiency
Gaucher's disease[a]	Glucocerebrosidase deficiency
Leukocyte adherence deficiency	CD18, CD11a, CD11b deficiency
Beta-thalassemia	Beta-globin deficiency
Sickle cell anemia	Beta-globin defect
Hurler's disease	Mucopolysaccharide deficiency
Hunter's disease[a]	Mucopolysaccharide deficiency (iduronato-s-sulfatase)
Fanconi's anemia[a]	Fanconi's anemia complementation group C
Multidrug resistance in stem cell transplantation[a]	MDR1, methyl transferase
Viral resistance or inactivation genes[a]	Ribozyme and HIV competitors and inhibitors (TAT decoy genes, antisense)
Gene marking in stem cell transplantation: myelogenous leukemia, neuroblastoma, chronic myelogenous leukemia	Neomycin phosphotransferase

HIV, human immunodeficiency virus; MDR1, multidrug resistance gene; NADH, Reduced nicotinamide adenine dinucleotide; TAT, transactivator gene.
[a] In trials or pending as per Office of Recombinant DNA Activities, National Institutes of Health, Feb, 1997.

of mixtures have been used, including mixtures of IL-3, IL-6, SCF, or PIXY321 [a fusion protein of IL-3/GM-CSF (Immunex Corp., Seattle, WA)] and G-CSF, or variations in mixes of these with other factors (51–55). Although the optimal mixture of factors may depend on the cell types desired, it is clear that placing cells in cycle leads to enhanced transduction efficiency with retrovirus. Currently, this is the most widely used vector in gene therapy trials.

An example of a gene therapy approach using a genetically modified CD34 cell population to treat a congenital deficiency is the work by Malech and colleagues, (56) in chronic granulomatous disease (CGD). In these studies, CD34 cells from patients with CGD having a p47 phox gene defect were transduced with a retroviral vector containing the p47 gene. In this disease, circulating granulocytes are defective in their ability to produce hydrogen peroxide owing to a defect in the nicotinamide adenine dinucleotide phosphate (NADPH)–dependent oxidase system. Patients were treated with G-CSF to mobilize CD34 cells to the peripheral circulation where they were harvested by apheresis. CD34 cells were selected using immunomagnetic CD34 cell selection technology [Isolex 300i (Nexell Therapeutics Inc., Irvine, CA)]. CD34 cells were then cultured with PIXY321 and G-CSF in a gas-permeable culture container system before three rounds of transduction with the MFGS retroviral vector. Cell culture and transduction were done over a 3-day period and CD34 cells were reinfused into the patient without myeloablation. As shown in Figure 2, when peripheral blood cells were analyzed using flow cytometry and a dihydrorhodamine assay for detection of oxidase-competent cells, small numbers of positive granulocytes were detected in the peripheral blood (56). These cells were morphologically granulocytes and appeared 2–3 weeks after infusion, peaking at 3–4 weeks. Circulating oxidase-positive cells then declined but could still be detected at low levels more than 100 days later. As with most gene therapy studies to date, a sus-

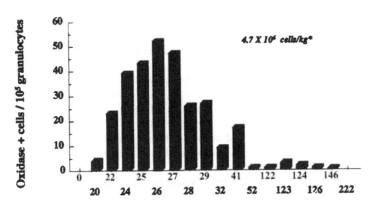

Figure 2   Presence of oxidase-positive neutrophils in peripheral blood of patient with CGD (p47 deficiency) following infusion of CD34 cells transduced with retroviral vector containing the p47 gene. CD34 cells were isolated from G-CSF–mobilized peripheral blood using the Isolex immunomagnetic cell separator. CD34 cells were transduced three times over a 3-day period and were reinfused at the concentration indicated above. Oxidase-positive cells were identified using flow cytometry and a dihydrorhodamine assay. Studies are described elsewhere (56). *Number of CD34 cells infused.

tained production of these cells was not achieved. However, these studies show that genetically modified CD34 cells can be delivered to an immunocompetent host without myeloablation with their functionally corrected progeny appearing in the peripheral blood.

The final application of stem cell expansion is one that is still far off in the future. This application is the large-scale production of blood cells for therapeutic use. Although it is possible to produce erythrocytes, platelets, granulocytes, monocytes, and other blood cells in vitro, the linkage between CD34 cell proliferation and differentiation toward lineage-committed cells makes the economics of this approach impractical. It is still more cost effective to collect and fractionate blood cells from donors than to produce them in sufficient quantity in vitro. However, if it becomes possible to dissociate stem cell differentiation from proliferation and to reduce the cost of culture, expansion of stem cells without differentiation followed by controlled differentiation could yield an affordable blood cell product.

III. CLINICAL USE OF NEUTROPHIL PROGENITORS AND PRECURSORS DERIVED FROM CD34 CELLS

Although achieving significant expansion of "stem cells" is difficult, it is possible to expand and differentiate CD34 cells into neutrophil progenitors [CFU-GM or granulocytes (G)] and neutrophil precursors (promyelocytes, myelocytes, and metamyelocytes) and/or mature neutrophils. This has been accomplished by many investigators using different growth factor mixes, although the final distribution of cell types varies with the factors used and the time of culture (13,23,24,38,40,43). Usually the mixes of growth factors to produce these cells include G-CSF or GM-CSF in some form to direct the differentiation of the CD34 cells down a neutrophil pathway (see Fig. 1). The potential clinical use of cell products containing large numbers of neutrophil lineage-committed cells includes. (1) conditions of neutrophil deficiency such as the neutropenia associated with high-dose chemotherapy, (2) conditions where neutrophils are dysfunctional such as CGD, and (3) conditions where the host may be overwhelmed by infectious agents that are normally destroyed by these cells. Such cells could be used in any situation where granulocyte transfusions would be recommended (57). One of the potential advantages of neutrophil progenitors and precursors clinically is that these cells, unlike mature granulocytes, have a longer life span and in the earlier stages through the myelocyte are still capable of proliferation. Furthermore, from the myelocyte stage on, these cells are capable of phagocytosis and bacterial killing. Neutrophil progenitors and precursors may also have another advantage over mature granulocytes in that they can be maintained in culture, whereas most studies show that a large percentage of mature neutrophils rapidly die off in vitro. In fact, one reason why neutrophil transfusions have been limited is that storing these cells for prolonged periods is extremely difficult (57).

An ever-increasing example of neutropenia that may be treatable with the infusion of neutrophil precursors is the neutropenia associated with high-dose chemotherapy or radiation therapy for cancer. In both allogeneic and autologous stem cell transplantation, even under the best conditions with posttransplant G-CSF or GM-CSF therapy, neutropenia cannot be reduced below approximately 9–10 days (4–6). This is despite the number of CD34 cells or CFU-GM given or G-CSF or GM-CSF delivered to the patient. It is believed that the reason for this delay is that it takes approximately 10 days for stem/progenitor cells to develop into mature neutrophils. Theoretically, if CD34 cells were allowed to mature to neutrophil precursor cells ex vivo before being transfused, they could potentially reach maturity more rapidly and reduce the period of neutropenia following high-dose chemotherapy. Indeed, studies (23) have shown that bone marrow cells cultured to mature granulocytes and then infused post–high-dose chemotherapy and stem cell transplantation eliminated neutropenia for 24–48 h. Similar studies have been done (58) where CD34 cells were cultured using SCF, IL-1, IL-3, IL-6, and erythropoietin (Epo) and infused in tandem with uncultured cells. In these studies, there was no toxicity associated with infusion. There also was no significant reduction in neutropenia which may be related to the dose or phenotype of cells used. Brugger and coworkers also utilized cultured CD34 cells to transplant high-dose chemotherapy patients (22). In this study, engraftment occurred in the usual time, with patients receiving only cultured cells. CD34 cells were cultured in SCF, IL-1, IL-3, IL-6, and Epo generating a median of 11.8×10^6 cells/kg in 12 days. In an earlier study (59), it was shown with bone marrow cells that a 3-day culture with GM-CSF and IL-3 reduced the engraftment time by 8 days. Engraftment, however, was not decreased below what is currently seen with a mobilized PBSC transplant. We and others have done similar studies using large-scale serum-free production of neutrophil precursors from selected peripheral blood CD34 cells (25,43,60). In these studies, peripheral blood CD34 cells were collected from patients with breast cancer undergoing high-dose chemotherapy and an autologous PBSC transplant. CD34 cells were cultured serum-free in the presence of PIXY321 for 12 days. CD34 cell mobilization in the patient was achieved with cytoxan/VP16/G–CSF as previously described (7). Apheresis products (one per day over 4 days) were collected when the peripheral cell count reached 1000/μL (generally around day 12). Three products were cryopreserved for transplantation and one was used for CD34 cell selection using the Isolex® (Nexell Therapeutics Inc., Irvine, CA) immunomagnetic cell selection system. CD34 cells were cultured for 12 days in gas-permeable culture containers. Cells were split and fed on days 5–7. Cells were then washed and reinfused 1 day after patients received the cryopreserved apheresis product to provide stem cells. Patients received between 0.8 and 157×10^6 cultured cells per kilogram of body weight. Figure 3 shows the characteristics of nine cultured patient CD34 cell products. As can be seen, apheresis products contained between 0.67 and 13.4% CD34 cells with a median of 2.93% before selection and a median purity of 90.7% after selection. Evaluation of the 12-day cultured cell product showed a reduction in CD34 cells to 2.2%, with the majority of cells being neutrophil precursors by Wright's Giemsa stain morphology. This preparation contained predominantly promyelocytes, myelocytes, and metamyelocytes. Flow cytometric analysis of these cultured cells for CD41 showed a median of 11.3% megakaryocyte lineage cells, although no mature megakaryocytes were observed. Overall, cell expansion in these cultures averaged 26-fold. Details of these studies are summarized elsewhere (7,25). When cultured cell products were infused into patients, no cell product–related toxicity was observed with infusions of up to 1×10^{10} cultured cells. Figure 4 shows neutrophil recovery and the correlation of decreased neutropenia with increased numbers of cultured cells infused. As shown in the example of two breast cancer patients (Fig. 4A), the degree and duration of neutropenia was decreased in the patients receiving the two indicated doses of cultured cells. Also shown is the median result of 10 control breast cancer patients not receiving cultured cells but undergoing similar chemotherapy and stem cell transplantation. In all 10 controls, neutrophil counts went to zero and remained there for 2–6 days. Figure 4B shows the results of studies where neutropenia (measured by the sum total number of neutrophils/μL below 500 at each day) was quantitated for each patient. As shown, there is a significant correlation between the number of

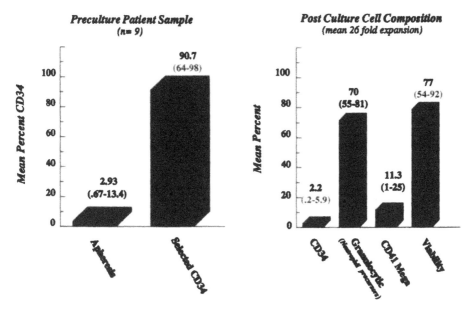

Figure 3   Characterization of cell preparations from clinical studies of cultured CD34 cells used as a supplement to a peripheral blood stem cell transplant in the treatment of breast cancer patients undergoing high-dose chemotherapy (7). Results with nine patient cultured cell products are shown.

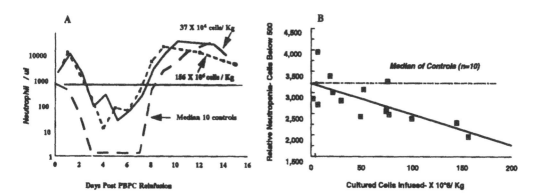

Figure 4   Results of studies using culture-derived myeloid progenitor/precursors as a supplement to cryopreserved peripheral blood stem cells in patients with breast cancer undergoing high-dose chemotherapy. (A) Neutrophil recovery in 2 of 10 patients receiving 37×10^6 and 156×10^6 cultured cells/kg following a 12-day culture of CD34 cells in PIXY321. Control line shows the median of 10 control patients who did not receive cultured cells but only cryopreserved stem cells. (B) Correlation of relative neutropenia (total neutrophils/day below 500) versus the number of cultured cells per kilogram infused. Details of this study are presented elsewhere (7). *Cultured cells given 24 hours post-cryopreserved stem cell infusion.

cultured cells/kg infused into each patient and relative neutropenia, suggesting that the cultured cells contributed to the decrease in neutropenia. It should be noted, however, that when greater numbers of cultured cells were obtained, it was generally related to a better harvest of CD34 cells and, therefore, the number of CD34 cells in the cyropreserved apheresis product. This increased number of CD34 cells in the cryopreserved sample is not likely the reason for decreased neutropenia, since the control patient apheresis products contained similar numbers of CD34 cells and all were totally neutropenic for several days.

One question that arises when using cultured cells is whether such cells can home to the appropriate sites of hematopoiesis. Previous studies (7,25) using [111]indium labeling of cultured CD34 cells followed by whole body scanning have been done to answer this question. In these studies, cells cultured under the same conditions as shown in Figures 3 and 4 were labeled with [111]indium and 1×10^9 cells were reinfused 1 h after the infusion of cryopreserved product (48 h after high-dose chemotherapy). Patients were scanned for [111]indium at various times after infusion. After 1 h, labeled cells appeared in the lung, whereas at 48 h, radiolabel was detected in the iliac crest, vertebral bodies, spleen, and liver—all sites of hematopoiesis. These studies show that not only can cells derived from CD34 cell culture be infused without toxicity, but that these cells can home to the marrow and remain there 48 h postinfusion.

These data show the feasibility of infusing cultured cells clinically and open the door to the future use of such cells in the treatment of neutropenia or other blood cell deficiencies. Such preparations of cells could be generated to treat not only high-dose chemotherapy induced neutropenia but also a variety of other diseases where granulocyte dysfunction or deficiency is an issue. The potential for longer in vivo survival of these cells versus mature granulocytes may be a significant advantage to this type of treatment. If these cells can be used in an allogeneic setting, this form of treatment could be extended even further to granulocyte dysfunction or ineffectiveness such as occurs in CGD or in patients with overwhelming infection.

IV. CLINICAL APPLICATIONS FOR PLATELET PROGENITORS AND PRECURSORS

With the discovery and production of growth factors that can direct CD34 differentiation down the platelet pathway, it is possible to consider the therapeutic potential for these cells. A number of growth factors and growth factor mixes have been shown to stimulate platelet production including PIXY321, IL-11, and thrombopoietin [Tpo, megakaryocyte growth factor (MGF),or c-*mpl*] (61–63). Studies have shown that both megakaryocytes and their progenitors can be produced in vitro. In some studies, it has even been possible to push differentiation to the point of platelet production (64). The ability to produce megakaryocyte progenitors in vitro makes it possible to consider the use of these cells in vivo for therapeutic purposes. Studies have shown that transplant patients receiving low doses of stem cells and G-CSF may have decreased platelet recovery (65). This suggests that the progenitors are driven to neutrophils at the expense of platelet recovery. It is also true that, like neutrophil recovery, there is a threshold at approximately 14 days for platelet recovery. Increasing the dose of stem cells has little effect on reducing this recovery time. This effect may be attributed to the fact that the duration of platelet recovery may be linked to the time it takes for stem cells to differentiate and produce platelets. In studies shown in Figure 3 using PIXY321, a low percentage of CD41$^+$ megakaryocyte progenitors were produced and present in the reinfused cell preparation. Although these cells were present in the cultured cell populations and reinfused into breast cancer patients following high-dose chemotherapy, no significant reduction in platelet recovery time was observed (7). However, the doses of megakaryocytes or their precursors in these studies were low. Another study (66) showed that ex vivo generated megakaryocytes and their precursors could be reinfused into high-dose chemotherapy patients without toxicity. Furthermore, there was some suggestion that patients receiving the higher doses of cells had fewer platelet transfusions. It is feasible that even higher doses of platelet progenitors may have an impact on platelet recovery. Studies to date have shown that in a radiation model of thrombocytopenia that platelet recovery can be enhanced with Tpo, although recovery still required many days (67,68). Even with the use of Tpo, it may be necessary to provide megakaryocyte precursors that can rapidly respond to the platelet growth factor and initiate platelet production at a faster rate in order to reduce thrombocytopenia.

V. GENERATION OF DENDRITIC CELLS FROM CD34 CELLS

One of the more recent potential applications of CD34 selection and culture is the generation of dendritic cells. Several investigators (69–74) have shown that functional dendritic cells can be generated from CD34 cells isolated from bone marrow, umbilical cord blood, thymus, and mobilized peripheral blood. The production of dendritic cells from CD34 cells in nearly all cases has been achieved using tumor necrosis factor (TNF) plus GM-CSF. In some cases, SCF has been used in combination with TNF and GM-CSF (72,74), although it clearly is not a requirement for the production of dendritic cells (72,75). Other studies have used IL-3 (69,76) and transforming growth factor-β1 (TGF-β1) (77). It has also been shown (78) that mobilization of CD34 cells to the peripheral blood using cyclophosphamide plus IL-3 and G-CSF dramatically enhances the number of dendritic cell precursors found in the blood. The dendritic cells generated from CD34 cells are functionally capable of presenting antigen and priming CD4$^+$T cells as well as stimulating T-cell proliferation in an human leukocyte antigen (HLA)–restricted manner (79). Figure 5 shows an example of studies using CD34 cells selected from G-CSF–mobilized normal donors using immunomagnetic beads and culturing these cells in the presence of TNF and GM-CSF for the production of dendritic cells. As shown, during cell culture the percentage of CD34 cells drops dramatically, whereas the percentage of cells bearing the dendritic cell marker CD86 increases. Morphologically and histochemically these cells appear to be dendritic cells and are capable of enhanced stimulation of a mixed lymphocyte reaction (80).

The ability to produce functional dendritic cells from human CD34 cells opens the possibility for a variety of new therapies using such cell populations. These include the development of autologous cellular vaccines for cancer or viral infections. This approach has worked successfully in animal models and is being evaluated in humans. Generation of dendritic cells ex vivo to stimulate naive T cells or augment the responses of primed T cells to antigen enables the ex vivo production of antigen specific T cells to virtually any T-cell antigen that the host is capable of responding to. This then makes it possible to use antigens from tumor cells or virus-infected cells or alternatively to utilize synthetic antigens to create antigen-specific T cells for a variety of therapeutic purposes. It may also be possible to generate enough dendritic cells to engineer them genetically to produce

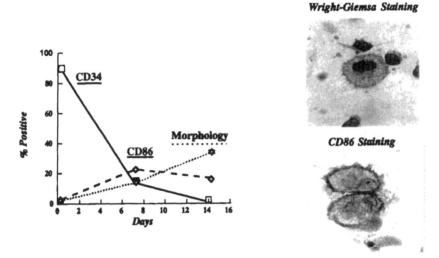

Figure 5   Generation of dendritic cells from selected CD34 cells. CD34 cells were selected using the Isolex immunomagnetic cell separator. Cells were cultured for the indicated time with GM-CSF (100 μg/mL) and TNF (100 μg/mL) (80). Graph on the left shows the loss of the CD34 antigen over time and the percentage of cells bearing the CD86 antigen found on dendritic cells or cells identified morphologically as dendritic cells after Wright-Giemsa staining. Photomicrographs on right show a Wright-Giemsa–stained dendritic cell (Top) and CD86 immunohistochemically stained dendritic cells (Bottom).

the antigen of choice and present it appropriately to stimulate an immune response. Finally, in some cases, such as chronic myelogenous leukemia or other leukemias where there is an intrinsic defect resulting in the expression of tumor antigens on the myeloid cell surface, it may be possible to generate dendritic cells which express this antigen from the host CD34 cells and use these for autologous immunization (81).

VI. CONCLUSION

In summary, the potential clinical applications for CD34 cell culture are extensive. Many of these therapeutic approaches are currently under investigation and at least some of these will be successful. In many cases, these cell-based therapies exploit natural defense and cell production mechanisms and provide some unique advantages which pharmaceutical approaches lack. Although some of these cell therapies may provide clinical benefit on their own, they may work best when used in tandem with conventional or new pharmaceutical approaches for the treatment of disease.

ACKNOWLEDGMENTS

I would like to thank Drs. Jim Bender, Harry Malech, Mona Vachula, Stephanie Williams, and Todd Zimmerman and individuals in their laboratories for their collaborative effort in generating the data presented here, and Ms. Donna Gaura for her expert secretarial and graphics support in preparing this chapter.

REFERENCES

1. Bezwoda WR, Seymour L, Dansey RD. High-dose chemotherapy with hematopoietic rescue as primary treatment for metastatic breast cancer: a randomized trial. J Clin Oncol 1995; 13: 2483–2489.

2. Attal M, Harousseau JL, Stoppa AM, Sotto JJ, Fuzibet JG, Rossi JF, Casassus P, Maisonneuve H, Facon T, Ifrah N, Payen C, Bataille R. A prospective, randomized trial of autologous bone marrow transplantation and chemotherapy in multiple myeloma. N Engl J Med 1996; 335: 91–97.

3. Gianni AM, Bregni M, Siena S, Brambilla C, Di Nicola M, Lombardi F, Gandola L, Tarella C, Pileri A, Ravagnani F, Valagussa P, Bonadonna G. High-dose chemotherapy and autologous bone marrow transplantation compared with MACOP-B in aggressive B-cell lymphoma. N Engl J Med 1997; 336:1290–1297.

4. Bender JG, To LB, Williams SF, Schwartzberg L. Defining a therapeutic dose of peripheral blood stem cells. J Hematother 1992; 1:329–341.

5. Sheridan WP, Begley CG, Juttner CA, Szer J, To LB, Maher D, McGrath KM, Morstyn G, Fox RM. Effect of peripheral blood progenitor cells mobilised by filgrastim (G-CSF) on platelet recovery after high-dose chemotherapy. Lancet 1992; 339:640–644.

6. To LB, Roberts MM, Haylock DN, Dyson PG, Branford AL, Thorp D, Ho JQK, Dart GW, Horvath N, Davy MLJ, Olweny CLM, Abdi E, Juttner CA. Comparison of haematological recovery times and supportive care requirements of autologous recovery phase peripheral blood stem cell transplants, autologous bone marrow transplants and allogeneic bone marrow transplants. Bone Marrow Transplant 1992; 9:277–284.

7. Williams SF, Lee WJ, Bender JG, Zimmerman T, Swinney P, Blake M, Carreon J, Schilling M, Smith S, Williams DE, Oldham F, Van Epps DE. Selection and expansion of peripheral blood CD34+ cells in autologous stem cell transplantation for breast cancer. Blood 1996; 87: 1687–1691.

8. Farley TJ, Ahmed T, Fitzgerald M, Preti RA. Optimization of CD34+ cell selection using immunomagnetic beads: implications for use in cryopreserved peripheral blood stem cell collections. J Hematother 1997; 6:53–60.

9. Sasaki DT, Tichenor EH, Lopez F, Combs J, Uchida N, Smith CR, Stokdijk W, Vardanega M, Buckle AM, Chen B, Tushinski R, Tsukamoto S, Hoffman R. Development of a clinically applicable high-speed flow cytometer for the isolation of transplantable human hematopoietic stem cells. J Hematother 1995; 4:503–514.

10. Shpall EJ, Jones RB. Editorial: Release of tumor cells from bone marrow. Blood 1994; 83: 623–625.

11. Widmer L, Pichert G, Jost LM, Stahel RA. Fate of contaminating t(14;18)+lymphoma cells during ex vivo expansion of CD34-selected hematopoietic progenitor cells. Blood 1996; 88: 3166–3175.

12. Moss TJ, Sanders DG, Lasky LC, Bostrom B. Contamination of peripheral blood stem cell harvests by circulating neuroblastoma cells. Blood 1990; 76:1879–1883.

13. Brugger W, Bross KJ, Glatt M, Weber F, Mertelsmann R, Kanz L. Mobilization of tumor cells and hematopoietic progenitor cells into peripheral blood of patients with solid tumors. Blood 1994; 83:636–640.

14. Vredenburgh JJ, Silva O, Tyer C, DeSombre K, Abou Ghalia A, Cook M, Layfield L, Peters WP, Bast RC Jr. A comparison of immunohistochemistry, two-color immunofluorescence, and flow cytometry with cell sorting for the detection of micrometastatic breast cancer in the bone marrow. J Hematother 1996; 5:57–62.

15. Mapara MY, Korner IJ, Hildebrandt M, Bargou R, Krahl D, Reichardt P, Dorken B. Monitoring of tumor cell purging after highly efficient immunomagnetic selection of CD34 cells from leukapheresis products in breast cancer patients: comparison of immunocytochemical tumor cell staining and reverse transcriptase-polymerase chain reaction. Blood 1997; 89:337–344.

16. Shpall EJ, Jones RB, Bearman SI, Franklin WA, Archer PG, Curiel T, Bitter M, Claman HN, Stemmer SM, Purdy M, et al. Transplantation of enriched CD34-positive autologous marrow into breast cancer patients following high-dose chemotherapy: influence of CD34-positive peripheral-blood progenitors and growth factors on engraftment. J Clin Oncology 1994; 12:28–36.

17. Collins NH, Gee AP, Henslee-Downey PJ. T cell depletion of allogeneic bone marrow transplants by immunologic and physical techniques. In: Lasky L, Warkentin P, eds. Stem Cell and Marrow Processing for Transplantation. Bethesda, MD: American Association of Blood Banks, 1994; 149–168.

18. O'Shaughnessy JA, Cowan KH, Nienhuis AW, et al. Retroviral mediated transfer of the human multidrug resistance gene (MDR-1) into hematopoietic stem cells during autologous transplantation after intensive chemotherapy for metastatic breast cancer. Hum Gene Ther 1994; 5:891–911.

19. Hanania EG, Kavanagh J, Hortobagyi G, Giles RE, Champlin R, Deisseroth AB. Recent advances in the application of gene therapy to human disease. Am J Med 1995; 99:537–552.

20. Liu L, Woffendin C, Yang ZY, Nabel GJ. Regulated expression of a dominant negative form of Rev improves resistance to HIV replication in T cells. Gene Ther 1994; 1:32–37.

21. Zhou C, Bahner IC, Larson GP, Zaia JA, Rossi JJ, Kohn EB. Inhibition of HIV-1 in human T-lymphocytes by retrovirally transduced anti-tat and rev hammerhead ribozymes. Gene 1994; 149:33–39.

22. Brugger W, Heimfeld S, Berenson RJ, Mertelsmann R, Kanz L. Reconstitution of hematopoiesis after high-dose chemotherapy by autologous progenitor cells generated ex vivo. N Engl J Med 1995; 333:283–287.

23. Gluck S, Chadderton T, Porter K, Dietz G, Maruyama M. Characterization and transfusion of in vitro cultivated hematopoietic progenitor cells. Transfus Sci 1995; 16:273–281.

24. Moore MA. Expansion of myeloid stem cells in culture. Semin Hematol 1995; 32:183–200.

25. Zimmerman TM, Bender JG, Lee WJ, Loudovaris M, Qiao X, Schilling M, Smith SL, Unverzagt KL, Van Epps DE, Blake M, Williams DE. Large scale selection of CD34+ peripheral blood progenitors and expansion of neutrophil precursors for clinical applications. J Hematother 1996; 5:247–254.

26. Peault B, Weissman IL, Buckle AM, Tsukamoto A, Baum C. Thy-1-expressing CD34+ human cells express multiple hematopoietic potentialities in vitro and in. Nouv Rev Fr Hematol 1993; 35:91–93.

27. Zanjani ED, Ascensao JL, Harrison MR, Tavassoli M. Ex vivo incubation with growth factors enhances the engraftment of fetal hematopoietic cells transplanted in sheep fetuses. Blood 1992; 79:3045–3049.

28. Zanjani ED, Ascensao JL, Flake AW, Harrison MR, Tavassoli M. The fetus as an optimal donor and recipient of hemopoietic stem cells. Bone Marrow Transplant 1992; 10(Suppl 1): 107–114.

29. Srour EF, Brandt JE, Briddell RA, Grigsby S, Leemhuis T, Hoffman R. Long-term generation and expansion of human primitive hematopoietic progenitor cells in vitro. Blood 1993; 81: 661–669.

30. Boswell HS, Wade J, Quesenberry PJ. Thy-1 antigen expression by murine high-proliferative capacity hematopoietic progenitor cells. J Immunol 1984; 133:2940–2940.

31. Briddell RA, Brandt JE, Straneva JE, Srour EF, Hoffman R. Characterization of the human burst-forming unit-megakaryocyte. Blood 1989; 74:145–151.

32. Sutherland HJ, Eaves CJ, Eaves AC, Dragowska W, Lansdorp PM. Characterization and partial purification of human marrow cells capable of initiating long-term hematopoiesis in vitro. Blood 1989; 74:1563–1570.

33. Brandt J, Srour EF, Van Besien K, Briddell RA, Hoffman R. Cytokine-dependent long-term culture of highly enriched precursors of hematopoietic progenitor cells from human bone marrow. J Clin Invest 1990; 86:932–941.

34. Sutherland HJ, Eaves CJ, Lansdorp PM, Phillips GL, Hogge DE. Peripheral blood long-term culture-initiating cell (LTC-IC) numbers rebound early after chemotherapy and GM-CSF. Blood 1991; 78:250a.

35. Udomsakdi C, Sutherland HJ, Eaves CJ, Lansdorp PM. Separation of functional subpopulations of primitive hemopoietic cells in normal human marrow using rhodamine-123. Exp Hematol 1990; 18:33a.

36. Hao QL, Shah AJ, Thiemann FT, Smogorzewska EM, Crooks GM. A functional comparison of CD34+ CD38- cells in cord blood and bone marrow. Blood 1995; 86:3745-3753.

37. Sutherland HJ, Lansdorp PM, Henkelman DH, Eaves AC, Eaves CJ. Functional characterization of individual human hematopoietic stem cells cultured at limiting dilution on supportive marrow stromal layers. Proc Natl Acad Sci (USA) 1990; 87:3584-3588.

38. Petzer AL, Zandstra PW, Piret JM, Eaves CJ. Differential cytokine effects on primitive (CD34+CD38-) human hematopoietic cells: Novel responses to flt3-ligand and thrombopoietin. J Exp Med 1996; 183:2551-2558.

39. Sandstrom CE, Bender JG, Papoutsakis ET, Miller WM. Effects of CD34+ cell selection and perfusion on ex vivo expansion of peripheral blood mononuclear cells. Blood 1995; 86:958-970.

40. Haylock DN, To LB, Dowse TL, Juttner CA, Simmons PJ. Ex vivo expansion and maturation of peripheral blood CD34+ cells into the myeloid lineage. Blood 1992; 80:1405-1412.

41. Koller MR, Bender JG, Papoutsakis ET, Miller WM. Effects of synergistic cytokine combinations, low oxygen, and irradiated stroma on the expansion of human cord blood progenitors. Blood 1992; 80:403-411.

42. Brugger W, Mocklin W, Heimfeld S, Berenson RJ, Mertelsmann R, Kanz L. Ex vivo expansion of enriched peripheral blood CD34+ progenitor cells by stem cell factor, interleukin-1 beta (IL-1 beta), IL-6, IL-3, interferon-gamma, and erythropoietin. Blood 1993; 81:2579-2584.

43. Smith SL, Bender JG, Maples PB, Unverzagt K, Schilling M, Lum L, Williams S, Van Epps DE. Expansion of neutrophil precursors and progenitors in suspension cultures of CD34+ cells enriched from human bone marrow. Exp Hematol 1993; 21:870-877.

44. Broxmeyer HE, Lu L, Cooper S, Ruggieri L, Li ZH, Lyman SD. Flt3 ligand stimulates/costimulates the growth of myeloid stem/progenitor cells. Exp Hematol 1995; 23:1121-1129.

45. Haylock DN, Makino S, Dowse TL, Trimboli S, Niutta S, To LB, Juttner CA, Simmons PJ. Ex vivo hematopoietic progenitor cell expansion. Immunomethods 1994; 5:217-225.

46. Shea TC, Mason JR, Storniolo AM, Bissent E, Breslin M, Mullen M, Taetle R. High-dose carboplatin chemotherapy with GM-CSF and peripheral blood progenitor cell support: a model for delivering repeated cycles of dose-intensive therapy. Cancer Treat Rev 1993; 19(Suppl C):11-20.

47. Broxmeyer HE, Hangoc G, Cooper S, Ribeiro RC, Graves V, Yoder M, Wagner J, Vadhan-Raj S, Benninger L, Rubinstein P, et al. Growth characteristics and expansion of human umbilical cord blood and estimation of its potential for transplantation in adults. Proc Natl Acad Sci (USA) 1992; 89:4109-4113.

48. Wagner JEJ. Umbilical cord and placental blood transplantation: analysis of the clinical results. J Hematother 1993; 2:265-268.

49. Kurtzberg J, Laughlin M, Graham ML, Smith C, Olson JF, Halperin EC, Ciocci G, Carrier D, Stevens CE, Rubinstein P. Placental blood as a source of hematopoietic stem cells for transplantation into unrelated recipients. N Engl J Med 1996; 335:157-166.

50. Brenner MK, Rill DR, Holladay MS, Heslop HE, Moen RC, Buschle M, Krance RA, Santana VM, Anderson WF, Ihle JN. Gene marking to determine whether autologous marrow infusion restores long-term haemopoiesis in cancer patients. Lancet 1993; 342:1134-1137.

51. Bregni M, Magni M, Siena S, Di Nicola M, Bonadonna G, Gianni AM. Human peripheral blood hematopoietic progenitors are optimal targets of retroviral-mediated gene transfer. Blood 1992; 80:1418-1422.

52. Nolta JA, Crooks GM, Overell RW, Williams DE, Kohn DB. Retroviral vector-mediated gene transfer into primitive human hematopoietic progenitor cells: Effects of mast cell growth factor (MGF) combined with other cytokines. Exp Hematol 1992; 20:1065–1071.

53. von Kalle C, Kiem HP, Goehle S, Darovsky B, Heimfeld S, Torok-Storb B, Storb R, Schuening FG. Increased gene transfer into human hematopoietic progenitor cells by extended in vitro exposure to a pseudotyped retroviral vector. Blood 1994; 84:2890–2897.

54. Conneally E, Bardy P, Eaves CJ, Thomas T, Chappel S, Shpall EJ, Humphries RK. Rapid and efficient selection of human hematopoietic cells expressing murine heat-stable antigen as an indicator of retroviral-mediated gene transfer. Blood 1996; 87:456–464.

55. Malech HL, Maples PB, Whiting-Theobald N, Linton GF, Sekhsaria S, Vowells SJ, Li F, Miller JA, DeCarlo E, Holland SM, Leitman SF, Carter CS, Butz RE, Read EJ, Fleisher TA, Schneiderman RD, Van Epps DE, Spratt SK, Maack CA, Rokovich JA, Cohen LK, Gallin JI. Prolonged production of NADPH oxidase-corrected granulocytes after gene therapy of chronic granulomatous disease. Proc Natl Acad Sci USA 1997; 94:12133–12138.

56. Malech HL, Sekhsaria N, Whiting-Theobold N, Linton GF, Vowells SJ, Li F, et al. Prolonged detection of oxidase-positive neutrophils in the peripheral blood of five patients following a single cycle of gene therapy for chronic granulomatous disease (abstr). Blood 1996; 88:486a.

57. Price TH, Dale DC. Neutrophil transfusion: the effect of storage and collection method on neutrophil blood kinetics. Blood 1978; 51:789–798.

58. Alcorn MJ, Holyoake TL, Richmond L, Pearson C, Farrell E, Kyle B, Dunlop DJ, Fitzsimons E, Steward WB, Pragnell IB, Franklin IM. CD34-positive cells isolated from cryopreserved peripheral blood progenitor cells can be expanded ex vivo and used for transplantation with little or no toxicity. J Clin Oncol 1996; 14:1839–1847.

59. Slavin S, Mumcuoglu M, Landesberg-Weisz A, Kedar E. The use of recombinant cytokines for enhancing immunohematopoietic reconstitution following bone marrow transplantation. I. Effects of in vitro culturing with IL-3 and GM-CSF on human and mouse bone marrow cells purged with mafosfamide (ASTA-Z). Bone Marrow Transplant 1989; 4:459–464.

60. Moore MA. Expansion of myeloid stem cells in culture. Semin Hematol 1995; 32:183–200.

61. Moriyama Y, Nikkuni K, Saito H, Aoki A, Furukawa T, Imanari A, Narita M, Kishi K, Takahashi M, Shibata A. In vitro sensitivity of human hematopoietic progenitor cells to hyperthermia: critical temperature for cells to survive and its application to in vitro purging. Bone Marrow Transplant 1990; 6:243–246.

62. Neben TY, Loebelenz J, Hayes L, McCarthy K, Stoudemire J, Schaub R, Goldman SJ. Recombinant human interleukin-11 stimulates megakaryocytopoiesis and increases peripheral platelets in normal and splenectomized mice. Blood 1993; 81:901–908.

63. Fanucchi M, Glaspy J, Crawford J, Garst J, Figlin R, Sheridan W, Menchaca D, Tomita D, Ozer H, Harker L. Effects of polyethylene glycol-conjugated recombinant human megakaryocyte growth and development factor on platelet counts after chemotherapy for lung cancer. N Engl J Med 1997; 336:404–409.

64. Choi ES, Nichol JL, Hokom MM, Hornkohl AC, Hunt P. Platelets generated in vitro from proplatelet-displaying human megakaryocytes are functional. Blood 1995; 85:402–413.

65. Bensinger W, Appelbaum F, Rowley S, Storb R, Sanders J, Lilleby K, Gooley T, Demirer T, Schiffman K, Weaver C. Factors that influence collection and engraftment of autologous peripheral-blood stem cells. J Clin Oncol 1995; 13:2547–2555.

66. Bertolini F, Battaglia M, Pedrazzoli P, Da Prada GA, Lanza A, Soligo D, Caneva L, Sarina B, Murphy S, Thomas T, Robustelli della Cuna G. Megakaryocytic progenitors can be generated ex vivo and safely administered to autologous peripheral blood progenitor cell transplant recipients. Blood 1997; 89:2679–2688.

67. Thibodeaux H, Mathias J, Eaton DL, Thomas GR, Stump DC. Evaluation of thrombopoietin (TPO) in murine models of thrombocytopenia induced by whole body irradiation and cancer chemotherapeutic agents (abstr). Blood 1995; 86:497a.

68. Grossman A, Lenox J, Ren HP, Humes JM, Forstrom JW, Kaushansky K, Sprugel KH. Throm-

bopoietin accelerates platelet, red blood cell, and neutrophil recovery in myelosuppressed mice. Exp Hematol 1996; 24:1238–1246.

69. Reid CDL, Stackpoole A, Meager A, Tikerpae J. Interactions of tumor necrosis factor with granulocyte-macrophage colony-stimulating factor and other cytokines in the regulation of dendritic cell growth in vitro from early bipotent CD34+ progenitors in human bone marrow. J Immunol 1992; 149:2681–2688.

70. Santiago-Schwarz F, Belilos E, Diamond B, Carsons SE. TNF in combination with GM-CSF enhances the differentiation of neonatal cord blood stem cells into dendritic cells and macrophages. J Leukoc Biol 1992; 52:274.

71. Caux C, Massacrier C, Dezutter-Dambuyant C, Vanbervliet B, Jacquet C, Schmitt D, Banchereau J. Human dendritic langerhans cells generated in vitro from CD34+ progenitors can prime naive CD4+ T cells and process soluble antigen. J Immunol 1995; 155:5427–5435.

72. Szabolcs P, Moore MAS, Young JW. Expansion of immunostimulatory dendritic cells among the myeloid progeny of human CD34+ bone marrow precursors cultured with c-kit-ligand, granulocyte-macrophage colony-stimulating factor, and TNF-α. J Immunol 1995; 154:5851–5861.

73. Res P, Martinez Caceres E, Cristina Jaleco A, Staal F, Noteboom E, Weijer K, Spits H. CD34+CD38 dim cells in the human thymus can differentiate into T, natural killer, and dendritic cells but are distinct from pluripotent stem cells. Blood 1996; 87:5196–5206.

74. Ye Z, Gee AP, Bowers WE, Lamb LS, Turner MW, Henslee-Downey PJ. In vitro expansion and characterization of dendritic cells derived from human bone marrow CD34+ cells. Bone Marrow Transplant 1996; 18:997–1008.

75. Young JW, Szabolcs P, Moore MAS. Identification of dendritic cells colony-forming units among normal human CD34+ bone marrow progenitors that are expanded by c-kit–ligand and yield pure dendritic cell colonies in the presence of granulocyte/macrophage colony-stimulating factor and tumor necrosis factor α. J Exp Med 1995; 182:1111–1120.

76. Caux C, Vanbervliet B, Massacrier C, Durand I, Banchereau J. Interleukin-3 cooperates with tumor necrosis factor α for the development of human dendritic/langerhans cells from cord blood CD34+ hematopoietic progenitor cells. Blood 1996; 87:2376–2385.

77. Strobl H, Riedl E, Scheinecker C, Bello-Fernandez C, Pickl WF, Rappersberger K, Majdic O, Knapp W. TGF-β1 promotes in vitro development of dendritic cells from CD34+ hemopoietic progenitors. J Immunol 1996; 157:1499–1507.

78. Siena S, Di Nicola M, Bregni M, Mortarini R, Anichini A, Lombardi L, Ravagnani F, Parmiani G, Gianni AM. Massive ex vivo generation of functional dendritic cells from mobilized CD34+ blood progenitors for anticancer therapy. Exp Hematol 1995; 23:1463–1471.

79. Caux C, Massacrier C, Dezutter-Dambuyant C, Vanbervliet B, Jacquet C, Schmitt D, Banchereau J. Human dendritic Langerhans cells generated in vitro from CD34+ progenitors can prime naive CD4+ T cells and process soluble antigen. J Immunol 1995; 155:5427–5435.

80. Kowalkowski KL, Berger CD, Aono FM, Van Epps DE, Vachula M. Dendritic cells culture-derived from Isolex CD34+ cells in serum-free media in PL2417 containers (abstr). Blood 1996; 88:111a.

81. Choudhury A, Gajewski JL, Liang JC, Popat U, Claxton DF, Kliche KO, Andreeff M, Champlin RE. Use of leukemic dendritic cells for the generation of antileukemic cellular cytotoxicity against Philadelphia chromosome-positive chronic myelogenous leukemia. Blood 1997; 89: 1133–1142.

19

Critical Parameters Influencing the Expansion and Differentiation of Cultured Human CD34$^+$ Cells

JANE S. LEBKOWSKI

Geron Corporation, Menlo Park, California

LISA R. SCHAIN

RPR Gencell, Hayward, California

I. INTRODUCTION

Patients undergoing high-or multiple-dose chemotherapies suffer periods of cytopenia which can be associated with infectious diseases, bleeding episodes, and other treatment-related complications. The use of cytokine-mobilized peripheral blood progenitor cell (PBPC) populations has significantly shortened such cytopenic periods. It has not completely eliminated them, however, especially in patients who have undergone multiple rounds of chemotherapy (1–4). It has been hypothesized that infusion of maturing populations of hematopoietic cells along with reconstituting grafts may minimize the magnitude and/or duration of these cytopenias (4–14).

One potential source of these maturing hematopoietic cells are human CD34$^+$ cells. Human CD34$^+$ cells, the precursors of cells of the hematopoietic lineage, can be isolated from a variety of source materials and expanded in vitro along multiple differentiative pathways (5,15–17). Large-scale isolation and expansion of CD34$^+$ cells from peripheral blood (PB), bone marrow (BM), or cord blood (CB) may provide sufficient numbers of differentiating cells and progenitors to maintain circulating hematopoietic cell numbers at engraftment levels until full hematopoiesis can be restored.

In order to establish reliable methods to expand hematopoietic progenitors, we studied several parameters which could influence the phenotype and quantity of cells in the final cell product. In this chapter, we review results showing that CD34$^+$ cells can be isolated and cultured from human BM, growth factor–mobilized PB and CB, and that different levels of cell and progenitor expansion are observed when CD34$^+$ cells from the alternative sources are used. We also show that PBPC mobilization conditions and the timing of collection of pheresis products can dramatically affect both the proliferative and differentiative capacity of the isolated CD34$^+$ cells. Lastly, we show that growth conditions, such as the media, growth factors, culture vessels, concentration of cells, and feeding schedules, profoundly influence the size and composition of the final cell product.

II. FACTORS INFLUENCING CD34$^+$ CELL CULTURE

A. Sources of CD34$^+$ Cells

Using both the RPR CELLector (RPR Gencell, Santa Clara, CA) CD34 and the soybean agglutinin (SBA) RPR CELLector SBA (18), we have isolated CD34$^+$SBA$^-$ cells from human BM cytokine-mobilized PB and CB. The purities and yields of CD34$^+$ cells for the experiments described in this chapter are listed in Table 1. After isolation, these CD34$^+$ cells were cultured in StemPro-34 (Life Technologies, Grand Island, NY) serum-free medium supplemented with 5% autologous plasma, interleukin-3 (IL-3) (10 ng/mL), IL-6 (10 ng/mL), G-CSF (10 ng/mL), and stem cell factor (SCF) (100 ng/mL) (19). Figure 1A shows the fold expansion of cell numbers at 7 and 14 days of culture. Likewise, Figures 1B and 1C show the fold increase in colony-forming units granulocyte-macrophage (CFU-GM) (Fig. 1B) and burst-forming units-erythroid (BFU-E) (Fig. 1C) progenitors in these same cultures. The data indicate that during the first week of culture, essentially equal fold increases of cells, CFU-GM, and BFU-E were observed from CB, granulocyte-colony stimulating factor (G-CSF) mobilized PB, and BM CD34$^+$ cells. The difference between the CD34$^+$ cell sources only truly became apparent at 2 weeks of incubation. With both PB and BM CD34$^+$ cells, the rate of expansion of cells slowed by the second week in culture and only two- to four fold increases in total cell numbers were observed between days 7 and 14 of culture. During that same time period, CFU-GM and BFU-E actually substantially decreased in absolute number as the cells matured to the myeloid lineage. Beyond 14 days, cell proliferation plateaued (data not shown), and essentially all of the cells expressed myeloid antigens. By contrast, CB CD34$^+$ cell numbers increased greater than 10-fold between days 7 and 14 of culture, and continued to increase through 28 days (Fig. 2). Unlike the BM and PB CD34$^+$ cell cultures, BFU-E and CFU-GM numbers in the CB CD34$^+$ cell cultures were elevated through 14 days of incubation and remained at detectable levels until 28 days (Fig. 2). Despite this difference in proliferative capacity, the phenotype of the expanded cells at the end of the culture period did not differ among the alternative sources of CD34$^+$ cells. The data are consistent with the presence of a higher percentage of more primitive CD34$^+$ cells in CB which can proliferate

Table 1 Purity and Yield of CD34$^+$SBA$^-$ Cells

Source material	N	% Purity (mean ± SD)	% Yield (mean ± SD)
Bone marrow	6	74.2 ± 12.4	12.4 ± 8.7
G-CSF–mobilized peripheral blood progenitors	21	55.9 ± 24.2	38.1 ± 51.0
Cord blood	8	35.6 ± 17.0	ND

G-CSF, granulocyte colony-stimulating factor; ND, not determined.

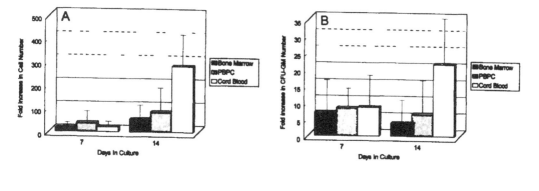

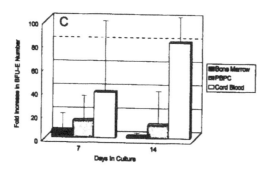

Figure 1 Fold increase in total cells, colony-forming units granulocyte-macrophage (CFU-GM), and burst-forming units-erythroid (BFU-E) in cultures of bone marrow, granulocyte colony-stimulating factor (G-CSF), mobilized normal healthy peripheral blood and cord blood. CD34+ cells were isolated from bone marrow (n = 6), G-CSF–mobilized peripheral blood progenitors cells (PBPC) (n = 21), and cord blood (n = 5) and cultured for up to 28 days in StemPro medium supplemented with 5% autologous plasma and interleukin (IL)–3, IL-6, G-CSF, and stem cell factor, at 10, 10, 10, and 100 ng/mL, respectively. Aliquots of the cultures were taken at the indicated time points and analyzed for total cell, CFU-GM, and BFU-E content. The bars indicate the mean (±SD)-fold increase over baseline of the particular cell type at the specified time in culture. (A) total cell numbers; (B) CFU-GM; (C) BFU-E.

and differentiate ex vivo for extended periods of time, leading to higher numbers of progeny per isolated CD34+ cell. Therefore, assuming equal yields of CD34+ cells during CD34+ cell purification and a 14- or 21-day culture period, expansion of standard BM, PB, or CB collections should produce approximately equal numbers of maturing myeloid cells (Table 2).

B. Peripheral Blood Progenitor Cell Collections

Because of its relative ease of collection, mobilized PB has become a routine source of engrafting stem cells and progenitors during suppressive or ablative cancer therapies. However, as a complicating factor to routine PBPC use, the mobilization agents, protocols, and collection times can all affect the subsequent proliferative and differentiative capacity of the collected CD34+ cells.

As an example, we have found that mobilization of normal healthy volunteers for

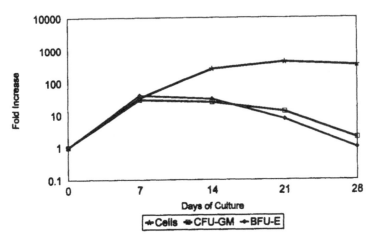

Figure 2 Fold increase in total cells, colony-forming units granulocyte-macrophage (CFU-GM), and burst-forming unit-erythroid (BFU-E) in cultures of cord blood CD34⁺ cells. The cultures of the cord blood CD34⁺ cells described in Figure 1 were extended for 28 days in the same growth conditions. The fold increase of total cells (*), CFU-GM (□), and BFU-E (◆) are plotted as a function of time in culture. The results shown here are from one of three representative experiments.

3 days with 500 µg/day of either granulocyte-macrophage colony-stimulating factor (GM-CSF) or G-CSF yielded CD34⁺ cells with different capacities for megakaryocytic differentiation. In these experiments, the pheresis products from G-CSF ($n = 4$) and GM-CSF ($n = 4$) donors had equivalent percentages ($P = $ NS) of CD34⁺ cells with a mean of 0.38 ± 0.14 and $0.37 \pm 0.31\%$ of the cells having the CD34 antigen, respectively. There were no statistically significant differences in the total number of cells collected with the two mobilization procedures. After CD34⁺ cell isolation, there were no differences in the

Table 2 Theoretical Yields of Expanded Cells from Bone Marrow, Peripheral Blood, or Cord Blood CD34⁺ Cells

	Bone marrow	Peripheral blood	Cord blood
Number of cells collected in the starting material	5×10^9	30×10^9	1×10^9
Purity of CD34⁺ cells in the starting material	0.5–2.0%	0.1–1.0%	0.5–2.0%
Assumed yield of CD34⁺ cells after purification	50%	50%	50%
Mean fold increase in cell number after 14 days of culture	82	95	283
Mean fold increase in cell number after 21 days of culture	160	180	811
Total number of expanded cells after 14 days of culture	$1–4 \times 10^9$	$5–50 \times 10^9$	$0.7–2.8 \times 10^9$
Total number of expanded cells after 21 days of culture	$2–8 \times 10^9$	$2.5–25.0 \times 10^9$	$2.1–8.0 \times 10^9$

purities of the final products (P = NS), although there was a trend (P = 0.06) toward higher yields of CD34+ cells from the G-CSF–mobilized products.

After culture using StemPro-34 media, autologous plasma, and 100 ng/mL PIXY321 (Immunex, Seattle, WA), CD34+ cells mobilized using either G-CSF or GM-CSF produced equal expansions of total cells at every point in culture. Likewise, BFU-E and CFU-GM expanded equivalently (data not shown). In contrast, in four of four experiments, the G-CSF–mobilized CD34+ cells produced higher numbers of CD41a+ megakaryocyte (MK) precursors at 14 days of culture (Fig. 3). In addition, three of four of the G-CSF–mobilized samples showed higher increases of CD41a+ megakaryocyte precursors at 21 days of culture (Fig. 3). The data indicate that G-CSF and GM-CSF may mobilize cells with different differentiative capacities or, alternatively, may bias progenitor maturation toward alternative lineages. Either mechanism has implications for the use of these mobilized PB cells and their cultured products in therapeutic applications.

The timing of PB collections after mobilization can be equally important for the harvest of CD34+ cells with the highest and broadest proliferative capacities. To analyze the effects of such cell harvest timing, we collected aliquots of PBPCs from the second and fourth daily phereses of patients with multiple myeloma who had been mobilized with both G-CSF and GM-CSF after treatment with cyclophosphamide. CD34+ cells were isolated from the aliquots and cultured in animal serum-free medium containing autologous plasma, IL-3, IL-6, G-CSF, and SCF for up to 10 days. The results from six experiments directly comparing CD34+ cells from the second (PH2) and fourth (PH4) pheresis

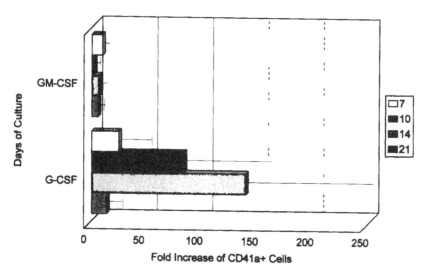

Figure 3 Fold increase of CD41a+ megakaryocyte precursors in cultures of CD34+ cells from peripheral blood progenitor cell (PBPC) collections from normal healthy volunteers. Volunteers were mobilized for 3 days using 500 µg/day granulocyte-colony-stimulating factor (G-CSF) (n = 4) or GM-CSF (n = 4). The next day, a PBPC collection was harvested using the Fenwal CS 3000. CD34+ cells were isolated from the individual pheresis collections and cultured in StemPro medium supplemented with 5% autologous plasma and 100 ng/mL PIXY321. CD41a+ cells were enumerated at different time points using flow cytometry. The figure plots the fold increase of CD41a+ cells from the cultured CD34+ cells from the different mobilization products as a function of the days of incubation.

products were analyzed. The percentage of CD34$^+$ cells and the actual number of collected cells in the original PH2 and PH4 products were not significantly different. Neither were the purities of CD34$^+$ cells after progenitor cell purification, although there was a trend toward higher CD34$^+$ cell recoveries after purification of the PH2 product. By contrast, the proliferative profiles of the CD34$^+$ cells differed substantially depending on the timing of the pheresis product collection, especially when normalized for the input CD34$^+$ cell number in the culture (Table 3). Each CD34$^+$ cell isolated from the PH2 product produced on average 6.4-fold more total cells, 5.2-fold more CD41a$^+$ MK precursors, 7.5-fold more CFU-GM, and 3.6-fold BFU-E than a given CD34$^+$ cell isolated from the PH4 product. The CD34$^+$ cells found in the earlier pheresis products may be in a more primitive state of differentiation compared to CD34$^+$ cells from the later pheresis products. Interestingly, these same results were not observed among patients who did not receive chemotherapy prior to steady-state mobilization with the growth factors (data not shown). These results indicate that the timing of PBPC collection can significantly impact the proliferative and differentiative state of the mobilized CD34$^+$ cells, and could significantly impact the utility of the collected cells for a variety of therapeutic applications.

C. CD34$^+$ Cell Culture Conditions

In order to improve the use and reproducibility of the CD34$^+$ cell culture procedures at scales sufficient for therapeutic application, several culture parameters were examined and optimized. To eliminate the requirements for fetal calf serum, CD34$^+$ cell expansion was carried out in an animal serum-free medium (StemPro-34), which was supplemented with 2–5% autologous plasma. In five experiments where BM CD34$^+$ cells were cultured under identical conditions in the presence or absence of 5% autologous plasma, cultures containing the autologous plasma supplement produced more progenitors and cells throughout a 14-day period. In these experiments, cultures without autologous plasma yielded 11.6 (SD = 3.9)–and 36.1 (SD = 36.1)–fold increases in total cell numbers on days 7 and 14 of culture, respectively. On the addition of autologous plasma, these cell expansions increased to 30.4 (SD = 11.9)–and 81.9 (SD = 41.5)–fold at days 7 and 14, respectively. Similar increases in CFU-GM and BFU-E number were observed on autologous plasma supplementation. These effects of autologous plasma were observed regardless of the growth factor combination used for expansion. Similar increases in cell (Fig. 4) and pro-

Table 3   Number of Total Cells, CD41a$^+$ Cells, CFU-GM, and BFU-E Generated per CD34$^+$ Cell Seeded into Culture from the PH2 and PH4 Pheresis Products

Mean number cells or progenitors generated per CD34$^+$ cell in the starting culture			
Time of pheresis harvest	Day 2	Day 4	P value
Total cells	91.4	14.3	0.11
CD41a$^+$ Cells	23.7	4.6	0.19
CFU-GM	1.3	0.2	0.07
BFU-E	2.8	0.8	0.03

CFU-GM, colony-forming units granulocyte-macrophage; BFU-E, burst-forming units-erythroid; PH2, second daily pheresis; PH4, fourth daily pheresis.

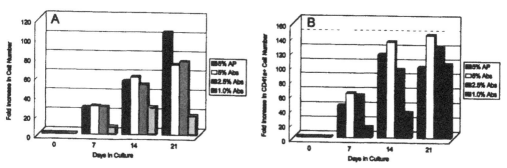

Figure 4 Cell and progenitor expansion with autologous plasma and pooled human AB serum supplements. CD34⁺ cells were isolated from peripheral blood progenitor cell (PBPC) collections from normal healthy volunteers who were mobilized for 3 days with 500 μg/day granulocyte colony-stimulating factor. The isolated CD34⁺ cells were cultured in StemPro-34 medium containing 100 ng/mL PIXY321 and 5% autologous plasma (■); 5% pooled human AB serum (□); 2.5% pooled human AB serum (■); or 1.0% pooled human AB serum (■). Fold increase of total cell numbers (A) and CD41a⁺ cells (B) were enumerated. The values are the results from one of three representative experiments.

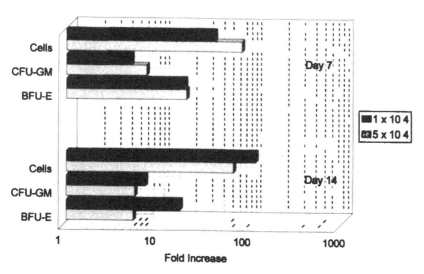

Figure 5 CD34⁺ cell seeding concentrations. CD34⁺ cells were isolated from peripheral blood progenitor cell collections from normal healthy volunteers who were mobilized for 3 days with granulocyte colony–stimulating factor (G-CSF). The isolated CD34⁺ cells were cultured in interleukin (IL)–3, IL-6, G-CSF, and stem cell factor at 10, 10, 10, and 100 ng/mL supplemented with 5% autologous plasma. The starting cell concentrations in the initial cultures were 1×10^4 (■) and 5×10^4 (■) cells/mL. The fold increase in total cells, colony-forming unit granulocyte-macrophage (CFU-GM), and burst-forming unit-erythroid (BFU-E) were measured at 7 and 14 days of culture. The values represent the mean (±SD) from five independent experiments.

genitor cell expansion were also observed when 2.5% pooled antibody (AB) serum re-placed autologous plasma as the media supplement.

In similar types of investigations, the culture vessels, feeding schedule, and the concentration of cells used for CD34$^+$ cell culture were evaluated and optimized, taking into consideration the practicalities of large-scale cell culture for clinical application. In these studies, Teflon cell culture bags (American Fluoroseal, Gaithersburg, MD) reproducibly yielded 2- to 10-fold higher increases in cell and progenitor proliferation when compared to other commercially available cell culture bags. Using these Teflon bags, cell expansions were equivalent to those observed at laboratory scale in conventional tissue culture flasks.

The seeding concentration of cells in the starting cultures were also optimized. Starting total cell concentrations of 1–20 × 10^4 CD34$^+$ cells/mL were tested using the animal serum-free conditions described above using IL-3, IL-6, G-CSF, and SCF. Cultures were fed at 7, 10, 14, and 21 days of incubation by adding an equal volume of fresh media supplemented with autologous plasma and growth factors. When seeded at concentrations greater than 1 × 10^5 cells/mL, cell and progenitor expansions were diminished, reaching a plateau by 7–10 days of incubation. By contrast, initial cell concentrations of 1–5 × 10^4 cells/mL led to the highest levels of cell expansion while providing total cell volumes which were still in the realm of practicality for routine clinical use (Fig. 5). As shown in

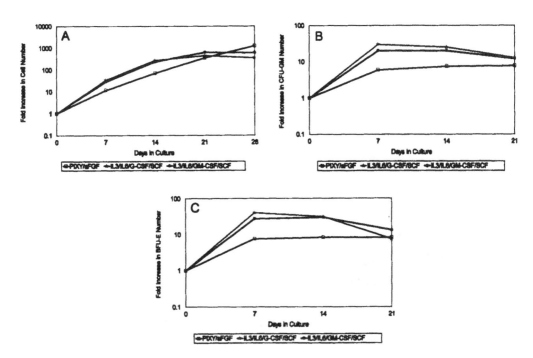

Figure 6 Cord blood CD34$^+$ cell culture with different growth factor combinations. CD34$^+$ cells were isolated from umbilical cord blood samples and cultured in StemPro-34 medium supplemented with 5% autologous plasma. The growth factor combinations interleukin (IL)-3, IL-6, granulocyte colony-stimulating factor (G-CSF), and stem cell factor (SCF) (*); interleukin (IL)-3, IL-6, GM-CSF, and SCF (●); and PIXY321 and aFGF (□) were all used at 10 ng/mL. SCF and PIXY321 were used at 100 ng/mL. The fold increase in total cells (A), CFU-GM (PlB), and BFU-E (PlC) were measured as a function of time in culture. The data are from one of three representative experiments.

Figure 5, starting cell concentrations of 1×10^4 and 5×10^4 cells/mL yielded equivalent expansions of cells and progenitors. Therefore, to restrict media consumption, concentrations of 5×10^4 starting cells per milliliter were adopted for all clinical scale CD34⁺ cell expansions.

The impact of different growth factors on CD34⁺ cell culture was also evaluated. IL-3 or GM-CSF was required for CD34⁺ cell proliferation. However, further additions of other factors such as SCF, flt3 ligand, IL-1, IL-6, IL-11, basic fibroblast growth factor (bFGF), and acidic fibroblast growth factor (aFGF) yielded varying increases in the magnitude of cell and progenitor expansion. None of these growth factor combinations altered the myeloid phenotype of the final expanded cell product. SCF consistently produced the largest increases in cell and progenitor expansion when combined with IL-3 and/or GM-CSF and on average produced 4.3 (SD = 5.0)–, 5.1 (SD = 2.5)–, and 11.0 (SD = 14.9)– fold further increases in total cell, CFU-GM, and BFU-E numbers when used with BM CD34⁺ cells. The largest increases in cells and progenitors were observed when IL-3, IL-6, SCF, and GM-CSF or G-CSF were used to supplement the animal serum-free media. However, growth factor combinations which led to the highest/fastest proliferation of the BM CD34⁺ cell cultures tended to produce the quickest plateauing and eventual senescence of the cultures. Similar results were also observed when CB CD34⁺ cells were cultured using various combinations of growth factors. Figure 6 shows the results from a representative experiment using CB CD34⁺ cells, where the expansion of cells and progenitors was monitored as a function of time and the growth factor combination. The use of IL-3, IL-6, SCF, and GM-CSF or G-CSF yielded the highest and fastest expansion

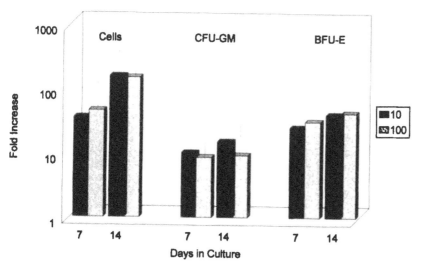

Figure 7 Peripheral blood progenitor cell (PBPC), CD34⁺ cell culture in different concentrations of interleukin (IL)–3, IL-6, granulocyte colony-stimulating factor (G-CSF), and stem cell factor (SCF). CD34⁺ cells were isolated from PBPC populations collected from normal healthy volunteers who were mobilized using G-CSF. The CD34⁺ cells were cultured in two different concentrations of IL-3, IL-6, and G-CSF for 14 days. SCF at 100 ng was added to both sets of cultures. Aliquots of the cultures were harvested at 7 and 14 days of incubation and cell, colony-forming unit-granulocyte-macrophage (CFU-GM), and burst-forming unit-erythroid (BFU-E) numbers were measured. (■), 10 ng/mL IL-3, IL-6, G-CSF; (■), 100 ng/mL IL-3, IL-6, G-CSF.

of cells and progenitors. However, these conditions also stimulated earlier terminal differentiation. CB CD34$^+$ cells culture initiated with PIXY321 and aFGF continued to proliferate and maintain progenitor expansions 1–2 weeks longer (Fig. 6).

Finally, the concentration of different growth factors used for culture was evaluated and optimized. When IL-3, IL-6, G-CSF, and SCF were used, concentrations of 10, 10, 10, and 100 ng/mL, respectively, were standardly utilized. Several experiments were performed to determine whether higher concentrations of the growth factors would yield greater cell or progenitor expansion. In five experiments using PBSC CD34$^+$ cells, where the standard and 10-fold higher concentrations of IL-3, IL-6, and G-CSF were directly compared, there were no statistically significant differences in the production of cells or progenitors at the higher growth factor concentrations (Fig. 7). As a result, 10 ng/mL was chosen as the standard concentration of IL-3, IL-6, and G-CSF for all experiments.

III. CONCLUSION

The ex vivo isolation and culture of hematopoietic stem cells could have numerous applications in the areas of cell transplantation and gene therapy. However, several factors influence the proliferative and differentiative potential of these cells. The source of the CD34$^+$ cells can affect the number and differentiative state of the CD34$^+$ cells themselves and influence their ability to proliferate in culture. Moreover, the procedures and timing used to collect these sources of CD34$^+$ cells can also dramatically affect their behavior in culture. With regard to the actual culture conditions themselves, the seeding concentrations, growth factors, media supplements, and culture vessels can also significantly affect the reproducibility and vigor of cultures, especially when clinical scale cultures are considered. As a result, careful design and optimization of CD34$^+$ cell expansion procedures must be performed before clinical applications are pursued, taking into special consideration the desired phenotype, number, and life span of the infused cell product.

REFERENCES

1. Kessinger A, Armitage JO. The evolving role of autologous peripheral stem cell transplantation following high-dose therapy for malignancies. Blood 1991; 77:211–213.
2. Chao NJ, Schriber JR, Grimes K, Long GD, Negrin RS. Raimondi CM, Horning SJ, Brown SL, Miller L, Blume KG. Granulocyte colony-stimulating factor "mobilized" peripheral blood progenitor cells accelerate granulocyte and platelet recovery after high-dose chemotherapy. Blood 1993; 81:2031–2035.
3. Elias AD, Ayash L, Tepler I, Wheeler C, Schwartz G, Mazanet R, Schnipper L, Frei II E, Antman K. The use of G-CSF or GM-CSF mobilized peripheral blood progenitor cells (PBPC) alone or to augment marrow as hematologic support of single or multiple cycle high-dose chemotherapy. J Hematol 1993; 2:377–382.
4. Spitzer G, Adkins DR. Persistent problems of neutropenia and thrombocytopenia with peripheral blood stem cell transplantation. J Hematol 1994; 3:193–198.
5. Haylock DN, To LB, Bowse TL, Juttner CA, Simmons PJ. Ex vivo expansion and maturation of peripheral blood CD34$^+$ cells into the myeloid lineage. Blood 1992; 80:1405–1412.
6. McAlister IB, Teepe M, Gillis S, Williams DE. Ex vivo expansion of peripheral blood progenitor cells with recombinant cytokines. Exp Hematol 1992; 20:626–688.
7. Biddle W, Lebkowski JL, Wysocki M, Dadey B, Pancook J, Donovan J, Schain L, Daley J. Cultivation and ex vivo expansion of human CD34$^+$ progenitor cells under serum-free culture conditions. In: Gee AP, Gross S, Worthington-White DA, eds. Advances in Bone Marrow

Purging and Processing: Fourth International Symposium, New York: Wiley-Liss, 1994:351–361.

8. Lill MC, Lynch M, Fraser JK, Chung GY, Schiller G, Giaspy JA, Souza L, Baldwin GC, Gasson JC. Production of functional myeloid cells from CD34-selected hematopoietic progenitor cells using a clinically relevant ex vivo expansion system. Stem Cells 1994; 12:626–637.

9. Brugger W, Heimfeld S, Berenson RJ, Mertelsmann R, Kanz L. Reconstitution of hematopoiesis after high-dose chemotherapy by autologous progenitor cells generated ex vivo. N Engl J Med 1995; 333:283–287.

10. Chang Q, Hanks S, Akard L, Thompson J, Harvey K, English D, Jansen J. Maturation of mobilized peripheral blood progenitor cells: preclinical and phase I clinical studies. J Hematother 1995; 4:289–297.

11. Glück S, Chadderton T, Porter K, Dietz G, Maruyama M. Characterization and transfusion of in vitro cultivated hematopoietic progenitor cells. Transfus Sci 1995; 16:273–281.

12. Emerson SG. Ex vivo expansion of hematopoietic precursors, progenitors, and stem cells: the next generation of cellular therapeutics. Blood 1996; 87:3082–3088.

13. Williams SF, Lee WJ, Bender JG, Zimmerman T, Swinney P, Blake M, Carreon J, Schilling M, Smith S, Williams DE, Oldham F, Van Epps D. Selection and expansion of peripheral blood CD34⁺ cells in autologous stem cell transplantation for breast cancer. Blood 1996; 87: 1687–1691.

14. Zimmerman TM, Bender JG, Lee WJ, Loudovaris M, Qiao X, Shilling M, Smith SL, Unverzagt K, Van Epps DE, Blake M, Williams DF, Williams SF. Large-scale selection of CD34⁺ peripheral blood progenitors and expansion of neutrophil precursors for clinical applications. J Hematother 1996; 5:247–253.

15. Broxmeyer HE, Hangoc G, Cooper S, Ribeiro RC, Graves V, Yoder M, Wagner J, Vadhan-Raj S, Benninger L, Rubinstein P, Broun ER. Growth characteristics and expansion of human umbilical cord blood and estimation of its potential for transplantation in adults. Proc Natl Acad Sci USA 1992; 89:4109–4113.

16. Brugger W, Möcklin W, Heimfeld S, Berenson RJ, Mertelsmann R, Kanz L. Ex vivo expansion of enriched peripheral blood CD34⁺ progenitor cells by stem cell factor, interleukin-1β(IL-1β), IL-6, IL-3, interferon-γ, and erythropoietin. Blood 1993; 81:2579–2584.

17. Dragowski W, Lansdorp PM. Cytokine-induced selective expansion and maturation of erythroid versus myeloid progenitors from purified cord blood precursor cells. Blood 1993; 81: 3252–3258.

18. Lebkowski JS, Schain LR, Okrongly D, Levinski R, Harvey MJ, Okarma TB. Rapid isolation of human CD34 hematopoietic stem cells—purging of human tumor cells. Transplantation 1992; 53:1011–1019.

19. Lebkowski JS, Schain, Hall M, Wysocki M, Dadey B, Biddle W. Rapid isolation and serum-free expansion of human CD34⁺ cells. Blood Cells 1994; 20:404–410.

20

Mobilization of Peripheral Blood Stem Cells from Normal Donors

THOMAS A. LANE and PING LAW

University of California, San Diego, La Jolla, California

I. INTRODUCTION

Mobilized peripheral blood stem cells (PBSCs) are increasingly used for allogeneic transplantation following myeloablative or nonmyeloblative therapies (1,2). PBSCs earned a well-deserved reputation for supporting rapid and durable trilineage hematological engraftment in transplantation. Other perceived advantages of autologous PBSCs included improved patient tolerance of the harvesting procedure (without general anesthesia) and possibly diminished tumor contamination (3–5). The ability of autologous and syngeneic mobilized PBSCs to provide long-term hematopoietic reconstitution suggested that PBSC grafting might also be successful in allogeneic transplantation. Allogeneic PBSC transplants in animals supported the hypothesis that long-term sustained engraftment was possible (6,7). Syngeneic transplants employing only mobilized PBSCs were successful in patients with malignancies (8). The first patient transplanted with allogeneic PBSCs from a human leukocyte antigen (HLA)–matched sibling donor engrafted, but sustained engraftment could not be evaluated, since the patient died of Aspergillus infection (9). Within the past 4 years, hundreds of patients have been transplanted using mobilized PBSC allografts instead of bone marrow. Reports on these patients have demonstrated that hematopoietic recovery using mobilized allogeneic PBSCs is rapid, complete (all lineages), and durable; the latter being demonstrated by cytogenetics or molecular markers (10–16). Neutrophil (>500/µL) and platelet recovery (>20,000/µL) is typically between 9 and 15 days (17,18) in HLA-matched sibling transplants, but longer engraftment times for neutrophils (16–33 days) have been reported in HLA-mismatched transplants (19). Only one graft failure was reported in 62 patients who received only mobilized PBSC allografts; in which case, the patient received PBSCs after failing an allogeneic marrow transplantation from the same donor (19). Thus, similar to the replacement of autologous marrow grafts with mobilized PBSC collections, allogeneic PBSCs from matched sibling donors are increasingly supplanting marrow as the graft of choice for hematopoietic recovery following myeloablative or nonmyeloablative therapies. Allogeneic PBSC transplants using matched unrelated donors are currently under clinical investigation. Intensive efforts have focused on methods to optimize the mobilization and collection of PBSCs from healthy individuals, since widespread successful utilization of allogeneic PBSCs is dependent on a variety of factors, including ethical considerations, which would impel physicians to harvest allogeneic PBSCs using regimens with the least possible risk, discomfort, and expense to the patient/donor, and quality of the grafts, which is determined by the content of primitive as well as committed hematopoietic cells. In this chapter, we will attempt to review the current practices and controversies regarding mobilization of PBSCs from normal donors. Important discussions are directed toward donor eligibility for PBSC versus marrow grafts; the dose and scheduling of cytokine regimens; the leukapheresis procedure, including processing volume and timing; the effects of growth factor administration and leukapheresis on the donor; and issues contributing to the choice between marrow and PBSCs for allogeneic transplantation.

II. DONOR ELIGIBILITY CONSIDERATIONS

Eligibility for PBSC donation does not differ from marrow collection in the requirements for infectious disease testing. All donors must be tested for hepatitis (hepatitis B surface antigen, hepatitis B core antibody, hepatitis C virus), human immunodeficiency virus (HIV)-1/2, HIV p24 antigen, human T cell lymphotropic virus-I/II, syphilis and cytomegalovirus. The list is mandated by national and international organizations, such as the American Association of Blood Banks (AABB), Foundation for the Accreditation of Hematopoietic Cell Therapy (FAHCT), and National Marrow Donor Program (NMDP). In contrast to blood donors, who are tested in the same fashion, the presence of a positive test result (especially a false positive) for one of these agents may not be a contraindication for donation, but this decision is made on an individual basis, with full disclosure to the recipient. However, whereas a history of active asthma may be a contraindication to bone marrow harvesting under general anesthesia, the same condition is not a contraindication for PBSC harvesting by leukapheresis after granulocyte colony-stimulating factor (G-CSF) mobilization. Likewise, the presence of severe low back pain increases the likelihood of prolonged recovery after marrow harvest; hence potential donors with this condition may be more suited to PBSC collection. In contrast, individuals with poor peripheral veins will require the placement of a central catheter for PBSC apheresis, and thus, harvesting of marrow may be preferred. A history of allergy to G-CSF is a contraindication for mobilization using this agent. Additional contraindications to mobilization and PBSC collection may include patients with inflammatory ocular conditions, autoimmune diseases with an inflammatory component, increased risk of thrombotic complications, or hematological malignancy. In general, persons who are eligible to donate blood or donate platelets by apheresis should be eligible for mobilization and collection of PBSCs.

III. MOBILIZATION AND APHERESIS COLLECTION REGIMENS

Hematopoietic stem cells are found in peripheral blood of healthy individuals. However, their numbers are insufficient to permit an adequate graft by leukapheresis (9,20).

Protocol/treatment procedures are employed to "mobilize" PBSCs from the marrow into the peripheral blood. In autologous transplantation, chemotherapeutic regimens that induce transient neutropenia have resulted in a marked PBSC increase as leukocytes reappear in the blood (21,22). Although a variety of such regimens are effective in mobilizing sufficient numbers of PBSCs for autografting, chemotherapeutic agents cannot be ethically administered to healthy individuals. Fortunately, several widely used hematopoietic growth factors also increase the level of blood PBSCs. An ideal regimen would, after a single administration of the drug, rapidly and reliably mobilize a sufficient number of primitive and committed stem cells to be collected, and on infusion into an allogeneic patient, result in both rapid and long-term engraftment. The number of contaminating mature leukocytes and platelets would be minimal. Harvesting would be accomplished with a single collection of a small volume (i.e., less than 500 mL) of blood from the donor, who would experience minimal discomfort and suffer no long-term effects. Such a regimen does not exist currently, but several possibilities are considered adequate, if imperfect, to accomplish this goal. Mobilization of PBSCs in healthy individuals for allogeneic transplants has most frequently been accomplished by administering recombinant human G-CSF.

A.   Dose of G-CSF

G-CSF administered subcutaneously for 4–6 days results in reliable mobilization of CD34-bearing cells and colony-forming units granulocyte-macrophage (CFU-GM) (both of which are used as surrogate assays for hematopoietic stem cells) (10–16,23–26). Several investigators have reported that mobilization of CD34$^+$ cells by G-CSF is dose dependent over the range of 2.5–10.0 µg G-CSF/kg/day given as a *single* dose subcutaneously, and that the higher peak levels of blood CD34$^+$ cells that resulted from the higher G-CSF doses were associated with a significantly higher apheresis yield of CD34$^+$ cells (23,25–29). The marked individual variation in CD34$^+$ cell mobilization is highlighted by Stroncek et al., who reported a significant relationship between G-CSF dose and the apheresis yield of CD34$^+$ cells. However, because of the wide variability, the investigators could not demonstrate any statistically significant difference in CD34$^+$ cell yields from healthy subjects treated with 7.5 µg G-CSF/kg/day for 5 days (4.1 ± 2.5 × 10^8 CD34$^+$ cells, N = 21) versus subjects treated with 10.0 µg G-CSF/kg/day for 5 days (4.7 ± 3.2 × 10^8 CD34$^+$ cells, N = 27) (23). Brown et al., reported that baseline blood CD34$^+$ cell counts varied over a 10-fold range in normal individuals (18). They also found that donors receiving less than 650 µg total G-CSF had only a 25% chance of achieving the targeted CD34$^+$ cell dose of 5 × 10^6/kg recipient weight in a single apheresis compared with a probability of 70% for donors receiving greater than 650 µg, and 86% for those receiving greater than 850 µg G-CSF. Since the patients who received the lower doses were also smaller in weight, and donor weight correlated poorly with CD34$^+$ cell yields, the investigators hypothesized that smaller donors may require higher doses of G-CSF per kilogram of body weight to achieve adequate mobilization (18). However, since the correlation between G-CSF dose (hence body weight) and preapheresis (or premobilization) blood levels of CD34$^+$ cells was poor (r^2 = 0.27), the likelihood that such a strategy will be successful is unclear. Administration of doses of G-CSF higher than 10 µg/kg/day have not been extensively studied in randomized trials with allogeneic donors. In a retrospective analysis of allogeneic PBSC donors, Luider et al., found that administration of more than 10 µg G-CSF/kg/day to 12 subjects for 3 days (apheresis on day 4 after G-CSF injection) did not lead to any increase in the yield of $CD34^+$ cells compared with 24 subjects treated with 4–10 µg G-CSF/kg/day (29). Duhrsen et al., studied the mobilization of colony-forming cells (CFCs) in groups of three cancer patients each treated with 1, 3, 10, 30, or 60 µg G-CSF/kg/day intravenously or 0.3–10 µg/kg/day subcutaneously (30). Maximal mobilization of PBSCs was observed with the 10 µg/kg/day dose subcutaneously and the 1 µg/kg dose intravenously, and no further increase was noted with higher doses administered intravenously. Waller et al., reported that twice-daily subcutaneous administration of 10 or 12 µg G-CSF/kg (total of 20 or 24 µg G-CSF/kg/day) to normal donors for 7 days was associated with a trend toward higher circulating leukocyte counts and higher apheresis yields of $CD34^+$ cells (per liter of blood processed) on days 4 through 7 than administration of 10 µg G-CSF/kg once daily, but the concentration of $CD34^+$ cells or CFCs in blood was not measured after mobilization and the differences in apheresis yields were not significant (31). The finding that the target value of 3.5×10^6 $CD34^+$ cells/kg was achieved after two aphereses in 11 of 14 subjects who received the 20–24 µg/kg dose compared with only 1 of 5 patients who received the 10 µg/kg/day dose suggests a benefit to the higher dose regimen. Majolino et al., administered 10 µg G-CSF/kg/day for 5 days to five normal donors and 16 µg G-CSF/kg bid to six donors for 4 days prior to apheresis collection (32). They found no difference between the two groups with respect to peak levels of blood $CD34^+$ cells, the apheresis yield of $CD34^+$ cells per liter of blood processed, or the total $CD34^+$ cells per kilogram of recipient weight, and that a single apheresis sufficed in 80% of all donors to reach the target dose of 4×10^6 $CD34^+$ cells/kg (32). Thus, doses of G-CSF higher than 10–12 µg/kg/d have been associated with higher peak circulating levels of $CD34^+$ cells and apheresis yields of $CD34^+$ cells in some, but not all, studies in healthy donors. In view of the large individual variability, it appears that additional randomized studies enrolling more donors will be required to resolve this issue. The routine use of high doses of G-CSF (>10 µg/kg/day) must be balanced against potential risks of growth factor administration to healthy subjects (33) and diminished donor tolerance, as Stroncek et al., have reported that side effects experienced by donors are also dependent on G-CSF dose (and to some extent donor gender; see below) (23). Kessinger found no difference in the mobilization of CFU-GM or their collection at leukapheresis in a heterogeneous group of 70 patients with hematological malignancy and solid tumors, who were mobilized with GM-CSF at a dose of 250 µg/m^2/day either by continuous intravenous infusion or by a single subcutaneous dose (33a).

B. Schedule of G-CSF

G-CSF is typically administered once each day by subcutaneous injection, but several centers have used twice daily dosing, presumably because of the short (3–4 hr) circulating half-life of G-CSF (34). However, many of the biological effects of G-CSF are prolonged for at least 24 hs (35), and it is not clear whether a twice-daily dosing schedule is advantageous as compared to single administration of the same total G-CSF dose. Grigg et al., reported no benefit in the level of blood $CD34^+$ cell by continuous infusion of G-CSF at 3 µg/kg/day compared with a single subcutaneous injection (27). Yano et al., reported no difference in the number of $CD34^+$ cells or CFCs collected by a single apheresis and in the tolerance of healthy subjects using two G-CSF dosing regimens: 5 µg/kg twice daily for 5 days versus a single injection of 10 µg/kg/day (36). Likewise, Majolino et al., treated normal donors with either a single dose of 10 µg/kg/day of G-CSF for 4 days or 16 µg G-CSF/kg/day in two equal doses (8 µg/kg bid) and found no difference in (1) the peak level of blood CD34$^+$ cells or CFCs, (2) the apheresis yield of CD34$^+$ cells, or (3) in donor tolerance (32). Recently, however, studies in breast cancer patients indicated an advantage to twice-daily doses of G-CSF at 5 μg/kg compared with a single dose of G-CSF at 10μg/kg with respect to circulating CD34$^+$ cells (37,38). The duration between G-CSF administration (a single daily subcutaneous dose) and apheresis collection has also been studied. In a preliminary report, Fischer et al., observed an up to 10-fold increase in blood CD34$^+$ cells within 4–7 hs following each injection of G-CSF in six autologous transplant patients, three of whom had been heavily pretreated. Surprisingly, they observed a return of CD34$^+$ cells to nearly baseline value by 12 hs after injection (39). It is not clear, however, to what extent the studies performed on autologous patients can be applied to healthy individuals with unperturbed hematopoietic function and who have not been exposed to chemotherapy/radiotherapy or marrow invasion. Sato et al., performed a systematic study of G-CSF administration to groups of seven normal subjects and observed changes in CFCs over 1, 2, 4, 6, 24, and 30 hs (40). They found that CFCs increased by day 3, and that the increases in CFCs occurred continuously during G-CSF dosing. CFCs were highest between 24 and 30 hs post–G-CSF injection after 5 days of treatment. Thus, these investigators concluded that the most appropriate time for PBSC collection was 24–30 hs following the last injection of G-CSF. However, since the difference between the 4- and 24-h postinjection CFC values was considered to be of little clinical significance after a 5-day regimen, apheresis can be started as early as 4 hs following 5 days of G-CSF dosing (40). In contrast, after only 3 days of G-CSF administration, the 4 hr postinjection CFC level was considerably lower than the level of CFC at 24 or 30 hs; hence apheresis should be delayed for 24 hs if a 3-day dosing regimen is used.

C. Duration of G-CSF

The optimal (minimum) duration of G-CSF administration prior to collection of mobilized PBSCs has been studied by several investigators. It is important to recognize that the kinetics of PBSC mobilization is distinctly different from the kinetics of granulocytosis caused by G-CSF administration. An elevated leukocyte count does not necessarily translate to an elevated level of blood CD34$^+$ cells. After a single injection of G-CSF, blood granulocytes increase as early as 2–4 hs, peak at 12–24 hs (40,41), and remain elevated for the duration of G-CSF administration (23,27). In contrast, an increase in CD34$^+$ cells and CFC generally occurs no earlier than 48–72 hs following the first G-CSF dose. The maximum level of blood CD34$^+$ cells is typically reached after 5 or 6 days of G-CSF administration (23,27,42). However, the day of peak blood CD34$^+$ cells varies considerably among individuals; for example, from day 4 to day 8. The increase in CD34$^+$ cells is typically paralleled by increases in CFCs over a similar time course (25,26,42,43). Matsunaga et al., studied the effect of prolonged administration of G-CSF in three healthy subjects given 2.5 μg G-CSF/kg/day for 6 days followed by 5 μg G-CSF for 4 days (for a total of 9 consecutive days of administration of G-CSF). The level of blood CD34$^+$ cells peaked on day 6 or 7, followed by a decline to baseline values, despite the continued administration of G-CSF. There were no differences in the kinetics of mobilization of CD34$^+$/CD33$^-$ and CD34$^+$/CD33$^+$ cells and no appreciable difference in the mobilization kinetics of CFU-GM and burst-forming units-erythroid (BFU-E). This small study thus suggested that PBSC mobilization occurred over a finite time course. In a later study, Stroncek et al., administered G-CSF to healthy individuals once daily in doses ranging from 2.0 to 7.5 µg/kg/day for up to 10 days (23). They reported that the level of blood CD34$^+$ cells peaked at day 6 (range from day 4 to 8 days) and began to decline in most subjects by day 8 despite continued G-CSF administration. Not surprisingly, the apheresis yield of CD34$^+$ cells also was also lower in the cohort of subjects when collection was performed after 10 days of G-CSF than in the cohort when cells were collected after 5 days of G-CSF. Similar results were reported by Grigg et al., who found that both CFCs and CD34$^+$ cells generally declined by day 6 despite continuous administration of 10 µg G-CSF/kg for 7 days (27). These studies indicated that (1) G-CSF results in maximal levels of blood CD34$^+$ cells and CFCs after 4–6 days of treatment and (2) prolonged administration of G-CSF did not enhance PBSC mobilization.

D. Factors Associated with CD34$^+$ Cell Mobilization

Despite receiving the same G-CSF dosing regimen, different individuals mobilize CD34$^+$ cells over a 10-fold range. The ability to define a predictable method to mobilize PBSCs increases the likelihood of collecting the target cell dose with a minimum number of apheresis procedures. Several groups have investigated potential factors that might account for the variability of mobilization and thereby to identify predictive correlation among PBSC collection, donor characteristics, drug and dosing regimens.

1. Age

The effect of age on PBSC mobilization in healthy donors has received attention. Older individuals are reported to have normal blood counts (44), but an age-dependent decrease in marrow cellularity has been reported (45) along with diminished yield of nucleated cells in harvested marrow (46) and responsiveness of myeloid precursors to hematopoietic cytokines (47). Bensinger studied 54 autologous transplant patients who received 16 µg/kg/day G-CSF for 4–7 days prior to two to six apheresis procedures targeted to collect≥ 10^9 mononuclear cells. They found that increasing age negatively influenced the number of CD34$^+$ cells collected (48). In contrast, a later publication by the same investigators failed to substantiate the correlation of CD34$^+$ cell mobilization with age, and other large retrospective studies have not identified the age dependence of PBSC mobilization or collection in autologous transplant patients mobilized with various doses and schedules of hematopoietic growth factors (49–54). However, factors affecting the mobilization of CD34$^+$ cell in autologous transplant patients may have limited predictive value for normal individuals who have not been exposed to prior myelotoxic therapy or bone marrow disease (see Ref. 55 for a review). Chatta et al. prospectively studied the effect of age on mobilization of PBSCs in normal subjects. Nineteen young (age 20–30 years) and elderly (age 70–80 years) healthy subjects were administered G-CSF 30 or 300 µg/day subcutaneously for 14 days. Young subjects mobilized two-fold more CFU-GM than older subjects ($P < .05$) after 5 days of G-CSF at the higher dose, and the older group did not respond to the lower dose at all (56). These data suggested that older individuals might require higher doses of G-CSF to achieve the same level of PBSC mobilization. Dreger et al. found that both the peak number of blood CD34$^+$ cells and the apheresis yield of CD34$^+$ cells from nine healthy donors (for allogeneic transplantation) ranging in age from 18 to 67 years (median 33 years) was inversely related to subject age (25). Anderlini et al. reported that significantly fewer CD34$^+$ cells were collected per liter blood processed by apheresis from 13 normal donors more than 55 years of age than the number collected from 106 donors less than 55 years of age; however, the yield of CD34$^+$ cells overlapped substantially among the two age groups (57). In contrast, other reports did not show that donor age negatively impacted on the apheresis yield of CD34$^+$ cells in mobilized normal donors. Stroncek et al., found no effect of age on the mobilization of CD34$^+$ cells in 102 subjects aged 20–55 years (mean 30 years) who were mobilized with varying doses of G-CSF for allogeneic transplantation (23). Bishop et al. mobilized 41 normal donors (for allogeneic transplantation) aged 18–69 years (median age 42 years) using 5 μg G-CSF/kg/day for 4 days and collected CD34$^+$ cells with three 12-L apheresis procedures. They could not identify any effect of age on the number of procedures required to achieve the target CD34$^+$ cell dose (58). There was no age-related effect in a series of 47 allogeneic PBSC donors (median 43 years; range 13–76 years) mobilized using 10 μg/kg G-CSF and whose CD34$^+$ cells were collected by one to three 18- to 20-L apheresis procedures (18). Taken together, these studies suggest that there may be a small age-dependent decrease in CD34$^+$ cell mobilization with growth factors, but this represents a minor portion of the variability in mobilization of CD34$^+$ cells among individuals, and donors over the age of 60 years can still effectively serve as PBSC donors (59).

2. Sex

Several studies have demonstrated a lack of association between donor sex and CD34$^+$ cells mobilization and collection (18,23,50,57,58). In contrast, Miflin et al. reported that, with the same G-CSF regimen (G-CSF, 10 μg/kg/day for 4 days), the apheresis yield of CD34$^+$ cells from 10 male donors (4.96 × 10^6/kg donor weight for a 12-L apheresis) was significantly higher than that from 7 female donors (2.79 × 10^6/kg donor weight (54). In addition, the target cell yield of 4 × 10^6 CD34$^+$ cells was achieved by a single apheresis in 9 of the 10 males but only 1 of the 7 females. Notably, the males were significantly heavier than the females (mean of 90 vs 60 kg), but the calculations of cell yield were corrected for this difference.

3. Obesity

In one study, a weak positive correlation was found between the presence of morbid obesity (>150% ideal body weight) and the apheresis yield of CD34$^+$ cells (57). This finding was attributed to the disproportionately smaller increase in extracellular fluid and hematopoietic tissue in obese subjects compared with body weight. This would result in obese subjects receiving a relatively higher dose of G-CSF per unit weight of hematopoietic tissue when G-CSF is administered on a per kilogram of body weight basis (57). Whether this effect might have also played a role in the improved cell yields achieved by Miflin et al. is unclear, since peak levels of blood CD34$^+$ cell were not reported (54).

4. Premobilization Characterization

The possibility that a readily available parameter measurable in the laboratory prior to mobilization might predict the apheresis yield of CD34$^+$ cells has been of great interest. Fruehauf et al. determined the level of blood and marrow CD34$^+$ cells in 15 patients prior to administration of chemotherapy and G-CSF (60), and they found a significant correlation between premobilization blood (but not bone marrow) CD34$^+$ cell levels and the apheresis yield of CD34$^+$ cells. Brown et al. reported that the level of premobilization blood CD34$^+$ cells correlated, but only poorly, with the apheresis yield of CD34$^+$ cells ($r^2 = 0.24$) and accounted for less than 50% of the variability in CD34$^+$ cell collection. Therefore, other, as yet unidentified factors play a more important role in mobilization efficacy (18). However, the relationship between premobilization blood CD34$^+$ cells and the apheresis yield of CD34$^+$ cells has not been confirmed by other groups. Specifically, Roberts et al., investigating 25 autologous patients mobilized with G-CSF (61), and Korbling et al., summarizing 41 normal donors mobilized with G-CSF for allogeneic transplantation (13), could not substantiate the correlation. Anderlini et al. retrospectively examined which premobilization characteristics might predict the apheresis yield of CD34$^+$ cells in normal individuals (57). Apart from the weak correlation in donor age (see above), they reported a small association ($r = 0.2$) in the baseline leukocyte count and could not confirm the correlation by multivariate analysis. A relationship between the percentage of marrow CD34$^+$ cells and the apheresis yield of CD34$^+$ cells has been reported in autologous transplant patients, but the correlation was too weak ($r^2 = 0.42$) to be of any practical value (62). Thus, at this time, there is no readily available laboratory or clinical parameter(s) which permits prediction of how an individual donor will respond to growth factor in the mobilization of CD34$^+$ cells.

5. Postmobilization Characterization

Attention has also been focused on the extent to which posttreatment measurements can predict either the level of mobilization or the apheresis yield of CD34$^+$ cells. As might be expected, there is extensive literature in the autologous transplant setting that demonstrates a consistent correlation between the level of blood CD34$^+$ cells or CFCs on the day of collection and the resultant number of PBSCs obtained by apheresis. Haas et al. studied PBSC mobilization in 61 lymphoma patients who received chemotherapy and G-CSF 300 µg/day subcutaneously followed by a sufficient number of apheresis procedures to collect either 4×10^8 nucleated cells or 5×10^6 CD34$^+$ cells/kg (50). They reported that the preleukapheresis level of circulating CD34$^+$ cells correlated significantly with the apheresis yield of CD34$^+$ cells; a result confirmed by several additional studies in autologous transplant patients (63–66). Excellent correlations have also been reported between the blood level of CD34$^+$ cells on the day of apheresis and the yield of CD34$^+$ cells in normal individuals mobilized with G-CSF for allogeneic transplantation in some (e.g., $r^2 = 0.73$) (14,26,27), but not all, studies ($r^2 = 0.32$) (29).

E. Timing of Apheresis Collections

Several investigators have proposed guidelines for the timing of apheresis after mobilization. One approach is to measure directly the level of blood CD34$^+$ cells on the day of apheresis. Schots et al. reported that a level of greater than 10 CD34$^+$ cells/µL predicted a yield of greater than 0.5×10^6 CD34$^+$ cells/kg after a single 10-L apheresis in 30 autologous transplant patients (63). In 60 autologous transplant patients, Remes et al. found that a level of less than 20 CD34$^+$ cells/µL predicted a poor collection ($<4 \times 10^6$ CD34$^+$ cells/kg) after a single 10-L apheresis, but if greater than 50 CD34$^+$ cells/µL, one or two apheresis procedures would be sufficient to collect the target CD34$^+$ cells (65). Luider et al. reported that a blood level of 20 CD34$^+$ cells/µL was reached 72 hs after initiation of G-CSF (after two doses; on the morning of the third scheduled injection) in 75 of 85 allogeneic PBSC donors treated with 4–10 µg G-CSF/kg/day and after 96 hs (after 3 doses of G-CSF) in 84 of 85 donors (29). Russell et al. employed a threshold of 20 blood CD34$^+$ cells/µL in 14 allogeneic PBSC donors mobilized with G-CSF as a guide to initiate leukapheresis (67). They reported collection of a sufficient number of CD34$^+$ cells (2.5×10^6/kg) after one to two apheresis procedures in 12 of 14 donors in whom the collection of CD34$^+$ cells was monitored periodically during apheresis. Similar thresholds have been used by others (65). In a retrospective analysis of mobilization and collection, Haas et al. reported that a peripheral blood count of 50 CD34$^+$ cells/μL on the day of apheresis was associated with a yield of 2.5 × 10^6 CD34$^+$ cells/kg after a single 10-L apheresis procedure (50). An additional benefit of the measuring CD34$^+$ cells daily is that timely identification of individuals who are not mobilizing sufficiently well (23) may permit (1) changes to enhance mobilization (such as G-CSF dose escalation or adding another cytokine), (2) cancellation of further G-CSF administration and the apheresis procedure to minimize donor exposure and inconvenience, or (3) avoiding delays to start a second course of mobilization or marrow collection. Alternatively, Luider et al. reported that the mobilization of CD34$^+$ cells is sufficiently reliable (see above) that apheresis can almost routinely be initiated on the morning after the third dose of G-CSF (29). These investigators have repeatedly measured CD34$^+$ cell yields during large-volume apheresis (see below) to guide directly the duration of collection toward the targeted cell dose (2.5 × 10^6 CD34$^+$ cells/kg recipient weight (29). In order to accomplish this, the flow cytometry laboratory was able to supply CD34$^+$ cell counts within 20 min. It is also noteworthy that, despite the investigators' attempts to quantitate directly the adequacy of CD34$^+$ cell collection on a real time basis, the collections were retrospectively found to be lower than predicted, presumably due to platelet clumping of test specimens, in 15% of the donors (29).

Protocols that employ direct measurements of circulating CD34$^+$ cells on the day of apheresis require a rapid laboratory turnaround. However, measurement of CD34$^+$ cells is time consuming, labor intensive, and requires an experienced staff to be available immediately, consequently investigators have attempted to identify more readily available and inexpensive predictors of CD34$^+$ cell yield. Although some investigators have identified a correlation between the preapheresis leukocyte count and the yield of CD34$^+$ cells (57), others have not (62), and, at best, the correlations are so weak that they are of no practical value (57,66). Others have proposed the measurement of circulating immature myeloid cells on the day of apheresis to predict the yield of CD34$^+$ cells, but the correlation with this parameter was much weaker ($r^2 = 0.59$) than with circulating CD34$^+$ cells and may be of limited practical value (68). Alternatively, measurement of blood CD34$^+$ cells on the day prior to apheresis has been reported to correlate nearly as well with the yield of CD34$^+$ cells ($r = 0.84$) as that the value measured on the day of apheresis ($r = 0.95$) and mitigates the need for rapid turnaround in the CD34$^+$ cell measurements (66). Since the day of peak blood CD34$^+$ cells varies between 4 and 8 days after G-CSF administration and is not predictable based on premobilization criteria or dosing schedule, and real time CD34$^+$ counts are not available in most institutions, the decision as to when to initiate leukapheresis in allogeneic PBSC donors is arbitrary and varies between institutions. In most centers, apheresis is initiated 3–4 hs after the fourth to fifth injection of G-CSF (approximately 72–96 hs after the initial injection) in order to permit a second procedure, if necessary, on the following day when the level of blood CD34$^+$ cells is still likely to be high. Anderlini et al. compared initiating leukapheresis on day 4 versus day 5 in similar groups of normal allogeneic donors who were mobilized with 6 μg G-CSF/kg twice daily (until completion of apheresis) and whose CD34$^+$ cells were collected using similar large-volume apheresis procedures (33). Peak blood CD34$^+$ cell levels were not measured, but the 5-day group had higher levels of blood mononuclear cells. The 5-day mobilization group was significantly more likely to achieve the target CD34$^+$ cell dose (4 × 10^6/kg recipient weight) after a single procedure (30 of 32 patients) than the 4-day group (30 of 45 patients). However, the 5-day group also had greater numbers of symptoms and higher leukocyte counts; consequently the investigators elected to use the 4-day regimen in order to minimize G-CSF exposure to the normal donors (33). Bishop et al. investigated the optimal timing of apheresis by mobilizing CD34$^+$ cells in 41 allogeneic donors using 5 µg G-CSF/kg/day until completion of apheresis, which was performed on days 4 through 6 (58). They found that collections on day 6 yielded the highest number of CD34$^+$ cells, and that 93% of the combined yields from days 5 and 6 apheresis procedures were adequate for transplantation (3 × 10^6 CD34$^+$ cells/kg recipient weight) compared with 83% of the combined days 4 and 5 yields. However, 15% of donors required a fourth apheresis to achieve the CD34$^+$ cell dose. Thus, the number of apheresis procedures in collecting allogeneic PBSCs typically varies from one to more than four, starting on days 3–5, and the amount of donor blood processed per procedure may vary from two to four times blood volumes depending on the efficacy of mobilization, the target dose of CD34$^+$ cells desired, the adequacy of venous access, donor tolerance of the procedure, the time of day apheresis is performed, and the need to perform ex vivo manipulations that will result in the loss of CD34$^+$ cells; for example, T-cell depletion.

F. Large-Volume Leukapheresis

Another technique to optimize the apheresis yield of CD34$^+$ cells is to increase the volume of blood processed during the procedure (69,70). Cull et al. performed sequential analysis of 24 leukapheresis products collected at 2-h intervals (mean of 7 L blood processed at each interval) from 17 autologous transplant patients mobilized with chemotherapy and/ or G-CSF (71). They reported that the apheresis yield of CD34$^+$ cells was constant between the 7th and 21st L of blood processed. Calculations showed that this result could only be achieved if CD34$^+$ cells were recruited into the circulation during the procedure. The investigators also reported that patients who had a blood CD34$^+$ count of greater than 10/ µL were likely to have an adequate apheresis yield of CD34$^+$ cells after a single procedure; however, their target cell dose, 1.5 × 10^6 CD34$^+$ cells/kg, was lower than those used by others (72).

G. Collection Devices

Differences among apheresis devices have been identified as a source of variability in CD34$^+$ cell yield. Morton et al. prospectively randomized 15 autologous transplant patients who were mobilized by chemotherapy and G-CSF to undergo consecutive apheresis procedures using COBE Spectra (Denver, CO) or Haemonetics MCS-3P (Braintree, MA), with the second procedure being performed on the alternative device (73). Preapheresis leukocyte counts were similar for groups starting on both instruments, but no measurements of preapheresis CD34$^+$ cells were made. Collection times were held constant, but the volume of blood collected, per manufacturers' suggestions, was nearly twofold higher on the Spectra than the MCS-3P. Not surprisingly, the total yield of CD34$^+$ cells collected was nearly twofold higher using the COBE; however, the number of CD34$^+$ cells collected per volume of blood processed on the two machines was similar. Thus, the improved collections with the Spectra could be attributed to the larger volume of blood processed than that of the MCS-3P.

In summary, the above studies showed that, despite the great individual variability in mobilization, most donors will mobilize CD34$^+$ cells sufficiently after administration of G-CSF in doses of 7.5–10.0 µg/kg for 4 to 6 days, and that one or two apheresis procedures would be adequate to collect the required number of CD34$^+$ cells for allogeneic transplantation (18,23,25,26,42,58). Recently, the National Marrow Donor Program has adopted a protocol which permits mobilization of matched unrelated allogeneic donors using G-CSF at 10 μg/kg/day for 4 to 5 days, with apheresis beginning on day 5 (74). If sufficient PBSCs are not collected, a second procedure may be performed the following day. Thus, the use of G-CSF has become a well-established, reliable method to mobilize PBSCs from normal donors. However, the optimal dose and schedule of G-CSF have not yet been defined (59), and not all normal individuals will have acceptable mobilization of CD34$^+$ cells after G-CSF administration at 10–12 μg G-CSF/kg/day for 4–6 days (16,18,33,58). The reported percentage of normal individuals who have inadequate mobilization after G-CSF administration varies from 1 to 33% (18,23,57,75). Obviously, the ease of collecting sufficient PBSCs depends on techniques of CD34$^+$ cell enumeration, the protocol for the apheresis procedure (see above), and the definition of an "adequate" mobilization. As noted above, some investigators define the adequacy of mobilization on the basis of the level of blood CD34$^+$ cells. A level of >20 CD34$^+$ cells/μL has been used by some (65,67). Others have defined inadequate mobilization based on the failure to collect a minimum number of CD34$^+$ cells per liter of blood processed during apheresis (e.g., >20 × 10^6/L) (57) or on the basis of failure to collect a targeted yield of CD34$^+$ cells (e.g., >4 × 10^6 CD34$^+$ cells/kg recipient weight) in one to three apheresis procedures (57). Since the minimum cell dose to engraft an allogeneic recipient has not been clearly defined, and may vary with the degree of HLA mismatch (72), these decisions are currently arbitrary; however, studies suggest that higher doses of CD34$^+$ cells are beneficial (76). The definition of an adequate mobilization may be further modified by the need to perform ex vivo manipulations on the cells, such as T-cell depletion, that will reduce the final number of CD34$^+$ cells for transplant.

The marked interdonor variability in mobilization after G-CSF remains a problem. A variety of clinical and investigational strategies has been suggested to mitigate this problem, including the use of higher doses of G-CSF (26), the use of different cytokines (42,77), or the use cytokine combinations (42,78–83), or in the investigational setting, the use monoclonal antibodies to PBSC adhesion molecules (84,85). There is little information available regarding alternative regimens to mobilize CD34$^+$ cells in allogeneic donors. Corringham and Ho described an allogeneic PBSC donor who failed to mobilize with 10 μg G-CSF/kg/day but mobilized well after administration of granulocyte-macrophage colony-stimulating factor (GM-CSF) 10 μg/kg/day for 3 days followed by G-CSF at the same dose until completion of apheresis (16). Recipient engraftment was rapid and durable. Lane et al. systematically investigated a variety of combinations of GM-CSF and G-CSF administration in normal individuals (42). They identified several alternative regimens employing combinations of GM-CSF and G-CSF that were as equally well tolerated by donors as G-CSF, yielded equal numbers of CD34$^+$ cells by apheresis, and mobilized greater numbers of primitive CD34$^+$ subsets than G-CSF alone (42,86). Additional investigation regarding optimal methods reliably to mobilize large numbers of hematopoietic stem cells from normal donors with tolerable side effects are needed.

IV. DONOR TOLERANCE AND SAFETY

The ability of healthy individuals to tolerate G-CSF administration and PBSC collection strongly influences the success achieving the target cell dose, which, in turn, influences the success of the transplant (18). Equally important, an optimal mobilization protocol should minimize adverse effects on short or long-term donor safety. Specific donor safety issues raised at a recent workshop included effects on donor tolerance, hematological parameters and function, organ function, complications of apheresis, possible contraindications to G-CSF administration, and the potential late effect of G-CSF for carcinogenesis or stem cell exhaustion (74).

A. Donor Tolerance

The administration of G-CSF in doses ranging from 5 to 10 μg/kg/day to normal individuals is associated with a predictable array of side effects (Table 1). The most common was bone pain, experienced by 77–90% of all subjects, and it was most commonly located in the back, hips, pelvis, or extremities, but may also be located in the chest. This could be alarming to some subjects (23). Headaches are the next most common symptom, found in 44–70% of subjects. Other common symptoms include body aches, fatigue, and "flu-like" symptoms, which occur in 15–50% of subjects. Less common are gastrointestinal abnormalities (anorexia, nausea, vomiting), fever and/or chills, inflammation at the injection site, and a variety of less common symptoms (23). Generalized skin rash was uncommon (2 of 241 reported subjects), but it is of considerable importance, since it might require discontinuation of G-CSF (23; T.A.L. unpublished data).

Symptoms appear in most subjects within hours of the first injection of G-CSF and tend to persist or increase throughout the course of G-CSF administration. Most donors (62–81%) require analgesics for symptomatic relief, and the treatment is at least partially effective in nearly all donors. One report suggested that an antihistamine drug prevented severe bone pain in an autologous patient mobilized with G-CSF (87). Prednisone, 1 mg/kg, has been reported to be of no benefit in preventing the side effects of G-CSF (18). Stroncek et al. performed a systematic study on the tolerability in 102 normal individuals mobilized using G-CSF in doses ranging from 2.5 to 10.0 μg/kg/day for 5–10 days (23). They found that increased doses of G-CSF were associated with an increased incidence of side effects (chiefly bone and body aches) as well as the use of analgesics. These data indicated a significant relationship between G-CSF dose and the severity of side effects. It is, therefore, noteworthy that Waller, who administered 20–24 μg G-CSF/kg/day for up to 7 days to allogeneic sibling PBSC donors, reported that most donors experienced

Table 1 Percentage of Subjects Reporting Symptoms During a Course of G-CSF Administration for PBSC Mobilization

				Symptoms				
Reference	n[a]	Bone pain[b]	Headache	Fever/ chills	Flu-like	GI	Fatigue	Local
25	9	77	n/a[c]	n/a	n/a	n/a	n/a	n/a
23	102	83	39	7	57	12	14	7
75	40	82	70	0	n/a	10	20	7
42	49	90	59	0	51	29	49	11
58	41	83	44	27	n/a	22	n/a	n/a

[a]Number of subjects in the trial.
[b]Percentage of subjects who reported the symptom during the course of growth factor administration.
[c]Data not available.

only mild to moderate bone pain (31). In addition, only 1 of 14 donors in Waller's report required G-CSF dose reduction for symptoms; a proportion similar to the 9 of 85 donors in Stroncek's group who received 5–10 µg G-CSF/kg/day for 5 days (31,23). This suggests that highly motivated family PBSC donors may tolerate doses of G-CSF higher than 10 µg/kg/day. Stroncek et al. also reported that women were more likely than men to experience side effects such as fatigue, gastrointestinal problems, fever, sweats, or flu-like symptoms; more likely to require dose reduction; or not able to complete the study (23). Symptoms were not affected by the age of the subject. Anderlini found that most symptoms lasted no longer than 2–4 days posttreatment, but some subjects complained of residual bone pain for up to a week (75). Taken together, these data indicated that a majority of healthy individuals can tolerate G-CSF in doses of 5–10 µg/kg/day for 4–6 days without the need for dose reduction or omission (23,25,27,42,58,75).

B. Hematological Effects

G-CSF administration results in a dose-dependent granulocytosis with a left shift (56,75,88). The leukocytosis peaks approximately 12 hs after each dose of G-CSF, but the leukocyte count tends to increase progressively during the course of G-CSF administration (27,41,74,89). In a preclinical study in which primates were treated with doses of G-CSF ≥ 1150 µg/kg/day for up to 18 days, the investigators observed 15- to 28-fold increases in peripheral leukocyte counts, neutrophil-infiltrated hemorrhagic foci in the cerebrum and cerebellum, neurological symptoms, and death in five of eight animals (Neupogen, package insert). In view of this, it has been recommended that the dose of G-CSF be reduced in normal donors if the leukocyte count exceeds 70,000/µL. Excessive leukocytosis is uncommonly observed in humans treated with 5–10 µg G-CSF/kg/day. Gabrilove reported that G-CSF administration to cancer patients increased the number of blood lymphocytes and monocytes as well as neutrophils (90). The finding has subsequently been confirmed by many investigators (8,43,91). A relationship between the dose of G-CSF administered to normal subjects and the extent of increase in peripheral blood T lymphocytes has been reported by one study (23) but not others (25,26). Most studies agreed on a lack of change in lymphocyte subsets with increasing doses of G-CSF (13,26,88). Eosinophils and basophils do not appear to be increased by G-CSF administration.

Depression of platelet counts has been observed in both patients (92) and healthy individuals during G-CSF administration (75). However, other investigators reported no change in platelet counts (23,25,42,88). More important from the perspective of donor safety is the predictable 30–50% decrease in platelet counts that accompanies large-volume apheresis collection of PBSCs after mobilization (93,94). Typically, platelet counts return to normal within 4–6 days after a single apheresis procedure for platelet collection (3). It has been reported that normal granulocyte donors receiving daily G-CSF treatment during a series of apheresis procedures have lower mean platelet counts than donors who did not receive G-CSF (95). In addition, a longer time is required for the platelet counts of allogeneic PBSC donors mobilized with G-CSF to return to the baseline value (approximately 7–10 days), suggesting that G-CSF may suppress platelet production (23,88). Moderate thrombocytopenia is a recognized (although occasional) complication in normal apheresis platelet donors and is not considered a cause for concern or deferral (98–99). During PBSC collection, both the physical loss of platelets and platelet activation may play a role in the thrombocytopenia (101). Likewise, thrombocytopenia was not severe enough to cause a delay in scheduling apheresis for allogeneic PBSC collection in G-

CSF–mobilized donors (25,75). Okamoto et al. reported an allogeneic PBSC donor who had a markedly depressed platelet count (47,000/μL) and prolonged thrombocytopenia (11 days) after mobilization with 10 μg G-CSF/kg/day for 5 days and two 6-L apheresis procedures (104). Luider et al., who employed large-volume apheresis reported that procedures were delayed or canceled in 3 of 85 allogeneic donors owing to postapheresis thrombocytopenia (30,000–50,000 platelets/μL) after one to three collections (29). It has been proposed to separate and reinfuse platelets from the PBSC products of donors whose postdonation platelet counts fall below 100,000/μL (105–106). All donors who are thrombocytopenic should be cautioned regarding activities and medications that might pose a bleeding risk, and apheresis should not be performed if the preapheresis platelet count is less than 70,000/μL (23,74).

Administration of G-CSF to normal subjects has been reported to activate platelets as indicated by increased platelet expression of P-selectin (107) and blood thromboxane B_2 and Antithrombin-III (AT-III) complex levels (108), and G-CSF enhances platelet aggregation to collagen and adenosine diphosphate (ADP) (24) presumably by a G-CSF receptor-mediated priming event (109). There have been two reports of arterial thrombosis in two cancer patients who were receiving G-CSF after chemotherapy (110,111). Concern has been expressed regarding induction of a possible prethrombic state in some normal donors (108,112), and such a risk was suggested in two cases. The first involved a 54-year-year-old, apparently healthy female PBSC donor mobilized with G-CSF who developed a cerebrovascular accident 2 days after an uneventful apheresis. The second involved a 64-year-old male with a history of coronary artery disease who developed a myocardial infarction after PBSC collection (74). The role of G-CSF and/or PBSC collection in these cases is unclear. The possible adverse effects of apheresis platelet collection on lymphocyte loss (1–50 $\times$ 10^6 per procedure) and immunological responsiveness after repeated procedures have been of some concern. Straus, et al. reported no long-term adverse effects of such procedures in normal donors, but they recommended limiting lymphocyte losses to less than 10^{11} and delaying apheresis when donor lymphocyte counts fell to less than 0.5 $\times$ 10^9/L (100). Korbling et al. investigated the effects of G-CSF mobilization (6 μg/kg, bid for 3–5 days, followed by apheresis on day 4 or 5) on lymphocyte subsets (113). They found that lymphocytes (and CD34$^+$ cells) decreased after apheresis to a nadir at day 7 after apheresis, returned to normal levels by day 30 after apheresis, and were slightly diminished at day 100. Kadar et al. studied 13 family donors for allogeneic PBSC transplantation mobilized with 5 μ/kg G-CSF bid and two large-volume apheresis procedures as well as bone marrow collection (114). They reported that the loss of T cells (3 $\times$ 10^{10} CD3$^+$ cells) was much greater as a result of the apheresis procedures than marrow harvesting, but they noted no long-term decrement in lymphocyte counts in seven of the donors who were followed for a mean of 209 days.

Transient neutropenia (absolute neutrophil count <1500/μL) persisting for at least 7–10 days has been reported in 2 of 13 allogeneic donors mobilized with 6 μg G-CSF/kg bid for 3 or 4 days followed by a three times blood volume apheresis. Neutropenia was asymptomatic and resolved within 8–45 days (34). The implications of this observation are unclear, and the investigators did not recommend routine monitoring of postapheresis leukocyte counts. Splenomegaly has been reported after high-dose G-CSF administration to primates and other species (Neupogen, package insert). Of note, Becker et al. reported a case of spontaneous splenic rupture in an allogeneic PBSC donor 4 days after a 6-day regimen of G-CSF (115).

C. Nonhematological Effects

Perhaps the most serious concern in mobilization and collection of PBSCs in normal individuals, apart from those relating to the administration of G-CSF or other cytokines, is the possible consequences of apheresis. Specifically, the placement of large-bore catheters into individuals who have inadequate venous access has raised medical and ethical issues. Apheresis for blood component production is reported to be at least as safe as blood donation and is occasionally associated with mild hypocalcemia due to the infusion of citrate (116). However, approximately 5–20% of healthy donors will have inadequate venous access for apheresis without a central venous catheter (18,58,74,75). Some institutions consider the requirement for catheter use to perform apheresis to be a contraindication to PBSC collection (49,75). The use of catheters appears to vary widely among institutions collecting PBSCs for allografting (11,12,15,16,18,23,25,28,58,75,117). For example Anderlini et al. reported that 3 of 43 allogeneic donors had inadequate venous access, a proportion similar to that reported by Urbano-Ispizua et al. who transplanted 30 patients using mobilized allogeneic PBSCs, 3 of whom required a central venous line (28). At the other end of the spectrum, the protocol employed by Russell et al. specified the use of central venous catheters for all 10 allogeneic PBSC donors (118). Although few complications and only one pneumothorax have been reported with catheter use in normal donors to date (28), catheter use has been associated with such complications as infection, pneumothorax, and bleeding up to 1% of autologous PBSC collections (119–121). Other apheresis complications, such as citrate toxicity or electrolyte disturbances, may be mitigated by electrolyte infusion or the addition of heparin to limit citrate use (122).

D. Adverse Reactions to G-CSF

The metabolic effects of G-CSF administration in both cancer patients and healthy individuals have been reported (23,25,75). G-CSF administration to normal subjects has been associated with transient two- to threefold increases in the serum levels of alkaline phosphatase (AP) and lactate dehydrogenase (LD), as well as smaller increases in alanine aminotransferase and uric acid. Serum gamma-glutamyl transferase and creatine phosphokinase remain unaltered, suggesting that the above changes in AP and LD are due to an expanding myeloid mass (74). Moderate decreases in blood urea nitrogen, glucose, bilirubin, potassium, and occasionally magnesium have been reported. These changes appear to be of no clinical consequence except for the possible need for electrolyte supplementation during large-volume leukapheresis (102).

E. Long-Term Safety Considerations

The use of G-CSF in normal donors for granulocyte collection has become a common practice (95,123). Despite the apparent safety of short-term courses of G-CSF in healthy individuals, there is minimal data regarding the long-term safety of G-CSF or other growth factors (74). Specific concerns have been raised regarding the potential for single or repeated courses of G-CSF and apheresis collection of PBSCs leading to "exhaustion" of hematopoietic stem cells in the donor. Although no large long-term studies are available, several small studies suggest that stem cell exhaustion does not occur with limited follow-up duration. Harada et al. found no abnormalities in the blood counts in nine donors 1.5 years after administration of 10 µg G-CSF/kg/day for 5 days (24). In a preliminary report,

Kunkel et al. reported no difference after 1 year in the baseline hematological values of 46 subjects who had been mobilized with G-CSF alone or in combination with GM-CSF (124). In a subgroup of 11 subjects who underwent a second course of mobilization using one of the three different regimens 1 year later, the apheresis yields of CD34$^+$ cells were not different between the first and the second collection. Anderlini et al. studied the results of a second mobilization performed in 13 normal donors (with a mean of 5 months after the first procedure), using the same regimen (6 μg G-CSF/kg/bid), until completion of collection of 4×10^6 CD34$^+$ cells/kg (103). They found no difference in baseline hematological values and no difference between the two mobilizations and collections with respect to adverse reactions during mobilization or the apheresis yield of CD34$^+$ cells per liter of blood processed. Stroncek et al. performed a second mobilization using G-CSF in doses of 7.5 or 10.0 μg/kg/day for 5 days, followed by apheresis, at least 12 months after the initial mobilization in 19 healthy subjects who were previously given G-CSF at 2–10 μg/kg/day for 5 days prior to apheresis (96). No differences were found in baseline hematological values or between the first and second mobilizations with respect to day 6 blood CD34$^+$ cell counts, the apheresis yield of mononuclear cells, or CD34$^+$ cells (total or per liter of blood processed) (96). Although 7 of the subjects were administered higher doses of G-CSF on the second mobilization, there were also no differences in the above parameters in the subgroup of 12 subjects who were administered the same G-CSF dose (7.5–10 μg/kg/day) on both occasions. In this subgroup, there was a good correlation between the apheresis yield of CD34$^+$ cells from a given donor on the first apheresis compared with the second one ($r^2 = 0.86$). Although these studies are encouraging, they are too small and of too short follow-up duration to provide assurances that no adverse effects on hematopoiesis will be encountered as a *rare* event after a longer time period. Given this uncertainty and the current lack of a central registry for allogeneic PBSC donors, it has been proposed that each institution periodically follow mobilized PBSC donors (74).

Because of its ability to stimulate the growth of leukemic cells ex vivo (125,126), another concern for normal PBSC donors is the leukemogenic or, more generally, the neoplastic potential for G-CSF. The peak serum levels of G-CSF after a single administration of 10 μg/kg subcutaneously (approximately 1 ng/mL) are reported to be approximately 1.5-fold higher than mean endogenous G-CSF levels during infection and equal to the upper quartile of values reported (approximately 1–3 ng/mL) (127,128). Thus, it seems doubtful that a short course of G-CSF would pose a significant risk. However, only anecdotal data are available attesting to the lack of leukemic potential in normals donors at this time (129). G-CSF has also been employed in patients with severe congenital neutropenia (SCN) for several years (130,131). Although cases of leukemia and myelodysplasia have been reported in patients with SCN and aplastic anemia (130,132,133–135), patients with these diseases appear to be predisposed to develop the malignancies (136,137), and it cannot be ascertained that the use of G-CSF has altered the natural history of the diseases. Thus, to date, there is insufficient data to evaluate the possible leukemogenic risk of G-CSF or even to indicate that such a risk exists. Moreover, it is doubtful that meaningful clinical data regarding the safety of G-CSF will become available in the near future. Hasenclever and Sextro have estimated that in order to ascertain even a 10-fold increase in leukemia risk in normal donors, it will be necessary to follow 2000 subjects for 10 years (138). The control group for such a study would require careful definition, since HLA-matched family members of patients with leukemia may also have an inherently increased risk of leukemia compared with the general population (138,139). A preliminary report on the follow-up of marrow donors supports this possibility (140).

F. Factors Influencing the Choice of Allogeneic Marrow Versus PBSCs

Donor preferences and safety considerations will play an important role in choosing marrow versus PBSCs. Kadar et al. studied the effect of combined PBSC mobilization with 5 μg/kg G-CSF bid and two large-volume leukapheresis procedures versus bone marrow collection from the same donors in 13 family donors for allogenic transplantation. Overall, 12 of the 13 donors preferred PBSC collection (114). For safety considerations, participants in a recent workshop concluded that the short-term safety profile of G-CSF appears to be acceptable for most healthy individuals to be PBSC donors, especially family donors (74). However, in view of our limited knowledge of possible unusual adverse effects of G-CSF, a variety of relative or possible contraindications to mobilization with G-CSF and PBSC apheresis should be considered. First, as noted above, some centers consider inadequate venous access to be a contraindication for PBSC collection owing to the risk of catheter-related complications. The decision to harvest marrow rather than inserting a catheter should include an assessment of all the possible risks for marrow harvesting; for example, general anesthesia, and the need for homologous transfusion. For example, PBSC collection might be safer for an HLA-matched sibling donor with poor veins who also has a higher anesthetic risk (e.g., active asthma). Likewise, for donors >65 years old, it might be preferred to collect PBSCs, since age has little effect on the apheresis yield of CD34$^+$ cells and a recent study reported a high rate (22%) of homologous blood transfusion in older allogeneic marrow donors (141). PBSC collection might be preferable in donors who have severe back pain, since exacerbations of this condition has been reported in marrow harvesting (97). Clearly, patients who have known allergy to G-CSF are candidates for marrow harvesting, as generalized allergic dermatitis after G-CSF has been observed (23; T.A.L. unpublished data). Marrow harvesting might be preferred in donors who have a history of inflammatory eye disorders, since cases of episcleritis and iritis during G-CSF administration have been reported (80,142). Potential donors who are at risk for venous or arterial thrombosis or those who have vascular disease may be at increased risk for complications due to PBSC mobilization in view of the effects of G-CSF on hemostasis. Whether marrow harvesting poses a lower risk than G-CSF administration and PBSC apheresis in such patients is also uncertain. Potential PBSC donors with a history of autoimmune disorders may be at increased risk for flare; for example systemic lupus erythematosus with serositis and or myalgia, rheumatoid arthritis, multiple sclerosis. Data regarding the possibility of excess risk in such patients may soon become available, as clinical trials of autologous PBSC transplantation after G-CSF mobilization are in progress for such autoimmune conditions. Preliminary studies showed that G-CSF did not cause unexpected inflammatory reactions (143). Whether bone marrow obtained from donors who have been administered G-CSF is equally as efficacious in promoting early engraftment is clear, but if this technique proves to be effective, then increasing numbers of normal morrow donors will also be exposed to G-CSF (144). PBSC mobilization and collection might be approached more cautiously in donors with a history of malignancy treated with chemotherapy/radiotherapy, premalignant conditions, or a strong family history of myelodysplasia or leukemia other than the intended recipient. Morbid obesity may also be a relative contraindication to marrow harvesting and would make PBSC collection preferable (54). Additional considerations should include the recipient conditions. Numerous studies have reported no significant difference in the incidence and severity of acute graft-versus-host disease (GVHD) in patients allografted with PBSCs (57%) compared with bone marrow (45%) despite the 10- to 20-fold higher numbers of T cells given with PBSCs (12,13,15,17,28). However, some preliminary reports suggested that the incidences of chronic GVHD were increased in recipients of PBSCs compared with marrow (14,145). Consequently, a patient considered to be at high risk for complications associated with chronic GVHD (and who has a disease that does not benefit from graft-versus-leukemia) might be a better candidate for marrow grafting. Alternatively, administration of T-cell–depleted PBSCs allografts has been associated with only mild acute GVHD and limited chronic GVHD (146).

The costs (approximately \$14,000–\$15,000) of PBSC mobilization and collection in 37 donors who did not require central venous lines were reported to be comparable to those associated with bone marrow harvesting in 33 donors (75). In the study, attempts were made to collect 2 U of autologous blood from the marrow donors prior to harvest, marrow donors were evaluated as outpatients the day prior to donation, they were admitted the morning of donation and discharged in the afternoon, and only three donors required overnight hospitalization. PBSC donors were mobilized using 6 µg G-CSF/kg bid (with self-injection at home) throughout the duration of apheresis, which was initiated on day 4 in nearly all subjects. Large-volume apheresis (approximately three times blood volume) was performed and a single procedure sufficed in 24 of 37 evaluable PBSC donors for the target dose of 4×10^6 CD34$^+$ cells/kg recipient weight. For these 24 donors, the costs of PBSC harvesting (approximately \$13,000) were less than that for marrow donation.

V. CONCLUSION

It is now possible reliably to obtain sufficient hematopoietic stem cells from most normal donors to perform allogeneic transplantation, with tolerable side effects, by the administration of a single daily dose of G-CSF at 7.5 to 10.0 µg/kg subcutaneously for 4–6 days followed by one to three apheresis procedures starting on days 3–5. However, there is wide variability among individuals with respect to the extent of mobilization achieved by the regimen and the optimal timing of apheresis. Studies suggest that the likelihood of obtaining an adequate harvest of CD34$^+$ cells, as defined locally, may be enhanced by employing higher doses or different schedules of G-CSF, monitoring the mobilization and/or collection of PBSCs, and using apheresis procedures processing two or more times blood volume. However, an optimal regimen for mobilization and harvesting for all donors has not yet been identified and a small percentage of donors may not mobilize adequately with G-CSF. Alternative regimens employing combinations of G-CSF and GM-CSF are available that may prove to be useful in such cases, and novel cytokines that are even more effective than G-CSF in mobilizing stem cells are eagerly awaited. Based on currently available experience with several hundred normal donors, the short-term safety of G-CSF appears to be acceptable; however, there exist several scenarios in which marrow harvesting may be preferable to G-CSF mobilization and apheresis collection of PBSCs. These include allergy to G-CSF, patients at risk for thrombotic phenomena, for example, cerebrovascular/cardiovascular disease, certain ocular (and perhaps other) inflammatory conditions, autoimmune diseases with an inflammatory component, and donors who may be at risk for development of myelodysplasia or leukemia. Whether marrow harvesting is preferable to PBSC mobilization in donors who require placement of large-lumen central venous catheters to provide adequate venous access will depend not only on the donor's health (e.g., asthma) but also on local protocols as well as the success rates and complications involving marrow harvesting, catheter insertion, and PBSC mobilization and collection. Since reliable information regarding the long-term safety of G-CSF is unlikely to be available for years, institutions should institute protocols for long-term donor follow-up and join in efforts to include donors' conditions in central registries.

REFERENCES

1. Lane TA. Allogeneic marrow reconstitution using peripheral blood stem cells: the dawn of a new era. Transfusion 1996; 36:585–589.
2. Giralt, S, Estey E, Albitar M, van Besien K, Rondón G, Anderlini P, O'Brien S, Khouri I, Gajewski J, Mehra R, Claxton D, Andersson B, Beran M, Przepiorka D, Koller C, Kornblau S, Kørbling M, Keating M, Kantarjian H, Champlin R. Engraftment of allogeneic hematopoietic progenitor cells with purine analog-containing chemotherapy: harnessing graft-versus-leukemia without myeloablative therapy. Blood 1997; 89:4531–6.
3. Lasky LC, Lin A, Kahn RA, McCullough J. Donor platelet response and product quality assurance in plateletpheresis. Transfusion 1981; 21(3):247–260.
4. Moss TJ, Sander, DG, Lasky LC, Bostrom B. Contamination of peripheral blood stem cell harvests by circulating neuroblastoma cells. Blood 1980; 76:1879–1883.
5. Sharp JG, Joshi SS, Armitage JO, Bierman P, Coccia PF, Harrington DS, Kessinger A, Crouse DA, Mann SL, Weisenburger DD. Significance of detection of occult non-Hodgkin's lymphoma in histologically uninvolved bone marrow by a culture technique. Blood 1992; 79:1074–1080.
6. Fliedner TM, Flad HD, Bruch C, Calvo W, Goldmann SF, Herbst E, Hugl E, Huget R, Korbling M, Krumbacher K, Nothdurft W, Ross WM, Schnappauf H-P, Steinbach J. Treatment of aplastic anemia by blood stem cell transfusion: a canine model. Haematological 1976; 61(2):141–156.
7. Molineux G, Pojda Z, Hampson IN, Lord BI, Dexter TM. Transplantation potential of peripheral blood stem cells induced by granulocyte colony-stimulating factor. Blood 1990; 76: 2153–2158.
8. Weaver CH, Buckner CD, Longin K, Appelbaum FR, Rowley S, Lilleby K, Miser J, Störb R, Hansen JA, Bensinger W. Syngeneic transplantation with peripheral blood mononuclear cells collected after the administration of recombinant human granulocyte colony-stimulating factor. Blood 1993; 82:1981–1984.
9. Kessinger A, Smith DM, Strandjord SE, Landmark JD, Dooley DC, Law P, Coccia PF, Warkentin PI, Weisenburger DD, Armitage JO. Allogeneic transplantation of blood-derived, T cell-depleted hemopoietic stem cells after myeloablative treatment in a patient with acute lymphoblastic leukemia. Bone Marrow Transplant 1989; 6:643–646.
10. Russell NH, Hunter A, Rogers S, Hanley J, Anderson D. Peripheral blood stem cells as an alternative to marrow for allogeneic transplantation (letter). Lancet 1993; 341(8858):1482.
11. Sasaki A, Tsukaguchi M, Hirai M, Ohira H, Nakao Y, Yamane T, Park K, Im T, Tatsumi N. Transplantation of Allogeneic peripheral blood stem cells after myeloablative treatment of a patient in blastic crisis of chronic myelocytic leukemia. Am J Hematology 1994; 47: 45–49.
12. Bensinger WI, Weaver CH, Appelbaum FR, Rowley S, Demirer T, Sanders J, Storb R, Buckner CD. Transplantation of allogeneic peripheral blood stem cells mobilized by recombinant human granulocyte colony-stimulating factor. Blood 1995; 85(6):1655–1658.
13. Korbling M, Huh YO, Durett A, Mizra N, Miller P, Engel H, Anderlini P, van Besien K,

Andreeff M, Przepiorka D, Deisseroth AB, Champlin R. Allogeneic blood stem cell transplantation: Peripheralization and yield of donor-derived primitive hematopoietic progenitor cells (CD34+ Thy-1 dim) and lymphoid subsets, and possible predictors of engraftment and graft-versus-host disease. Blood 1995; 86:2842–2848.

14. Korbling M, Przepiorka D, Huh YO, Engel H, van Besien K, Giralt S, Andersson B, Kleine HD, Seong D, Deisseroth AB, Andreeff M, Champlin R. Allogeneic blood stem cell transplantation for refractory leukemia and lymphoma: potential advantage of blood over marrow allografts. Blood 1995; 85(6):1659–1565.

15. Schmitz N, Dreger P, Suttorp M, Rohwedder EB, Haferlach T, Löffler H, Hunter A, Russell NH. Primary transplantation of allogeneic peripheral blood progenitor cells mobilized by filgrastim (granulocyte colony-stimulating factor). Blood 1995; 85(6):1666–1672.

16. Corringham RET, Ho AD. Rapid and sustained allogeneic transplantation using immuno-selected CD34+ selected peripheral blood progenitor cells mobilized by recombinant granulocyte- and granulocyte-macrophage colony stimulating factors. Blood 1995; 86:2052–2054.

17. Pavletic ZS, Bishop MR, Tarantolo SR, Martin-Algarra S, Bierman PJ, Vose JM, Reed EC, Gross TG, Kollath J, Nasrati K, et al. Hematopoietic recovery after allogeneic blood stem-cell transplantation compared with bone marrow transplantation in patients with hematologic malignancies. J Clin Oncol 1997; 4:1608–1616.

18. Brown RA, Adkins D, Goodnough LT, Haug JS, Todd G, Wehde M, Hendricks D, Ehlenbeck C, Laub L, DiPersio J. Factors that influence the collection and engraftment of allogeneic peripheral-blood stem cells in patients with hematologic malignancies. J Clin Oncol 1997; 15(9):3067–3074.

19. Russell JA, Desai S, Herbut B, Brown C, Luider J, Ruether JD, Stewart D, Chaudhry A, Booth K, Jorgenson K, et al. Partially mismatched blood cell transplants for high-risk hematologic malignancy. Bone Marrow Transplant 1997; 19(9):861–866.

20. Bender JG, Unverzagt KL, Walker DE, Lee W, Van Epps DE, Smith DH, Stewart CC, To LB. Identification and comparison of CD34-positive cells and their subpopulations from normal peripheral blood and bone marrow using multicolor flow cytometry. Blood 1991; 77:2591–2596.

21. Richman, CM, Weiner, RS, Yankee, RA. Increase in circulating stem cells following chemotherapy in man. Blood 1976; 47:1031–1039.

22. To LB. Mobilizing and collecting blood stem cells. In: Gale, RP, Juttner CA, Henon P, eds. Blood Stem Cell Transplants. Cambridge, UK: Cambridge: University Press, 1994:56–74.

23. Stroncek DF, Clay ME, Petzoldt ML, Smith J, Jaszcz W, Oldham F, McCullough J. Treatment of normal individuals with G-CSF: donor experiences and the effects on peripheral blood CD34+ cell counts and the collection of peripheral blood stem cells. Transfusion 1996; 36:601–610.

24. Harada M, Nagafuji K, Fujisaki T, Kubota A, Mizuno S-I, Takenaka K, Miyamoto T, Ohno Y, Gondo H, Kuriowa M, Okamura T, Inaba S, Niho Y. G-CSF-induced mobilization of peripheral blood stem cells from healthy adults for allogeneic transplantation. J Hematother 1996; 5:63–72.

25. Dreger P, Haferlach T, Eckstein V, Jacobs S, Suttorp M, Loffler H, Muller-Ruchholtz W, Schmitz N. G-CSF-mobilized peripheral blood progenitor cells for allogeneic transplantation: safety, kinetics of mobilization, and composition of the graft. Br J Haematol 1994; 87(3):609–613.

26. Hoglund M, Smedmyr B, Simonsson B, Totterman T, Bengtsson M. Dose-dependent mobilisation of haematopoietic progenitor cells in healthy volunteers receiving glycosylated rHuG-CSF. Bone Marrow Transplant 1996; 18:19–27.

27. Grigg AP, Roberts AW, Raunow H, Houghton S, Layton JE, Boyd AW, McGrath KM, Maher D. Optimizing dose and scheduling of filgrastim (granulocyte colony-stimulating factor) for mobilization and collection of peripheral blood progenitor cells in normal volunteers. Blood 1995; 86(12):4437–4445.

28. Urbano-Ispizua A, Solano C, Brunet S, Hernandez F, Sanz G, Alegre A, et al. Allogeneic peripheral blood progenitor cell transplantation: analysis of short-term engraftment and acute GVHD incidence in 33 cases. Bone Marrow Transplant 1996; 18:35–40.

29. Luider J, Brown C, Selinger S, Quinaln D, Karlsson L, Ruether D, Stewart D, Klassen J, Russell JA. Factors influencing yields of progenitor cells for allogeneic transplantation: Optimization of G-CSF dose, day of collection, and duration of leukapheresis. J Hematother 1997; 6:575–580.

30. Duhrsen U, JL Villeval, J Boyd, G Kannourakis, G Morstyn, and D Metcalf. Effects of recombinant human granulocyte colony-stimulating factor on hematopoietic progenitor cells in cancer patients. Blood 1988; 72:2074–2081.

31. Waller CF, Bertz H, Wenger MK, Fetscher S, Hardung M, Engelhardt M, Behringer D, Lange W, Mertelsmann R, Finke J. Mobilization of peripheral blood progenitor cells for allogeneic transplantation: efficacy and toxicity of a high-dose rhG-CSF regimen. Bone Marrow Transplant 1996; 18(2):279–283.

32. Majolino I, Scime R, Vasta S, Cavallaro AM, Fiandaca T, Indovina A, Catania P, Santoro A. Mobilization and collection of PBSC in healthy donors: comparison between two schemes of rhG-CSF administration. Eur J Haematol 1996; 57(3):214–221.

33. Anderlini P, Przepiorka D, Huh Y, Lauppe J, Miller P, Sundberg J, Seong D, Champlin R, Korbling M. Duration of filgrastim mobilization and apheresis yield of CD34+ progenitor cells and lymphoid subsets in normal donors for allogeneic transplantation. Br J Haematol 1996; 93(4):940–942.

33a. Kessinger A, Bishop MR, Anderson JR, Armitage JO, Bierman PJ, Reed EC, Tarantolo S, Tempero MA, Vose JM, Warkentin PI. Comparison of subcutaneous and intravenous administration of recombinant human granulocyte-macrophage colony-stimulating factor for peripheral blood stem cell mobilization. J Hematother 1995; 4:81–84.

34. Anderlini P, Przepiorka D, Seong D, Champlin R, Korbling M. Transient neutropenia in normal donors after G-CSF mobilization and stem cell apheresis. Br J Haematol 1996; 94(1):155–158.

35. Pollmacher T, Korth C, Mullington J, Schreiber W, Sauer J, Vedder H, Galanos C, Holsboer F. Effects of granulocyte colony-stimulating factor on plasma cytokine and cytokine receptor levels and on the in vivo host response to endotoxin in healthy men. Blood 1996, 87(3):900–905.

36. Yano T, Katayama Y, Sunami K, Deguchi S, Nawa Y, Hiramatsu Y, Nakayama H, Arakawa T, Ishimaru F, Teshima T, et al. G-CSF–induced mobilization of peripheral blood stem cells for allografting: comparative study of daily single versus divided dose of G-CSF. Int J Hematol 1997; 66(2):169–178.

37. Somlo G, Sniecinski I, Odom-Maryon T, Nowicki B, Chow W, Hamasaki V, Leong L, Margolin K, Morgan R Jr, Raschko J, et al. Effect of CD34+ selection and various schedules of stem cell reinfusion and granulocyte colony-stimulating factor priming on hematopoietic recovery after high-dose chemotherapy for breast cancer. Blood 1997; 89(5):1521–1528.

38. Kröger N, W Zeller, T Hassan, W Krüger, K Hummel, C Goepfert, C Löliger, B Biermann, AR Zander. 10μg versus 2 × 5μg G-CSF in steady-state mobilisation of CD34+ progenitor cells in high risk breast cancer patients: higher yield by splitting the dose (abstr). Blood 1997; 90(suppl 1):592a.

39. Fischer J, Unkrig C, Ackermann M at al. Intra-day CD34+ cell counts depend on the time to application and correlate with the resulting G-CSF plasma level after steady-state mobilization of PBPC by filgrastim (abstr). Blood 1994; 84(suppl 1):23a.

40. Sato N, Sawada K, Takahashi TA, Mogi Y, Asano S, Koike T, Sekiguchi S. A time course study for optimal harvest of peripheral blood progenitor cells by granulocyte colony-stimulating factor in health volunteers. Exp Hematol. 1994; 22:973–978.

41. de Haas M, Kerst JM, van der Schoot CE, Calafat J, Hack CE, Nuijens JH, Roos D, van Oers

RH, von dem Borne AE. Granulocyte colony-stimulating factor administration to healthy volunteers: analysis of the immediate activating effects on circulating neutrophils. Blood 1994, 84(11):3885–3894.

42. Lane TA, Law P, Maruyama M, Young D, Burgess J, Mullen M, Mealiffe M, Terstappen LWMM, Hardwick A, Moubayed M, Oldham F, Corringham RET, and Ho AD. Harvesting and enrichment of hematopoietic stem cells mobilized into the peripheral blood of normal donors by granulocyte-macrophage colony stimulating factor (GM-CSF) or G-CSF: potential role in allogeneic marrow transplantation. Blood 1995, 85:275–282.

43. Matsunaga T, Sakamaki S, Kohgo Y, Ohi S, Hirayama Y, Nitsu Y. Recombinant human granulocyte colony stimulating factor can mobilize sufficient amounts of peripheral blood stem cells in healthy volunteers for allogeneic transplantation. Bone Marrow Transplant. 1993; 11:103–108.

44. Zaino EC. Blood counts in the nonagenarian. NY State J Med 1981; 81(8):1199–1200.

45. Lipschitz DA, Udupa KB, Milton KY, Thompson CO. Effect of age on hematopoiesis in man. Blood 1984; 63(3):502–509.

46. Buckner CD, Clift RA, Sanders JE, Stewart P, Bensinger WI, Doney KC, Sullivan KM, Witherspoon RP, Deeg HJ, Appelbaum FR, et al. Marrow harvesting from normal donors. Blood 1984; 64(3):630–634.

47. Chatta GS, Andrews RG, Rodger E, Schrag M, Hammond WP, Dale DC. Hematopoietic progenitors and aging: alterations in granulocytic precursors and responsiveness to recombinant human G-CSF, GM-CSF, and IL-3. J Geronto 1993; 48(5):M207–212.

48. Bensinger WI, Longin K, Appelbaum F, Rowley S, Weaver C, Lilleby K, Gooley T, Lynch M, Higano T, Klarnet J, Chauncey T, Storb R, Buckner CD. Peripheral blood stem cells (PBSCs) collected after recombinant granulocyte colony stimulating factor (rhG-CSF): an analysis of factors correlating with the tempo of engraftment after transplantation. Br J Haematol. 1994; 87(4):825–831.

49. Bensinger W, Appelbaum F, Rowley S, Storb R, Sanders J, Lilleby K, Gooley T, Demirer T, Schiffman K, Weaver C, et al. Factors that influence collection and engraftment of autologous peripheral-blood stem cells. J Clin Oncol 1995; (10):2547–2555.

50. Haas R, Mohle R, Fruhauf S, Goldschmidt H, Witt B, Flentje M, Wannenmacher M, Hunstein W. Patient characteristics associated with successful mobilizing and autografting of peripheral blood progenitor cells in malignant lymphoma. Blood 1994; 83(12):3787–3794.

51. Kotasek D, Shepherd KM, Sage RE, Dale BM, Norman JE, Charles P, Gregg A, Pillow A, Bolton A. Factors affecting blood stem cell collections following high-dose cyclophosphamide mobilization in lymphoma, myeloma and solid tumors. Bone Marrow Transplant 1992; 9(1):11–17.

52. Henon PR. Blood stem cell autografts in malignant blood disease: The French experience with a special focus on myeloma. The France Autogreffe Group (FAG). Haematologica 1990; 75(1):53–59.

53. Bolwell BJ, Goormastic M, Yanssens, T, Dannley R, Baucco P, Fishleder A. Comparison of G-CSF with GM-CSF for mobilizing peripheral blood progenitor cells and for enhancing marrow recovery after autologous bone marrow transplant. Bone Marrow Transplant 1994; 14:13–18.

54. Miflin G, Charley C, Stainer C, Anderson S, Hunter A, Russell N. Stem cell mobilization in normal donors for allogeneic transplantation: analysis of safety and factors affecting efficacy. Br J Haematol 1996; 95(2):345–348.

55. Lane TA. Mobilization of hematopoietic progenitor cells. In: Brecher M, Lasky L, Sacher R, Issitt L, eds. Hematopoietic Progenitor Cells; Processing, Standards, and Practice. American Association of Blood Banks. Bethesda, MD: 1995:59–108.

56. Chatta GS, Price TH, Allen RC, Dale DC. Effects of in vivo recombinant methionyl human granulocyte colony-stimulating factor on the neutrophil response and peripheral blood colony-forming cells in healthy young and elderly adult volunteers. Blood 1994; 84:2923–2929.

57. Anderlini P, Przepiorka D, Seong D, Smith TL, Huh YO, Lauppe J, Champlin R, Korbling M. Factors affecting mobilization of CD34+ cells in normal donors treated with filgrastim. Transfusion 1997; 37:507–512.

58. Bishop MR, Tarantolo SR, Jackson JD, Anderson JR, Schmit-Pokorny K, Zacharias D, Pavletic ZS, Pirruccello SJ, Vose JM, Bierman PJ, et al. Allogeneic-blood stem-cell collection following mobilization with low-dose granulocyte colony-stimulating factor. J Clin Oncol 1997; 15(4):1601–1607.

59. Anderlini P, Przepiorka D, Lauppe J, Seong D, Giralt S, Champlin R, Korbling M. Collection of peripheral blood stem cells from normal donors 60 years of age or older. Br J Haematol 1997; 97(2):485–487.

60. Fruehauf S, Haas R, Conradt C, Murea S, Witt B, Mohle R, Hunstein W. Peripheral blood progenitor cell (PBPC) counts during steady-state hematopoiesis allow to estimate the yield of mobilized PBPC after filgrastim (R-metHuG-CSF)–supported cytotoxic chemotherapy. Blood 1995; 85:2619–2626.

61. Roberts A, Begley C, Grigg A, Basser R. Do steady-state peripheral blood progenitor cell (PBPC) counts predict the yield of PBPC mobilized by filgrastim alone? (letter). Blood 1995; 86:2451.

62. Passos-Coelho JL, Braine HG, Davis JM, Huelskamp AM, Schepers KG, Ohly K, Clarke B, Wright SK, Noga SJ, Davidson NE, et al. Predictive factors for peripheral-blood progenitor-cell collections using a single large-volume leukapheresis after cyclophosphamide and granulocyte-macrophage colony-stimulating factor mobilization. J Clin Oncol 1995; 13(3): 705–714.

63. Schots R, Van Riet I, Damiaens S, Flament J, Lacor P, Staelens Y, Steenssens L, van Camp B: De Waele M. The absolute number of circulating CD34+ cells predicts the number of hematopoietic stem cells that can be collected by apheresis. Bone Marrow Transplant 1996; 17(4):509–515.

64. Papadopoulos KP, Ayello J, Tugulea S, Heitjan DF, Williams C, Reiss RF, Vahdat LT, Suciu-Foca N, Antman KH, Hesdorffer CS. Harvest quality and factors affecting collection and engraftment of CD34+ cells in patients with breast cancer scheduled for high-dose chemotherapy and peripheral blood progenitor cell support. J Hematother 1997; 6(1):61–68.

65. Remes K, Matinlauri I, Grenman S, Itala M, Kauppila M, Pelliniemi TT, Salminen E, Vanharanta R, Rajamaki A. Daily measurements of blood CD34+ cells after stem cell mobilization predict stem cell yield and posttransplant hematopoietic recovery. J Hematother 1997, 6(1): 13–19.

66. Elliott C, Samson DM, Armitage S, Lyttelton MP, McGuigan D, Hargreaves R, Giles C, Abrahamson G, Abboudi Z, Brennan M, et al. When to harvest peripheral-blood stem cells after mobilization therapy: prediction of CD34-positive cell yield by preceding day CD34-positive concentration in peripheral blood. J Clin Oncol 1996; 14(3):970–973.

67. Russell JA, Luider J, Weaver M, Brown C, Selinger S, Railton C, Karlsson, Klassen J. Collection of progenitor cells for allogeneic transplantation from peripheral blood of normal donors. Bone Marrow Transplant 1995; 15:111–115.

68. Teshima T, Sunami K, Bessho A, Shinagawa K, Omoto E, Ueoka H, Harada M, Ohno Y, Miyoshi T, Miyamoto T, et al. Circulating immature cell counts on the harvest day predict the yields of CD34+ cells collected after granulocyte colony-stimulating factor plus chemotherapy-induced mobilization of peripheral blood stem cell [letter]. Blood 1997; 89(12): 4660–4661.

69. Hillyer CD. Large volume leukapheresis to maximize peripheral blood stem cell collection. J Hematother 1993; 2(4):529–532.

70. Gillespie TW, Hillyer CD. Peripheral blood progenitor cells for marrow reconstitution: mobilization and collection strategies. Transfusion. 1996; 36(7):611–624.

71. Cull G, Ivey J, Chase P, Picciuto R, Herrmann R, Cannell P. Collection and recruitment of CD34+ cells during large-volume leukapheresis. J Hematother 1997; 6:309–314.

72. Bender JG, To LB, Williams S, Schwartzberg LS. Defining a therapeutic dose of peripheral blood stem cells. J Hematother 1992; 1(4):329–341.

73. Morton JA, Baker DP, Hutchins CJ, Durrant ST. The COBE Spectra cell separator is more effective than the Haemonetics MCS-3P cell separator for peripheral blood progenitor cell harvest after mobilization with cyclophosphamide and filgrastim. Transfusion 1997; 37(6): 631–633.

74. Anderlini P, Korbling M, Dale D, Gratwohl A, Schmitz N, Stroncek D, Howe C, Leitman S, Horowitz M, Gluckman E, et al. Allogeneic blood stem cell transplantation: considerations for donors (editorial). Blood 1997; 90(3):903–908.

75. Anderlini P, Przepiorka D, Seong D, Miller P, Sundberg J, Lichtiger B, Norfleet F, Chan K-W, Champlin R, Korbling M. Clinical toxicity, laboratory effects and analysis of charges for filgrastim mobilization and blood stem cell apheresis from normal donors. Transfusion 1996; 36:590–595.

76. Mavroudis D, Read E, Cottler-Fox M, Couriel D, Molldrem J, Carter C, Yu M, Dunbar C, Barrett J. CD34+ cell dose predicts survival, posttransplant morbidity, and rate of hematologic recovery after allogeneic marrow transplants for hematologic malignancies. Blood 1996; 88(8):3223–3229.

77. Moskowitz CH, Stiff P, Gordon MS, McNiece I, Ho AD, Costa JJ, Broun ER, Bayer RA, Wyres M, Hill J, et al. Recombinant methionyl human stem cell factor and filgrastim for peripheral blood progenitor cell mobilization and transplantation in non-Hodgkin's lymphoma patients–results of a phase I/II trial. Blood 1997; 89(9):3136–3147.

78. Mauch P, Lamont C, Neben TY, Quinto C, Goldman SJ, Witsell A. Hematopoietic stem cells in the blood after stem cell factor and interleukin-11 administration: evidence for different mechanisms of mobilization. Blood 1995; 86(12):4674–4680.

79. Glaspy, JA, Shpall, EJ, LeMaistre, CF, Briddell, RA, and others. Peripheral blood progenitor cell mobilization using stem cell factor in combination with filgrastim in breast cancer patients. Blood 1997; 90:2939–2951.

80. Huhn RD, Yurkow EJ, Tushinski R, Clarke L, Sturgill MG, Hoffman R, Sheay W, Cody R, Philipp C, Resta D, et al. Recombinant human interleukin-3 (rhIL-3) enhances the mobilization of peripheral blood progenitor cells by recombinant human granulocyte colony-stimulating factor (rhG-CSF) in normal volunteers. Exp Hematol 1996; 24(7):839–847.

81. Basser RL, Rasko JE, Clarke K, Cebon J, Green MD, Grigg AP, Zalcberg J, Cohen B, O'Byrne J, Menchaca DM, et al. Randomized, blinded, placebo-controlled phase I trial of pegylated recombinant human megakaryocyte growth and development factor with filgrastim after dose-intensive chemotherapy in patients with advanced cancer. Blood 1997; 89(9): 3118–3128.

82. Papayannopoulou T, Nakamoto B, Andrews RG, Lyman SD, Lee MY. In vivo effects of Flt3/Flk2 ligand on mobilization of hematopoietic progenitors in primates and potent synergistic enhancement with granulocyte colony-stimulating factor. Blood 1997; 90(2):620–629.

83. Geissler K, Peschel C, Niederwieser D, Strobl H, Goldschmitt J, Ohler L, Bettelheim P, Kahls P, Huber C, Lechner K, et al. Potentiation of granulocyte colony-stimulating factor-induced mobilization of circulating progenitor cells by seven-day pretreatment with interleukin-3. Blood 1996; 87(7):2732–2739.

84. Papayannopoulou T, Nakamoto B. Peripheralization of hemopoietic progenitors in primates treated with anti-VLA4 integrin. Proc Natl Acad Sci USA 1993; 90(20):9374–9378.

85. Craddock CF, Nakamoto B, Andrews RG, Priestley GV, Papayannopoulou T. Antibodies to VLA4 integrin mobilize long-term repopulating cells and augment cytokine-induced mobilization in primates and mice. Blood 1997; 90:4779–4788.

86. Ho AD, Young D, Maruyama M, Corringham RET, Mason JR, Grenier K, Law P, Terstappen LWMM, Lane T. Pluripotent and lineage committed CD34+ subsets in leukapheresis products mobilized by G-CSF, GM-CSF versus a combination of both. Exp Hematol 1996; 24: 1460–1468.

87. Gudi R. Astimizole in the treatment of granulocyte colony-stimulating factor–induced pain. Ann Intern Med 1995; 123:236–237.

88. Stroncek DF, Clay ME, Smith J, Ilstrup S, Oldham F, McCullough J. Changes in blood counts following the administration of G-CSF and the collection of peripheral blood stem cells from healthy donors. Transfusion 1996; 36:596–600.

89. Liles WC, Huang JE, Llewellyn C, SenGupta D, Price TH, Dale DC. A comparative trial of granulocyte-colony-stimulating factor and dexamethasone, separately and in combination, for the mobilization of neutrophils in the peripheral blood of normal volunteers. Transfusion 1997; 37(2):182–187.

90. Gabrilove JL, Jakubowski A, Fain K, Grous J, Scher H, Sternberg C, Yagoda A, Clarkson B, Bonilla MA, Oettgen HF, et al. Phase I study of granulocyte colony-stimulating factor in patients with transitional cell carcinoma of the urothelium. J Clin Invest 1988; 82(4): 1454–1461.

91. Sica S, Rutella S, Di Mario A, Salutari P, Rumi C, Ortu la Barbera E, Etuk B, Menichella G, D'Onofrio G, Leone G. rhG-CSF in healthy donors: mobilization of peripheral hemopoietic progenitors and effect on peripheral blood leukocytes. J Hematother 1996; 5(4):391–397.

92. Lindemann A, F Herrmann, W Oster, G Haffner, W Meyenburg, LM Souza, and R Mertels-mann. Hematologic effects of recombinant human granulocyte colony-stimulating factor in patients with malignancy Blood 1989; 74:2644–2651.

93. Hillyer CD. Tiegerman KO, Berkman EM: Increase in circulating colony-forming units-granulocyte-macrophage during large-volume leukapheresis: evaluation of a new cell separator. Transfusion 1991; 31:327.

94. Malachowski ME, Comenzo RL, Hillyer CD, Tiegerman KO, Berkman EM. Large-volume leukapheresis for peripheral blood stem cell collection in patients with hematologic malignancies. Transfusion 1992; 32:732.

95. Bensinger WI, Price TH, Dale DC, Appelbaum FR, Clift RC, Lilleby K, Williams B, Storb R, Thomas ED, Buckner CD. The effects of daily recombinant human granulocyte colony-stimulating-factor administration on normal granulocyte donors undergoing leukapheresis. Blood 1993; 81:1883–1888.

96. Stroncek D, Clay ME, Herr G, Smith J, Ilstrup S, McCullough J: Blood counts in healthy donors one year following the collection of granulocyte-colony-stimulating factor-mobilized progenitor cells and the results of a second mobilization and collection. Transfusion 1997; 37:304–308.

97. Stroncek DF, Holland PV, Bartch G, Bixby T, Simmons RG, Antin JH, Anderson KC, Ash RC, Bolwell BJ, Hansen JA, et al. Experiences of the first 493 unrelated marrow donors in the National Marrow Donor Program. Blood 1993; 81(7):1940–1946.

98. Rogers RL, Johnson H, Ludwig G, Winegarden D, Randels MJ, Strauss RG. Efficacy and safety of plateletpheresis by donors with low-normal platelet counts. J Clin Apheresis 1995; 10(4): 194–197.

99. Strauss RG. Mechanisms of adverse effects during hemapheresis. J Clin Apheresis 1996; 11(3):160–164.

100. Strauss RG. Effects on donors of repeated leukocyte losses during plateletpheresis. J Clin Apheresis 1994; 9(2):130–134.

101. Gutensohn K, Maerz M, Kuehnl P. Alteration of platelet-associated membrane glycoproteins during extracorporeal apheresis of peripheral blood progenitor cells. J Hematother 1997; 6(4): 315–321.

102. Anderlini P, Przepiorka D, Champlin R, Korbling M. Biologic and clinical effects of granulocyte colony-stimulating factor in normal individuals. Blood 1996; 88(8):2819–2825.

103. Anderlini P, Lauppe J, Przepiorka D, Seong D, Champlin R, Korbling M. Peripheral blood stem cell apheresis in normal donors: feasibility and yield of second collections. Br J Haemat 1997; 96(2):415–417.

104. Okamoto S, Ishida A, Wakui M, Tanosaki R, Oda A, Ikeda Y. Prolonged thrombocytopenia

after administration of granulocyte colony-stimulating factor and leukapheresis in a donor for allogeneic peripheral blood stem cell transplantation (letter). Bone Marrow Transplant 1996; 18(2):482–483.

105. Link H, Arseniev L, Bähre O, Kadar JG, Diedrich H, Poli-E H. Transplantation of allogeneic CD34/cells. Blood 1996; 87:4903.

106. Bensinger WI, Buckner CD, Shannon-Dorcy K, Rowley S, Appelbaum FR, Benyunes M, Clift R, Martin P, Demirer T, Storb R, Lee M, Schiller G. Transplantation of allogeneic CD34+ peripheral blood stem cells in patients with advanced hematologic malignancy. Blood 1997; 88:4132–4138.

107. Avenarius HJ, Freund M, Kleine HD, Heussner P, Poliwoda H. Granulocyte colony-stimulating factor enhances the expression of CD62 on platelets in vivo. Int J Hematol 1993; 58(3): 189–196.

108. Kuroiwa M, Okamura T, Kanaji T, Okamura S, Harada M, Niho Y. Effects of granulocyte colony-stimulating factor on the hemostatic system in healthy volunteers. Int J Hematol 1996; 63(4):311–316.

109. Shimoda K, Okamura S, Harada N, Kondo S, Okamura T, Niho Y. Identification of a functional receptor for granulocyte colony-stimulating factor on platelets. J Clin Invest 1993; 91(4):1310–1313.

110. Conti JA, Scher HI. Acute arterial thrombosis after escalated-dose methotrexate, vinblastine, doxorubicin, and cisplatin chemotherapy with recombinant granulocyte colony-stimulating factor. A possible new recombinant granulocyte colony-stimulating factor toxicity. Cancer 1992; 70(11):2699–2702.

111. Kawachi Y, Watanabe A, Uchida T, Yoshizawa K, Kurooka N, Setsu K. Acute arterial thrombosis due to platelet aggregation in a patient receiving granulocyte colony-stimulating factor. Br J Haematol 1996; 94(2):413–416.

112. Falanga A, Marchetti M, Oldani E, Giovanelli S, Barbui T: Changes of hemostatic parameters in healthy donors administered G-CSF for peripheral blood progenitor cells (PBPC) collection (abstr). Bone Marrow Transplant 1996; 17:S72.

113. Korbling M, Anderlini P, Durett A, Maadani F, Bojko P, Seong D, Giralt S, Khouri I, Andersson B, Mehra R, et al. Delayed effects of rhG-CSF mobilization treatment and apheresis on circulating CD34+ and CD34+ Thy-1dim CD38– progenitor cells, and lymphoid subsets in normal stem cell donors for allogeneic transplantation. Bone Marrow Transplantat 1996; 18(6):1073–1079.

114. Kadar JG, Arseniev L, Schnitger K, Sudmeier I, Zaki M, Battmer K, Jacobs R, Diedrich H, Poliwoda H, Stangel W, et al. Technical and safety aspects of blood and marrow transplantation using G-CSF mobilized family donors. Transfus Sci 1996; (4):611–618.

115. Becker PS, Wagle M, Matous S, Swanson RS, Pihan G, Lowry PA, Stewart FM, Heard SO. Spontaneous splenic rupture following administration of granulocyte colony-stimulating factor (G-CSF): occurrence in an allogeneic donor of peripheral blood stem cells. Biol Blood Marrow Transplant 1997; 3(1):45–49.

116. Huestis DW. Adverse effects in donors and patients subjected to hemapheresis. J Clin Apheresis 1984; 2(1):81–90.

117. Bensinger WI, Clift R, Martin P, Appelbaum FR, Demirer T, Gooley T, Lilleby K, Rowley S, Sanders J, Storb R, et al. Allogeneic peripheral blood stem cell transplantation in patients with advanced hematologic malignancies: a retrospective comparison with marrow transplantation. Blood 1996; 88(7):2794–2800.

118. Russell JA, Bowen T, Brown C, Luider J, Ruether JD, Stewart D, Jorgenson K, Coppes MJ, Turner AR, Larratt L, et al. Second allogeneic transplants for leukemia using blood instead of bone marrow as a source of hemopoietic cells. Bone Marrow Transplantation 1996; 18(3): 501–505.

119. Goldberg SL, Mangan KF, Klumpp TR, Macdonald JS, Thomas C, Mullaney MT, Au FC.

Complications of peripheral blood stem cell harvesting: review of 554 PBSC leukaphereses. J Hematother 1995: 4(2):85–90.

120. Alegre A, Requena MJ, Fernandez-Villalta MJ, Orts M, Gilsanz F, Tomas JF, Arranz R, Gil-Fernandez JJ, Granda A, Bernardo MR, et al. Quinton-Mahurkar catheter as short-term central venous access for PBSC collection: single-center experience of 370 aphereses in 110 patients. Bone Marrow Transplant 1996; 18(5):865–869.

121. Meisenberg BR, Callaghan M, Sloan C, Sampson L, Miller WE, McMillan R. Complications associated with central venous catheters used for the collection of peripheral blood progenitor cells to support high-dose chemotherapy and autologous stem cell rescue. Support Care Cancer 1997; 5(3):223–227.

123. Caspar CB, Seger RA, Burger J, Gmur J: Effective stimulation of donors for granulocyte transfusions with recombinant methionyl granulocyte colony-stimulating factor. Blood 1993; 81:2866–2871.

124. Kunkel LA, Samia SA, Ioli M, Tillman T, Chlebowski J, Schwartz M, Liggett A, Oldham FB. Normal donor follow-up after second cytokine mobilization of peripheral blood stem cells (abstr) Blood 1996; 88(suppl 1):398a.

125. Baer MR, Bernstein SH, Brunetto VL, Heinonen K, Mrozek K, Swann VL, Minderman H, Block AMW, Pixley LA, Christiansen NP, Fay JW, Barcos M, Rustum Y, Herzig GP, Bloomfield CD. Biological effects of recombinant human granulocyte colony-stimulating factor in patients with untreated acute myeloid leukemia. Blood 1996; 87:1484–1494.

126. Matsushita K, Arima N, Ohtsubo H, Fujiwara H, Hidaka S, Kukita T, Suruga Y, Fukumori J, Matsumoto T, Kanzaki A, et al. Granulocyte-colony stimulating factor-induced proliferation of primary adult T-cell leukaemia cells. Bri J Haematol 1997; 96(4):715–723.

127. Morstyn, G, Lieschke GJ, Sheridan W, Layton J, Cebon J, Fox RM. Clinical experience with recombinant human granulocyte colony-stimulating factor and granulocyte-macrophage colony -stimulating factor. Semin Hematol 1989; 26(suppl 2):9–13.

128. Kawakami M, Tsutsumi H, Kumakawa T, Abe H, Hirai M, Kurosawa S, Mori M, Fukushima M. Levels of serum granulocyte colony-stimulating factor in patients with infections. Blood 1990; 76:1962–1964.

129. Sakamaki S, Matsunaga T, Hirayama Y, Kuga T, Niitsu Y. Haematological study of healthy volunteers 5 years after G-CSF (letter). Lancet 1995; 346(8987):1432–1433.

130. Imashuku S, Hibi S, Nakajima F, Mitsui T, Yokoyama S, Kojima S, Matsuyama T, Nakahata T, Ueda K, Tsukimoto I, Hanawa Y, Takaku F. A review of 125 cases to determine the risk of myelo-dysplasia and leukemia in pediatric neutropenic patients after treatment with recombinant human granulocyte colony-stimulating factor (letter). Blood 1994; 84:2380–2381.

131. Freedman MH, Bonilla MA, Boxer L, Catalano P, Cham B, Fier C, Kannourakis G, Kinsey S, Mori PG, Shannon K, Touw I, Welte K, Dale DC. MDS/AML in patients with severe chronic neutropenia (SCN) receiving G-CSF (abstr). Blood 1996; 88(suppl 1):448a.

132. Kojima S, Tsuchida M, Matsuyama T. Myelodysplasia and leukemia after treatment of aplastic anemia with G-CSF (letter). N Engl J Med 1992; 326(19):1294–1295.

133. Bonilla MA, Dale D, Zeider C, et al. Long-term safety of treatment with recombinant human granulocyte colony-stimulating factor (R-metHuG-CSF) in patients with severe congenital neutropenias. Br J Haematol 1994; 88:723–730.

134. Dong F, Brynes RK, Tidow N, Welte K, Lowenberg B, Touw IP. Mutations in the gene for the granulocyte colony-stimulating-factor receptor in patients with acute myeloid leukemia preceded by severe congenital neutropenia (see comments). N Engl J Med 1995; 333(8): 487–493.

135. Imashuku S, Hibi S, Kataoka-Morimoto Y, Yoshihara T, Ikushima S, Morioka Y, Todo S. Myelodysplasia and acute myeloid leukaemia in cases of aplastic anaemia and congenital neutropenia following G-CSF administration. Br J Haematol 1995; 89(1):188–90.

136. Gilman, PA, Jackson, DP, Guild, HG. Congenital agranulocytosis: prolonged survival and terminal acute leukemia. Blood 1970; 36(5):576–585.

137. de Planque MM, Bacigalupo A, Wursch A, Hows JM, Devergie A, Frickhofen N, Brand A, Nissen C. Long-term follow-up of severe aplastic anaemia patients treated with antithymocyte globulin. Severe Aplastic Anaemia Working Party of the European Cooperative Group for Bone Marrow Transplantation (EBMT). Br J Haematol 1989; 73(1):121–126.

138. Hasenclever D, Sextro M. Safety of AlloPBPCT donors: biometrical considerations on monitoring long term risks. Bone Marrow Transplant 1996; 17(suppl 2):S28–30.

139. Bortin MM, D'Amaro J, Bach FH, Rimm AA, van Rood JJ. HLA associations with leukemia. Blood 1987; 70:227–232.

140. Gluckman E, Socie G, Guivarch C, Rabannes F, Meresse V, Henry-Amar. The long time forgotten HLA identical bone marrow donor: Result of a survey on 818 patients (abstr) Blood 1996; 88(suppl 1):612a.

141. Doney K, Buckner CD, Storb R. Marrow harvesting from donors >65 years of age (abstr). Exp Hematol 1995; 23:861a.

142. Parkkali T, Volin L, Siren MK, Ruutu T. Acute iritis induced by granulocyte colony-stimulating factor used for mobilization in a volunteer unrelated peripheral blood progenitor cell donor. Bone Marrow Transplant 1996; 7(3):433–434.

143. Fassas A, Anagnostopoulos A, Kazis A, Kapinas K, Sakellari I, Kimiskidis V, Tsompanakou A. Peripheral blood stem cell transplantation in the treatment of progressive multiple sclerosis: first results of a pilot study. Bone Marrow Transplant 1997; 20:631–638.

144. Damiani D, Fanin R, Silvestri F, Grimaz S, Infanti L, Geromin A, Cerno M, Michieli M, Rinaldi C, Savignano G, et al. Randomized trial of autologous filgrastim-primed bone marrow transplantation versus filgrastim-mobilized peripheral blood stem cell transplantation in lymphoma patients. Blood 1997; 90(1):36–42.

145. Majolino I, Saglio G, Scime R, Serra A, Cavallaro AM, Fiandaca T, Vasta S, Pampinella M, Catania P, Indovina A, et al. High incidence of chronic GVHD after primary allogeneic peripheral blood stem cell transplantation in patients with hematologic malignancies. Bone Marrow Transplant 1996; 17(4):555–560.

146. Urbano-Ispizua A, Rozman C, Martinez C, Marin P, Briones J, Rovira M, Feliz P, Viguria MC, Merino A, Sierra J, et al. Rapid engraftment without significant graft-versus-host disease after allogeneic transplantation of CD34+ selected cells from peripheral blood. Blood 1997; 89(11):3967–3973.

21

Innovative Approaches for Allogeneic
Blood and Marrow Transplantation for
Treatment of Hematological
Malignancies
Graft Engineering and Nonmyeloablative
Preparative Regimens

RICHARD E. CHAMPLIN

University of Texas M.D. Anderson Cancer Center, Houston, Texas

I. INTRODUCTION

The biological effects of allogeneic hematopoietic transplantation depend on the cellular composition of the graft. Hematopoietic stem and progenitor cells for transplantation can be obtained from bone marrow, mobilized peripheral blood, or cord blood. The goal for patients transplanted for malignancies is to achieve engraftment, develop the immune-mediated graft-versus-malignancy effect, whereas avoiding graft-versus-host disease (GVHD). This is a major challenge, since T cells participate in each of these processes and altering the composition of the graft may produce both positive and negative effects. Innovative technology is under evaluation to reduce the alloreactivity of the graft and for the later infusion of immunocompetent cells to enhance immunoreconstitution and graft-versus-leukemia (GVL).

GVHD results from reactivity of immunocompetent donor cells present in the hematopoietic graft against recipient (host) tissues. The pathophysiology is incompletely described, but it involves sensitization and expansion of donor alloreactive T cells, recruitment of natural killer (NK) cells and macrophages, and a final effector phase in which cytokine as well as cell-mediated tissue injury occurs (1). The development of GVHD requires T lymphocytes. CD4 and CD8$^+$ T cells initiate this process, with subsequent recruitment of NK cells and macrophages within affected tissues (2–4). The skin, liver, and gastrointestinal tract are the primary target tissues of GVHD. The thymus is also effected, and defective thymic function may contribute to the pathophysiology of GVHD. Cytokines produced by the infiltrating cells enhance the afferent and efferent phase of the graft-versus-host response, as well as contributing directly to tissue injury. Inflammatory cytokines, including interleukin-1, tumor necrosis factor, and interferon-γ appear to be important in this process (1,5).

II. T-CELL–DEPLETED HEMATOPOIETIC TRANSPLANTS

A logical approach to prevent GVHD is removal of the putative effector cells, immuno-competent T lymphocytes, from the donor bone marrow. In animals, pan–T-cell depletion effectively prevents GVHD across major or minor histocompatibility differences (2). Techniques which deplete CD3$^+$ T cells alone without targeting NK cells appear sufficient to prevent GVHD (6). Selective depletion of NK cells has also been reported to reduce GVHD in animals, but this has not been tested in humans (7).

A. Methods of T-Cell Depletion

Several techniques have been proposed for ex vivo depletion of T lymphocytes from human bone marrow transplants (6). These include physical depletion using soybean lectin agglutination or elutriation or immunological methods with monoclonal anti–T-cell antibodies either with complement, magnetic beads, or as immunotoxins. Ex vivo treatment of donor bone marrow with single or multiple anti–T-lymphocyte antibodies alone has been ineffective to reduce the incidence of GVHD indicating that opsonization of T cells, at least with the antibodies studied, is insufficient to prevent GVHD. Techniques that lyse or physically eliminate T lymphocytes from the donor bone marrow without damaging hematopoietic progenitors have been more effective (reviewed in Ref. (6). These antibodies are selected to be nonreactive with hematopoietic progenitors. Combinations of multiple antibodies have generally produced a greater reduction of T lymphocytes than single antibody treatments. Optimal physical or immunological techniques are capable of a 3- to 4-log reduction (99.9–99.99%). Antibody-based depletion methods which include or exclude NK cells have had similar results in the reduction of GVHD, although no controlled studies have been performed to address directly this issue (8). Recently, techniques for positive selection of CD34$^+$ cells have been developed as a means to eliminate passively T lymphocytes whereas retaining stem and progenitor cells necessary for reconstitution (9–13).

B. Results of T-Cell–Depleted Transplants

Depletion of T cells from the transplanted marrow is effective to prevent GVHD across both major and minor histocompatibility barriers (6). When engraftment occurs, hematopoietic recovery is prompt and immune reconstitution occurs from undifferentiated progenitors or pre–T cells present within the graft. The kinetics of immune reconstitution are similar as with unmodified transplants (14). Pan–T-cell depletion markedly reduces the incidence and severity of both acute and chronic GVHD. The incidence of acute GVHD is related to the number of residual T cells or their precursors present in the transplanted marrow (15). Its occurrence in some studies probably relates to incomplete reduction in the number of T cells. Acute GVHD generally does not occur if less than 10^5 T cells/kg are infused in patients with an HLA-identical sibling donor. With transplantation of unmodified bone marrow, approximately 35% of patients receiving optimal immunosuppressive therapy develop moderate to severe acute GVHD (16). In contrast, 0–15% of patients develop acute GVHD after T-cell–depleted transplants; if GVHD occurs, it is usually mild in severity. Addition of posttransplant immunosuppression such as cyclosporine and methotrexate further reduces acute GVHD (8); this is probably necessary if subtotal T-cell depletion is used. T-cell depletion is a notable advance, since no other form of treatment has effectively prevented the development of both acute and chronic GVHD. Acute GVHD is more common in recipients of HLA-nonidentical and unrelated donor transplants and is inadequately controlled by systemic immunosuppressive therapy; T-cell depletion significantly reduces the risk of GVHD in these patients (17).

The risk of graft rejection is increased in T-cell–depleted transplants (18,19). High doses of total body irradiation do not completely ablate host immunity; viable T and NK cells persist after the preparative regimen which can mediate graft rejection (20). Rejection can often be overcome by higher doses of CD34$^+$ cells or intensification of the immunosuppressive conditioning regimen (21). In humans, it is not possible to increase substantially the cell dose harvested from volunteer donors; most centers attempt to collect >1500 mL prior to T-cell depletion to optimize the cell dose. Recently, the use of mobilized peripheral blood has been studied as a means to increase the CD34$^+$ cell dose (22,23). Peripheral blood contains approximately 1 log more T cells than marrow, and more efficient depletion of T cells is required to avoid GVHD. Ideally CD34$^+$ cell doses should exceed 6×10^6/kg (22). Engraftment is also favored with more intensive radiotherapy, such as higher doses of external radiation, administration of single-dose or large fractions, or addition of splenic radiation (24). Addition of busulfan or thiotepa enhance engraftment of T-cell–depleted transplants; these agents provide little immunosuppression but produce more complete ablation of host hematopoiesis. There is an interaction between the intensity of conditioning, the transplanted stem/progenitor cell dose, and the T-cell content of the marrow. Low cell doses are sufficient in the presence of T cells or with very intensive conditioning. Higher cell doses are required if the marrow is thoroughly depleted of T lymphocytes.

Engraftment is enhanced by the presence of facilitating cells in the graft. Transplantation of purified stem cells in the mouse generally fail to engraft across a major histocompatibility barrier (18). T cells are important facilitators of engraftment. The mechanisms by which T cells enhance engraftment are not completely understood. T cells may act via a graft-versus-host effect ablating residual host T cells and NK cells. However, T cells enhance engraftment even in F1 mice transplanted into parental strains in which GVHD does not occur (25,26). CD8$^+$ cells appear to be important to facilitate engraftment (27,28). Growth factors or lymphokines produced by T cells may contribute to engraftment, although the T-cell effect cannot be replaced with any known cytokine. A novel cell population of CD8$^+$ cells which do not express alpha/beta or gamma/delta T-cell receptors has been shown to facilitate engraftment in mice without producing GVHD (29); similar cells have been identified in humans (30), and clinical trials are ongoing to determine if this cell population can enhance engraftment of T-cell–depleted human hematopoietic transplants.

In humans, the risk of graft failure is approximately 2% in recipients transplanted for leukemia using unmodified bone marrow from an HLA-identical sibling donor. In contrast, 10–20% of patients receiving T-lymphocyte–depleted bone marrow transplants have had graft failure (8). Graft failure has occurred in two clinical patterns; some patients fail to have any evidence of engraftment, whereas others have hematological recovery only to experience graft failure leading to marrow aplasia. Most cases of graft failure following T-cell–depleted transplants are due to immunological rejection. Host T lymphocytes have been described that react against donor major or minor histocompatibility antigens. Less commonly, NK cells have been implicated (31–33). Single dose or large-fraction total body irradiation (TBI), higher doses of radiation, or addition of total lymphoid radiation, cytarabine (ara-C), or thiotepa in combination cyclophosphamide/TBI preparative regimen are reported to favor engraftment. It is not well established that the commonly used busulfan-cyclophosphamide preparative regimen will reliably allow engraftment of T-cell–depleted transplants.

C. Innovative Approaches to Improve Results of T-Cell–Depleted Transplants

A number of novel approaches to ex vivo treatment have been proposed to improve the results of transplants for leukemia (Table 1). The major problems which need to be addressed are graft failure, GVHD, and recurrent leukemia. One approach is to employ an intensified more effective pretransplant preparative regimen in hope of overcoming resistance to engraftment and providing a greater antileukemic activity. Preliminary data suggest that administration of a higher dose of TBI (13.5–15.75 Gy) or addition of total lymphoid irradiation may be associated with a lower risk of graft failure (6,34,35). Intensification of the conditioning therapy is limited by nonhematopoietic toxicity, and although many centers are actively evaluating this approach, no intensified regimen has been documented to improve overall results. Preliminary data suggest that addition of antithymocyte globulin or thiotepa to the preparative regimen may reduce graft failure (36).

It is possible that a less complete depletion technique which spares a small number of T lymphocytes may allow engraftment and still reduce GVHD (37). It is likely that the threshold dose of T cells will vary among patients depending on the degree of genetic disparity and the major and minor histocompatibility differences present. Thus, it seems unlikely that an optimal T-cell dose for all patients can be defined in the absence of a more thorough understanding of the pathogenesis of GVHD, engraftment, and GVL. Subtotal depletion of T cells might be beneficial if combined with posttransplant immunosuppressive therapy. Preliminary studies suggest favorable results with a 1.5- to 2-log T-cell depletion followed by systemic therapy with cyclosporine in patients with matched sibling donors or HLA-matched unrelated donors (38,39). More complete T-cell depletion is necessary to prevent GVHD for HLA-mismatched blood stem cell or marrow transplants.

Table 1 Innovative Approaches for Ex Vivo Treatment of Allogeneic Transplants to Prevent GVHD

Prevent rejection of T-cell–depleted transplants by intensified conditioning or biological therapies.

Transplant high doses of T-cell–depleted hematopoietic stem/progenitor cells to enhance engraftment.

Induce anergy in the allograft against recipient tissue antigens.

Add or retain graft facilitating cells to enhance engraftment.

T-cell–depleted transplants followed by delayed add back of T cells to mediate GVL.

Bone marrow harvest results in a suboptimal cell dose for T-cell–depleted transplants. One can markedly increase the cell dose by combining marrow with cytokine-mobilized peripheral blood cells collected by apheresis. Following granulocyte colony-stimulating factor (G-CSF) treatment, normal donors markedly mobilize progenitor cells into the peripheral blood (40,41). The most encouraging approach for haploidentical transplantation utilizes high doses of allogeneic peripheral blood stem cells to maximize the progenitor dose with T-cell depletion and/or CD34 selection to achieve engraftment, whereas reducing T cells below the threshold to produce GVHD. This strategy has been effective to achieve engraftment with a low rate of GVHD (21,22). An alternative strategy for HLA-mismatched transplants involves inducing anergy in the donor graft. Cocultivation of irradiated host cells with the donor bone marrow graft in the presence of CTLA4-Ig blocks costimulation through the CD28-B7 pathway act to induce anergy against host but not third-party antigens (42,43).

D. Cord Blood Transplantation

Cord blood transplants have been proposed as an alternative to bone marrow or peripheral blood. Cord blood contains a relatively small fraction of cells, but the stem/progenitor cells have a high proliferative potential (44,45). The numbers of T cells are relatively low and may have a reduced potential to induce GVHD. Preliminary studies of cord blood transplantation has been successful in achieving engraftment and reconstitution with a relatively low rate of GVHD even in recipients mismatched for one or two HLA loci (46–49). The tempo of hematological recovery is dependent on the dose of CD34$^+$ cells and is substantially slower than with marrow or peripheral blood stem cell grafts. Survival has been largely dependent on the cell dose and CD34$^+$ dose/kg recipient body weight and have been substantially better in children than in adult recipients.

III. GRAFT-VERSUS-MALIGNANCY EFFECT

An immune-mediated graft-versus-malignancy effect may after allogeneic hematopoietic transplants. This is best established against hematological malignancies and is often referred to generically as graft-versus-leukemia (GVL). Considerable data support the presence of a GVL effect (Table 2). This includes the reduced risk of leukemia relapse in

Table 2 Evidence Supporting an Allogeneic Graft-Versus-Leukemia Effect

Demonstration of minimal residual disease present
  early after high-dose therapy
Reduced risk of relapse in patients with acute and
  chronic GVHD
Increased risk of relapse after syngeneic transplants
Increased risk of relapse after T-cell–depleted
  transplants
Induction of remission by donor lymphocyte infusion
  in patients relapsing post-BMT
Demonstration of reactivity of donor-derived T-cell
  clones against malignant cells

BMT, bone marrow transplantation.

patients with acute and chronic graft-versus-host disease (50–53), a higher risk of leukemia relapse after syngeneic bone marrow transplantation (54–56), and higher relapse rates after T-cell–depleted transplants (8,52). The most direct evidence of GVL is the observation that many patients who relapse after allogeneic transplantation can be reinduced into complete remission by infusing additional donor lymphocytes (57–59).

Hematological malignancies differ in their susceptibility to GVL effects. The risk of relapse is increased with syngeneic transplants in both acute myclogenous leukemia (AML) and chronic myclogenous leukemia (CML) suggesting that allogeneic target antigens are involved (52). T lymphocytes appear most important in CML where T-cell–depleted transplants are associated in a fivefold increase in the risk of leukemia relapse (8,52,60,61). GVL has been best studied in patients with CML. High-dose chemoradiotherapy generally does not eradicate the malignancy; minimal residual disease can be detected in most patients by polymerase chain reaction analysis of *bcr-abl* gene rearrangement or by cytogenetic techniques (62–66). These cells are later eliminated in most patients receiving unmodified marrow transplants, presumably due to the GVL effect. In patients receiving syngeneic or T-cell–depleted transplants, the residual leukemia generally proliferates, producing relapse. Patients relapsing can be reinduced into bcr-abl–negative complete remissions with donor lymphocyte infusions (67,68).

In AML, the relapse rate is only minimally affected by T-cell depletion and NK cells have been suggested as mediators of antileukemic activity (8,69). Acute lymphocytic leukemia (ALL) appears to be least affected by GVL (8,52,55), possibly due to the limited capacity of the leukemic lymphoblasts to stimulate an effective immune response (70,71).

Approximately 70% patients relapsing into chronic phase achieve complete remission following donor lymphocyte infusion (57,58,72,73). Similar results have been achieved with HLA-identical sibling or matched unrelated donors (74). The best results occur with relapses into the chronic phase and when infusions are administered early in the course of relapse (67). In responding patients, residual leukemia becomes undetectable by polymerase chain reaction analysis for bcr-abl rearrangement, and these responses are generally durable. Approximately one third of AML or myelodysplasia patients respond, but these remissions are generally transient, and patients typically recur within the following year. Only rare patients with ALL have benefited. Small numbers of patients with juvenile CML (75) or myelodysplastic syndrome have been reported to respond (76,77). Graft-vs-malignancy responses also affect lymphoid malignancies. Selected patients with CLL (78), lymphoma (79,80), and multiple myeloma (81–83) have also responded to donor lymphocyte infusions or modification of immunosuppressive therapy.

Following engraftment of an allogeneic transplant, immune reconstitution generally occurs exclusively from donor-derived immunocompetent cells. In patients who relapse, there is no effective immune suppression of the malignancy. This may be in part due to immunosuppressive therapy, an inadequate number of cytotoxic precursors in the original graft or induction of tolerance during the period of immune reconstitution. This unresponsive state can be overcome by infusion of fresh donor lymphocytes capable of responding against the malignant cells.

A. Target Antigens of Graft-Versus-Malignancy

The target antigens of graft-vs-malignancy responses are not clearly defined. The relationship between GVL and GVHD suggests that these may be alloantigens shared by the malignant cells and the visceral tissues involved with GVHD. Patients may achieve a

GVL response, that is, remission of their leukemia, without developing GVHD following donor lymphocyte infusion. Although this is consistent with the premise that different target antigens may be involved with each process, it could also result from greater sensitivity of leukemic cells than visceral tissues to a common immunological mechanism.

Selective GVL activity could also be due to reactivity against polymorphic hematopoietic lineage-related antigens or leukemia-specific targets. Minor histocompatibility antigens restricted to hematopoietic tissues have been described (84–91). Donor-derived T-cell clones from allogeneic chimeras typically react against both host normal hematopoietic cells and the leukemia (92–96). Although candidate leukemia-specific target antigens have been proposed, for example, such as the fusion peptides bcr-abl in CML, promyelocytic leukemia (PML)/retinoic acid receptor-alpha in PML leukemia, there is little evidence to suggest that a leukemia-specific response in GVL reactions after allogeneic transplantation. Over- or abnormally expressed cellular constituents could also serve as a target antigen for GVL. Proteinase-3, a serine protease present in myeloid primary granules, is overexpressed in CML and in some cases of AML; it may serve as a target for an antileukemic immune response. Peptide antigens derived from proteinase-3 can stimulate generation of autologous or allogeneic T-cell cytotoxicity against the leukemia (97,98).

It is uncertain whether graft-versus-tumor effects occur against nonhematopoietic malignancies. Pilot studies in patients with breast cancer have reported antitumor responses in patients with graft-versus-host disease suggesting a graft-versus-adenocarcinoma effect (99,100). Further studies are required to determine if immunodominant tissue-restricted minor histocompatibility antigens are present in nonhematopoietic tumors and whether a clinically meaningful graft-versus-tumor effect will occur in order to justify the added morbidity related to allogeneic transplantation.

B. Effector Cells of Graft-Versus-Malignancy

The effector cells involved with GVHD and GVL are incompletely defined. Both $CD4^+$ and $CD8^+$ T cells participate in the initiation of GVHD; other cell populations, including NK cells, are subsequently recruited and cytokines participate as mediators of tissue injury (1–3, 101–103). In animal models of leukemia, both $CD4^+$ and $CD8^+$ effectors have been described. In many systems, $CD8^+$ cells appear to be the principal effectors of GVL (92,96,104–107). In human bone marrow transplantation (BMT) recipients, both $CD4^+$ and $CD8^+$ cytotoxic antileukemic T-cell lines or clones have been described. In patients transplanted for CML, several recent studies have identified $CD4^+$ T-cell lines or clones which either inhibit the growth of leukemia progenitors or are directly lytic (94,96,108,109). NK cells have also been implicated as mediators of GVL effects (107,110–113).

C. Donor Lymphocyte Infusion to Induce Graft-Versus-Malignancy

In patients relapsing after bone marrow transplantation, the leukemia typically recurs in host-derived cells, but residual normal hematopoiesis and immunity remain largely donor derived. The infused donor lymphocytes are, therefore, not subject to rejection, but acute GVHD is a major problem. In initial studies, patients generally received large doses of T cells, generally $>5 \times 10^7$ T cells/kg and acute GVHD developed in 50–80% of cases, with mortality in up to 20% of recipients. After infusion of donor lymphocytes, there is initially little change in peripheral blood counts, but after a median of 4 months, responding patients may suddenly become hypoplastic followed by recovery from donor-derived hematopoietic cells and return to complete chimerism (57,58,114). Antileukemic effectors presumably proliferate in vivo following the infusion and presumably must reach a threshold level to eradicate the leukemia and normal hematopoietic cells that are host derived (115). Marrow aplasia may occur unless sufficient donor-derived normal progenitors are present to restore hematopoiesis (116) Consistent with this premise, CML patients with advanced relapse more frequently develop marrow aplasia than patients treated in cytogenetic or early hematological relapse (67). Patients developing aplasia generally recover after a second infusion of donor hematopoietic stem cells from either marrow of mobilized peripheral blood. A critical factor following donor lymphocyte infusion is the kinetics of growth of the leukemia; rapid regrowth may out pace the development of an effective immune antileukemic response.

A major challenge is to separate the beneficial GVL effect from the adverse manifestations of GVHD. A number of approaches have been studied, as indicated in Table 3.

There is a dose-response effect with higher rates of GVHD as well as antileukemia responses with increasing doses of T cells (68). MacKinnon et al. performed a study administering graded doses of T cells to patients with CML relapsing into chronic phase after an allogeneic transplant from an HLA-identical sibling. A starting dose of 10^5 T cells/kg was administered. Patients failing to respond received progressively higher doses after a median of 2 months. Antileukemic responses and GVHD did not occur at doses of 10^5 to 5×10^6 T cells/kg. Of 21 patients receiving 10^7 T cells/kg, 8 achieved clinical remission (CR) and only one developed acute GVHD. At higher doses there were additional responses but a much increased risk of GVHD. Thus, it may be possible to induce antileukemic responses at a T-cell dose below the threshold necessary to product GVHD. This general approach has been confirmed by others (73,117).

An alternative strategy is to infuse T-cell subpopulations which can mediate GVL with a reduced potential for GVHD. Selective depletion of $CD8^+$ cells from the allogeneic donor marrow transplants reduces the incidence of GVHD without increasing the risk of relapse in CML (118–120). Donor lymphocyte infusions using CD8-depleted cells have also been effective to reinduce remission in patients with CML and multiple myeloma with a low rate of GVHD (121,122). At the M.D. Anderson Cancer Center, 18 patients with relapsed CML have been treated. At the time of the original transplant, 15 were in chronic phase and 3 in blast crisis. Thirteen patients received marrow from their HLA-identical sibling and five received marrow from matched unrelated donors. The median time from relapse to donor lymphocyte infusion (DLI) was 138 days (range 14–2876). Eleven patients had failed prior interferon with or without other agents. At the time of infusion, five patients were in isolated cytogenetic relapse, seven in chronic phase, three in clinical accelerated phase, and three in blast crisis. The median number of mononuclear cells infused was 0.6×10^8 mononuclear cells/kg. After depletion of $CD8^+$ cells, the

Table 3 Separation of Graft-Versus-Leukemia from Graft-Versus-Host Disease

Administration of repeated low doses of T cells
Separate GVL from GVHD effector cells, depletion of
  $CD8^+$ cells
Transduction of donor lymphocytes with suicide gene
Administration of nonalloreactive T cells
Administration of antigen specific T cells

median lymphocyte content infused was 3.14×10^7 CD3$^+$ cells/kg, 3.08×10^7 CD4$^+$ cells/kg, 3.0×10^5 CD8$^+$ cells/kg, and 4.7×10^6 CD56$^+$ cells/kg. Eleven patients achieved complete hematological and cytogenetic remissions a median of 98 days post-DLI. One patient relapsed after 14 months and responded to a second CD8-depleted infusion. Acute GVHD occurred in two patients, both grade 3 and responding to steroids. Two patients developed chronic GVHD. Eleven patients are alive a median of 2.5 years postinfusion. These data indicate that donor lymphocyte infusions depleted of CD8$^+$ cells are effective to induce remission in patients with CML relapsing posttransplant with a relatively low rate of acute GVHD. Further study is required to determine the optimal cell dose and to compare the relative effectiveness of CD8-depleted DLI with graded doses of unfractionated lymphocytes.

GVHD is initiated by alloreactive T cells. A novel strategy to prevent GVHD is to transduce donor T cells with a suicide gene, such as Herpes simplex virus thymidine kinase (TK), which renders the cells sensitive to ganciclovir treatment. This approach has been successful in pilot studies using TK-transduced T cells for donor lymphocyte infusions (123) or combining TK-transduced lymphocytes with T-cell–depleted marrow transplants (124,125). In each setting, acute GVHD could be successfully treated with ganciclovir. The ex vivo transduction and expansion procedure may change the composition and immune reactivity of the cells and the ultimate therapeutic efficacy must be established. This approach requires further evaluation in both animal models and human clinical trials.

Generation of nonalloreactive T cells is another potential approach to separate GVL from GVHD. Alloreactive cells stimulated in a mixed lymphocyte culture can be depleted by treatment of the cells with an immunotoxin targeting activation antigens such as the IL-2 receptor or CD69 (126–128). The remaining nonactivated cells have a reduced potential to produce GVHD, yet may retain reactivity against infectious organisms and, possibly, the malignancy. Another strategy involves generation of nonalloreactive cells by sublethal radiation treatment; in preliminary studies, this prevents their proliferation, yet retention of cytokine production and some function (129).

An ideal cellular therapy would consist of antigen-specific effectors, reactive with the malignancy or relevant infections, but devoid of graft-versus-host activity. T-cell clones or lines have been successfully used for treatment of Epstein-Barr virus (130) and cytomegalovirus (131) infections after allogeneic bone marrow transplantation. Falkenburg et al. reported a single case of a patient with CML who relapsed after allogeneic transplantation and failed to respond to donor lymphocyte infusions (85,132). As an alternative strategy, cytotoxic T lymphocytes specific for malignancy-related peptide antigens could be selected, expanded, and parenterally administered as adoptive cellular therapy. Finally, generation of T cells reactive with hematopoietic lineage restricted minor histocompatibility antigens may selectively eliminate host normal and leukemic cells without impairing donor-derived hematopoiesis or immunity (133).

The effectiveness of donor lymphocyte infusions in patients susceptible to GVL suggests a strategy of an initial T-cell–depleted transplant to achieve engraftment without GVHD with subsequent infusion of effector cells to induce GVL effects. Clinical trials using this approach are ongoing (134,135).

D. Induction of GVL Using Nonmyeloablative Preparative Regimens

The high-dose chemotherapy and radiation typically used as the preparative regimen for bone marrow transplantation produces considerable morbidity and mortality and limits the use of this modality to a minority of patients who are young and in good general medical condition. The data described above indicate that the GVL effect alone can cure susceptible diseases. An alternative strategy is to utilize a lower dose, nonmyeloablative, preparative regimen designed to provide sufficient immunosuppression to achieve engraftment of an allogeneic hematopoietic transplant, allowing for subsequent development of a graft-versus-malignancy effect.

At the M.D. Anderson Cancer Center, we evaluated this strategy by using relatively nontoxic, "standard dose" chemotherapy as a nonmyeloablative preparative regimen for allogeneic marrow or blood progenitor cell transplantation using chemotherapy regimens active against the patient's malignancy which are only modestly myelosuppressive without marrow transplantation. This approach allows treatment of older patients and those with comorbidities who were considered ineligible for high-dose myeloablative preparative regimens. Following engraftment, patients may receive additional donor lymphocytes as necessary to augment the graft-versus-malignancy effects.

The hypothesis underlying this treatment strategy is that less intensive preparative regimens would be associated with decreased regimen related toxicity. This would also be expected to produce less severe acute GVHD, since the clinical manifestations partly result from the toxicity of the preparative regimen and subsequent cytokine production in addition to the alloreactivity of the transplanted cells (136,137). In the initial studies, standard posttransplant immunosuppression using cyclosporine or tacrolimus-based immunosuppression was used; 3 of 15 patients transplanted from an HLA-identical sibling developed grade $\geq$ 2 acute GVHD (138). Chronic GVHD may also occur. Separation of graft-versus-malignancy effects from GVHD remains a major challenge.

Purine analogue (fludarabine or cladribine) containing nonmyeloablative chemotherapy is sufficiently immunosuppressive to allow engraftment of HLA-compatible hematopoietic progenitor cells, and extended remissions were observed in some patients with CML (139) or recurrent AML (138). Giralt et al. reported a study combining melphalan (180 mg/m^2) and either fludarabine (125 mg/m^2) or cladribine (60 mg/m^2) for treatment of advanced acute leukemia; patients with refractory relapse usually recurred rapidly, but 56% of patients with chemotherapy-sensitive disease remained in continuous remission beyond 1 year (140). Storb et al. reported an alternative strategy using a nonablative, low-dose total body irradiation regimen followed by cyclosporine and mycophenolate mofetil as a means to achieve engraftment and mixed chimerism (141), which can be converted to complete chimerism with GVL effects by subsequent donor lymphocyte infusion.

Indolent lymphoid malignancies also appear to be amenable to this strategy. Khouri et al. treated 15 heavily pretreated patients with chronic lymphocytic leukemia (CLL) or lymphoma using a nonmyeloablative regimen of fludarabine/cyclophosphamide or fludarabine, cytarabine, and cisplatin (142). Eleven of the 15 patients had durable engraftment, with 50–100% donor cells at 1 month posttransplant, typically converting to 100% over the next 2 months spontaneously or after infusion of additional donor lymphocytes. Hematopoietic recovery was prompt and nonhematological toxicity of greater than grade 2 did not occur. Patients failing to engraft recovered endogenous hematopoiesis promptly. All 11 patients with engraftment have responded, and 8 achieved complete remission. Maximal responses were slow to develop and gradually occur over a period of several months to 1 year.

Allogeneic bone marrow transplantation is associated with a high risk of treatment-related mortality in multiple myeloma; up to 70% in some series (143,144). The strategy of a nonablative preparative regimen may reduce this morbidity while still harnessing a graft-versus-myeloma effect while reducing regimen related toxicities. We are exploring this using a regimen of melphalan (140 mg/m^2) and fludarabine (30 mg/m^2 for 4 days). This appears to be a promising strategy; 7 of 13 patients with far advanced myeloma have achieved complete remission (145).

The use of nonablative regimens is not appropriate in many settings. This strategy is only useful in diseases susceptible to graft-versus-malignancy effects. Success also requires development of an effective GVL effect before the underlying disease can progress. This approach has generally been unsuccessful in patients with active, aggressive malignancies such as refractory acute leukemias. In these cases, the malignancy may recur rapidly after a nonablative regimen, out pacing generation of graft-versus-malignancy effects. Nonablative regimens may be useful, however, for consolidation of remission in AML patients at high risk to relapse. Indolent malignancies which are not immediately life threatening appear to be the best candidates for this strategy; responses developing over several months can be effective in relatively stable patients with CML in chronic phase or low-grade lymphoid malignancies.

Slavin and coworkers reported the use of a more intensive preparative regimen consisting of busulfan 8 mg/kg, fludarabine, and antithymocyte globulin with encouraging preliminary results (146). Although less intensive and less toxic than commonly used ablative preparative regimens, this regimen produces marked myelosuppression and has not been administered without hematopoietic transplantation. Other lower dose or nonablative regimens have been proposed (147).

The optimal intensity of the preparative regimen depends on several factors, including aggressiveness of the underlying malignancy, immunocompetence of the recipient, and genetic disparity between donor and recipient. Immunocompromised patients, such as those with advanced CLL, require less intensive immunosuppressive therapy to achieve engraftment than a fully immunocompetent recipient. Nonablative regimens have generally been studied in patients with an HLA-identical related or unrelated donor. Greater immunosuppression will be required for engraftment of HLA-nonidentical or unrelated transplants, and nonablative regimens have not been effective in achieving engraftment in histoincompatible recipients. Indolent malignancies may not require major cytoreduction, but more cytoreduction is necessary to achieve at least a short-term remission in patients with highly proliferative malignancies, such as acute leukemias and aggressive lymphomas, to allow development of an effective GVL response. The optimal posttransplant immunosuppressive therapy is also uncertain. Acute GVHD does occur with these nonablative regimens but has been relatively mild and controllable. Immunosuppressive therapy given early posttransplant to prevent GVHD likely also inhibits GVL (148). Effective strategies to separate GVHD from GVL are critical for the success of this approach to treatment.

IV. CONCLUSION

Allogeneic hematopoietic transplants are an effective treatment for a broad range of hematological malignancies. Hematopoietic transplantation allows administration of high-dose myelosuppressive therapy, and the allograft also produces an immune graft-versus-malignancy effect. The cellular composition of the allograft determines its biological effects. The goal of ongoing research is to improve the efficacy, whereas reducing the morbidity of allogeneic transplantation procedures. T-cell depletion strategies are a promising approach for patients lacking an HLA-identical sibling. The use of less toxic, nonmyeloablative preparative regimens allows engraftment and generation of graft-versus-malignancy effects. This approach allows the use of allotransplantation for older patients and those with comorbidities which preclude high-dose chemoradiotherapy. Further clinical trials are required to define the relative efficacy of these strategies versus alternative forms of treatment.

REFERENCES

1. Ferrara JLM, Deeg HJ. Mechanisms of disease: graft-versus-host disease. N Engl J Med 1991; 324:667–674.
2. Korngold R, Sprent J. T cell subsets and graft-versus-host disease. Transplantation 1987; 44:335–339.
3. Ferrara JLM, Guillen FJ, vanDijken PJ, Marion A, Murphy GF, Burakoff SJ. Evidence that large granular lymphocytes of donor origin mediate acute graft-versus-host disease. Transplant 1989; 47:50–54.
4. Ferrara JLM. Advances in GVHD: novel lymphocyte subsets and cytokine dysregulation. Bone Marrow Transplant 1992; 10(Suppl)1:10–12.
5. Ferrara JLM. Cytokine dysregulation as a mechanism of graft versus host disease. Curr Opin Immunol. 1993; 5:794–799.
6. Champlin RE. T-cell depletion for allogeneic bone marrow transplantation: impact on graft-versus-host disease, engraftment, and graft-versus-leukemia. J Hematother 1993; 2:27–42.
7. Johnson BD, Truitt RL. A decrease in graft-vs.-host disease without loss of graft-vs.-leukemia reactivity after MHC-matched bone marrow transplantation by selective depletion of donor NK cells in vivo. Transplantation 1992; 54:104–112.
8. Marmont AM, Horowitz MM, Gale RP, Sobocinski K, Ash RC, van Bekkum DW, Champlin RE, Dicke KA, Goldman JM, Good RA, Herzig RH, Hong R, Masaoka T, Rimm AA, Ringdén O, Speck B, Weiner RS, Bortin MM. T-cell depletion of HLA-identical transplants in leukemia. Blood 1991; 78:2120–30.
9. Andrews RG, Bryant EM, Bartelmez SH, Muirhead DY, Knitter GH, Bensinger W, Strong DM, Bernstein ID, CD34+ marrow cells, devoid of T and B lymphocytes, reconstitute stable lymphopoiesis and myelopoiesis in lethally irradiated allogeneic baboons. Blood 1992; 80: 1693–1701.
10. Bensinger WI, Buckner CD, Shannon-Dorcy K, Rowley S, Appelbaum FR, Benyunes M, Clift R, Martin P, Demirer T, Storb R, Lee M, Schiller G. Transplantation of allogeneic CD34+ peripheral blood stem cells in patients with advanced hematologic malignancy. Blood 1996; 88(11):4132–4138.
11. Civin CI, Almeida-Porada G, Lee MJ, Olweus J, Terstappen LWMM, Zanjani ED. Sustained, retransplantable, multilineage engraftment of highly purified adult human bone marrow stem cells in vivo. Blood 1996; 88:4102–4109.
12. Berenson RJ, Bensinger WI, Hill RS, Andrews RG, Garcia-Lopez J, Kalamasz DF, Still BJ, Spitzer G, Buckner CD, Bernstein ID. Engraftment after infusion of CD34+ marrow cells in patients with breast cancer or neuroblastoma. Blood 1991; 77:1717–1722.
13. Urbano-Ispizua A, Rozman C, Martínez C, Marín P, Briones J, Rovira M, Féliz P, Viguria MC, Merino A, Sierra J, Mazzara R, Carreras E, Montserrat E. Rapid engraftment without significant graft-versus-host disease after allogeneic transplantation of CD34+ selected cells from peripheral blood. Blood 1997; 89:3967–3973.
14. Keever CA, Small TN, Flomenberg N, Heller G, Pekle K, Black P, Pecora A, Gillio A, Kernan NA, O'Reilly RJ. Immune reconstitution following bone marrow transplantation: Comparison of recipients of T-cell depleted marrow with recipients of conventional marrow grafts. Blood 1989; 73:1340–1350.
15. Kernan NA, Collins NH, Juliano L, et al. Cloneable T-lymphocytes in t-cell depleted bone

marrow transplants correlate with development of graft-versus-host disease. Blood 1986; 68: 770.

16. Storb R, Pepe M, Deeg HJ, Anasetti C, Appelbaum FR, Bensinger W, Buckner CD, Clift RA, Doney K, Hansen J, Martin P, Pettinger M, Sanders JE, Singer J, Stewart P, Sullivan KM, Thomas ED, Witherspoon RP. Long-term follow-up of a controlled trial comparing a combination of methotrexate plus cyclosporine with cyclosporine alone for prophylaxis of graft-versus-host disease in patients administered HLA-identical marrow grafts for leukemia. Blood 1992; 80:560–561.

17. Gajewski J, Gjertson D, Cecka M, Tonai R, Przepiorka D, Giralt S, Chan KW, Feig S, Territo M, Andersson B, Van Besien K, Khouri I, Fischer H, Babbitt L, Hunt L, Schiller G, Petz L, Terasaki P, Champlin RE. Impact of molecular subtype of HLA DR and DQ alleles on acute graft-vs.-host disease and relapse free survival in HLA serologically identical unrelated donor bone marrow transplants: effect of T-cell depletion. Biol Blood Marrow Transplant 1997; 3:76–82.

18. Shizuru JA, Jerabek L, Edwards CT, Weissman IL. Transplantation of purified hematopoietic stem cells: requirements for overcoming the barriers of allogeneic engraftment. Biol Blood Marrow Transplant. 1996; 2:3–14.

19. Mitsuyasu R, Champlin RE, Gale RP, Ho WG, Lanarsky C, Winston D, Selch M, Elashoff R, Giorgi JV, Wells J, Terasaki P, Billing R, Feig S. Depletion of T-lymphocytes from donor bone marrow for the prevention of graft-versus-host disease following bone marrow transplantation. Ann Intern Med 1986; 105:20–26.

20. Reisner Y, Ben-Bassat B, Douer D, Kaploon A, Schwartz E, Ramot B. Demonstration of clonable alloreactive host T cells in a primate model for bone marrow transplantation. Proc Natl Acad Sci USA 1986; 83:4012–4015.

21. Bachar-Lustig E, Rachamim N, Li HW, Lan FS, Reisner Y. Megadose of T cell–depleted bone marrow overcomes MHC barriers in sublethally irradiated mice. Nature Med 1995; 1: 1268–1273.

22. Aversa F, Tabilio A, Terenzi A, Velardi A, Falzetti F, Giannoni C, Iacucci R, Zei T, Martelli MP, Gambelunghe C, Rossetti M, Caputo P, Latini P, Aristei C, Raymondi C, Reisner Y, Martelli MF. Successful engraftment of T-cell–depleted haploidentical "three-loci" incompatible transplants in leukemia patients by addition of recombinant human granulocyte colony-stimulating factor-mobilized peripheral blood progenitor cells to bone marrow inoculum. Blood 1994; 84:3948–55.

23. Friedrich W, Goldmann SF, Vetter U, Fliedner TM, Heymer B, Peter HH, Reisner Y, Kleihauer E. Immunoreconstitution in severe combined immunodeficiency after transplantation of HLA-haploidentical T-cell–depleted bone marrow. Lancet 1984; 1:761–764.

24. Lapidot T, Singer TS, Salomon O, Terenzi A, Schwartz E, Reisner Y. Booster irradiation to the spleen following total body irradiation: a new immunosuppressive approach for allogeneic bone marrow transplantation. J Immunol 1988; 141:2619–24.

25. Faktorowich Y, Lapidot T, Lubin I, Reisner Y. Enhancement of BM allografting from C57BL/6 'nude' mice into C3H/HeJ recipients by tolerized T cells from (C57BL/6 → C3H/ HeJ) and (C3H/HeJ → C57BL/6) chimeras. Bone Marrow Transplant 1993; 12:15–20.

26. Lapidot T, Lubin I, Terenzi A, Faktorowich Y, Erlich P, Reisner Y. Enhancement of bone marrow allografts from nude mice into mismatched recipients by T cells void of graft-versus-host activity. Proc Natl Acad Sci USA 1990; 87:4595–4599.

27. Martin PJ. Donor CD8 cells prevent allogeneic marrow graft rejection in mice: potential implications for marrow transplantation in humans. J Exp Med 1993; 178:703–712.

28. Iemura A, Tsai M, Ando A, Wershil BK, Galli SJ. The c-kit ligand, stem cell factor, promotes mast cell survival by suppressing apoptosis. Am J Pathol 1994; 144:321–328.

29. Kaufman CL, Colson YL, Wren SM, Watkins S, Simmons RL, Ildstad ST. Phenotypic characterization of a novel bone marrow-derived cell that facilitates engraftment of allogeneic bone marrow stem cells. Blood 1994; 84:2436–2446.

30. Yaroslavskiy B, Colson Y, Ildstad S, Parrish D, Boggs SS. Addition of a bone marrow "facilitating cell" population increases stem cell-derived cobblestone area formation in impaired long-term bone marrow culture stroma. Expl Hematoly 1998; 26:604–611.

31. Kernan NA, Flomenberg N, Dupont B, O'Reilly RJ. Graft rejection in recipients of T-cell–depleted HLA-nonidentical marrow transplants for leukemia. Transplantation 1987; 43:842.

32. Kernan NA, Bordignon C, Heller G, Cunningham I, Castro-Malaspina H, Shank B, Flomenberg N, Burns J, Yang SY, Black P, Collins NH, O'Reilly RJ. Graft failure after T-cell–depleted human leukocyte antigen identical marrow transplants for leukemia: I. Analysis of risk factors and results of secondary transplants. Blood 1989; 74:2227–2236.

33. Bordignon C, Keever CA, Small TN, Flomenberg N, Dupont B, O'Reilly RJ, Kernan NA. Graft failure after T-cell–depleted human leukocyte antigen identical marrow transplants for leukemia: II. In vitro analyses of host effector mechanisms. Blood 1989; 74:2237–2243.

34. Uharek L, Glass B, Gassmann W, Eckstein V, Steinmann J, Loeffler H, Mueller-Ruchholtz W. Engraftment of allogenic bone marrow cells: Experimental investigations on the role of cell dose, graft-versus-host reactive T cells and pretransplant immunosuppression. Transplant Proc 1992; 24:3023–3025.

35. Vallera DA, Blazar BR. T cell depletion for graft-versus-host disease prophylaxis: a perspective on engraftment in mice and humans. Transplantation 1989; 47:751–760.

36. Mackinnon S, Barnett L, Bourhis JH, Black P, Heller G, O'Reilly RJ. Myeloid and lymphoid chimerism after T-cell–depleted bone marrow transplantation: Evaluation of conditioning regimens using the polymerase chain reaction to amplify human minisatellite regions of genomic DNA. Blood 1992; 80:3235–3241.

37. Verdonck LF, Dekker AW, de Gast GC, Van Kempen ML, Lokhorst HM, Nieuwenhuis HK. Allogenic bone marrow transplantation with a fixed low number of T cells in the marrow graft. Blood 1994; 83:3090–3096.

38. Ash RC, Casper JT, Chitambar CR, Hansen R, Bunin N, Truitt RL, Lawton C, Murray K, Hunter J, Baxter-Lowe LA, Gottschall JL, Oldham K, Anderson T, Camitta B, Menitove J. Successful allogenic transplantation of T-cell–depleted bone marrow from closely HLA-matched unrelated donors. N Engl J Med 1990; 322:485–494.

39. Henslee-Downey PJ, Abhyankar SH, Parrish RS, Pati AR, Godder KT, Neglia WJ, Goon-Johnson KS, Geier SS, Lee CG, Gee AP. Use of partially mismatched related donors extends access to allogeneic marrow transplant. Blood 1997; 89:3864–3872.

40. Korbling M, Przepiorka D, Huh YO, Engel H, Van Besien K, Giralt S, Andersson B, Kleine HD, Seong D, Deisseroth AB, Andreeff M, Champlin R. Allogeneic blood stem cell transplantation for refractory leukemia and lymphoma: potential advantage of blood over marrow allografts. Blood 1995; 85:1659–1665.

41. Korbling M, Huh YO, Durett A, Mirza N, Miller P, Engel H, Anderlini P, Van Besien K, Andreeff M, Przepiorka D, Deisseroth AB, Champlin RE. Allogeneic blood stem cell transplantation: peripheralization and yield of donor-derived primitive hematopoietic progenitor cells (CD34$^+$ Thy-1^{dim}) and lymphoid subsets, and possible predictors of engraftment and graft-versus-host disease. Blood 1995; 86:2842–2848.

42. Gribben JG, Guinan EC, Boussiotis VA, Ke XY, Linsley L, Sieff C, Gray GS, Freeman GJ, Nadler LM. Complete blockade of B7 family-mediated costimulation is necessary to induce human alloantigen-specific anergy: a method to ameliorate graft-versus-host disease and extend the donor pool. Blood 1996; 87:4887–4893.

43. Guinan EC, Boussiotis VA, Neuberg D, Brennan LL, Hirano N, Nadler LM, Gribben JG. Transplantation of anergic histoincompatible bone marrow allografts. N Engl of Med 1999; 340:1704–1714.

44. Broxmeyer HE, Hangoc G, Cooper S, Ribeiro RC, Graves V, Yoder M, Wagner J, Vadhan-Raj S, Benninger L, Rubinstein P, Broun ER. Growth characteristics and expansion of human umbilical cord blood and estimation of its potential for transplantation in adults. Proc Natl Acad Sci USA 1992; 89:4109–4113.

45. Cairo MS, Wagner JE. Placental and/or umbilical cord blood: an alternative source of hematopoietic stem cells for transplantation. Blood 1997; 90:4665–4678.

46. Gluckman E, Broxmeyer HE, Auerbach AD, Friedman HS, Douglas GW, Devergie A, Esperou H, Thierry D, Socie G, Lehn P, Cooper S, English D, Kurtzberg J, Bard J, Boyse EA. Hematopoietic reconstitution in a patient with Fanconi's anemia by means of umbilical-cord blood from an HLA-identical sibling. N Engl J Med 1989; 321:1174–1178.

47. Kurtzberg J, Laughlin M, Graham ML, Smith C, Olson JF, Halperin EC, Ciocci G, Carrier C, Stevens CE, Rubinstein P. Placental blood as a source of hematopoietic stem cells for transplantation into unrelated recipients. N Engl J Med 1996; 335:157–166.

48. Rubinstein P, Carrier C, Scaradavou A, Kurtzberg J, Adamson J, Migliaccio AR, Berkowitz RL, Cabbad M, Dobrila NL, Taylor PE, Rosenfield RE, Stevens CE. Outcomes among 562 recipients of placental-blood transplants from unrelated donors. N Engl J Med 1998; 339: 1565–1577.

49. Wagner JE, Rosenthal J, Sweetman R, Shu XO, Davies SM, Ramsay NKC, McGlave PB, Sender L, Cairo MS. Successful transplantation of HLA-matched and HLA-mismatched umbilical cord blood from unrelated donors: analysis of engraftment and acute graft-versus-host disease. Blood 1996; 88:795–802.

50. Weiden PL, Flournoy N, Thomas ED, Prentice R, Fefer A, Buckner CD, Storb R. Antileukemic effect of graft-versus-host disease in human recipients of allogeneic marrow grafts. N Engl J Med 1979; 300:1068.

51. Weiden PL, Sullivan KM, Flournoy N, Storb R, Thomas ED, The Seattle Marrow Transplant Team. Antileukemic effect of chronic graft-versus-host disease: contribution to improved survival after allogeneic marrow transplantation. N Engl J Med 1981; 304:1529–1532.

52. Horowitz MM, Gale RP, Sondel PM, Goldman JM, Kersey J, Kolb H-J, Rimm AA, Ringdén O, Rozman C, Speck B, Truitt RL, Zwaan FE, Bortin MM. Graft-versus-leukemia reactions after bone marrow transplantation. Blood 1990; 75:555–562.

53. Sullivan KM, Storb R, Buckner CD, Fefer A, Fisher L, Weiden PL, Witherspoon RP, Appelbaum FR, Banaji M, Hansen J, Martin P, Sanders JE, Singer J, Thomas ED. Graft-versus-host disease as adoptive immunotherapy in patients with advanced hematologic neoplasms. N Engl J Med. 1989; 320:828–834.

54. Gale RP, Champlin RE. How does bone marrow transplantation cure leukemia? Lancet 1984; 2:28–30.

55. Gale RP, Horowitz MM, Ash RC, Champlin RE, Goldman JM, Rimm AA, Ringdén O, Stone JAV, Bortin MM. Identical-twin bone marrow transplants for leukemia. Ann Intern Med 1994; 120:646–652.

56. Fefer A, Cheever MA, Greeberg PD. Identical-twin (syngeneic) marrow transplantation for hematologic cancers. J Nat Cancer Inst 1986; 76:1269–1271.

57. Kolb HJ, Schattenberg A, Goldman JM, Hertenstein B, Jacobsen N, Arcese W, Ljungman P, Ferrant A, Verdonck L, Niederwieser D, Van Rhee F, Mittermueller J, de Witte T, Holler E, Ansari H. Graft-vs.-leukemia effect of donor lymphocyte transfusions in marrow grafted patients. Blood 1995; 86:2041–2050.

58. Collins RH, Jr., Shpilberg O, Drobyski WR, Porter DL, Giralt S, Champlin R, Goodman SA, Wolff SN, Hu W, Verfaillie C, List A, Dalton W, Ognoskie N, Chetrit A, Antin JH, Nemunaitis J. Donor leukocyte infusions in 140 patients with relapsed malignancy after allogeneic bone marrow transplantation. J Clin Oncol 1997; 15:433–444.

59. Drobyski WR, Keever CA, Roth MS, Koethe S, Hanson G, McFadden P, Gottschall JL, Ash RC, Van Tuinen P, Horowitz MM, Flomenberg N. Salvage immunotherapy using donor leukocyte infusions as treatment for relapsed chronic myelogenous leukemia after allogeneic bone marrow transplantation: Efficacy and toxicity of a defined T-cell dose. Blood 1993; 82:2310–2318.

60. Apperley JF, Jones L, Hale G, Waldmann H, Hows J, Rombos Y, Tsatalas C, Marcus RE, Goolden AWG, Gordon-Smith EC, Catovsky D, Galton DAG, Goldman JM. Bone marrow

transplantation for patients with chronic myeloid leukaemia: T-cell depletion with Campath-1 reduces the incidence of graft-versus-host disease but may increase the risk of leukaemic relapse. Bone Marrow Transplant 1986; 1:53–68.

61. Mackinnon S, Barnett L, Heller G, O'Reilly RJ. Minimal residual disease is more common in patients who have mixed T-cell chimerism after bone marrow transplantation for chronic myelogenous leukemia. Blood 1994; 83:3409–3416.

62. Offit K, Burns JP, Cunningham I, Jhanwar SC, Black P, Kernan NA, O'Reilly RJ, Chaganti RSK. Cytogenetic analysis of chimerism and leukemia relapse in chronic myelogenous leukemia patients after T cell–depleted bone marrow transplantation. Blood 1990; 75:1346–1355.

63. Radich JP, Gehly G, Gooley T, Bryant E, Clift RA, Collins S, Edmands S, Kirk J, Lee A, Kessler P, Schoch G, Buckner CD, Sullivan KM, Appelbaum FR, Thomas ED. Polymerase chain reaction detection of the BCR-ABL fusion transcript after allogeneic marrow transplantation for chronic myeloid leukemia: results and implications in 346 patients. Blood 1995; 85:2632–2638.

64. Hughes TP, Morgan GJ, Martiat P, Goldman JM. Detection of residual leukemia after bone marrow transplant for chronic myeloid leukemia: role of polymerase chain reaction in predicting relapse. Blood 1991; 77:874–878.

65. DeLage R, Soiffer RJ, Dear K, Ritz J. Clinical significance of bcr-abl gene rearrangement detected by polymerase chain reaction after allogeneic bone marrow transplantation in chronic myelogenous leukemia. Blood 1991; 78:2759–2767.

66. Lee M, Khouri I, Champlin R, Kantarjian H, Talpaz M, Trujillo J, Freireich E, Deisseroth A, Stass S. Detection of minimal residual disease by polymerase chain reaction of bcr/abl transcripts in chronic myelogenous leukaemia following allogeneic bone marrow transplantation. Br J Haematol 1992; 82:708–714.

67. Van Rhee F, Lin F, Cullis JO, Spencer A, Cross NCP, Chase A, Garicochea B, Bungey J, Barrett J, Goldman JM. Relapse of chronic myeloid leukemia after allogeneic bone marrow transplant: the case for giving donor leukocyte transfusions before the onset of hematologic relapse. Blood 1994; 83:3377–3383.

68. Mackinnon S, Papadopoulos EB, Carabasi MH, Reich L, Collins NH, Boulad F, Castro-Malaspina H, Childs B, Gillio A, Kernan NA, Small T, Young J, O'Reilly RJ. Adoptive immunotherapy evaluating escalating doses of donor leukeocytes for relapse of chronic myeloid leukemia after bone marrow transplantation: separataiton of graft-versus-leukemia responses from graft-versus-host disease. Blood 1995; 86:1261–1268.

69. Papadopoulos EB, Carabasi MH, Castro-Malaspina H, Childs BH, Mackinnon S, Boulad F, Gillio AP, Kernan NA, Small TN, Szabolcs P, Taylor J, Yahalom J, Collins NH, Bleau SA, Black PM, Heller G, O'Reilly RJ, Young JW. T-cell–depleted allogeneic bone marrow transplantation as postremission therapy for acute myelogenous leukemia: freedom from relapse in the absence of graft-versus-host disease. Blood 1998; 91:1083–1093.

70. Cardoso AA, Seamon MJ, Afonso HM, Ghia P, Boussiotis VA, Freeman GJ, Gribben JG, Sallan SE, Nadler LM. Ex vivo generation of human anti-pre-B leukemia-specific autologous cytolytic T cells. Blood 1997; 90:549–561.

71. Brenner M, Porcelli S. Antigen presentation: a balanced diet. Science 1997; 277:332.

72. Raanani P, Dazzi F, Sohal J, Szydlo RM, Van Rhee F, Reiter A, Lin F, Goldman JM, Cross NCP. The rate and kinetics of molecular response to donor leucocyte transfusions in chronic myeloid leukaemia patients treated for relapse after allogeneic bone marrow transplantation. Br J Haematol 1997; 99:945–950.

73. Bacigalupo A, Soracco M, Vassallo F, Abate M, Van Lint MT, Gualandi F, Lamparelli T, Occhini D, Mordini N, Bregante S, Figari O, Benvenuto F, Sessarego M, Fugazza G, Carlier P, Valbonesi M. Donor lymphocyte infusions (DLI) in patients with chronic myeloid leukemia following allogeneic bone marrow transplantation. bone Marrow Transplant 1997; 19:927–932.

74. Van Rhee F, Savage D, Blackwell J, Orchard K, Dazzi F, Lin F, Chase A, Bungey J, Cross

NCP, Apperley J, Szydlo R, Goldman JM. Adoptive immunotherapy for relapse of chronic myeloid leukemia after allogeneic bone marrow transplant: equal efficacy of lymphocytes from sibling and matched unrelated donors. Bone Marrow Transplant 1998; 21:1055–1061.

75. Orchard PJ, Miller JS, McGlennen R, Davies SM, Ramsay NKC. Graft-versus-leukemia is sufficient to induce remission in juvenile myelomonocytic leukemia. Bone Marrow Transplant 1998; 22:201–203.

76. Porter DL, Roth MS, Lee SJ, McGarigle C, Ferrara JLM, Antin JH. Adoptive immunotherapy with donor mononuclear cell infusions to treat relapse of acute leukemia or myelodysplasia after allogeneic bone marrow transplantation. Bone Marrow Transplant 1996; 18:975–980.

77. Okumura H, Takamatsu H, Yoshida T. Donor leucocyte transfusions for relapse in myelodysplastic syndrome after allogeneic bone marrow transplantation. Br J Haematol 1996; 93:386–388.

78. Rondón G, Giralt S, Huh Y, Khouri I, Andersson B, Andreeff M, Champlin R. Graft-versus-leukemia effect after allogeneic bone marrow transplantation for chronic lymphocytic leukemia. Bone Marrow Transplant 1996; 18:669–672.

79. Van Besien KW, De Lima M, Giralt SA, Moore DF, Jr., Khouri IF, Rondón G, Mehra R, Andersson BS, Dyer C, Cleary K, Przepiorka D, Gajewski JL, Champlin RE. Management of lymphoma recurrence after allogeneic transplantation: the relevance of graft-versus-lymphoma effect. Bone Marrow Transplant 1997; 19:977–982.

80. Khouri I, Keating MJ, Przepiorka D, O'Brien S, Giralt S, Korbling M, Champlin R. Engraftment and induction of GVL with fludarabine-based non-ablative preparative regimen in patients with chronic lymphocytic leukemia. Blood 1996; 88(suppl 1):301a.

81. Lokhorst HM, Schattenberg A, Cornelissen JJ, Thomas LLM, Verdonck LF. Donor leukocyte infusions are effective in relapsed multiple myeloma after allogeneic bone marrow transplantation. Blood 1997; 90:4206–4211.

82. Tricot G, Vesole DH, Jagannath S, Hilton J, Munshi N, Barlogie B. Graft-versus-myeloma effect: proof of principle. Blood 1996; 87:1196–1198.

83. Verdonck LF, Lokhorst HM, Dekker AW, Nieuwenhuis HK, Petersen EJ. Graft-versus-myeloma effect in two cases. Lancet 1996; 347:800–801.

84. Goulmy E, Voogt P, Van Els C, De Bueger M, van Rood J. The role of minor histocompatibility antigens in GVHD and rejection: a mini-review. Bone Marrow Transplant 1991; 7(suppl)1:49–51.

85. Falkenburg JHF, Goselink HM, Van der Harst D, Van Luxemburg-Heijs SAP, Kooy-Winkelaar EMC, Faber LM, De Kroon JFEM, Brand A, Fibbe WE, Willemze R, Goulmy E. Growth inhibition of clonogeneic leukemic precursor cells by minor histocompatibility antigen specific cytotoxic T lymphocytes. J Exp Med 1991; 174:27–33.

86. Beatty PG. National Heart, Lung, And Blood Institute (NHLBI) workshop on the importance of minor histocompatibility antigens in marrow transplantation. Exp Hematol 1997; 25:548–558.

87. De Beuger M, Bakker A, van Rood JJ, Van Der Woude F, Goulmy E. Tissue distribution of human minor histocompatibility antigens. Ubiquitous versus restricted tissue distribution indicates heterogeneity amon human cytotoxic T lymphocyte defined non-MHC antigens. J Immunol 1992; 149:1788–1794.

88. Kernan NA, Dupont B. Minor histocompatibility antigens and marrow transplantation. N Engl J Med 1996; 334:323–324.

89. Beatty PG. Minor histocompatibility antigens. Exp Hematol 1993; 21:1514–1516.

90. Perreault C, Décary F, Brochu S, Gyger M, Bélanger R, Roy D. Minor histocompatibility antigens. Blood 1990; 76:1269–1280.

91. Marijt WAF, Veenhof WFJ, Brand A, Goulmy E, Fibbe WE, Willemze R, van Rood JJ, Falkenburg JHF. Minor histocompatibility antigen-specific cytotoxic T cell lines, capable of lysing human hematopoietic progenitor cells, can be generated in vitro by stimulation with HLA-identical bone marrow cells. J Exp Med 1991; 173:101–109.

92. Faber LM, Van der Hoeven J, Goulmy E, Hooftman-den Otter AL, Van Luxemburg-Heijs SAP, Willemze R, Falkenburg JHF. Recognition of clonogenic leukemic cells, remission bone marrow and HLA-identical donor bone marrow by CD8+ or CD4+ minor histocompatibility antigen-specific cytotoxic T lymphocytes. J Clin Invest 1995; 96:877–883.

93. Jiang Y-Z, Kanfer EJ, Macdonald D, Cullis JO, Goldman JM, Barrett AJ. Graft-versus-leukaemia following allogeneic bone marrow transplantation: Emergence of cytotoxic T lymphocytes reacting to host leukaemia cells. Bone Marrow Transplant. 1991; 8:253–258.

94. Sosman JA, Oettel KR, Smith SD, Hank JA, Fisch P, Sondel PM. Specific recognition of human leukemic cells by allogeneic T cells: II. Evidence for HLA-D restricted determinants on leukemic cells that are crossreactive with determinants present on unrelated nonleukemic cells. Blood 1990; 75:2005–2016.

95. Marijt WAF, Veenhof WFJ, Goulmy E, Willemze R, van Rood JJ, Falkenburg JHF. Minor histocompatibility antigens HA-1-, -2-, and -4-, and HY-specific cytotoxic T-cell clones inhibit human hematopoietic progenitor cell growth by a mechanism that is dependent on direct cell-cell contact. Blood 1993; 82:3778–3785.

96. Van der Harst D, Goulmy E, Falkenburg JHF, Kooij-Winkelaar YMC, Van Luxemburg-Heijs SAP, Goselink HM, Brand A. Recognition of minor histocompatibility antigens on lymphocytic and myeloid leukemic cells by cytotoxic T-cell clones. Blood 1994; 83:1060–1066.

97. Molldrem JJ, Clave E, Jiang YZ, Mavroudis D, Raptis A, Hensel N, Agarwala V, Barrett AJ. Cytotoxic T lymphocytes specific for a nonpolymorphic proteinase 3 peptide preferentially inhibit chronic myeloid leukemia colony-forming units. Blood 1997; 90:2529–2534.

98. Molldrem J, Dermime S, Parker K, Jiang YZ, Mavroudis D, Hensel N, Fukushima P, Barrett AJ. Targeted T-cell therapy for human leukemia: Cytotoxic T lymphocytes specific for a peptide derived from proteinase 3 preferentially lyse human myeloid leukemia cells. Blood 1996; 88:2450–2457.

99. Ueno NT, Rondón G, Mirza NQ, Geisler DK, Anderlini P, Giralt SA, Andersson BS, Claxton DF, Gajewski JL, Khouri IF, Körbling M, Mehra RC, Przepiorka D, Rahman Z, Samuels BI, Van Besien K, Hortobagyi GN, Champlin RE. Allogeneic peripheral-blood progenitor-cell transplantation for poor-risk patients with metastatic breast cancer. J Clin Oncol 1998; 16:986–993.

100. Eibl B, Schwaighofer H, Nachbaur D, Marth C, Gächter A, Knapp R, Böck G, Gassner C, Schiller L, Petersen F, Niederwieser D. Evidence for a graft-versus-tumor effect in a patient treated with marrow ablative chemotherapy and allogeneic bone marrow transplantation for breast cancer. Blood 1996;88:1501–1508.

101. Korngold R, Sprent J. Variable capacity of L3 T4 + T cells to cause lethal graft versus host disease across minor histocompatibility barriers in mice. J Exp Med 1987; 165:52–64.

102. Sakamoto H, Michaelson J, Jones WK, Bhan AK, Abhyankar S, Silverstein M, Golan DE, Burakoff SJ, Ferrara JLM. Lymphocytes with a CD4$^+$CD8$^-$CD3$^-$ phenotype are effectors of experimental cutaneous graft-versus-host disease. Proc Natl Acad Sci USA 1991; 88:10890–10894.

103. Ferrara JLM, Abhyankar S, Gilliland DG. Cytokine storm of graft-versus-host disease: a critical effector role for interleukin-1. Transplant Proc 1993; 25:1216–1217.

104. Faber LM, Van Luxemburg-Heijs SAP, Willemze R, Falkenburg JHF. Generation of leukemia-reactive cytotoxic T lymphocyte clones from the HLA-identical bone marrow donor of a patient with leukemia. J Exp Med 1992; 176:1283–1289.

105. Truitt RL, Atasoylu AA. Contribution of CD4+ and CD8+ T cells to graft-versus-host disease and graft-versus-leukemia reactivity after transplantation of MHC-compatible bone marrow. Bone Marrow Transplant. 1991; 8:51–58.

106. Okunewick JP, Kociban DL, Machen LL, Buffo MJ. The role of CD4 and CD8 T cells in the graft-versus-leukemia response in Rauscher murine leukemia. Bone Marrow Transplant. 1991; 8:445–452.

107. Okunewick JP, Kociban DL, Machen LL, Buffo MJ. Evidence for a possible role of Asialo-GM1-positive cells in the graft-versus-leukemia repression of a murine type-C retroviral leukemia. Bone Marrow Transplant 1995; 16:451–456.

108. Jiang Y-Z, Barrett AJ. Cellular and cytokine mediated effects of CD4-positive lymphocyte lines generated in vitro against chronic myelogeneous leukemia. Exp Hematol 1995; 23: 1167–1172.

109. Jiang YZ, Mavroudis D, Dermime S, Hensel N, Couriel D, Molldrem J, Barrett AJ. Alloreactive CD4$^+$ T lymphocytes can exert cytotoxicity to chronic myeloid leukaemia cells processing and presenting exogenous antigen. Br J Haematol 1996; 93:606–612.

110. Jiang YZ, Barrett AJ, Goldman JM, Mavroudis DA. Association of natural killer cell immune recovery with a graft-versus-leukemia effect independent of graft-versus-host disease following allogenic bone marrow transplantation. Ann Hematol 1997; 74:1–6.

111. Zeis M, Uharek L, Glass B, Gaska T, Steinmann J, Gassmann W, Löffler H, Müller-Ruchholtz W. Allogeneic NK cells as potent antileukemic effector cells after allogeneic bone marrow transplantation in mice. Transplantation 1995; 59:1734–1736.

112. Glass B, Uharek L, Zeis M, Loeffler H, Mueller-Ruchholtz W, Gassmann W. Graft-versus-leukaemia activity can be predicted by natural cytotoxicity against leukaemia. Br J Haematol 1996; 93:412–420.

113. Hauch M, Gazzola MV, Small T, Bordignon C, Barnett L, Cunningham I, Castro-Malaspinia H, O'Reilly RJ, Keever CA. Anti-leukemia potential of interleukin-2 activated natural killer cells after bone marrow transplantation for chronic myelogenous leukemia. Blood 1990; 75: 2250–2262.

114. Giralt SA, Champlin RE. Leukemia relapse after allogeneic bone marrow transplantation: a review. Blood 1994; 84:3603–3612.

115. Hoffman T, Theobald M, Bunjes D, Weiss M, Heimpel H, Heit W. Frequency of bone marrow T cells responding to HLA-identical non-leukemic and leukemic stimulator cells. Bone Marrow Transplant. 1993; 12:1–8.

116. Keil F, Haas OA, Fritsch G, Kalhs P, Lechner K, Mannhalter C, Reiter E, Niederwieser D, Hoecker P, Greinix HT. Donor leukocyte infusion for leukemic relapse after allogeneic marrow transplantation: lack of residual donor hematopoiesis predicts aplasia. Blood 1997; 89: 3113–3117.

117. Rahman SL, Mahendra P, Nacheva E, Sinclair P, Arno J, Marcus RE. Achievement of complete cytogenetic remission after two very low-dose donor leucocyte infusions in a patient with extensive cGVHD relapsing in accelerated phase post allogeneic BMT for CML. Bone Marrow Transplant 1998; 21:955–956.

118. Champlin R, Ho W, Gajewski J, Feig S, Burnison M, Holley G, Greenberg P, Lee K, Schmid I, Giorgi J, Yam P, Petz L, Winston D, Warner N, Reichert T. Selective depletion of CD8$^+$ T lymphocytes for prevention of graft-versus-host disease after allogeneic bone marrow transplantation. Blood 1990; 76:418–423.

119. Champlin RE, Jansen J, Ho W, Gajewski J, Nimer S, Lee K, Territo M, Winston D, Tricot G, Reichert T. Retention of graft-versus-leukemia using selective depletion of CD8 positive T lymphocytes for prevention of graft versus host disease following bone marrow transplantation for chronic myelogenous leukemia. Transplant Proc 1991; 23:1695–1696.

120. Nimer SD, Giorgi J, Gajewski JL, Ku N, Schiller GJ, Lee K, Territo M, Ho W, Feig S, Selch M, Isacescu V, Reichert TA, Champlin RE. Selective depletion of CD8$^+$ cells for prevention of graft-versus-host disease after bone marrow transplantation: A randomized controlled trial. Transplantation 1994; 57:82–87.

121. Giralt S, Hester J, Huh Y, Hirsch-Ginsberg C, Rondon G, Guo J, Lee M, Gajewski J, Talpaz M, Kantarjian H, Fischer H, Deisseroth A, Champlin R. CD8+ depleted donor lymphocyte infusion as treatment for relapsed chronic myelogenous leukemia after allogeneic bone marrow transplantation: graft vs leukemia without graft vs. host disease. Blood 1995; 86:4337–4343.

122. Alyea EP, Soiffer RJ, Canning C, Neuberg D, Schlossman R, Pickett C, Collins H, Wang YL, Anderson KC, Ritz J. Toxicity and efficacy of defined doses of CD4$^+$ donor lymphocytes for treatment of relapse after allogeneic bone marrow transplant. Blood 1998; 91:3671–3680.

123. Bonini C, Ferrari G, Verzeletti S, Servida P, Zappone E, Ruggieri L, Ponzoni M, Rossini S, Mavilio F, Traversari C, Bordignon C. HSV-TK gene transfer into donor lymphocytes for control of allogeneic graft-versus-leukemia. Science 1997; 276:1719–1724.

124. Munshi NC, Govindarajan R, Drake R, Ding LM, Iyer R, Saylors R, Kornbluth J, Marcus S, Chiang Y, Ennist D, Kwak L, Reynolds C, Tricot G, Barlogie B. Thymidine kinase (TK) gene-transduced human lymphocytes can be highly purified, remain fully functional, and are killed efficiently with ganciclovir. Blood 1997; 89:1334–1340.

125. Tiberghien P, Reynolds CW, Keller J, Spence S, Deschaseaux M, Certoux J-M, Contassot E, Murphy WJ, Lyons R, Chiang Y, Hervé P, Longo DL, Ruscetti FW. Ganciclovir treatment of herpes simplex thymidine kinase-transduced primary T lymphocytes: An approach for specific in vivo donor T-cell depletion after bone marrow transplantation. Blood 1994; 84: 1333–1341.

126. Cavazzana-Calvo M, Stephan JL, Sarnacki S, Chevret S, Fromont C, De Coene C, Le Deist F, Guy-Grand D, Fischer A. Attenuation of graft-versus-host disease and graft rejection by ex vivo immunotoxin elimination of alloreactive T cells in an H-2 haplotype disparate mouse combination. Blood 1994; 83:288–298.

127. Mavroudis DA, Dermime S, Molldrem J, Jiang YZ, Raptis A, Van Rhee F, Hensel N, Fellowes V, Eliopoulos G, Barrett AJ. Specific depletion of alloreactive T cells in HLA-identical siblings: a method for separating graft-versus-host and graft-versus-leukaemia reactions. Br J Haematol 1998; 101:565–570.

128. Garderet L, Snell V, Przepiorka D, Schenk T, Lu JG, Marini F, Gluckman E, Andreeff M, Champlin RE. Effective depletion of alloreactive lymphocytes from peripheral blood mononuclear cell preparations. Transplantation 1999; 67:124–130.

129. Ship AM, Carter R, Murray T, Guerriero A, Waller EK. Irradiated donor lymphocyte infusion, a novel approach to prevent graft failure during allogeneic bone marrow transplant. Proc Am Assoc Clin Oncol 1998; 17:74a.

130. Rooney CM, Smith CA, Ng CYC, Loftin S, Li C, Krance RA, Brenner MK, Heslop HE. Use of gene-modified virus-specific T lymphocytes to control Epstein-Barr virus-related lymphoproliferation. Lancet 1995; 345:9–13.

131. Walter EA, Greenberg PD, Gilbert MJ, Finch RJ, Watanabe KS, Thomas ED, Riddell SR. Reconstitution of cellular immunity against cytomegalovirus in recipients of allogeneic bone marrow by transfer of T-cell clones from the donor. N Engl J Med 1995; 333:1038–1044.

132. Falkenburg JHF, Faber LM, Van den Elshout M, Van Luxemburg-Heijs SAP, Hooftman-den Otter A, Smit WM, Voogt PJ, Willemze R. Generation of donor-derived antileukemic cytotoxic T-lymphocyte responses for treatment of relapsed leukemia after allogeneic HLA-identical bone marrow transplantation. J Immunother 1993; 14:305–309.

133. Mutis T, Verdijk R, Schrama E, Esendam B, Brand A, Goulmy E. Feasibility of immunotherapy of relapsed leukemia with ex vivo-generated cytotoxic T lymphocytes specific for hematopoietic system–restricted minor histocompatibility antigens. Blood 1999; 93:2336–2341.

134. Barrett AJ, Mavroudis D, Tisdale J, Molldrem J, Clave E, Dunbar C, Cottler-Fox M, Phang S, Carter C, Okunnieff P, Young NS, Read EJ. T cell-depleted bone marrow transplantation and delayed T cell add-back to control acute GVHD and conserve a graft-versus-leukemia effect. Bone Marrow Transplant 1998; 21:543–551.

135. Slavin S, Naparstek E, Nagler A, Ackerstein A, Kapelushnik J, OR R. Allogeneic cell therapy for relapsed leukemia after bone marrow transplantation with donor peripheral blood lymphocytes. Exp Hematol 1995; 23:1553–1562.

136. Antin JH, Ferrara JLM. Cytokine dysregulation and acute graft-versus-host disease. Blood 1992; 80:2964–2968.

137. Hill GR, Crawford JM, Cooke KR, Brinson YS, Pan LY, Ferrara JLM. Total body irradiation

and acute graft-versus-host disease:the role of gastrointestinal damage and inflammatory cytokines. Blood 1997; 90:3204–3213.

138. Giralt S, Estey E, Albitar M, Van Besien K, Randon G, Anderlini P, O'Brien S, Khouri I, Gajewski J, Mehra R, Claxton D, Andersson B, Beran M, Przepiorka D, Koller C, Kornblau S, Körbling M, Keating M, Kantarjian H, Champlin R. Engraftment of allogeneic hematopoietic progenitor cells with purine analog-containing chemotherapy: harnessing graft-versus-leukemia without myeloablative therapy. Blood 1997; 89:4531–4536.

139. Giralt S, Gajewski J, Khouri I, Korbling M, Claxton D, Mehra R, Przepiorka D, Andersson B, Talpaz M, Kantarjian H, Champlin R. Induction of graft-versus-leukemia as primary treatment of chronic myelogenous leukemia. Blood 1997; 90(suppl 1):1857a.

140. Giralt S, Cohen A, Mehra R, Gajewski J, Andersson B, Przepiorka D, Khouri I, Korbling M, Davis M, Van Besien K, Ippoliti C, Bruton J, Anderlini P, Ueno N, Champlin R. Preliminary results of fludarabine/melphalan or 2CDA/melphalan as preparative regimens for allogeneic progenitor cell transplantation in poor candidates for conventional myeloablative conditioning. Blood 1997; 90:1853a.

141. Storb R, Yu C, Wagner JL, Deeg HJ, Nash RA, Kiem HP, Leisenring W, Shulman H. Stable mixed hematopoietic chimerism in DLA-identical littermate dogs given sublethal total body irradiation before and pharmacological immunosuppression after marrow transplantation. Blood 1997; 89:3048–3054.

142. Khouri I, Keating M, Korbling M, Przepiorka D, Anderlini P, O'Brien S, Von Wolff B, Giralt S, Gajewski JG, Mehra R, Ippoliti C, Claxton D, Champlin RE. Transplant Lite: induction of graft-versus-leukemia using fludarabine-based nonablative chemotherapy and allogeneic blood progenitor cell transplantation as treatment for lymphoid malignancies. J Clin Oncol 1998; 16:2817–2824.

143. Bensinger WI, Buckner CD, Anasetti C, Clift R, Storb R, Barnett T, Chauncey T, Shulman H, Appelbaum FR. Allogeneic marrow transplantation for multiple myeloma: an analysis of risk factors on outcome. Blood 1996; 88:2787–2793.

144. Gahrton G, Tura S, Ljungman P, Bladé J, Brandt L, Cavo M, Façon T, Gratwohl A, Hagenbeek A, Jacobs P, De Laurenzi A, Van Lint M, Michallet M, Nikoskelainen J, Reiffers J, Samson D, Verdonck L, de Witte T, Volin L. Prognostic factors in allogeneic bone marrow transplantation for multiple myeloma. J Clin Oncol 1995; 13:1312–1322.

145. Bertucci F, Viens P, Gravis G, Blaise D, Faucher C, Oziel-Taoeb S, Bardou VJ, Jacquemier J, Delpero JR, Maraninchi D. High-dose chemotherapy with hematopoietic stem cell support in patients with advanced epithelial ovarian cancer: analysis of 67 patients treated in a single institution. Anticancer Res 1999; 19:1455–1461.

146. Slavin S, Nagler A, Naparstek E, Kapelushnik Y, Aker M, Cividalli G, Varadi G, Kirschbaum M, Ackerstein A, Samuel S, Amar A, Brautbar C, Ben-Tal O, Eldor A, Or R. Nonmyeloablative stem cell transplantation and cell therapy as an alternative to conventional bone marrow transplantation with lethal cytoreduction for the treatment of malignant and nonmalignant hematologic diseases. Blood 1998; 91:756–763.

147. Kelemen E, Masszi T, Reményi P, Barta A, Pálóczi K. Reduction in the frequency of transplant-related complications in patients with chronic myeloid leukemia undergoing BMT preconditioned with a new, non-myeloablative drug combination. Bone Marrow Transplant 1998; 21:747–749.

148. Bacigalupo A, Van Lint MT, Occhini D, Gualandi F, Lamparelli T, Sogno G, Tedone E, Frassoni F, Tong J, Marmont AM. Increased risk of leukemia relapse with high-dose cyclosporine A after allogeneic marrow transplantation for acute leukemia. Blood 1991; 77: 1423–1428.

22

Peripheral Blood Stem Cells for Allogeneic Transplantation

LUTZ UHAREK and MATTHIAS ZEIS

University of Leipzig, Leipzig, Germany

PETER DREGER, BERTRAM GLASS, and NORBERT SCHMITZ

Christian Albrechts University of Kiel, Kiel, Germany

I. INTRODUCTION

In the late 1960s, Epstein et al. and Storb et al. reported on a canine model set up to investigate the possibility of transplanting allogeneic blood stem cells (1,2). These series of experiments, later followed by transplant studies in nonhuman primates gave the first evidence that hematopoietic stem cells circulate in the peripheral blood and can engraft in allogeneic recipients (3). A unique and successful attempt to transplant T-cell–depleted blood stem cells from a normal donor to an human leukocyte antigen (HLA)–identical recipient with acute lymphoblastic leukemia was published in 1989 (4).

The broader utilization of allogeneic peripheral blood progenitor cells (PBPCs), however, was hindered by two major problems. First, PBPCs normally circulate in very low numbers. Thus, harvesting of a sufficient number of PBPCs was cumbersome, time-consuming, and expensive until recombinant human hematopoietic growth factors (HGFs) became available (5,6). Second, PBPC collection products contain high numbers of T lymphocytes, and it was therefore anticipated that the transplantation of allogeneic PBPCs instead of bone marrow would induce more frequent and/or severe graft-versus-host disease (GVHD). The first successful transplants using allogeneic PBPCs mobilized by granulocyte colony-stimulating factor (G-CSF) were therefore performed in emergency situations like the inability of the donor to undergo general anesthesia or failure of previous bone marrow grafts (7,8). Surprisingly, these case reports and subsequent pilot studies from Houston, Seattle, and Kiel did not show that transplantation of allogeneic PBPCs was followed by the development of devastating GVHD (9–11). On the contrary, the mostly favorable outcome of these early patients induced a surge of allogeneic peripheral blood progenitor transplants. More than 500 allogeneic peripheral blood progenitor cell transplants were reported to the European Group for Blood and Marrow Transplantation (EBMT) for 1995, and there is good reason to believe that this trend will continue when the first results of the currently running randomized trials will be communicated (12).

This chapter will attempt to review the rapidly accumulating knowledge on clinical allogeneic peripheral blood progenitor cell transplantation (PBPCT) and summarize our current understanding of this new technology. It must be stressed, however, that large areas of uncertainty still exist. In such a situation, experimental data from the laboratory can corroborate clinical observations and—more importantly—help to predict some of the consequences of allogeneic PBPCT which have not yet been fully addressed in the clinical situation. Finally, animal experiments are useful to produce new ideas on how to proceed in this new and exciting field of clinical research.

II. EXPERIMENTAL APPROACHES TO ALLOGENEIC PERIPHERAL BLOOD PROGENITOR CELL TRANSPLANTATION

Although animal models will always have limitations, and results of such experiments can never be directly translated into clinical consequences, they offer the opportunity to investigate basic biological problems in a systematic way.

Whereas some work on the possibilities of transplanting unmanipulated blood cells was done in Seattle, experimental data on allogeneic transplants performed with growth factor–mobilized PBPCs, however, are scarce (1–3).

A. Mobilization of Peripheral Blood Progenitor Cells and Composition of the Collection Products

In order to avoid pooling of PBPCs in the spleen, it is necessary to splenectomize rodents prior to mobilization. Subcutaneous injection of G-CSF then results in an immediate increase in the number of circulating progenitor cells, which peak around day 5 after administration of G-CSF (13). Comparable results can be obtained with stem cell factor (SCF) as the mobilizing agent (14). The combination of both cytokines synergistically enhances the mobilization of murine progenitor cells into the circulation (15,16).

Table 1 shows the number of colony-forming units granulocyte-macrophage (CFU-GM) found in the peripheral blood of mice treated with optimal doses of either recombinant human (rhu)–G-CSF or recombinant rat (rr)-SCF alone or in combination. Animals treated with a combination of both HGFs exhibited significantly higher concentrations of progenitor cells (147 CFU-GM/µL) in the blood as compared to animals treated with G-CSF alone (52 CFU-GM/µL). Although such results may be of particular interest for the mobilization of autologous PBPCs in heavily pretreated patients, they may also have a bearing in allogeneic transplantation in situations when very high progenitor cell numbers are required to minimize the risk of graft rejection [i.e., for ex vivo manipulated major histocompatibility complex (MHC)–mismatched transplants]. Another issue, namely, the variation in the cellular composition of the graft depending on the growth factor or the combination of HGFs used for mobilization, may be even more important. The major subsets of lymphoid and myeloid cells that can be found in murine PBPC harvests after 5 days of treatment with G-CSF and SCF are shown in Table 1.

Whereas myeloid (Gr-1$^+$) cells are predominant in the PBPC collection products of animals treated with the combination of both cytokines or with G-CSF alone, the myeloid

Table 1 Cellular Composition of PBPC Grafts Mobilized by G-CSF, SCF, or a Combination of Both Cytokines

Growth factor	WBC/nl	CFU-GM/μL[a]	Percentage of nucleated cells positive for						
			CD3	CD4	CD8	NK 1.1[b]	Gr-1	CD19
None	14,9 (2,5)	0 (0,0)	55,3 (11,2)	44,9 (10,3)	11,7 (2,6)	7,8 (3,0)	28,7 (10,9)	7,9 (4,8)
G-CSF	67,2 (5,9)	53 (4,5)	20,2 (4,8)	18,7 (6,3)	6,2 (1,8)	6,0 (3,6)	67,9 (7,5)	4,8 (2,1)
SCF	32,2 (10,8)	16 (2,3)	38,6 (11,2)	29,8 (12,4)	8,9 (1,7)	11,5 (1,8)	43,0 (12,8)	11,7 (5,9)
G-CSF+SCF	102,2 (15,1)	147 (16,5)	17,4 (4,8)	13,0 (2,3)	5,3 (2,0)	3,8 (2,3)	74,1 (6,0)	4,7 (2,3)

PBPC, peripheral blood progenitor cell; G-CSF, granulocyte colony-stimulating factor; SCF, stem cell factor; WBC, white blood cells; CFU-GM, colony-forming units granulocyte-macrophage; NK, natural killer.

[a]CFU-GM were counted on day +12 postseeding.

[b]The monoclonal antibody 5E6 marks a subpopulation of NK cells.

cell fraction in the peripheral blood is not significantly affected by treatment with SCF. PBPC collection products of SCF-treated animals therefore contain particularly high numbers of lymphoid elements, especially $CD3^+$ T cells but also natural killer (NK) and B cells.

Neither the expression of activation markers like B220 nor of the α or β chain of the interleukin-2 (IL-2) receptor on NK cells is significantly altered by treatment with G-CSF or SCF. Similarly, we did not observe a difference in the relationship of $CD4^+$ and $CD8^+$ T cells or the number of $CD3^+$, $CD4^+$, or $CD8^+$ T cells.

Pan et al. detected a functional difference between resting T cells and T cells from G-CSF–treated mice (17). They were able to demonstrate that T cells from G-CSF–treated mice produced significantly more IL-4 but less IL-2 and interferon-γ. Thus, pretreatment of donors with G-CSF seemed to polarize donor T cells toward the production of type 2 cytokines—a situation which is associated with reduced type 1 cytokine production and reduced severity of acute graft-versus-host disease (GVHD) (17,18). These findings may help to explain why the incidence and severity of acute GVHD after transplantation of allogeneic, G-CSF–mobilized PBSCs appears to be no worse than after bone marrow transplantation (see Sect. III.C).

The functional activity of T cells and NK cells has also been evaluated in a canine model (19). The T lymphocytes of dogs treated with recombinant (rc)G-CSF for 7 days were found to be hyporesponsive in the mixed lymphocyte culture and their response to concanavalin A (Con A) was also impaired. These findings raised hopes that the alloreactivity of these cells might be reduced and these T cells might thus cause less GVHD. Canine NK cells, on the other hand, were not affected in their functional activity by treatment with G-CSF, suggesting that NK-mediated graft-versus-leukemia (GVL) activity should be preserved.

B. Engraftment

The two most important factors influencing the incidence of graft failure and the kinetics of hematopoietic recovery after allogeneic bone marrow transplantation (BMT) are the number of transplanted progenitor cells and the intensity of immunosuppression in the recipient (20–22). In contrast to BMT, where harvesting of substantially higher cell numbers is usually not feasible, allogeneic PBPCs can be harvested in virtually unlimited numbers. Following transplantation of T-cell–depleted bone marrow grafts, the benefit of reduced GVHD was counterbalanced by increased frequencies of leukemic relapse and graft failure (23); the latter problem being a consequence of the loss of progenitor cells associated with the technical maneuvers necessary to deplete the T cells (20,21). This problem should be avoidable with the high numbers of progenitor cells continued in PBPC harvest products.

Figure 1 shows the incidence of primary graft failure after transplantation of increasing numbers of syngeneic and allogeneic PBPCs. Following syngeneic PBPCT, no animal died as a result of engraftment failure after administration of at least 5×10^8 mononuclear cells (MNCs)/kg body weight (BW), and a prompt recovery of leukocyte and granulocyte counts was demonstrated (Fig. 2). The percentage of animals dying with graft failure increased with decreasing numbers of nucleated cells in the graft.

The transfer of increasing doses of allogeneic MHC-matched G-CSF–mobilized peripheral blood stem cells also resulted in a decreasing percentage of graft rejections. Compared to the syngeneic situation, however, significantly higher cell doses (1×10^9 cells/

graft failure (%)

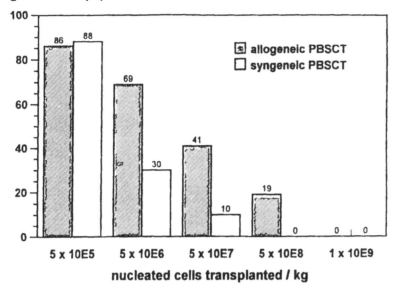

Figure 1 Comparison of graft failure rates after syngeneic or allogeneic major histocompatibility complex (MHC)–matched peripheral blood progenitor cell transplantation (PBPCT). Recipients were BALB/c mice; donors were BALB/c or DBA/2 mice, respectively. Donors were pretreated with $2 \times 5/\mu g$ filgastrim subcutaneously for 5 consecutive days prior to stem cell harvest. Experiments were done in a head-to-head manner with six repeated single experiments. The total number of animals in each group ranged from 8 to 27.

kg BW) were necessary to achieve fast and durable engraftment. As depicted in Figure 2, transplantation of low cell numbers led to delayed recovery from cytopenia.

When the engraftment potential of bone marrow (BM) cells and PBPCs was compared on the basis of the number of nucleated cells contained in the grafts, BM cells resulted in faster and more reliable engraftment—a situation contradictory to the clinical experience (24). This seemingly unusual finding can easily be explained if one keeps in mind that, in the clinical situation, the highest possible (and not a fixed) number of nucleated cells is harvested and transferred to the recipient. The average number of nucleated cells contained in a PBPCT collection product, however, is three to four times higher than in a typical BM graft and thus can more than compensate for the relative scarcity of colony-forming cells in the peripheral blood.

Data obtained in dogs also indicated that rapid engraftment can be achieved with G-CSF–mobilized progenitor cells. Sandmaier and coworkers (19) transferred a median of 17.1×10^8 PBPCs/kg (containing 27×10^4 CFU-GM/kg) from littermate donors after 9.2 Gy of total body irradiation (TBI) to the recipient. Prompt engraftment was documented in all animals even after transplantation of dog leukocyte antigen (DLA)–haploidentical grafts. In contrast, Storb and Deeg more than a decade ago had reported a rejection rate of 92% after transplantation of bone marrow cells in a similar canine model (25).

Taken together, present animal data demonstrate that the problem of graft rejection can be overcome by transplantation of increased numbers of progenitor cells as provided by a PBPC collection product. This is an important finding, because it offers two interest-

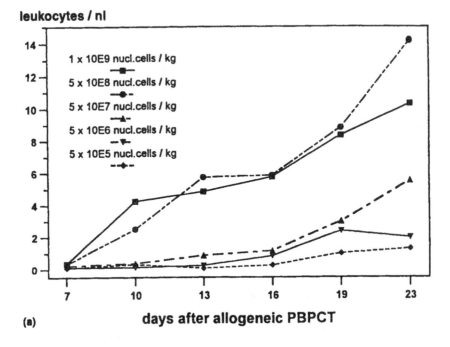

(a)

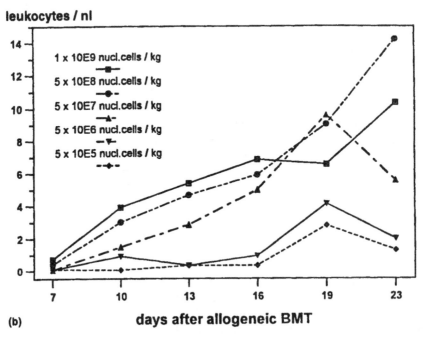

(b)

Figure 2 Leukocyte recovery in murine recipients of allogeneic major histocompatibility complex (MHC)–matched peripheral blood progenitor cells (PBPCs) or bone marrow grafts. Lethally irradiated BALB/c mice received increasing numbers of PBPCs (a) or bone marrow cells (b) from DBA/2 donors. PBPCT, peripheral blood progenitor cell transplantation; BMT, bone marrow transplantation.

ing new perspectives. First, it may be possible to lower the intensity of pretransplant immunosuppression, for example, the dose of TBI, in patients where complete and irreversible myeloablation is not the primary goal of conditioning therapy (i.e., patients with autoimmune disorders or severe combined immunodeficiency). Second, the possibility to collect high numbers of progenitor cells from the peripheral blood allows for extensive manipulation of the graft, because the cell loss usually associated with such procedures is better tolerated.

C. Graft-Versus-Host Reactivity

One major concern related to transplantation of allogeneic PBPCs was the assumption that the large numbers of T cells contained in PBPC grafts might give rise to an increased incidence or severity of graft-versus-host reactions (GVHRs) (26). It is very difficult to address this question in animal models, because acute and chronic GVHD are not easy to define and quantitate in such models. Sublethal forms of GVHD are especially difficult to assess. Moreover, GVHRs in rodents may have a partly different pathogenesis (27) as compared to nonhuman primates and humans (28), and the different numbers and functional status of T cells contained in grafts from rodents and humans preclude direct comparison of GVHD reactions occurring in both species.

Animal data therefore must be interpreted with caution. Our results in lethally irradiated BALB/c mice receiving MHC-identical PBPCs do not provide any evidence for an increased incidence of GVH-related mortality following PBPCT as compared to BMT. In these experiments, death due to GVHD was defined as death after recovery of hematopoiesis (leukocytes >3/nL and platelets >50/nL) with clinical signs of GVHD such as weight loss, rough fur, hair loss, and gibbus. Roughly the same rates of mortality due to GVHD (25%) were observed after allogeneic BMT and PBPCT (Fig. 3). With approximately three times more T cells in a PBPC graft as compared to marrow, this is a surprising yet unexplained finding which is in line, however, with clinical observations (29). As expected, T-cell depletion of PBPC grafts can also reduce GVHD-related mortality in mice (see below).

In the canine model, the incidence and severity of acute GVHD after transplantation of mobilized PBPCs into lethally irradiated dogs was not different than previously reported for nonmobilized PBPCs or marrow grafts (19). All DLA-haploidentical recipients of PBPCs, however, developed hyperacute and fatal GVHD. Owing to the limited numbers of animals treated per group, it seems impossible to draw definite conclusions from these data.

In summary, there is no experimental evidence for an increased incidence of acute and chronic GVHD after transplantation of G-CSF-mobilized PBPCs. On the other hand, the beneficial effect of G-CSF treatment on the alloreactivity of donor T cells, which has been observed in vitro, obviously does not translate into a reduced incidence of GVHD in vivo (17,19,30).

D. Graft-Versus-Leukemia Effect

It has been suggested that the high numbers of T and NK cells contained in a typical PBPC collection product (31) (see Table 1) not only induce more GVHD but also may exert a more vigorous GVL effect, reduce the risk of relapse, and improve disease-free survival after allogeneic PBPCT.

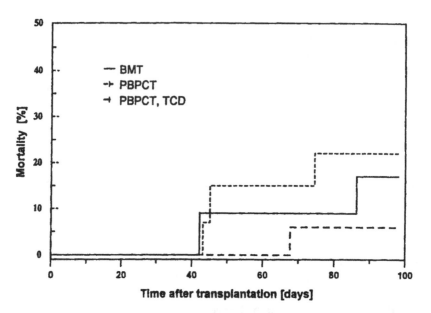

Figure 3 Mortality of lethally irradiated, nonleukemic BALB/c mice after transfer of 2×10^7 unmanipulated allogeneic bone marrow cells, peripheral blood progenitor cells (PBPCs), or CD3-depleted allogeneic PBPCs (n = 12–16). T-cell depletion was done by immunomagnetic removal of these cells by anti-CD3 coated magnetic beads, resulting in less than 1% CD3$^+$ cells as shown by flow cytometry. PBPCT, peripheral blood progenitor cell transplantation: BMT, bone marrow transplantation; TCD, T-cell depletion.

We addressed this issue in an experimental model with BALB/c mice bearing the B-lymphoblastic leukemia A20 (32). Our data indicate a superior antileukemic activity of G-CSF–mobilized allogeneic PBPCs over bone marrow cells (Fig. 4).

BALB/c mice were injected with 1×10^5 leukemia cells 2 days prior to transplantation of allogeneic or syngeneic BM and PBPC grafts. Whereas untreated animals died of leukemia after a median of 28 days, TBI with a dose of 7.5 Gy and subsequent syngeneic BMT resulted in a prolongation of the time to relapse up to 43 days. Twenty percent of the animals remained free from leukemia. Transplantation of allogeneic MHC-matched PBPCs after identical pretreatment of the recipient was followed by a significantly lower relapse rate: Freedom from leukemia was 66% in mice grafted with PBPCs (median time to relapse 58 days) as opposed to 40% after allogeneic BMT ($P < .05$) (see Fig. 4). Transplantation of SCF-mobilized cells showed a tendency toward even lower relapse rates. These findings, however, need confirmation by further experiments.

These data suggest a significant advantage of PBPC over BM grafts with respect to their antileukemic activity, whereas within the limitations of the model, an increased incidence of GVHD was not observed (see Fig. 3). The enhanced GVL effect of PBPC grafts may be explained by the transfer of higher numbers of T cells and NK cells as compared to a marrow graft (see Fig. 1) if one assumes that all of the donor's GVHD potential but only part of the GVL potential is transferred with the number of T cells contained in a marrow graft. Yet another explanation could be that peripheral and marrow-derived T cells differ with regard to subtype and functional properties which might also be altered by treatment with HGFs.

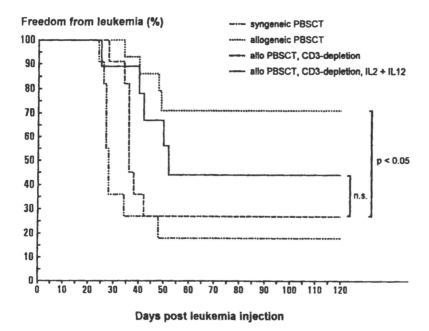

Freedom from leukemia (%)

---- syngeneic PBSCT
······ allogeneic PBSCT
--- allo PBSCT, CD3-depletion
— allo PBSCT, CD3-depletion, IL2 + IL12

Days post leukemia injection

Figure 4 Freedom from leukemia of lethally irradiated BALB/c mice after transplantation of syngeneic peripheral blood progenitor cell (PBPC), allogeneic bone marrow (BM) cells, or allogeneic PBPCs mobilized by recombinant human granulocyte colony-stimulating factor (rh-G-CSF) or recombinant rat (rr)-stem cell factor (rr-SCF). Two days prior to transplantation, the recipients were injected with 1×10^5 cells of the B-lymphoblastic leukemia cell line A20. Allogeneic peripheral blood progenitor cell transplantation (PBPCT) resulted in a significantly lower relapse rate as compared to allogeneic bone marrow transplantation (BMT) or syngeneic PBPCT ($P < .05$). Allo, allogeneic; IL, interleukin.

E. T-Cell Depletion

Following the transplantation of T-cell–depleted bone marrow grafts, the benefit of reduced GVHD was counterbalanced by increased frequencies of graft failure and leukemia relapse (23). The problem of an increased graft failure risk should be avoidable provided that high numbers of progenitor cells as contained in PBPC collection products are available (see Sect. II.B).

The second problem that emerged after lymphocyte depletion of marrow grafts, namely, the increased risk of leukemia relapse (23), may also be positively affected by the use of peripheral progenitor cells instead of marrow cells. Because leukapheresis products contain up to 20 times more NK cells than a bone marrow harvest (26), the number of NK cells remains significantly higher in T-cell–depleted PBPC grafts as compared with T-cell–depleted marrow grafts. GVL activity may therefore be partly conserved if peripheral progenitor cells are selectively depleted from CD3$^+$ T cells.

Experimental data, however, do not support this hypothesis. After depletion of CD3$^+$ cells from allogeneic PBPC transplants, only one animal (6%) died as a result of GVHD, but the results shown in Figure 5 clearly indicate that the depletion of CD3$^+$ T cells resulted in complete loss of antileukemic activity exerted by allogeneic (MHC-matched) G-CSF–mobilized PBPCs. Obviously, the remaining NK cells were not able to exert significant

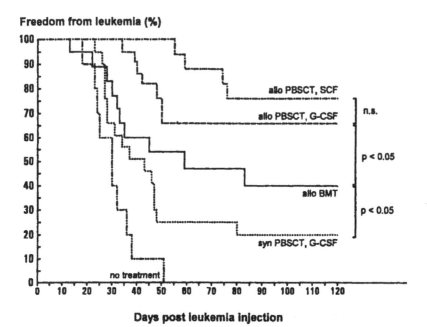

Freedom from leukemia (%)

Days post leukemia injection

Figure 5 Freedom from leukemia of BALB/c mice injected with 1×10^5 cells of the B-lympho-blastic leukemia cell line A20. Two days after leukemia cell injection, recipients were treated with 7.5 Gy of total body irradiation (TBI) followed by transplantation of either syngeneic or allogeneic peripheral blood progenitor cells (PBPCs). In some experimental groups, allogeneic grafts were T-cell depleted and activated with interleukin (IL)–2 (500 U/mL) and IL-12 (100 U/mL). Transplanta-tion of untreated allogeneic PBPCs resulted in a significantly lower relapse rate as compared to syngeneic or T-cell–depleted allogeneic PBPCs ($P < .05$). Allo PBPCT, allogeneic peripheral blood progenitor cell transplantation; SCF, stem cell factor; G-CSF, granulocyte colony-stimulating factor; Allo BMT, allogeneic bone marrow transplantation.

antileukemic activity in vivo. Since this may be due to the lack of T-cell–derived stimula-tory signals, we tested the antileukemic effectiveness of allogeneic CD3⁻ effector cells incubated with NK-stimulatory cytokines prior to grafting. Although the treatment of T-cell–depleted peripheral progenitor cells with IL-2 and IL-12 resulted in some enhance-ment of natural cytotoxicity in vitro, it was not able to restore the GVL effect to a level comparable to that of unmanipulated PBPC grafts (Fig. 5).

T-cell depletion was not associated with an increased rate of graft rejection in this preclinical model. All animals receiving a sufficient number of CD3-depleted PBPC (2 × 10⁷/kg) engrafted with prompt reconstitution of leukocytes and platelets. Tests for a donor-type chimerism revealed long-term engraftment.

III. CLINICAL ASPECTS OF ALLOGENEIC PERIPHERAL BLOOD STEM CELL TRANSPLANTATION

In the autologous setting, BMT has largely been replaced by the transplantation of PBPCs (12). In contrast, clinical experience with allogeneic PBPCT is still limited. This obvious discrepancy has multiple reasons. On the recipient's side it was anticipated that transplantation of allogeneic PBPCs would cause more frequent and/or severe acute and/or chronic GVHD. Furthermore, formal proof that PBPCs would ensure long-term hematopoietic recovery was lacking. For the donors, harvesting of PBPCs necessitated the administration of G-CSF. It was largely unknown which acute toxicities and long-term risks would be associated with the administration of this HGF to healthy volunteers. On the other hand, there were obvious benefits to be expected with the transplantation of allogeneic PBPCs. The donors could be spared the risks and discomfort of general anesthesia, and the local problems sometimes associated with the marrow harvest procedure could be avoided. Data obtained after autologous PBPCT suggested that a more rapid recovery of platelets, granulocytes, and the immune system could occur (29). Because the earlier hematopoietic recovery seen after autologous PBPCT resulted in earlier discharge of the patients, it was hoped that a similar posttransplant course after allogeneic PBPCT could make the procedure less expensive. The large number of lymphocytes transferred with a PBPC graft could possibly enhance the GVL effect exerted by allogeneic transplants.

A. The Donors and the Graft

A number of studies have addressed the question of how allogeneic PBPCs can best be mobilized, at what time leukaphereses should be performed, and which factors would influence the yield of harvesting PBPCs in healthy donors (31,33–37). G-CSF is the only HGF which has been used to mobilize allogeneic PBPCs. Doses between 10 and 16 µg/kg administered for 5 or 6 consecutive days seem optimal for effective mobilization of PBPCs. Lower or higher doses of G-CSF have occasionally been administered to healthy volunteers but have not been used in larger cohorts of donors. Doses below 10 µg/kg of G-CSF per day result in mobilization of significantly lower numbers of CD34$^+$ cells, which then necessitates additional leukaphereses. Higher doses of G-CSF are more expensive and have been reported to cause more frequent side effects. It is not clear if higher doses of G-CSF would allow an increase in the fraction of patients who have sufficient numbers of CD34$^+$ cells harvested with one leukapheresis procedure. At the University of Kiel, we administered 10 µg/kg of filgrastim subcutaneously to 35 consecutive donors of allogeneic PBPCs and were able to show that 43% of the donors achieved the target number of >4 × 10^6/kg CD34$^+$ cells after one leukapheresis (38). It can be anticipated that less than 10% of healthy donors will need more than two leukapheresis procedures if G-CSF at a dose between 10 and 16 µg/kg/day is administered for 5 days and leukapheresis is performed on days 5 and 6. Other groups have reported similar results.

Although phenotypic and functional differences between CD34$^+$ cells obtained from mobilized peripheral blood or BM surely exist, there is convincing evidence that immature stem cells as well as more mature progenitor cells committed to the various myeloid lineages are contained in mobilized peripheral blood. Meanwhile, detailed investigations on the development of chimerism after allogeneic PBPCT prove the existence of cells with long-term repopulating capacity in the peripheral blood (39). Compared to a typical marrow graft, PBPC harvests contain approximately 10 times more T cells and 20 times more NK cells (9,31). The frequency of T-cell subsets and of CD3$^+$, CD4$^-$, and CD8$^-$ cells in particular is more controversial (9,40,41).

The acute toxicities encountered with the administration of G-CSF to healthy donors and the subsequent leukapheresis procedures are well described.

Table 2 lists side effects prospectively documented in healthy donors who were treated at several European institutions with 10 µg/kg/day of G-CSF for 5 or 6 consecutive

Table 2 Side Effects of G-CSF Administration to Healthy Family Donors

Adverse event	No. of donors	Severity (WHO)			
		Grade 1	Grade 2	Grade 3	Grade 4
Muscularskeletal pain	16	8	7	1	
Headache	3	2	1		
Chills	1		1		
Elevation of AP	1	1			
Elevation of GGT and LDH	1		1		
Hypocalcemia	1		1		
Thrombocytopenia	1		1		
Hyperthermia	1	1			
Hot flushes	1	1			
"Common cold"	1	1			
Dyspnea	1	1			
Thoracic pain	1	1			
Circulatory distress	1	1			
Periorbital exanthema	1	1			
Hysteria during apheresis procedure	1		1		

Results from a prospective randomized trial carried out by the European Group for Blood and Marrow Transplantation.
G-CSF, granulocyte colony-stimulating factor; WHO, World Health Organization; AP, alkaline phosphatase; GGT, gamma-glutamyl transferase; LDH, lactic acid dehydrogenase.

days. The side effects largely resemble those seen in patients who received G-CSF to harvest autologous PBPCs. The predominant side effect of G-CSF administration was bone pain, which occurred in the vast majority of donors receiving G-CSF at doses >5 μg/kg/day. Leukapheresis procedures carry a low risk of severe complications if carried out in an appropriate setting. One myocardial infarction and two donors with angina pectoris–like symptoms have been reported to date. The true denominator of these figures is unknown, and it therefore seems difficult to comment reliably on the incidence of severe complications of G-CSF administration and leukapheresis procedures. Most investigators feel that monitoring of volunteer donors is necessary to recognize potential acute problems and, more importantly, to exclude long-term adverse effects of G-CSF administration (42). Although there is no evidence so far that short-term administration of G-CSF may cause any late effects, the laboratory finding that G-CSF is able to stimulate growth of leukemic blast cells under certain experimental conditions has created fears that G-CSF administration might induce leukemia in volunteer donors. Experimental findings as well as the observation of strongly elevated G-CSF levels associated with severe infections may temper against these fears. Nevertheless, international activities aimed at the long-term monitoring of both blood and marrow donors are ongoing.

B. Engraftment

Table 3 shows the times needed to reach an absolute neutrophil count (ANC) >0.5 × 10^9/L and a platelet count >20 × 10^9/L after transplantation of unmanipulated allogeneic PBPCs, as recently reported by major centers in the United States and Europe. Although

Table 3 Hematopoietic Recovery After
Transplantation of Unmodified Allogeneic PBPCs

Reference	N	ANC > 0.5	Platelets > 20
43	33	14[a]	14
44	31	14	—
24	59	15[a]	16
45	61	16	18
46	37	14	11

PBPCs, peripheral blood progenitor cells; ANC, absolute
neutrophil count; G-CSF, granulocyte colony-stimulating
factor.
[a]Some patients received G-CSF posttransplant.

these patient cohorts varied with respect to the use of G-CSF posttransplant, the administration of methotrexate for prophylaxis of GVHD and other variables potentially influencing hematopoietic recovery, the times to neutrophil recovery ($\geq 0.5 \times 10^9$/L) were surprisingly consistent (days 14–16), whereas platelet recovery ($\geq 20 \times 10^9$/L) seemed somewhat more variable. This is not too surprising, because severe GVHD and other typical complications of allogeneic transplantation, such as cytomegalovirus (CMV) infection and veno-occlusive disease of the liver, affect platelet recovery after allogeneic transplantation of hematopoietic stem cells. A retrospective study comparing the hematopoietic recovery following allogeneic PBPCT and BMT reported a significant difference in favor of the PBPCT group with regard to neutrophil and platelet engraftment (thresholds as above) (14 vs 16 and 11 vs 15 days, respectively). Moreover, the proportion of patients not achieving a durable platelet recovery tended to be lower after PBPCT (14 vs 32%; $P = .097$) (47). Several investigators have provided data on hematopoietic chimerism developing after allogeneic PBPCT (39; M. Suttorp, et al., unpublished data). These data generally show the rapid development of full donor chimerism in the marrow and blood of the recipients of allogeneic PBPCs. There are no data available which support earlier fears that allogeneic PBPCs might be unable to sustain long-term hematopoiesis in a recipient grafted with such cells.

C. Acute Graft-Versus-Host Disease

Since T lymphocytes represent the main effector cells of acute GVHD, there were major concerns that the large numbers of T cells transferred with a PBPC collection product might lead to an increased incidence or severity of GVHD. Surprisingly, pilot trials on allogeneic PBPCT suggested that the incidence of GVHD might be even lower after allogeneic PBPCT as compared to BMT (9–11).

The retrospective comparison performed by Bensinger and colleagues (10) seems to confirm these findings. The risks to develop acute GVHD grades II–IV or grades III–IV after transplantation of BM or PBPCs were 37 and 14% versus 56 and 33%, $P = .05$ and $P = .077$, respectively. Other investigators have reported somewhat higher incidences of moderate to severe GVHD (24), and it might therefore be more appropriate to state that without any prospective data being available at this time, the incidence and severity of acute GVHD seen after allogeneic PBPCT or BMT may not largely differ.

D. Chronic Graft-Versus-Host Disease

Table 4 shows the incidence and severity of chronic GVHD as reported by the Seattle Group and in a recent paper published by the EBMT. Again, it seems impossible to judge if the percentages given in Table 4 represent an increase of chronic GVHD after allogeneic PBPCT if compared to BMT.

The data on chronic GVHD is particularly limited, because the follow-up of patients reported by most transplant teams was short and the development of chronic GVHD therefore was not fully evaluable. Although most investigators did not report more frequent or severe chronic GVHD after transplantation of allogeneic PBPCs, other groups did claim a higher incidence of extensive chronic GVHD after allogeneic PBPCT (48,49; M. Körbling et al., unpublished data). Although it is far from clear whether chronic GVHD will be a particular problem after allogeneic PBPCT, this question surely deserves further study as early clinical experience with the infusion of donor buffy coat in order to prevent graft rejection in multiply transfused patients with aplastic anemia suggests that the infusion of large amounts of T cells contained in buffy coat preparations can cause an increase in chronic GVHD (50). Again, the results of prospective randomized trials are needed to settle this issue.

E. T-Cell Depletion

Although exact numbers are unavailable today, acute and chronic GVHD will remain a major problem after allogeneic PBPCT. It is therefore logical to investigate the clinical consequences of T-cell depletion of allogeneic PBPC harvests. Although T-cell depletion in the narrower sense is possible, clinical results are only available for patients who have been transplanted with CD34$^+$ selected PBPCs. CD34$^+$ selection can result in 2- to 3-log T-cell depletion leaving between 1×10^5 and 1×10^6 T cells/kg in the PBPC graft. Obviously, this extent of T-cell depletion is not sufficient to avoid reliably the occurrence of moderate to severe acute GVHD (Table 5).

As shown in Table 5, all investigators except for Urbano-Ispizua et al. (54) reported on the occurrence of grades III–IV acute GVHD in a substantial fraction of patients grafted with CD34$^+$–selected PBPCs. Further efforts to reduce the T-cell content of PBPC collec-

Table 4   Incidence and Severity of Chronic GVHD After Allogeneic PBPCT from HLA-Identical Siblings

Chronic GVHD	Seattle[a] (%)	EBMT[b] (%)
None	7/17 (41)	22/49 (45)
Subclinical	3/17 (18)	—
Limited	3/17 (18)	17/49 (35)
Extensive	4/17 (24)	10/49 (20)

GVHD, graft-versus-host disease; PBPCT, peripheral blood progenitor cell transplantation; HLA, human leukocyte antigen; EBMT, European Group for Blood and Marrow Transplantation.
[a] Ref. 46.
[b] Ref. 24.

Table 5 Clinical Experience with T-Cell Depletion of Allogeneic PBPC Harvests Using CD34$^+$ Selection

Reference	N	Device	CD34$^+$ ($\times10^6$/kg)	CD3$^+$ ($\times10^5$/kg)	GVHD prophylaxis	GVHD (II–IV)
51	10	CellPro	7.5	11.9	CyA (+MTX)	5/5 (1/5)
52	10	CellPro	4.1	4.2	CyA	3/10
47	16	CellPro	9.0	7.3	CyA (+MTX)	4/8 (8/10)
53	7	Isolex	7.1	2.0	CyA	6/6
54	16	CellPro	3.3	4.5	CyA + Pred	0/16

PBPC, peripheral blood progenitor cell; GVHD, graft-versus-host disease; CyA, cyclosporine A; MTX, methotrexate; Pred, Prednisone.

tion products seem therefore necessary to abrogate GVHD in this setting. Whereas an increased frequency of graft failure or graft rejection has not been reported so far after transplantation of CD34$^+$–selected PBPC grafts because of the huge numbers of CD34$^+$ cells contained in a normal PBPC collection product (see above), there is no reason to believe that the loss of GVL activity noticed after transplantation of T-cell–depleted BM will not also occur after transplantation of T-cell–depleted (or CD34$^+$–selected) allogeneic PBPCs. Clinical results supporting this hypothesis are not available. However, the experimental data presented in Figure 4 strongly suggest that the loss of GVL activity is more than of theoretical concern.

Nevertheless, the transplantation of highly selected CD34$^+$ cells remains an attractive possibility, because it may allow the transplantation from HLA partly matched family or unrelated donors (55). Late T-cell add backs or the infusion of allogeneic NK cells early after the transplant may be able to compensate for the loss of GVL activity without reintroducing severe GVHD.

F. Graft-Versus-Leukemia Activity

There are no clinical data available which might support the experimental data reported earlier in this chapter that allogeneic peripheral blood stem cell transplantation confers an improved GVL effect. Allogeneic transplantation of PBPCs has preferably been used in patients with advanced hematological malignancies. The relapse rates reported for these patients have been relatively low. However, patients have usually been very heterogeneous with respect to disease, conditioning regimen, GVHD prophylaxis, and other variables which are known to influence the risk of relapse. Thus, larger cohorts of patients with longer follow-up will be necessary to answer reliably the question of an improved GVL effect after allogeneic PBPCT. International organizations like the International Bone Marrow Transplant Registry (IBMTR) and EBMT have set out to address this problem and are currently performing retrospective and prospective analyses which hopefully will help to answer this important question in the near future. Whereas leukemia-free survival and overall survival as the most important endpoints to be analyzed after allogeneic BMT and PBPCT are the result of transplant-related mortality, acute and chronic GVHD, relapse incidence, and other variables, it is surely true that currently available data do not allow comparison of the merits or disadvantages of allogeneic PBPCT or BMT.

IV. FUTURE DIRECTIONS

According to the currently available data, there is no obvious advantage of allogeneic PBPCT over BMT with regard to the development of GVHD. The induction of T-cell hyporeactivity and/or a polarization of T cells toward Th2-type cytokine secretion by G-CSF, however, may at least counterbalance the aggravation of GVHD to be expected after transferring 5–10 times more T cells to the recipient with the graft.

The availability of high numbers of hematopoietic progenitor cells allows the depletion of T cells from PBPC grafts without negative effects on engraftment. This has been demonstrated in the experimental setting (20) as well as by recent clinical experience. Our animal data, however, anticipate that T-cell depletion (or CD34+ selection) will result in the loss of most, if not all, of the GVL potential exerted by an allogeneic graft. Based on these findings, T-cell depletion of PBPC collection products may be advantageous if the loss of antileukemic activity is irrelevant (i.e., in the treatment of patients with aplastic anemia or autoimmune disorders), but it should be used with caution in patients whose clinical outcomes largely depend on the presence of a vigorous GVL effect.

The main advantage of allogeneic PBPCs over BM appears to be their excellent suitability for extensive graft engineering. Thus, T-cell depletion will not be the end but the beginning of a new era of transplantation of hematopoietic cells made possible by the availability of PBPCs. Further progress will make necessary attempts to identify which cell fractions in the graft carry the clinically important activities. Selection, expansion, and genetic engineering of these populations hopefully will result in the production of a graft individually tailored to the needs of the patient. Among other possibilities, such manipulations could allow the transplantation of highly selected hematopoietic progenitor cells from haploidentical donors or family donors without the problems currently seen in these situations. The subsequent infusion of leukemia-specific T cells or MHC-mismatched NK cells could elicit an immunological reaction against residual tumor cells and diminish the relapse rates in patients grafted with "pure" stem cell preparations.

REFERENCES

1. Epstein RB, Graham TC, Buckner CD, Bryant J, Thomas ED. Allogeneic marrow engraftment by cross circulation in lethally irradiated dogs. Blood 1966; 28:692–707.
2. Storb R, Epstein RB, Ragde H, Bryant J, Thomas ED. Marrow engraftment by allogeneic leukocytes in lethally irradiated dogs. Blood 1967; 30:805–811.
3. Storb R, Graham TC, Epstein RB, Sale GE, Thomas ED. Demonstration of hemopoietic stem cells in the peripheral blood of baboons by cross circulation. Blood 1977; 50:537–542.
4. Kessinger A, Smith DM, Strandjord SE, Landmark JD, Dooley DC, Law P, Coccia PF, Warkentin PI, Weisenburger DD, Armitage JO. Allogeneic transplantation of blood-derived, T cell–depleted hemopoietic stem cells after myeloablative treatment in a patient with acute lymphoblastic leukemia. Bone Marrow Transplant 1989; 4:643–646.
5. Socinski MA, Elias A, Schnipper L, Cannistra SA, Antman KH, Griffin JD. Granulocyte-macrophage colony stimulating factor expands the circulation haemopoietic progenitor cell compartment in man. Lancet 1989; 1:1194–1198.
6. Sheridan WP, Begley CG, Juttner CA, Szer J, To LB, Mahel D, McGrath KM, Morstyn G, Fox RM. Effect of peripheral-blood progenitor cells mobilised by filgrastim (G-CSF) on platelet recovery after high-dose chemotherapy. Lancet 1992; 339:640–644.
7. Russell NH, Hunter A, Rogers S, Hanley J, Anderson D. Peripheral blood stem cells as an alternative to marrow for allogeneic transplantation (letter). Lancet 1993; 341:1482.
8. Dreger P, Suttorp M, Haferlach T, Löffler H, Schroyens W, Schmitz N. Allogeneic granulocyte

colony-stimulating factor-mobilized peripheral blood progenitor cells for treatment of engraftment failure after bone marrow transplantation. Blood 1993; 81:1404–1407.

9. Körbling M, Huh YO, Durett A, Mirza N, Miller P, Engel H, Anderlini P, van Besien K, Andreeff M, Przepiorka D, Deisseroth AB, Champlin RE. Allogeneic blood stem cell transplantation: Peripheralization and yield of donor-derived primitive hematopoietic progenitor cells (CD34⁺ Thy-1-dim) and lymphoid subsets, and possible predictors of engraftment and graft-versus-host disease. Blood 1995; 86:2842–2848.

10. Bensinger WI, Weaver CH, Appelbaum FR, Rowley S, Demirer T, Sanders J, Storb R, Buckner CD. Transplantation of allogeneic peripheral blood stem cells mobilized by recombinant human granulocyte colony-stimulating factor. Blood 1995; 85:1655–1658.

11. Schmitz N, Dreger P, Suttorp M, Rohwedder EB, Haferlach T, Löffler H, Hunter A, Russell NH. Primary transplantation of allogeneic peripheral blood progenitor cells mobilized by filgrastim (granulocyte colony-stimulating factor). Blood 1995; 85:1666–1672.

12. Gratwohl A, Hermans J, Baldomero H for the European Group for Blood and Marrow Transplantation (EBMT). Blood and marrow transplantation activity in Europe 1995. Bone Marrow Transplant 1997; 19:407–419.

13. Molineux G, Pojda Z, Hampson IN, Lord BI, Dexter TM. Transplantation potential of peripheral blood stem cells induced by granulocyte colony-stimulating factor. Blood 1990; 76:2153–2158.

14. Yan XQ, Briddell R, Hartley C, Stoney G, Samal B, McNiece, I. Mobilization of long-term hematopoietic reconstituting cells in mice by the combination of stem cell factor plus granulocyte colony-stimulating factor. Blood 1994; 84:795–799.

15. Briddell RA, Hartley CA, Smith KA, McNiece, IK. Recombinant rat stem cell factor synergizes with recombinant human granulocyte colony-stimulating factor in vivo in mice to mobilize peripheral blood progenitor cells that have enhanced repopulating potential. Blood 1993; 82:1720–1723.

16. Drize N, Chertkov J, Samoilina N, Zander A. Effect of cytokine treatment (granulocyte colony-stimulating factor and stem cell factor) on hematopoiesis and the circulating pool of hematopoietic stem cells in mice. Exp Hematol 1996; 24:816–822.

17. Pan L, Delmonte J, Jalonen CK, Ferrara JL. Pretreatment of donor mice with granulocyte colony-stimulating factor polarizes donor T lymphocytes toward type-2 cytokine production and reduces severity of experimental graft-versus-host disease. Blood 1995; 86:4422–4429.

18. Krenger W, Snyder KM, Byon JC, Falzarano G, Ferrara JL. Polarized type 2 alloreactive CD4⁺ and CD8⁺ donor T cells fail to induce experimental acute graft-versus-host disease. J Immunol 1995; 155:585–593.

19. Sandmaier BM, Storb R, Santos EB, Krizanac-Bengez L, Lian T, McSweeney PA, Yu C, Schuening FG, Deeg HJ, Graham T. Allogeneic transplants of canine peripheral blood stem cells mobilized by recombinant canine hematopoietic growth factors. Blood 1996; 87:3508–3513.

20. Uharek L, Gassmann W, Glass B, Steinmann J, Loeffler H, Müller-Ruchholtz W. Influence of cell dose and graft-versus-host reactivity on rejection rates after allogeneic bone marrow transplantation. Blood 1992; 79:1612–1621.

21. Uharek L, Glass B, Gaska T, Gassmann W, Loeffler H, Mueller-Ruchholtz W. Influence of donor lymphocytes on the incidence of primary graft failure after allogeneic bone marrow transplantation in a murine model. Br J Haematol 1994; 88:79–87.

22. Reisner Y, Martelli MF. Bone marrow transplantation across HLA barriers by increasing the number of transplanted cells. Immunol Today 1995; 16:437–440.

23. Maraninchi D, Gluckman E, Blaise D, Guyotat D, Rio B, Pico JL, Leblond V, Michallet M, Dreyfus F, Ifrah N. Impact of T-cell depletion on outcome of allogeneic bone marrow transplantation for standard-risk leukemias. Lancet 1987; 2:175–178.

24. Schmitz N, Bacigalupo A, Labopin M, Majolino I, Laporte JP, Brinch L, Cook G, Lambertenghi Deliliers G, Lange A, Rozman C, Garcia-Conde J, Finke J, Domingo-Albos A, Gratwohl

A for the European Group for Blood and Marrow Transplantation (EBMT). Transplantation of peripheral blood progenitor cells from HLA-identical sibling donors. Br J Haematol 1996; 95:715–23.

25. Storb R, Deeg HJ. Failure of allogeneic canine marrow grafts after total body irradiation: allogeneic "resistance" vs transfusion induced sensitization. Transplantation 1985; 42:571–578.

26. Dreger P, Viehmann K, Steinmann J, Eckstein V, Müller-Ruchholtz W, Löffler H, Schmitz N. G-CSF-mobilized peripheral blood progenitor cells for allogeneic transplantation: Comparison of T cell depletion strategies using different CD34+ selection systems or CAMPATH-1. Exp Hematol 1995; 23:147–154.

27. Vallera DA, Soderling CCB, Carlson GJ, Kersey JH. Bone marrow transplantation across major histocompatibility barriers in mice. Effect of elimination of T cells from donor grafts by treatment with monoclonal Thy-1.2 plus complement or antibody alone. Transplantation 1981; 31:218–222.

28. Ferrara JL, Deeg HJ. Graft-versus-host disease. N Engl J Med 1991; 324:667–669.

29. Schmitz N, Linch DC, Dreger P, Goldstone AH, Boogaerts MA, Ferrant A, Demuynck HMS, Link H, Zander A, Barge A, Borkett K. Randomised trial of filgrastim-mobilised peripheral blood progenitor cell transplantation versus autologous bone-marrow transplantation in lymphoma patients. Lancet 1996; 347:353–357.

30. Fowler DH, Kurasawa K, Smith R, Gress RE. Donor lymphoid cells of Th2 cytokine phenotype reduce lethal graft versus host disease and facilitate fully allogeneic cell transfers in sublethally irradiated mice. Prog Clin Biol Res 1994; 389:533–540.

31. Dreger P, Haferlach T, Eckstein V, Jacobs S, Suttorp M, Löffler H, Müller-Ruchholtz W, Schmitz N. G-CSF-mobilised peripheral blood progenitor cells for allogeneic transplantation: safety, kinetics of mobilisation, and composition of the graft. Br J Haematol 1994; 87:609–613.

32. Glass B, Uharek L, Zeis M, Dreger P, Löffler H, Steinmann J, Schmitz N. Allogeneic peripheral blood progenitor cell transplantation in a murine model: evidence for an improved graft-versus-leukemia effect. Blood 1997; 90:1694–1700.

33. Matsunaga T, Sakamaki S, Kohgo Y, Ohi S, Hirayama Y, Niitsu Y. Recombinant human granulocyte colony-stimulating factor can mobilize sufficient amounts of peripheral blood stem cells in healthy volunteers for allogeneic transplantation. Bone Marrow Transplant 1993; 11:103–108.

34. Grigg AP, Roberts AW, Raunow H, Houghton S, Layton JE, Boyd AW, McGrath KM, Maher D. Optimizing dose and scheduling of filgrastim (granulocyte colony-stimulating factor) for mobilization and collection of peripheral blood progenitor cells in normal volunteers. Blood 1995; 86:4437–4445.

35. Körbling M, Przepiorka D, Huh YO, Engel H, van Besien K, Giralt S, Andersson B, Kleine HD, Seong D, Deisseroth AB, Andreef M, Champlin R. Allogeneic blood stem cell transplantation for refractory leukemia and lymphoma: potential advantage of blood over marrow allografts. Blood 1995; 85:1659–1665.

36. Anderlini P, Przepiorka D, Huh Y, Lauppe J, Miller P, Sundberg J, Seong D, Champlin R, Körbling M. Duration of filgrastim mobilization and apheresis yield of CD34+ progenitor cells and lymphoid subsets in normal donors for allogeneic transplantation. Br J Haematol 1996; 93:940–942.

37. Harada M, Nagafuji K, Fujisaki T, Kubota A, Mizuno S-I, Takenaka K, Miyamoto T, Ohno Y, Gondo H, Kuriowa M, Okamura T, Inaba S, Niho Y. G-CSF–induced mobilization of peripheral blood stem cells from healthy adults for allogeneic transplantation. J Hematother 1996; 5:63–71.

38. Dreger P, Glass B, Uharek L, Zeis M, Schmitz N. Allogeneic transplantation of mobilized peripheral blood progenitor cells: towards tailored cell therapy. Int J Hematol 1997; 66:1–11.

39. Elmaagacli AH, Beelen DW, Becks HW, Mosbacher A, Stockova J, Tzrensky S, Schaefer UW. Molecular studies of chimerism and minimal residual disease after allogeneic peripheral blood progenitor cell or marrow transplantation. Ann Hematol 1996; 73:A84.

40. Dreger P, Oberböster K, Schmitz N. PBPC grafts from healthy donors: analysis of CD34$^+$ and CD3$^+$ subpopulations. Bone Marrow Transplant 1996; 17:S22–S27.

41. Negrin RS, Kusnierz-Glaz C, Blume KG, Strober S. Enrichment of allogeneic CD34$^+$ cells and T cell depletion by percoll density gradient centrifugation. Bone Marrow Transplant 1996; 17:S31–S33.

42. Anderlini P, Körbling M, Dale D, Gratwohl A, Schmitz N, Stroncek D, Howe C, Leitman S, Horowitz M, Gluckman E, Rowley S, Przepiorka D, Champlin R. Allogeneic blood stem cell transplantation: considerations for donors. Blood 1997; 90:903–908.

43. Urbano-Ispizua A, Solano C, Brunet S, Hernández F, Sanz G, Alegre A, Petit J, Besalduch J, Vivancos P, Díaz MA, Moraleda JM, Carreras E, Ojeda E, de la Rubia J, Benet I, Domingo-Albós A, García-Conde J, Rozman C for the Spanish Group of Allo-PBPCT. Allogeneic peripheral blood progenitor cell transplantation: analysis of short-term engraftment and acute GVHD incidence in 33 cases. Bone Marrow Transplant 1996; 18:35–40.

44. Bacigalupo A, Van Lint MT, Valbonesi M, Lercari G, Carlier P, Lamparelli T, Gualandi F, Occhini D, Bregante S, Valeriani A, Piaggio G, Pitto A, Benvenuto F, Figari O, De Stefano G, Caimo A, Sessarego M. Thiotepa cyclophosphamide followed by granulocyte colony-stimulating factor mobilized allogeneic peripheral blood cells in adults with advanced leukemia. Blood 1996; 88:353–357.

45. Blaise D, Rossi JF, Jourdan E, Michallet M, Reiffers J, Jouet JP, Michel G, Faucher C, Fortainer C, Hua A, Schuller MP, Badri N, Chabannon C, Maraninchi D. A pilot study of allogeneic stem cell transplantation after priming with lenograstim. Blood 1996; 88:617a.

46. Bensinger WI, Clift R, Martin P, Appelbaum FR, Demirer T, Gooley T, Lilleby K, Rowley S, Sanders J, Storb R, Buckner CD. Allogeneic peripheral blood stem cell transplantation in patients with advanced hematologic malignancies: a retrospective comparison with marrow transplantation. Blood 1996; 88:2794–2800.

47. Bensinger WI, Buckner CD, Shannon-Dorcy K, Rowley S, Appelbaum FR, Benyunes M, Clift R, Martin P, Demirer T, Storb R, Lee M, Schiller G. Transplantation of allogeneic CD34$^+$ peripheral blood stem cells in patients with advanced hematologic malignancy. Blood 1996; 88:4132–4138.

48. Urbano-Ispizua A, Garcia-Conde J, Brunet S, Hernández F, Sanz G, Alegre A, Petit J, Bargay J, Vivancos P, Solano C, Ojeda E, Domingo A, Rozman C for the Spanish Group of Allo PBPCT. High incidence of chronic graft versus host disease (GVHD) after allogeneic peripheral blood progenitor cell transplantation (allo-PBPCT) from matched related donors. Blood 1996; 88(suppl 1):617a.

49. Majolino I, Saglio G, Scimé R, Serra A, Cavallaro AM, Fiandaca T, Vasta S, Pampinella M, Catania P, Indovina AS, Marcenò R, Santoro A. High incidence of chronic GVHD after primary allogeneic peripheral blood stem cell transplantation in patients with hematologic malignancis. Bone Marrow Transplant 1996; 17:555–560.

50. Storb R, Etzioni R, Anasetti C, Appelbaum FR, Buckner CD, Bensinger W, Bryant W, Clift R, Deeg HJ, Doney K, Hansen H, Martin P, Pepe M, Sale G, Sanders J, Singer J, Sullivan KM, Thomas ED, Witherspoon RP. Cyclophosphamide combined with antithymocyte globulin in preparation for allogeneic marrow transplants in patients with aplastic anemia. Blood 1994; 84:941–949.

51. Link H, Arseniev L, Bähre O, Kadar JG, Diedrich H, Poliwoda H. Transplantation of allogeneic CD34+ blood cells. Blood 1996; 87:4903–4909.

52. Finke J, Brugger W, Bertz H, Behringer D, Kunzmann R, Weber-Nordt RM, Kanz L, Mertelsmann R. Allogeneic transplantation of positively selected peripheral blood CD34$^+$ progenitor cells from matched related donors. Bone Marrow Transplant 1996; 18:1081–1086.

53. Bensinger WI, Rowley S, Appelbaum FR, Mills B, Oldham F, Chauncey T, Buckner CD.

CD34 selected allogeneic peripheral blood stem cell (PBSC) transplantation in older patients with advanced hematologic malignancies. Blood 1995; 86:97a.

54. Urbano-Ispizua A, Rozman C, Martinez C, Marin P, Briones J, Rovira M, Féliz P, Viguria MC, Merino A, Sierra J, Mazzara R, Carreras E, Montserrat E. Rapid engraftment without significant GVHD after allogeneic transplantation of CD34$^+$ selected cells from peripheral blood. Blood 1997; 89:3967–3973.

55. Aversa F, Tabilio A, Terenzi A, Velardi A, Falzetti F, Giannoni C, Iacucci R, Zei T, Martelli MP, Gambelunghe C, Rossetti M, Caputo P, Latini P, Aristei C, Raymondi C, Reisner Y, Matelli MF. Successful engraftment of T-cell–depleted haploidentical "three-loci" incompatible transplants in leukemia patients by addition of recombinant human granulocyte colony-stimulating factor-mobilized peripheral blood progenitor cells to bone marrow inoculum. Blood 1994; 84:3948–3955.

23

Mechanisms of Cure of Acute Myeloid Leukemia with Allogeneic Transplantation

FREDERICK R. APPELBAUM

Fred Hutchinson Cancer Research Center, Seattle, Washington

I. INTRODUCTION

Although the precise role of allogeneic transplantation in the treatment of acute myeloid leukemia (AML) continues to be discussed and refined, there is no argument that this therapeutic technique is able to cure patients who are incurable by any other means. The clearest examples are patients who fail initial induction chemotherapy. Such patients are incurable with any nontransplant approach, yet several studies have documented long-term disease-free survival in approximately 20% of induction-failure patients if treated with allogeneic transplantation (1,2). Similarly, many studies have demonstrated that 15–20% of patients who have relapsed from an initial remission and have failed attempts at reinduction can still be cured with transplantation (3). Recently, the question of the appropriate timing of allogeneic transplantation in AML has tended to dominate most discussions, and although it is important to define which patients are best served by being treated with allogeneic transplantation in first remission versus those who may better benefit by withholding transplantation until first relapse, this debate should not obscure the fact that allogeneic transplantation cures otherwise incurable patients. Understanding the mechanisms by which transplantation achieves this result should allow for further improvements in transplantation and may have relevance for other approaches as well.

II. GRAFT VERSUS ACUTE MYELOID LEUKEMIA

Credit for the first demonstration that a graft-versus-leukemia (GVL) effect might exist is usually given to Barnes and Loutit, who reported in 1957 that CBA mice bearing a

Table 1 Evidence for a Graft-Versus-Leukemia Effect in Acute Myeloid Leukemia

1. Relapse rates following syngeneic transplantation are higher than after allogeneic transplantation.
2. Relapse is less likely in patients who develop graft-versus-host disease.
3. The risk of relapse is increased with T-cell depletion of marrow.
4. Donor lymphocyte infusions can induce complete remission in patients who recur posttransplant.

syngeneic leukemia could not be cured by total body irradiation and infusion of syngeneic marrow, whereas infusion of allogeneic marrow resulted in death with graft-versus-host disease (GVHD) but without leukemia (4). In the decades since, the immunotherapeutic effects of allogeneic marrow transplantation have been increasingly well defined and dissected in numerous animal models.

At least four lines of evidence suggest that a GVL effect exists in patients treated for AML (Table 1). First, the incidence of AML recurrence is far greater following identical twin transplantation than following allogeneic transplantation. In a recent publication from the International Bone Marrow Transplant Registry (IBMTR), the 3-year probability of relapse among 45 twins transplanted for AML in first remission was 52% compared to 16% in 450 human leukocyte antigen (HLA)–identical sibling transplants selected to match the twins for known pretransplant prognostic factors ($P < .001$) (5). A second body of evidence supporting a graft-versus-AML effect in humans includes the repeated observation that among recipients of allogeneic grafts, the likelihood of relapse is reduced in those who develop GVHD. This phenomenon was first reported by Weiden et al. in 1979 and has been reconfirmed in a number of studies since (6,7). For example, in 1990, the IBMTR reported an analysis of the association of GVHD and outcome in 2254 patients with various forms of leukemia (8). Among 1046 patients transplanted for AML in first remission, the actuarial probability of relapse was $49 \pm 21\%$ among recipients of syngeneic marrow, $24 \pm 7\%$ for allogeneic recipients with no GVHD, $27 \pm 18\%$ among patients who developed only acute GVHD, $11 \pm 10\%$ among those who developed chronic GVHD, and $7 \pm 4\%$ among those who developed both acute and chronic GVHD (Table 2). Thus,

Table 2 Probability of Relapse After Transplantation for Acute Myeloid Leukemia in First Clinical Remission

Study group	N	Probability of relapse (%)
Syngeneic	34	49 ± 21
Allogeneic		
No GVHD	228	24 ± 7
Acute only	330	27 ± 8
Chronic only	54	11 ± 10
Acute and chronic	237	7 ± 4
T-cell depleted	163	35 ± 12

GVHD, graft-versus-host disease.
Source: Ref. 8.

in this study, chronic GVHD appeared to have the greatest association with a reduction in leukemia recurrence. Of interest, in the same study, the major GVL effect in acute lymphoblastic leukemia (ALL) appeared to be associated with acute GVHD where the incidence of recurrence dropped from 44 ± 17% in those without GVHD to 17 ± 9% in those with acute GVHD. No further drop was seen in those who developed both acute and chronic GVHD. Thus, although a GVL effect is seen in most settings of allogeneic transplantation for leukemia, there may be differences among leukemia subtypes as to the strength of this effect and the relative contributions of acute and chronic GVHD.

A third observation supporting a GVL effect in AML is the observed trend toward more leukemic recurrence in recipients of T-cell–depleted marrow. In the IBMTR report noted above, the risk of disease recurrence was 35 ± 12% in recipients of T-cell–depleted marrow compared to 24 ± 7% in recipients of non–T-cell–depleted marrow who did not develop GVHD (8). Although the relative increased risk of relapse associated with T-cell depletion in AML was far less than that seen in chronic myelogenous leukemia (CML), the trend was consistent with the other observations noted above in favor of a graft-versus-AML effect.

A final group of observations supporting the existence of a graft-versus-AML effect are those involving attempts to reestablish remissions in patients who have relapsed following allogeneic transplantation. A number of case reports have documented that complete remissions can be achieved in some patients who have relapsed after allogeneic transplantation by stopping immunosuppression and allowing GVHD to develop (9). In an attempt to induce an increased GVL effect, a number of investigators have initiated studies involving infusion of viable donor buffy coat cells in such patients. In a recent review by Kolb et al., 26% of patients with AML who had relapsed after allogeneic transplantation and were treated with buffy coat infusions without concomitant chemotherapy achieved a subsequent remission (10).

Although all these lines of evidence support the existence of a graft-versus-AML effect, it has been difficult to translate this association into improved cure rates. Attempts to increase the antileukemic effects of allogeneic transplantation by nonspecifically increasing the extent of GVHD have not led to convincing successes. In a prospective randomized trial, eliminating or diminishing the amount of GVHD prophylaxis or adding viable donor buffy coat immediately posttransplant led to an increased incidence of GVHD, but any gain in diminished recurrence was more than balanced by an increased incidence of severe or fatal complications resulting from GVHD and its treatment (11). Studies examining the use of interferon-α after transplant to upregulate the expression of class I human leukocyte antigens (HLAs) or the use of low-dose interleukin-2 (IL-2) are being conducted (12,13–13b).

As noted earlier, there is general agreement that both CD8$^+$ T cells, which recognize endogenously processed peptides presented by class I molecules, and CD4$^+$ T cells, which react with peptides presented by HLA class II molecules, contribute to the GVL effect, at least in animal models. The exact peptides recognized by T cells responsible for the graft-versus-AML effect in humans are unknown, but they can be thought of as being in three possible categories. First, there are peptides that differ between HLA-matched donor and recipient and which are expressed on most, if not all, cells. After HLA-matched allogeneic transplantation, donor-derived cytotoxic T cells can be isolated from the recipients' circulation with specificity against such peptides and with the capability of recognizing and lysing a broad range of host cells, including host leukemia cells. Such broadly expressed HLA–minor histocompatibility antigens, being present on both leukemic cells as well as on cells that are the targets of GVHD, may help explain the association of GVHD with a reduced risk of relapse, but they would not appear to represent obvious targets for specifically increasing a GVL effect. There are, however, HLA–minor antigens that are relatively tissue specific. The existence of such tissue-specific antigens is not surprising given that the types of proteins in different tissues differ greatly and such proteins are the source of the peptides presented by HLA class I molecules. The observation of GVHD or autoimmune diseases affecting predominantly one tissue type is consistent with the existence of such tissue-specific antigens and, hence, tissue-specific T cells. Although the majority of CD8[+] T cells with reactivity against minor histocompatibility antigens lyse cells from all recipient tissues tested, several investigators have now demonstrated that it is possible to isolate allogeneic T cells with reactivity to host minor histocompatibility antigens that are relatively tissue specific; lysing, for example, hematopoietic cells but not epithelial cells, endothelial cells, or fibroblasts (14–16). A third category of peptide which, at least theoretically, could be the target of a GVL effect are true tumor-specific antigens, such as the unique peptides resulting from translocations or mutation associations with malignant transformation. T cells reactive with the unique peptides produced by, for example, t(9;22) or t(15;17), have been isolated by in vitro stimulation of lymphocytes with antigen-presenting cells pulsed with the unique peptide, but such cells have been found in only a minority of patients (17), and target antigens have not been identified for the majority of patients.

The observation of the existence of allogeneic T cells with reactivity to host antigens that are relatively tissue specific suggests one approach to elicit a GVL effect without necessarily inducing GVHD. Recently, it has been convincingly demonstrated that donor-derived antigen-specific T cells can be isolated, cloned, expanded, and infused to HLA-matched siblings following transplantation without toxicity and with therapeutic effects. As one example, Riddell et al. demonstrated that cytomegalovirus (CMV)–specific T cells from marrow donors can be isolated, expanded to large numbers, and given to patients posttransplant restoring immunity to CMV infection and protecting patients against the development of CMV disease (18,19). Similarly, T cells reactive with the Epstein-Barr virus (EBV) have been obtained from donors, expanded, and successfully used to treat EBV-associated lymphoproliferative disorders developing posttransplant. Based on these experiences, it may be possible to isolate T cells with the desired specificity against, for example, a minor histocompatibility antigen restricted to host hematopoietic tissue, and use these cells posttransplant as specific adoptive immunotherapy.

III. DOSE RESPONSE

In addition to providing a GVL effect, allogeneic transplantation enables patients to be cured of AML, because transplantation allows the administration of far higher doses of chemoradiotherapy than would be possible with transplantation. The observation that some patients are cured following autologous or syngeneic transplantation without an obvious or easily explained GVL effect is probably the clearest evidence for the curative potential of the higher doses of therapy permitted with transplantation (5). In addition, there is at least some evidence that within the dose range generally used in transplantation, there is a relationship between the dose delivered and the risk of relapse. Evidence for this dose response in AML is best provided by a prospective randomized trial comparing cyclophosphamide and 12 Gy total body irradiation (TBI) versus cyclophosphamide and 15.75 Gy TBI as the preparative regimen for patients with AML in first remission (20). The incidence of relapse was 34% with the lower TBI dose versus 13% with the higher TBI dose. Although there are few, if any, other randomized trials in AML addressing the dose effect of the preparative regimen, several studies in CML in chronic phase provide similar results. In a randomized trial similar to that described above, the relapse rate for patients with CML in chronic phase undergoing transplantation from HLA-identical siblings was 30% at 12 Gy of TBI compared with 7% at the higher TBI dose (21). Although these two randomized trials demonstrate the dose-response relationship with relapse, they also demonstrate a similar relationship between dose and toxicity in this same dose range. In both of these randomized trials, the incidence of nonrelapse mortality was increased in the high-dose arm with the result that the overall disease-free survival was similar in the two arms of the trials. Thus, although there is evidence for a steep dose-response in AML within the doses possible with transplantation, new approaches are needed to take advantage of this phenomenon.

There are several approaches under study attempting to capitalize on the dose-response relationship seen in transplantation. One approach is to ensure that patients' tumor cells are exposed to the appropriate dose of therapy. For many chemotherapeutic agents, considerable variability in pharmacokinetics among patients exists leading to the likelihood that, without appropriate adjustments, some patients may be undertreated, whereas others may be exposed to toxic doses of drugs. In the transplant setting, the most extensively studied chemotherapeutic agent is busulfan. Initial studies found that there was considerable variability in the pharmacokinetics of this agent with the result that, at a given oral dose, there was as much as a threefold difference in the plasma concentrations of the drug among patients (22). In a study of 44 patients transplanted for chronic phase CML after a fixed preparative regimen of 16 mg/kg busulfan and 120 mg/kg cyclophosphamide, the median steady-state concentration of busulfan was 917 ng/mL. After 2 years of follow-up, 7 of the 44 patients had relapsed, including 0 of 23 in the group with busulfan values above the median versus 7 of 21 in those with levels below the median ($P < .001$) (Fig. 1) (23). This study demonstrates a remarkable dependence of tumor eradication on the blood level of busulfan achieved. Other studies have shown that by measuring busulfan blood levels after an initial dose, subsequent doses can be adjusted to achieve a target level. These studies thus suggest that by monitoring busulfan levels and adjusting subsequent doses appropriately to achieve a steady-state level of 900 ng/mL or greater, relapse

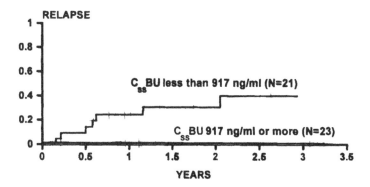

Figure 1   Shown are the cumulative incidences of relapse following allogeneic marrow transplantation for CML in chronic phase among patients with a median steady-state plasma concentration of busulfan of less than and more than 917 ng/mL ($P<.001$).

in CML can be substantially reduced. No similar studies have yet been reported in AML, but several are underway.

A second approach to capitalize potentially on the dose-response effect of the preparative regimen is physically to target therapy to sites of disease and away from critical normal organs such as the lungs, liver, and gastrointestinal tract. One strategy for achieving this aim is to employ monoclonal antibodies reactive with leukemia and other hematopoietic cells as carriers of radionuclides that deliver their energy locally. The feasibility of such an approach in humans gained support from a number of studies in animal models demonstrating that it is possible to radiolabel monoclonal antibodies with high levels of radionuclides without diminishing immunoreactivity. In tumored mice, administration of such antibodies can result in the delivery of at least fourfold more radiation to sites of tumor than to normal organs (24). These animal studies further showed that the exact ratio of radiation delivered to the tumor versus normal organs depends on a number of factors, including the immunoreactivity of the antibody, the dose of antibody delivered, the choice of radiolabel, the size of the tumor, the number of antigenic sites per tumor cell, and whether the cell surface antigen internalizes after antibody binding, among others. In a canine model, it was further shown that marrow was a particularly easy organ to target, perhaps because of its blood supply, and that using a monoclonal antibody directed against an antigen on early hematopoietic progenitor cells radiolabeled with ^{131}I, it was possible to ablate normal marrow, and further that this marrow-ablative effect could be reversed with subsequent marrow transplantation (25).

Based on these findings and similar observations by others, a number of clinical trials exploring targeted radiotherapy as part of a transplant-preparative regimen were initiated. In an initial attempt, we explored the use of an antibody directed against CD33 as a carrier for [131]I (26). CD33 is expressed on normal myeloid cells up to the metamyelocyte stage and in 90% of cases of AML, but it is not expressed on nonhematopoietic tissues. [131]I was chosen as the first radionuclide for study because the techniques for conjugation of antibody with ^{131}I are well worked out, ^{131}I has a gamma component which allows for accurate imaging making determination of its biodistribution possible thus allowing for accurate dosimetry, and because the half-life of ^{131}I is long enough for practical labeling and administration and short enough to be cleared over several days, allowing for subsequent transplantation. In this initial study, a dose of the antibody trace labeled with ^{131}I was given to patients with AML scheduled to undergo transplantation. The distribution of the radionuclide over time was determined by imaging and marrow biopsies, and if it was determined that more radiation would be delivered to marrow than to normal organs, the patient was entered on a dose-escalation study employing increasing doses of radiation delivered by the radioconjugate combined with a standard preparative regimen including cyclophosphamide 120 mg/kg plus 12 Gy TBI. The results of the study were disappointing. Among the first nine patients studied, in only four was more radiation delivered to marrow than to liver and lungs with the radioconjugate. Major limitations of the use of CD33 as a target using radioiodinated antibody appeared to be that relatively few antigenic sites exist per target cell, which limits the amount of initial uptake, and that there is short retention of the isotope at the target site. Further studies suggested that the short retention is likely the result of rapid internalization of the antigen-antibody complex with subsequent metabolism and excretion of the radioiodine from the cell (27). These studies suggest several alternative approaches, including the use of new radiolabeling techniques that allow stabilization of internalized complexes or targeting alternative antigens that are cell surface stable and more abundant.

In Seattle, we have been focusing on the latter alternative. CD45 is an antigen expressed on most hematopoietic cells, including approximately 90% of all cases of AML and ALL. Unlike CD33, CD45 remains cell surface stable after antibody binding and is expressed in numbers 5- to 10-fold greater per cell than CD33. In murine models of subcutaneously implanted human leukemia, which expresses both CD33 and CD45 antigens, antibodies against CD45 conventionally labeled with radioiodine led to substantially greater concentrations of the radionuclide within the tumor than did radioiodinated anti-CD33 antibodies (27). Studies in macaques likewise predicted that an anti-CD45 antibody should allow for favorable biodistribution of the radionuclide in human patients (28). Accordingly, a trial of radiolabeled anti-CD45 antibody in patients with acute leukemia, analogous to that described earlier for anti-CD33, was initiated (29). Twenty-eight patients have so far been studied. The trace-labeled infusions have been accompanied by fever, chills, and occasional nausea and vomiting, all lasting no more than several hours. In 25 of the 28 trace-labeled studies, the results predicted that more radiation would be delivered to sites of leukemia than to any normal organ, and these patients were therefore defined as having "favorable" biodistribution. Patients with AML in relapse tended to have more favorable biodistribution than those in remission, presumably because with hypercellular marrows there is more antigen to target in the marrow space. The 25 patients with favorable biodistribution were then entered into a dose-escalation treatment study in which increased doses of radiation delivered by ^{131}I–anti-CD45 were combined with cyclophosphamide and 12 Gy TBI. Among the 25 patients so far treated were 18 with recurrent AML or advanced myelodysplasia (MDS) and 7 with ALL. These 25 patients received between 10 and 28 Gy of radiation delivered to marrow by the radiolabeled antibody along with the conventional preparative regimen. Dose-limiting toxicity has not yet been reached. Of the 18 patients with AML or advanced MDS, 12 remain in remission for 2–53 months, 3 have died of GVHD and/or infection, and 3 have relapsed (Fig. 2). This rate of relapse and overall survival is superior to what one would predict from our historical experience in similar patients. Among the seven patients with ALL, two remain disease-free, one died of infection, and three relapsed.

Given the encouraging results in patients with myeloid malignancies, a similar study has been initiated in patients with AML in first remission combining a standard busulfan (16 mg/kg)/cyclophosphamide (120 mg/kg) regimen with ^{131}I anti–CD45 (29). The amount of radiolabel added to the antibody is calculated to deliver 5.2 Gy to liver, resulting in the delivery of 10–15 Gy to marrow in addition to the standard preparative regimen.

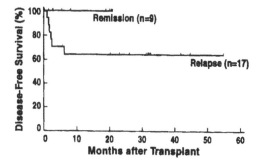

Figure 2 Disease-free survival of the first 26 patients with AML entered onto the ^{131}I–anti CD45 trials described in this text.

Among 17 patients with AML entered onto the study to date, 1 died of a transplant-related infection, and the other 16 remain alive and disease-free at 4–48 months posttransplant. No patient has yet relapsed.

These studies demonstrate the possibility of using monoclonal antibodies to target radiotherapy to the marrow and other sites of leukemia with relative specificity in an effort to take advantage of the dose-response relationship of radiotherapy in AML. The experiments so far performed are only the initial attempts, and a large number of variations are possible. Other antigens might be considered as targets and other conjugation techniques or other radionuclides are yet to be tested. Instead of antibodies, it might be possible to use myeloid growth factors as carriers of radionuclides. Instead of targeting the cells in the marrow, it might be possible to target the stroma or the surrounding bone. Radioactive iron has been proposed as a method to deliver radiotherapy specifically to the marrow. With time, it is hoped that a number of these approaches will be shown to improve further on our ability to take advantage of the steep dose-response of AML to therapy.

ACKNOWLEDGMENT

This work was supported, in part, by grants CA-18029, CA-18221 and CA-26386 from the National Institutes of Health, DHHS.

REFERENCES

1. Biggs JC, Horowitz MM, Gale RP, Ash RC, Atkinson K, Helbig W, Jacobsen N, Phillips GL, Rimm AA, Ringden O, Rozman C, Sobocinski K, Zeum J, Bortin M. Bone marrow transplants may cure patients with acute leukemia never achieving remission with chemotherapy. Blood 1992; 80:1090–1093.
2. Forman SJ, Schmidt GM, Nademanee AP, Amylon MD, Chao NJ, Fahey JL, Konrad PN, Margolin KA, Niland JC, O'Donnell MR, Parker PM, Smith EP, Snyder DS, Somlo G, Stein AS, Blume KG. Allogeneic bone marrow transplantation as therapy for primary induction failure for patients with acute leukemia. J Clin Oncol 1991; 9:1570–1574.
3. Clift RA, Buckner CD, Thomas ED, Kopecky KJ, Appelbaum FR, Tallman M, Storb R, Sanders J, Sullivan K, Banaji M, Beatty PS, Bensinger W, Cheever M, Deeg J, Doney K, Fefer A, Greenberg P, Hansen JA, Hackman R, Hill R, Martin P, Meyers J, McGuffin R, Neiman P, Sale G, Shulman H, Singer J, Stewart P, Weiden P, Witherspoon R. The treatment of acute non-lymphoblastic leukemia by allogeneic marrow transplantation. Bone Marrow Transplant 1987; 2:243–258.
4. Barnes DWH, Corp MJ, Loutit JF, Neal FE. Treatment of murine leukaemia with x-rays and homologous bone marrow. Preliminary communication. Br Med J 1956; 2:626–627.
5. Gale RP, Horowitz MM, Ash RC, Champlin RE, Goldman JM, Rimm AA, Ringden O, Stone JAV, Bortin MM. Identical twin bone marrow transplants for leukemia. Ann Intern Med 1994; 120:646–652.
6. Weiden PL, Flournoy N, Thomas ED, Prentice R, Fefer A, Buckner CD, Storb R. Antileukemic effect of graft-versus-host disease in human recipients of allogeneic-marrow grafts. N Engl J Med 1979; 300:1068–1073.
7. Weiden PL, Sullivan KM, Flournoy N, Storb R, Thomas ED, and the Seattle Marrow Transplant Team. Antileukemic effect of chronic graft-versus-host disease. Contribution to improved survival after allogeneic marrow transplantation. N Engl J Med 1981; 304:1529–1533.
8. Horowitz MM, Gale RP, Sondel PM, Goldman JM, Kersey J, Kolb H-J, Rimm AA, Ringden O, Rozman C, Speck B, Truitt RL, Zwaan FE, Bortin MM. Graft-versus-leukemia reactions after bone marrow transplantation. Blood 1990; 75:555–562.

9. Higano CS, Brixey M, Bryant EM, Durnam DM, Doney K, Sullivan KM, Singer JW. Durable complete remission of acute non-lymphocytic leukemia associated with discontinuation of immunosuppression following relapse after allogeneic bone marrow transplantation: a case report of a graft-versus-leukemia effect. Transplantation 1990; 50:175–177.

10. Kolb HJ, Schattenberg A, Goldman JM, Hertenstein B, Jacobsen N, Arcese W, Ljungman P, Ferrant A, Verdonck L, Niederwieser D, van Rhee F, Mittermueller J, De Witte T, Holler E, Ansari H. Graft-versus-leukemia effect of donor lymphocyte transfusions in marrow grafted patients. European Group for Blood and Marrow Transplantation Working Party Chronic Leukemia. Blood 1995; 86:2041–2050.

11. Sullivan KM, Storb R, Buckner CD, Fefer A, Fisher L, Weiden PL, Witherspoon RP, Appelbaum FR, Banaji M, Hansen J, Martin P, Sanders JE, Singer J, Thomas ED. Graft-versus-host disease as adoptive immunotherapy in patients with advanced hematologic neoplasms. N Engl J Med 1989; 320:828–834.

12. Soiffer RJ, Murray C, Gonin R, Ritz J. Effect of low-dose interleukin-2 on disease relapse after T-cell depleted allogeneic bone marrow transplantation. Blood 1994; 84:964–971.

13. Robinson N, Sanders JE, Benyunes MC, Beach K, Lindgren C, Thompson JA, Appelbaum FR, Fefer A. Phase I trial of interleukin-2 after unmodified HLA-matched sibling bone marrow transplantation for children with acute leukemia. Blood 1996; 87:1249–1254.

13a. Singhal S. Leuk Lymphoma 1999; 32:505–512.

13b. Mehta J. Bone Marrow Transplant 1997; 2:129–135.

14. de Bueger M, Bakker A, van Rood JJ, Van der Woude F, Goulmy E. Tissue distribution of human minor histocompatibility antigens. Ubiquitous versus restricted tissue distribution indicates heterogeneity among human cytotoxic T lymphocyte–defined non-MHC antigens. J Immunol 1992; 149:1788–1794.

15. van der Harst D, Goulmy E, Falkenburg JH, Kooij-Winkelaar YM, van Luxemburg-Heijs SA, Goselink HM, Brand A. Recognition of minor histocompatibility antigens on lymphocytic and myeloid leukemic cells by cytotoxic T-cell clones. Blood 1994; 83:1060–1066.

16. Goulmy E, Schipper J, Pool J, Blokland E, Falkenburg JHF, Vossen J, Gratwohl A, Vogelsang GB, van Houwelingen HC, van Rood JJ. Mismatches of minor histocompatibility antigens between HLA-identical donors and recipients and the development of graft-versus-host disease after bone marrow transplantation. N Engl J Med 1996; 334:281–285.

17. Chen W, Peace DJ, Rovira K, You SG, Cheever MA. T-cell immunity to the joining region of p210[bcr-abl] protein. Proc Natl Acad Sci 1992; USA 89:1468.

18. Riddell SR, Watanabe KS, Goodrich JM, Li CR, Agha ME, Greenberg PD. Restoration of viral immunity in immunodeficient humans by the adoptive transfer of T cell clones. Science 1992; 257:238–241.

19. Walter EA, Greenberg PD, Gilbert MJ, Finch RJ, Watanabe KS, Thomas ED, Riddell SR. Reconstitution of cellular immunity against cytomegalovirus in recipients of allogeneic bone marrow by transfer of T-cell clones from the donor. N Engl J Med 1995; 333:1038–1044.

20. Clift RA, Buckner CD, Appelbaum FR, Bearman SI, Petersen FB, Fisher LD, Anasetti C, Beatty P, Bensinger WI, Doney K, Hill R, McDonald G, Martin P, Sanders J, Singer J, Stewart P, Sullivan KM, Witherspoon R, Storb R, Hansen J, Thomas ED. Allogeneic marrow transplantation in patients with acute myeloid leukemia in first remission: a randomized trial of two irradiation regimens. Blood 1990; 76:1867–1871.

21. Clift RA, Buckner CD, Appelbaum FR, Bryant E, Bearman SI, Petersen FB, Fisher LD, Anasetti C, Beatty P, Bensinger WI, Doney K, Hill RS, McDonald GB, Martin P, Meyers J, Sanders J, Singer J, Stewart P, Sullivan KM, Witherspoon R, Storb R, Hansen JA, Thomas ED. Allogeneic marrow transplantation in patients with chronic myeloid leukemia in the chronic phase: a randomized trial of two irradiation regimens. Blood 1991; 77:1660–1665.

22. Slattery JT, Clift RA, Buckner CD, Radich J, Storer B, Bensinger WI, Soll E, Anasetti C, Bowden R, Bryant E, Chauncey T, Deeg HJ, Doney KC, Flowers M, Gooley T, Hansen JA, Martin PJ, McDonald GB, Nash R, Petersdorf EW, Sanders JE, Schoch G, Stewart P, Storb

R, Sullivan KM, Thomas ED, Witherspoon RP, Appelbaum FR. Marrow transplantation for chronic myeloid leukemia: the influence of plasma busulfan levels on the outcome of transplantation. Blood 1997; 89:3055–3060.

23. Slattery JT, Sanders JE, Buckner CD, Schaffer RL, Lambert KW, Langer FP, Anasetti C, Bensinger WI, Fisher LD, Appelbaum FR, Hansen JA. Graft-rejection and toxicity following bone marrow transplantation in relation to busulfan pharmacokinetics. Bone Marrow Transplant 1995; 16:31–42.

24. Badger CC, Krohn KA, Shulman H, Flournoy N, Bernstein ID. Experimental radioimmunotherapy of lymphoma with ^{131}I-labelled anti–T-cell antibodies. Cancer Res 1986; 46:6223–6228.

25. Appelbaum FR, Brown P, Sandmaier B, Badger C, Schuening F, Graham TC, Storb R. Antibody-radionuclide conjugates as part of a myeloblative preparative regimen for marrow transplantation. Blood 1989; 73:2202–2208.

26. Appelbaum FR, Matthews DC, Eary JF, Badger CC, Kellogg M, Press OW, Martin PJ, Fisher DR, Nelp WB, Thomas ED, Bernstein ID. Use of radiolabeled anti-CD33 antibody to augment marrow irradiation prior to marrow transplantation for acute myelogenous leukemia. Transplantation 1992; 54:829–833.

27. van der Jagt RHC, Badger CC, Appelbaum FR, Press OW, Matthews DC, Eary JF, Krohn KA, Bernstein ID. Tumor localization of radiolabeled anti-myeloid antibodies in a human acute leukemia xenograft tumor model. Cancer Res 1992; 52:89–94.

28. Matthews DC, Appelbaum FR, Eary JF, Hui TE, Fisher DR, Martin PJ, Durack LD, Nelp WB, Press OW, Badger CC, Bernstein ID. Radiolabeled Anti-CD45 monoclonal antibodies target lymphohematopoietic tissue in the macaque. Blood 1991; 78:1864–1874.

29. Matthews DC, Appelbaum FR, Eary JF, Fisher DR, Durack LD, Bush SA, Hui TE, Martin PJ, Mitchell D, Press OW, Badger CC, Storb R, Nelp WB, Bernstein ID. Development of a marrow transplant regimen for acute leukemia using targeted hematopoietic irradiation delivered by ^{131}I-labeled anti-CD45 antibody, combined with cyclophosphamide and total body irradiation. Blood 1995; 85:1122–1131.

24

Late Complications of Hematopoietic Stem Cell Transplantation

EMIN KANSU

Hacettepe University, Hacettepe, Ankara, Turkey

KEITH M. SULLIVAN

Duke University Medical Center, Durham, North Carolina

I. INTRODUCTION

Stem cell transplantation of peripheral blood or bone marrow has evolved into an accepted treatment for a variety of life-threatening hematological, neoplastic, and immunological disorders. The numbers and types of transplants have increased as unrelated and mismatched related individuals are now used as alternative donors, as different sources of hematopoietic stem cells are employed, and as new disease indications are considered for transplantation (Kernan et al., 1993; Kurtzberg et al., 1996; Walters et al., 1996). As transplant outcomes improve with advances in supportive care, new treatment protocols are being developed to extend the application of stem cell transplantation to nonmalignant conditions such as sickle cell disease, thalassemia, and selected autoimmune disorders (Lucarelli et al., 1993; Sullivan and Furst, 1997). As shown in Fig. 1, there has been a steady increase in the number of transplant centers and an increasing number of long-term survivors (Armitage, 1994). Thousands of patients worldwide are currently alive more than 5 years following bone marrow transplantation and increasing attention is being directed to potential late complications (Sullivan et al., 1991).

In this chapter, we will review the key areas for long-term follow-up care of hematopoietic cell recipients, including:

Ambulatory care and long-term monitoring
Regimen-related toxicities
Immunodeficiency and immunization
Infection

413

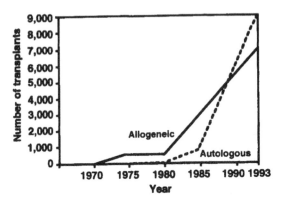

Figure 1 Growth of hematopoietic stem cell transplantation (annual number from 1970 to 1993). (From Armitage, 1994.)

Chronic graft-versus-host disease
Bone disease
Secondary malignancy
Recurrent malignancy
Quality of life

II. AMBULATORY CARE AND LONG-TERM MONITORING

The role of ambulatory care of the stem cell transplant recipient is expanding, and many services traditionally provided in the hospital can now be provided in an ambulatory setting (Flowers and Sullivan, 1992; Peters et al., 1994; Rowe et al., 1994). Careful follow-up monitoring and reliable reporting of the results of all transplants are essential for accurate assessment of outcome (Clift et al., 1989; Jones and Shpall, 1994). It is especially important to follow transplant recipients actively for potential late complications (Table 1). Figures 2 and 3 depict interrelationships and times of onset of the late events following stem cell transplantation (Nims, 1990; Sullivan et al., 1992).

Table 1 Late Complications
of Stem Cell Therapy

Regimen-related toxicity
  Cataracts
  Neurological conditions
  Gonadal conditions
  Endocrine conditions
  Growth and development
Immunodeficiency
Infection
Chronic graft-versus-host disease
Bone disease
Relapse of malignancy
Secondary malignancy

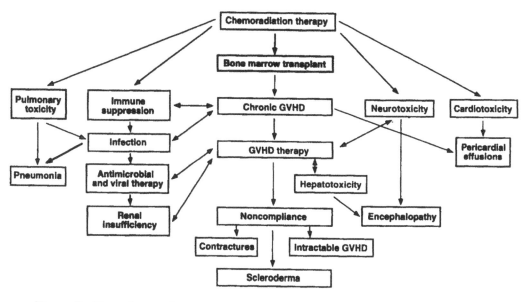

Figure 2 Time of onset of late complications. (From Nims, 1990.)

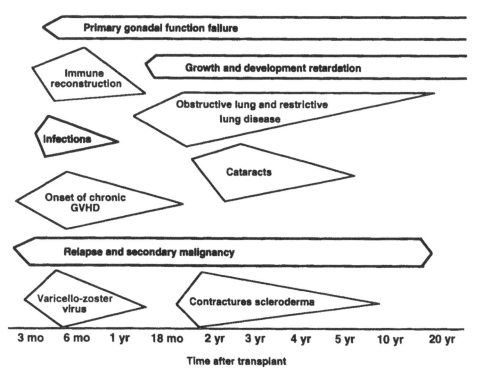

Figure 3 Interrelationship of late complications after stem cell transplantation. (From Nims, 1990.)

Over the past two decades, the Long-Term Follow-Up Program at the Fred Hutchinson Cancer Research Center has developed methods for posttransplant evaluation and research (Flowers and Sullivan, 1992; Sullivan and Saidak, 1997). Currently, over 2500 patients given stem cell transplants are monitored after discharge from the Center.

Tracking is performed in several ways. On-site evaluation of returning patients is conducted at the first and selected subsequent anniversaries of transplantation. On-site examination includes detailed medical, hematological, and immunological evaluations. Initially at 6 months and then yearly thereafter, medical questionnaires are sent to referring physicians. These questionnaires are focused to ensure a high return on the first mailing. Survival data are reported to the date of last contact, including a standardized rating of the Karnofsky and Lansky functional performance scores (Table 2). Yearly questionnaires are also mailed to patients to obtain additional information about functional performance symptoms and medical complications (Sullivan and Saidak, 1997).

Table 2 Karnofsky Performance Scale and Lansky Play-Performance Scale

---

Karnofsky Performance Scale[a]
(For use with persons ages >17 years)

100% = Normal; no complaints; no evidence of disease
 90% = Able to carry on normal activity; minor signs or symptoms of disease
 80% = Normal activity with effort; some signs or symptoms of disease
 70% = Cares for self; unable to carry on normal activity or to do active work
 60% = Requires occasional assistance, but is able to care for most of own
            needs
 50% = Requires considerable assistance and frequent medical care
 40% = Disabled; requires special care and assistance
 30% = Severely disabled; hospitalization is indicated although death is not
            imminent
 20% = Hospitalization necessary; very sick; active supportive treatment
            necessary
 10% = Moribund; fatal processes progressing rapidly
  0% = Dead

Modified Lansky Play-Performance Scale[b]
(For use with persons ages 1 through 16 years)

100% = Fully active, normal
 90% = Minor restrictions in physically strenuous activity
 80% = Active, but tires more quickly
 70% = Both greater restriction of, and less time spent in, play activities
 60% = Up and around, but minimal active play; keeps busy with quieter
            activities
 50% = Gets dressed but lies around much of the day; no active play; able to
            participate in all quiet play and activities
 40% = Mostly in bed; participates in quiet activities
 30% = Often sleeping; play entirely limited to very passive activities
 20% = No play; does not get out of bed
 10% = Unresponsive
  0% = Dead

---

[a] From Karnofsky and Burchenal, 1949.
[b] From Lansky et al. 1987.

This broad-based approach, combined with patients and physicians who are highly interested in remaining in contact with the Transplant Center, has resulted in reliable life-long medical updates. Consistently, no more than 4–9% of the surviving patients have been lost to follow-up, and all the other patients were contacted for updates within the last 2-year period.

III. REGIMEN-RELATED TOXICITIES

Late events after autologous and allogeneic stem cell transplantation may arise from chemoradiation-associated organ toxicity, and standardized criteria for grading regimen-related toxicities have been reported (Bearman et al., 1988). Potential late effects of high-dose conditioning are listed in Table 1.

A. Cataract Formation

Cataract formation is a known consequence of corticosteroids and total body irradiation (TBI). Benyunes et al. reported an analysis of 492 adults followed a median of 6 (range 1–18) years after marrow transplantation (Benyunes et al., 1995). During this period of the study, cataracts developed in 159 patients (32%). The probability of cataract formation at 11 years after transplantation was 85%, 50%, 34% and 19% for patients receiving 10-Gy single-dose TBI; greater than 12-Gy fractionated TBI, 12-Gy fractionated TBI, and no TBI, respectively (P < .0001). In the cohort developing cataracts, the severity was greater in patients given single-dose TBI (59% probability of surgical extraction) than those given 12 Gy or more fractionated TBI or no TBI (33%, 22% and 23%, respectively).

Corticosteroids given after day 100 further increased the incidence/risk of cataract formation associated with TBI, as shown in Figure 4. Patients given corticosteroids after transplantation had a significantly higher probability of cataracts (45%) than those who did not receive steroids (38%). In all groups under study, cataract formation appeared to reach a plateau at 7 years after transplantation, and the median time for cataract formation was 2–5 years (Benyunes et al., 1995). Our group is currently studying the use of "quasi-elastic light scattering" technology for early detection of cataracts in older individuals and those given TBI (Thurston et al., 1997).

B. Neurological Complications

Late neurological complications may result from previous cranial radiation, recurrence of the primary disease, intrathecal chemotherapy, and other drug toxicities. Progressive leukoencephalopathy has been noted in 7% of patients who received either cranial irradiation or intrathecal chemotherapy before TBI and transplantation (Thompson et al., 1986). Mechlorethamine used as a preparative regimen and cyclosporine administered as prophylaxis or treatment of graft-versus-host disease (GVHD) have been associated with neurotoxicity (Sullivan et al., 1982; Atkinson et al., 1984).

C. Endocrine and Growth Abnormalities

Growth and development and endocrine function can be affected by myeloablative conditioning. Overt hypothyroidism, compensated hypothyroidism, thyroiditis, and thyroid neoplasms may develop after irradiation of the thyroid gland (Sanders, 1991). Thyroid defi-

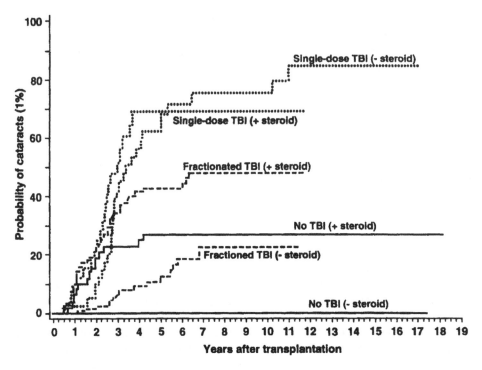

Figure 4   Probability of cataracts in patients who received 10 Gy total body irradiation (TBI). TBI as a single dose (bulleted line) (+) with steroids (n = 33) or (−) without steroids (n = 41); ≥12 Gy of fractionated TBI (broken line) (+) with steroids (n = 250) or (−) without steroids (n = 128); no TBI (solid line) (+) with steroids (n = 60) or (−) without steroids (n = 25). (From Benyunes et al., 1995.)

ciency was noted in 31–43% of patients after single fraction TBI (Sanders, 1991). Hypothyroidism in children is now less frequent following fractionated irradiation (Sanders, 1991). In adult transplant recipients, two thirds of the individuals may have elevated thyroid-stimulating hormone (TSH) with normal T3 and T4 levels, and between one fourth and one fifth of patients will have definite hypothyroidism (Schimpff et al., 1980). Fractionated TBI has decreased the incidence of "compensated" hypothyroidism from between 30 and 60% to between 15 and 25% (Sklar et al., 1982; Sanders, 1991).

When the diagnosis of hypothyroidism is made, thyroid hormone replacement should be given in order to normalize the TSH levels. Graves' disease is rare after marrow transplantation, but clinical hyperthyroidism has been reported with subacute or chronic thyroiditis. Accordingly, transplant recipients should be evaluated yearly with physical examination and thyroid function tests.

Growth hormone deficiency has been reported after TBI and may exceed 90% in children prepared with TBI who received prior additional cranial irradiation for control of central nervous system leukemia (Sanders, 1994). In contrast, growth hormone deficiency has not been observed after high-dose cyclophosphamide conditioning (Sanders, 1991). Some children with chronic GVHD treated with corticosteroids may have growth arrest followed by normal growth after resolution of chronic GVHD and discontinuation of corticosteroid therapy.

Busulfan is an agent known to cross the blood-brain barrier, and children who are prepared with this agent may develop growth hormone deficiency. They require early diagnosis and appropriate growth hormone replacement (Wingard et al., 1992; Sanders, 1994). Follow-up monitoring is critical so that hormone deficiencies can be detected at an early phase, since final height achieved with growth hormone replacement is inversely related to patient age at the onset of therapy.

D. Gonadal Dysfunction and Fertility

Gonadal dysfunction is a frequent result of myeloablative chemoradiotherapy. Females may have anovulation, low estrogen levels, and elevation of serum gonadotropins with or without menopausal symptoms (Heimpel et al., 1991). Following cyclophosphamide-containing regimens, most postpubertal females and males less than 26 years of age will regain gonadal function (Sanders et al., 1988) In contrast, patients who received TBI containing preparative regimens rarely have return of fertility (Sanders et al., 1983). Among men receiving busulfan-containing regimens, return of gonadal function has been seen in rare individuals as early as 2 years after transplantation. In contrast, no return of gonadal function has been noted to date in women receiving busulfan-containing regimens (Sanders, 1994).

Children aged 8 years and older should be examined annually and assessed by Tanner Development Scores for grading of secondary sexual development (Tanner and Whitehouse, 1976). Those with gonadal failure and delayed development of secondary sexual characteristics appear to benefit from sex hormone–replacement therapy. Women who conceive after transplant require careful attention to potential obstetrical complications (Sanders et al., 1996).

E. Gynecological and Obstetrical Care

Gynecological follow-up of postpubertal females studied 1–13 years after allogeneic transplantation showed atrophic abnormalities in 33 of 36 recipients of TBI-containing regimens (Schubert et al., 1990). Recognition of these climacteric abnormalities can lead to early hormone replacement with long-term estrogen and progestrone supplements, thereby alleviating unnecessary discomfort, reducing the risk of osteoporosis, and improving the well-being of the transplant recipient. Obstetrical monitoring of stem cell transplant recipients requires careful attention to potential complications (Hinterberger-Fischer et al., 1991). Preterm delivery and low birth weight children were observed at a higher than expected rate after marrow grafting. However, the incidence of congenital abnormalities did not appear to differ from that reported for the general population (Sanders et al., 1996).

IV. IMMUNODEFICIENCY AND IMMUNIZATION

Although the peripheral blood of marrow recipients may have normal numbers of white blood cells within the first months posttransplant, both allogeneic and autologous hematopoietic cell recipients experience immunological impairment for 6–12 months after transplantation (Witherspoon et al., 1984). The recapitulation of normal immune and lymphoid ontogeny is prolonged by increasing human leukocyte antigen (HLA) disparity with the allogeneic donor and development of chronic GVHD leading to both cellular and humoral immune defects (Atkinson et al., 1982; Olsen et al., 1988). Reconstitution of CD3[+] T cells in allogeneic transplants is seen within 12 weeks and recovery of CD8[+] suppressor

Table 3 Recommended Immunizations After
Hematopoietic Transplantation

Year 1[a]
  Diphtheria-pertussis-tetanus
  Haemophilus influenzae conjugate
  Hepatitis B
  Influenza (repeat every November)
  Salk poliovirus (inactivated vaccine)
Year 2[b]
  Measles-mumps-rubella
Family member
  No Sabin poliovirus during year 1
  (Measles-mumps-rubella does not pass to others)

---

[a] Patients with chronic graft-versus-host disease may not benefit.
[b] Only in patients free of chronic graft-versus-host disease and immunosuppressive treatment.

T cells is earlier than that of CD4$^+$ helper T-cell subpopulations. Significantly low levels of CD4$^+$ T cells may be present within the first 6 months after transplantation. Normal numbers of CD20$^+$ B lymphocytes are detected in the peripheral blood 1–2 months after marrow transplantation. Usually, if patients do not develop chronic GVHD, they may be expected to normalize serum IgG levels in 2–3 months, IgM levels in 9–12 months, and IgA levels in 2–3 years. Individuals with serum IgG levels below 400 mg/dL in the first 3 months after transplant should be repleted with intravenous immunoglobulin (IVIg) to decrease the risk of infection (Aucouturier et al., 1987; Sullivan et al., 1990).

Recovery of T- and B-lymphocyte populations following stem cell transplantation can also permit adoptive transfer of allergen-specific IgE-mediated hypersensitivity reactions, such as food or drug allergies (Agosti et al., 1988). Vaccination of stem cell recipients during the first 3 months does not usually lead to adequate synthesis of tetanus or diphtheria antibodies. In patients without chronic GVHD, antigen-specific functional T-cell clones develop after day 100, and augmentation of disease-specific protective immunity should be given as booster immunizations for patients with low or absent antibody titers at 1 year after transplantation. During the first year, patients without chronic GVHD are most likely to respond to booster immunizations with pneumococcal, inactivated poliomyelitis, influenza, diphtheria, pertussis, tetanus toxoid, hepatitis B, and *Haemophilus influenzae* type B vaccines (Table 3). Live viral vaccines are to be avoided until the second year when patients are free of chronic GVHD and off immunosuppressive therapy (Ljungman et al., 1989).

V. INFECTION

Prior studies have shown that chronic GVHD is the major determinant of late infection after allogeneic transplantation and that encapsulated gram-positive organisms are common pathogens (Atkinson et al., 1979; Winston et al., 1979). The Seattle group reviewed their experience during the period from 1985 to 1989 and reported the incidence of late infection in 364 patients given HLA-identical sibling marrow and 79 patients given autolo-

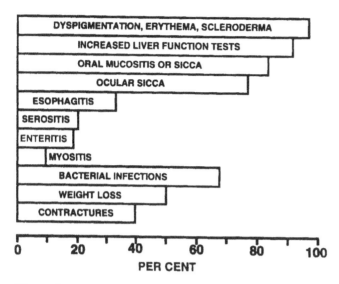

Figure 5 Frequency of clinical manifestations in extensive chronic GVHD. (From Sullivan et al., 1991.)

gous marrow grafts (Sullivan et al., 1992). The time to the first pulmonary infection or sinusitis/otitis media after discharge home is illustrated in Figures 5, 6, and 7. Among the viral infections, cytomegalovirus infection is uncommon after day 100, but varicella-zoster infection is seen in 30–45% of patients within the first year after stem cell transplantation (Locksley et al., 1985; Schuchter et al., 1989).

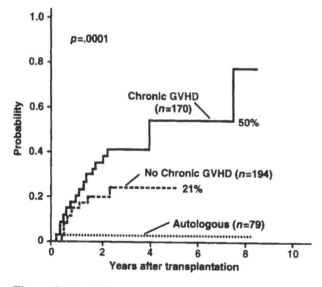

Figure 6 Probability of pulmonary infection after discharge home. Between 1985 and 1989, 364 human lymphocyte antigen–identical and 79 autologous marrow recipients returned home a median of 99 days after transplantation. GVHD, graft-versus-host-disease. (From Sullivan et al., 1992.)

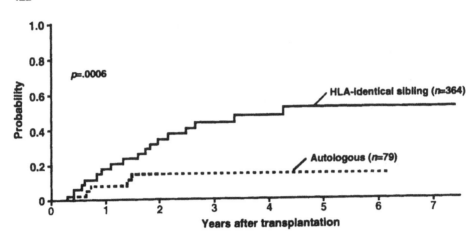

Figure 7 Probability of sinusitis or otitis media infection after discharge home. Between 1985 and 1989, 364 human lymphocyte antigen–identical and 79 autologous marrow recipients returned home a median of 99 days after transplantation. (From Sullivan et al., 1992.)

VI. CHRONIC GRAFT-VERSUS-HOST DISEASE

A. Incidence

Chronic GVHD is a clinicopathological syndrome which is the major determinant of long-term outcome (mortality) and quality of life (morbidity) after allogeneic bone marrow transplantation. Chronic GVHD may develop within 3–18 months after allografting and occurs in approximately 33% of HLA-identical sibling recipients and 50–70% of recipients of unrelated or mismatched-related marrow grafts (Sullivan et al., 1991). Increasing patient age and degree of prior acute GVHD are known risk factors for developing chronic GVHD (Sullivan, 1994). Although most patients have had preceding acute GVHD, 20–30% have a de novo late onset without preceding acute GVHD. In addition, allogeneic peripheral blood stem cell recipients appear to have a higher incidence of chronic GVHD than bone marrow recipients (Storek et al., 1997).

Chronic GVHD may manifest in two ways. "Limited disease" is defined as the presence of signs and symptoms of GVHD limited to skin and/or liver involvement. "Extensive disease" is defined as the presence of signs and symptoms consistent with GVHD involving multiple organ systems with at least one biopsy showing characteristic pathological GVHD findings. Individuals with extensive chronic GVHD have an unfavorable natural history (18% disability-free survival without treatment) compared to individuals with the limited form, who have a favorable course without immunosuppressive treatment (Sullivan, 1994; Sullivan et al., 1981).

There are three typical patterns of onset of chronic GVHD. *Progressive* chronic GVHD is defined as direct continuation of signs and symptoms of acute GVHD, and it is associated with the highest mortality rate. A *quiescent* onset of chronic GVHD is observed after the complete resolution of prior acute GVHD. *De novo* onset of chronic GVHD is defined as onset of the disease without any prior history of acute GVHD. *De novo* onset of chronic GVHD has the best prognosis (Sullivan et al., 1981; Wingard et al., 1989; Atkinson, 1990).

Chronic GVHD is a pleiotropic disease with clinical and pathological signs and symptoms similar to several naturally occurring autoimmune disorders. As shown in Figure 5, organ involvement in extensive and chronic GVHD affects the skin, mouth, eyes, sinuses, gastrointestinal tract, lungs, muscles, tendons, serous surfaces, and vagina (Sullivan, 1994; Sullivan et al., 1981).

B. Clinical Manifestations

1. Dermal

Dermal involvement is the most frequent clinical feature of chronic GVHD. Erythema, dyspigmentation, poikiloderma, and violaceous papules resembling lichen planus may be observed. Lichenoid lesions can be generalized and coalesce to form plaques. If no therapeutic intervention is given, the skin becomes progressively indurated and sclerotic, leading to joint contractures and profound disability. The sclerosis can be associated with skin ulcers, alopecia, and anhidrosis. Progressive hair loss with scarring alopecia can be observed in patients with chronic GVHD.

2. Oral

Oral lesions associated with chronic GVHD include erythema, atrophy, and lichen planus–like findings. Severe mucous membrane involvement with chronic GVHD may lead to a Sjögren's syndrome–like disease with xerostomia and xerophthalmia. The presence of the "oral sicca" syndrome in these patients may lead to poor oral hygiene and dental caries.

3. Ocular

Ocular abnormalities associated with chronic GVHD include keratoconjuctivitis sicca, conjuctivitis, and uveitis. Schirmer's testing of lacrimal gland function may show wetting <5 mm at 5 min or <10 mm with signs of keratitis diagnosed with slit-light examination. Other symptoms will include blurring, dryness, "gritty eyes," and/or photophobia. Artificial tear replacements may be required to prevent corneal abrasion.

4. Pulmonary

Chronic GVHD may be associated with recurrent sinopulmonary infection and progressive obstructive lung defects. Clinical and pathological features are characterized by the presence of bronchiolitis obliterans (Clark et al., 1987, 1989). Progressive bronchiolitis obliterans affects 5–10% of all patients with active chronic GVHD.

5. Hepatic

Liver function abnormalities associated with chronic GVHD are common and are predominantly cholestatic in nature, but hepatocellular dysfunction may make it difficult to distinguish chronic GVHD from viral or drug-induced hepatitis. Ursodeoxycholic acid may be of benefit as bile displacement therapy (Fried et al., 1992).

6. Musculoskeletal

Arthralgias, synovial effusions, arthritis, tendonitis, and fasciitis have been associated with chronic GVHD (Janin et al., 1994). Proximal muscle weakness with increased creative phosphokinase (CPK), aldolase and electromyographic findings are consistent with myositis. Muscle cramping can also occur. Muscle biopsy may be required to confirm the diagnosis if the muscle is the only organ involved.

7. Gastrointestinal

Chronic GVHD rarely involves the intestine. Weight loss often is related to loss of appetite and increased metabolic needs. Esophageal complications may include desquamative esophagitis causing web formation and gastroesophageal reflux. Classic findings of malabsorption may be noted owing to bacterial overgrowth in the gut or pancreatic or hepatic disease.

8. Other Sites

Vaginal stenosis, dryness, and inflammation can all be seen during the course of chronic GVHD. Peripheral neuropathy and myesthenia gravis are less common manifestations.

9. Infections

Owing to the prolonged time to immunological recovery, infections may be common in patients with chronic GVHD. Treatment of chronic GVHD with corticosteroids and associated hypogammaglobulinemia contribute to this risk. Infections with encapsulated grampositive bacteria are most common and require daily penicillin or trimethoprim-sulfamethaxazole prophylaxis (Sullivan et al., 1986). Figure 6 illustrates the risk of pulmonary infection associated with chronic GVHD.

10. Outcome

In an analysis of 164 consecutive patients with extensive chronic GVHD, older patient age, progressive onset of GVHD, failure to respond to 9 months of therapy, and continued thrombocytopenia (platelets <100,000/mL), hyperbilirubinemia, and lichenoid histology have been reported to be associated with an increased nonrelapse mortality and poor prognosis. Among unrelated donor marrow transplants, a prolonged course of interferon-α given before transplant in patients with chronic myeloid leukemia (CML) resulted in poorer survival due to chronic GVHD which was refractory to immunosuppressive treatment (Morton et al., 1997a, 1997b).

C. Treatment

As noted above, without treatment only 18% of patients with extensive chronic GVHD survived free of major disability. In standard-risk patients (i.e., those with a platelet count >100,000/μL, de novo, or quiescent type of onset), early treatment with prednisone alone significantly improved outcome (21% mortality) compared to prednisone and azathioprine (40% mortality) (Sullivan et al., 1988). In high-risk patients (i.e., those with platelet counts <100,000/μL or the progressive type of onset), survival after prednisone treatment was only 10–26%. Subsequently, the addition of cyclosporine to an alternating-day regimen of prednisone has improved the survival to 52% in high-risk patients (Sullivan et al., 1988). However, transplant-related mortality still continues to be higher (35%) in high-risk patients than in standard-risk patients (20%) because of increased rates of infection.

New treatment approaches include the use of FK506, thalidomide, mycophenolate mofetil, and rapamycin (Vogelsang et al., 1992; Nash et al., 1997). Supportive care includes correction of hypogammaglobulinemia and administration of trimethoprim-sulfa-methoxazole to reduce the risk of infection (Sullivan et al., 1996).

VII. BONE DISEASE

Bone disease is a well-known complication of solid organ transplantation; however, the development of avascular necrosis, osteoporosis, and fractures following stem cell transplantation is less well characterized (Kelly et al., 1990; Socie et al., 1994). Recently, adult patients treated with prednisone and cyclosporine for chronic GVHD were evaluated for biochemical factors associated with skeletal turnover at initiation of immunosuppressive therapy and 9 months later (Stern et al., 1996). Single and dual photon absorptiometry of the wrist and spine and dual energy x-ray absorptiometry (DEXA) were used to evaluate bone mineral density. Results showed a significant (>2.5 times the test precision) decrease over 9 months in bone mineral density in three of five evaluable males and all three females who were receiving prednisone and cyclosporine treatment. The results of the study indicated increased collagen and bone turnover, increased urinary magnesium and calcium excretion, and a significant risk of osteoporosis in patients receiving corticosteroids for chronic GVHD.

VIII. SECONDARY MALIGNANCY

Secondary neoplasms may arise in the oncogenic milieu of genetically determined factors, infection, immunodeficiency, and cytotoxic conditioning regimens, including TBI (Witherspoon et al., 1989, 1992). The Seattle team reported the cumulative incidence of secondary cancers in 330 patients with aplastic anemia who received cyclophosphamide alone as pretransplant conditioning (Witherspoon et al., 1992). As illustrated in Figure 8, the cumulative incidence at 5 years was 0.4% (95% confidence interval 0–1.1), at 10 years

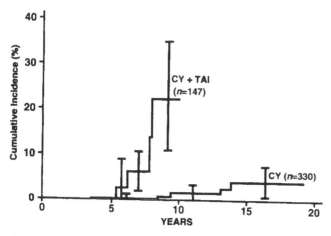

Figure 8 Cumulative incidence of secondary malignancy in 330 patients with aplastic anemia given marrow transplantations from family members. Brackets indicate the 5th through 95th percentile confidence intervals. Cy, cyclophosphamide; TAI, thoracoabdominal irradiation. (From Witherspoon et al., 1992.)

Table 4 Solid Cancers and Age at Bone
Marrow Transplantation[a] (80 cases among
19,229 transplants)

Age at BMT (years)	Relative risk (95% CI)
<10	36.6 (22.9–55.4)
10–19	4.6 (2.0–9.1)
20–29	4.6 (2.8–7.0)
30–39	1.4 (0.7–2.4)
>40	1.2 (0.7–1.9)

[a] Cumulative incidence: 1.5% at 10 years and 6.7% at
15 years.
Source: Curtis et al., 1997.

was 1.4% (0–3.4), and at 15 years was 4.2% (0.9–8.6). The rate was less than reported by the Paris team in patients with aplastic anemia given cyclophosphamide and thoracoabdominal irradiation as conditioning (N = 147).

European studies confirm that pretransplantation irradiation is a major determinant of late malignancies in patients with aplastic anemia (Socie et al., 1993). To further define these interactions, 700 patients with severe aplastic anemia treated with allogeneic marrow transplantation in Seattle or in Paris were reviewed (Deeg et al., 1996). A malignancy developed in 23 patients 1.4–221.0 (median 91) months after transplantation, for a Kaplan-Meir estimate of 14% (confidence interval 4–24%) at 20 years. Proportional hazards models indicated that azathioprine therapy ($P < .0001$) and the diagnosis of Fanconi's anemia ($P < .0001$) were significant factors for development of secondary malignancies for all patients. Irradiation was a significant factor ($P = .004$) only if the time-dependent variable azathioprine was not included in the analysis. If only nonFanconi patients were considered, azathioprine ($P = .0043$), age ($P = .025$), and irradiation ($P = .042$) were independent risk factors for development of late secondary neoplasms.

In a recent report, a multi-institutional data base including 19,229 recipients of allogeneic marrow transplants was analyzed to determine the risk of developing late solid cancers (Curtis et al., 1997). The risk of new solid cancers was 8.3 times higher than expected for the general population among those who survived 10 or more years after transplantation. The cumulative incidence rate of solid cancers was 2.2% (95% confidence interval, 1.5–3.0%) at 10 years and 6.7% (3.7–9.6%) at 15 years. In this study, the risk of developing a new solid cancer was also found to be higher for recipients who were younger at the time of transplantation. Table 4 presents this relationship. Radiogenic tumors (especially of brain and thyroid) were noted in children, most of whom had cranial irradiation given before referral for transplantation.

IX. RECURRENT MALIGNANCY

Prior experience has indicated poor survival after recurrence of the original malignancy after marrow cell transplantation (Mortimer et al., 1989). In some patients, recurrent leukemia has been successfully treated with second transplantations, but resistant disease and regimen-related toxicities contribute to high mortality (Radich et al., 1993). In recent years, the development of highly sensitive molecular biology techniques has helped detect minimal residual disease. For patients with CML, long-term monitoring includes cytogenetics for the Philadelphia chromosome and bone marrow and peripheral blood molecular determinations for the *bcr/abl* transcripts every 6 months after transplantation through year 3, then annual evaluations through year 5. Positive *bcr/abl* studies 6 months or more after transplantation appears to predict the risk of subsequent hematological relapse (Radich et al., 1995). Patients with residual disease could be eligible for treatment with interferon-α during early molecular or cytogenetic relapse (Higano et al., 1992).

Recurrent leukemia following stem cell transplantation may also be successfully treated with donor leukocyte infusions. This beneficial effect derives from an apparent graft-versus-leukemia effect associated with allogeneic stem cells that recognize and destroy host histocompatibility antigens and/or tumor-associated antigens (Weiden et al., 1981; Sullivan et al., 1989). Donor leukocyte infusions have been used successfully to treat patients with recurrent leukemia and Epstein-Barr virus–associated lymphoproliferative disorders (Kolb, 1990; Papadopoulos et al., 1994).

X. QUALITY OF LIFE

Recovery from transplantation is a dynamic process blending physical and psychosocial aspects. Quality of life is a multidimensional construct composed of at least four domains: physical function, psychological function, social role function, and disease and treatment symptoms. Recent studies examining the medical and psychosocial sequelae of stem cell or marrow transplantation have reported that most survivors do relatively well, whereas a smaller group continues to experience a less than optimal quality of life (Wingard et al., 1991; Chao et al., 1992; Schmidt et al., 1993). We conducted a prospective analysis of 67 adults with quality of life measures taken before and after allogeneic transplantation (Syrjala et al., 1993). Physical function was most impaired at 90 days posttransplant, with a return to pretransplant levels of functioning in most areas by 1 year. By 2 years, 68% of patients had returned to full-time work, and only 9% of 4-year survivors failed to return to full-time occupations. Before transplantation, 27% of patients reported elevated anxiety. Mean levels of anxiety and depression did not change over the first year. In a multivariate analysis, greater emotional distress at 1 year was predicted by pretransplantation family conflict and nonmarried status. Impaired physical recovery at 1 year was predicted by more severe chronic GVHD, pretransplant physical impairment, and family conflict. Family relationships therefore appear to be important determinants of recovery.

Another study used a cross-sectional analysis of 125 adults surviving a mean of 10 (range 6–18) years after allogeneic (87%) or autologous/syngeneic (13%) transplantation (Bush et al., 1995). Seven wide-ranging tests measured physical, psychological, social functioning, and disease and treatment symptoms. Eighty percent of individuals rated their quality of life as good to excellent, and 5% rated it as poor. The most frequently cited problem during recovery was a perceived lack of social support from family and friends. Although complaints such as fatigue, sexual dysfunction, and sleep disturbances were noted, most survivors judged these to be of low severity, and 88% of the 125 patients said the benefits of transplantation outweighed the side effects.

XI. CONCLUSION

Bone marrow and peripheral blood stem cell transplantation is now considered the treatment of choice for a variety of nonmalignant and malignant disorders. In some patients, the impact of late complications determines the success of the procedure and efforts directed at preventing rare events are vital. Knowledge of late complications and follow-up care by the specialist and general practioner will enhance the outcome of recipients of allogeneic and autologous hematopoietic cell transplantation.

ACKNOWLEDGMENT

Supported by Grants CA 18029, CA 18221, and HL 36444 from the National Institutes of Health, Department of Health and Human Services. E.K. is supported by a grant from the Turkish Scientific and Technical Research Council, TUBITAK, Ankara-Turkey.

REFERENCES

Agosti JM, Sprenger JD, Lum LG, Witherspoon RP, Storb R, Henderson WR. Transfer of allergen-specific IgE mediated hypersensitivity with allogeneic bone-marrow transplantation. N Engl J Med 1988; 319:1623–1628.

Armitage JO. Research potential of the ABMTR Database. Autologous Blood and Marrow Transplant Registry–North America 1994; 1:2.

Atkinson K. Chronic graft-versus-host disease (review). Bone Marrow Transplant 1990; 5:69–82.

Atkinson K, Storb R, Prentice RL, Weiden PL, Witherspoon RP, Sullivan KM, Noel D, Thomas ED. Analysis of late infections in 89 long-term survivors of bone marrow transplantation. Blood 1979; 53:720–731.

Atkinson K, Farewell V, Storb R, Tsoi M-S, Sullivan KM, Witherspoon RP, Fefer A, Clift R, Goodell B, Thomas ED. Analysis of late infections after human bone marrow transplantation: role of genotypic nonidentity between marrow donor and recipient and of non-specific suppressor cells in patients with chronic graft-versus-host disease. Blood 1982; 60:714–720.

Atkinson K, Biggs J, Darveniza P, Boland J, Concannon A, Dodds A. Cyclosporine-associated central nervous system toxicity after allogeneic bone marrow transplantation. Transplantation 1984; 38:34–37.

Aucouturier P, Barra A, Intrator L, Cordonnier C, Schulz D, Duarte F, Vernant J-P, Oreud'homme J-L. Long lasting IgG subclass and anti-bacterial polysaccharide antibody deficiency after allogeneic bone marrow transplantation. Blood 1987; 70:779–785.

Bearman SI, Appelbaum FR, Buckner CD, Peterson FB, Fisher LD, Clift RA, Thomas ED. Regimen-related toxicity in patients undergoing bone marrow transplantation. J Clin Oncol 1988; 6: 1562–1568.

Benyunes MC, Sullivan KM, Deeg HJ, Mori M, Meyer W, Fisher L, Bensinger W, Jack MK, Hicks J, Witherspoon R, Buckner CD, Hansen JA, Appelbaum FR, Storb R. Cataracts after bone marrow transplantation: long-term follow-up of adults treated with fractionated total body irradiation. Int J Radiat Oncol Biol Phys 1995; 32:661–670.

Bush NE, Haberman M, Donaldson G, Sullivan KM. Quality of life of 125 adults surviving 6–18 years after bone marrow transplantation. Soc Sci Med 1995; 40:479–490.

Chao NJ, Tierney DK, Bloom JR, Long GD, Barr TA, Stallbaum BA, Wong RM, Negrin RS, Horning SJ, Blume KG. Dynamic assessment of quality of life after autologous bone marrow transplantation. Blood 1992; 80:825–830.

Clark JG, Schwartz DA, Flournoy N, Sullivan KM, Crawford SW, Thomas ED. Risk factors for airflow obstruction in recipients of bone marrow transplants. Ann Intern Med 1987; 107:648–656.

Clark JG, Crawford SW, Madtes DK, Sullivan KM. Obstructive lung disease after allogeneic marrow transplantation. Ann Intern Med 1989; 111:368–376.

Clift R, Goldman J, Gratwohl A, Horowitz M. Proposals for standardized reporting of results of bone marrow transplantation for leukemia. Bone Marrow Transplant 1989; 4:445–448.

Curtis RE, Rowlings PA, Deeg HJ, Shriner DA, Socie G, Travis LB, Horowitz MM, Witherspoon RP, Hoover RN, Sobocinski KA, Fraumeni JF, Boice JD. Solid cancers after bone marrow transplantation. N Engl J Med 1997; 336:897–904.

Deeg HJ, Socie G, Schoch G, Henry-Amar M, Witherspoon RP, Devergie A, Sullivan KM, Gluckman E, Storb R. Malignancies after marrow transplantation for aplastic anemia and Fanconi anemia: a joint Seattle and Paris analysis of results in 700 patients. Blood 1996; 87:386–392.

Flowers ME, Sullivan KM. Pre-admission procedures, marrow transplant hospitalization, and post-transplant outpatient monitoring. In: Atkinson K, ed. Textbook on Bone Marrow Transplantation, London: Cambridge University Press, 1992:75–86.

Fried RH, Murakami CS, Fisher LD, Wilson RA, Sullivan KM, McDonald GB. Ursodeoxycholic acid treatment of refractory chronic graft-versus-host of the liver. Ann Intern Med 1992; 116:624–629.

Heimpel H, Arnold R, Hetzel WD, Hueske D, Kreuser ED, Wirthenson EF, Voss AC, Slanina J. Gonadal function after bone marrow transplantation in adult male and female patients. Bone Marrow Transplant 1991; 8(suppl 1):21–24.

Higano CS, Raskind WH, Singer JW. Use of alpha-interferon for treatment of relapse of chronic myelogenous leukemia in chronic phase after allogeneic bone marrow transplantation. Blood 1992; 80:1437–1442.

Hinterberger-Fisher M, Kier P, Kalhs P, Marosi C, Geissler K, Schwarzinger I, Pabinger I, Huber J, Spona J, Kolbabek H, Koren H, Muller G, Hawliczek R, Lechner K, Hayek-Rosenmayr A, Hinterberger W. Fertility, pregnancies and offspring complications after bone marrow transplantation. Bone Marrow Transplant 1991; 7:5–9.

Janin A, Socie G, Devergie A, Aractingi S, Esperou H, Verola O, Gluckman E. Fasciitis in chronic graft-versus-host disease. Ann Intern Med 1994; 120:993–998.

Jones RB, Shpall EJ. Dissemination and commercialization of hematopoietic progenitor cell transplantation (editorial). Hematotherapy 1994; 3:93–94.

Karnofsky DA, Burchenal JH. The clinical evaluation of chemotherapeutic agents in cancer. In: MacLeod CM, ed. Evaluation of Chemotherapeutic Agents. New York: Columbia Press, 1949:199–205.

Kelly PJ, Atkinson K, Ward RL, Sambrook PN, Biggs JC, Eisman JC. Reduced bone mineral density in men and women with allogeneic bone marrow transplantation. Transplantation 1990; 50:881–883.

Kernan NA, Bartsch G, Ash RC, Beatty PG, Champlin R, Filipovich A, Gajewski J, Hansen JA, Henslee-Downey J, McCullough J, McGlave P, Perkins HA, Phillips GL, Sanders J, Stroncek D, Thomas ED, Blume KG. Analysis of 462 transplantations from unrelated donors facilitated by the National Marrow Donor Program. N Engl J Med 1993; 328:593–602.

Kolb HJ, Mittermuller J, Clemm C, Holler E, Ledderose G, Brehm G, Heim M, Wilmanns W. Donor leukocyte transfusions for treatment of recurrent chronic myelogenous leukemia in marrow transplant patients. Blood 1990; 76:2462–2465.

Kurtzberg J, Laughlin M, Graham ML, Smith C, Olson JF, Halperin EC, Ciocci G, Carrier C, Stevens CE, Rubinstein P. Placental blood as a source of hematopoietic stem cell for transplantation into unrelated recipients. N Engl J Med 1996; 335:157–166.

Lansky SB, List MA, Lansky LL, Ritter-Sterr C, Miller DR. The measurement of performance in childhood cancer patients. Cancer 1987; 60:1651–1656.

Ljungman P, Fridell E, Lonnqvist B, Bolme P, Bottiger M, Gahrton G, Linde A, Ringden O, Wahren B. Efficacy and safety of vaccination of marrow transplant recipients with a live attenuated measles, mumps, and rubella vaccine. J Infect Dis 1989; 159:610–615.

Locksley RM, Flournoy N, Sullivan KM, Meyers JD. Infection with varicella-zoster virus after marrow transplantation. J Infect Dis 1985; 152:1172–1181.

Lucarelli G, Galimbeti M, Pochi P, Angelucci E, Baronciani D, Giardini C, Andreani M, Agostinelli F, Albertini F, Clift RA. Marrow transplantation in patients with thalassemia responsive to iron chelation therapy. N Engl J Med 1993; 329:840–844.

Mortimer J, Blinder MA, Schulman S, Appelbaum FR, Buckner CD, Clift RA, Sanders JE, Storb R, Thomas ED. Relapse of acute leukemia after marrow transplantation: natural history and results of subsequent therapy. J Clin Oncol 1989; 7:50–57.

Morton AJ, Anasetti C, Gooley T, Flowers MED, Deeg HJ, Hansen JA, Martin PJ, Sullivan KM. Chronic graft-versus-host disease (GVHD) following unrelated donor transplantation (abstr). Blood 1997a; 90:590a.

Morton AJ, Gooley T, Hansen JA, Appelbaum FR, Bjerke JW, Clift R, Martin PJ, Petersdorf EW, Sanders JE, Storb R, Sullivan KM. Impact of pretransplant interferon-alpha on outcome of unrelated donor marrow transplants for chronic myeloid leukemia (CML) in first chronic phase (abstr). Blood 1997b; 90:105a.

Nash RA, Furlong T, Storb R, Anasetti C, Appelbaum FR, Deeg HJ, Doney K, Martin R, Witherspoon R, Sullivan KM. Mycophenolate mofetil (MMF) as salvage treatment for graft-versus-host disease (GVHD) after allogeneic hematopoietic stem cell transplantation (HSCT): safety analysis (abstr). Blood 1997; 90(suppl. 1):459a.

Nims JW. Late effects of bone marrow transplantation: a nursing perspective. In: Kasprisin CA, ed. Bone Marrow Transplantation: A Nursing Perspective. Arlington, VA: American Association of Blood Banks, 1990:45–57.

Olsen GA, Gockerman JP, Bast RC Jr, Borowitz M, Peters WP. Altered immunologic reconstitution after standard-dose chemotherapy or high-dose chemotherapy with autologous bone-marrow support. Transplantation 1988; 46:57–60.

Papadopoulos EB, Ladanyi M, Emanuel D, Mackinnon S, Boulad F, Carabasi MH, Castro-Malaspina H, Childs BH, Gillio AP, Small TN, Young JW, Kernan NA, O'Reilly RJ. Infusions of donor leukocytes to treat Epstein-Barr virus-associated lymphoproliferative disorders after allogeneic bone marrow transplantation. N Engl J Med 1994; 330:1185–1191.

Peters WP, Ross M, Vredenburgh JJ, Hussein A, Rubin P, Dukelow K, Cavanaugh C, Beauvais R, Kasprzak S. The use of intensive clinic support to permit outpatient autologous bone marrow transplantation for breast cancer. Semin Oncol 1994; 21(Suppl 7):25–31.

Radich JP, Sanders JE, Buckner CD, Martin PJ, Peterson FB, Bensinger W, McDonald GB, Moro M, Schoch G, Hansen JA. Second allogeneic marrow transplantation for patients with recurrent leukemia after initial transplant with total-body irradiation-containing regimens. J Clin Oncol 1993; 11:304–313.

Radich JP, Gehly G, Gooley T, Bryant E, Clift RA, Collins S, Edmands S, Kirk J, Lee A, Kessler P, Schoch G, Buckner CD, Sullivan KM, Appelbaum FR, Thomas ED. Polymerase chain reaction detection of the BCR-ABL fusion transcript after allogeneic marrow transplantation for chronic myeloid leukemia: results and implications in 346 patients. Blood 1995; 85:2632–2638.

Rowe JM, Ciobanu N, Ascensao J, Stadtmauer EA, Weiner RS, Schenkein DP, McGlave P, Lazarus HM, ECOG. Recommended guidelines for the management of autologous and allogeneic bone marrow transplantation: a report from the Eastern Cooperative Oncology Group (ECOG). Ann Intern Med 1994; 120:143–158.

Sanders JE. Growth and development after bone marrow transplantation. In: Forman FSJ, Blume KG, Thomas ED, eds. Bone Marrow Transplantation. Boston: Blackwell, 1994:527–537.

Sanders JE, Buckner CD, Leonard JM, Sullivan KM, Witherspoon RP, Deeg HJ, Storb R, Thomas ED. Late effects on gonadal function of cyclophosphamide total-body irradiation, and marrow transplantation. Transplantation 1983; 36:252–255.

Sanders JE, Buckner CD, Amos D, Levy W, Appelbaum FR, Doney K, Storb R, Sullivan KM, Witherspoon RP, Thomas ED. Ovarian function following marrow transplantation for aplastic anemia or leukemia. J Clin Oncol 1988; 6:813–818.

Sanders JE, and the Seattle Transplant Team. The impact of marrow transplant preparative regimens on subsequent growth and development. Semin Hematol 1991; 28:244–249.

Sanders JE, Hawley J, Levy W, Gooley T, Buckner CD, Deeg HJ, Doney K, Storb R, Sullivan KM, Witherspoon R, Appelbaum FR. Pregnancies following high-dose cyclophosphamide with or without high-dose busulfan or total body irradiation and bone marrow transplantation. Blood 1996; 87:3045–3052.

Schimpff SC, Diggs CH, Wiswell JG, Salvatore PC, Wiernik PH. Radiation-related thyroid dysfunction: Implications for the treatment of Hodgkin's disease. Ann Intern Med 1980; 92:91–98.

Schmidt GM, Niland JC, Forman SJ, Fonbuena PP, Dagis AC, Grant MM, Ferrell BR, Barr TA, Stallbaum BA, Chao NJ, Blume KG. Extended follow-up of 212 long-term allogeneic bone marrow transplant survivors. Transplantation 1993; 55:551–557.

Schubert MA, Sullivan KM, Schubert MM, Nims J, Hansen M, Sanders JE, O'Quigley J, Witherspoon RP, Buckner CD, Storb R, and Thomas ED. Gynecological abnormalities following allogeneic bone marrow transplantation. Bone Marrow Transplant 1990; 5:425–430.

Schuchter LM, Wingard JR, Piantadosi S, Burns WH, Santos GW, Saral R. Herpes zoster infection after autologous bone marrow transplantation. Blood 1989; 74:1424–1427.

Sklar CA, Kim TH, Ramsay NK. Thyroid dysfunction among long-term survivors of bone-marrow transplantation. Am J Med 1982; 73:688–694.

Socie G, Henry-Amar M, Bacigalupo A, Hows J, Tichelli A, Ljungman P, McCann SR, Frickhofen N, Veer-Kirthof EV, Gluckman E. Malignant tumors occurring after treatment of aplastic anemia. N Engl J Med 1993; 329:1152–1157.

Socie G, Selimi F, Sedel L, Frija J, Devergie A, Esperou-Bourdeau H, Ribaud P, Gluckman E. Avascular necrosis of bone after allogeneic bone marrow transplantation: clinical findings, incidence and risk factors. Br J Haematol 1994; 86:624–628.

Stern JM, Chesnut CH, Bruemmer B, Sullivan KM, Lenssen PS, Aker SN, Sanders J. Bone density loss during treatment of chronic GVHD. Bone Marrow Transplant 1996; 17:395–400.

Storek J, Gooley T, Siadak M, Bensinger WI, Maloney DG, Chauncey TR, Flowers M, Sullivan KM, Witherspoon RP, Rowley SD, Hansen JA, Storb R, Appelbaum FR. Allogeneic peripheral blood stem cell transplantation may be associated with a high risk of chronic graft-versus-host disease. Blood 1997; 90:4705–4709.

Sullivan KM. Long-term follow-up and quality of life after hematopoietic stem cell transplantation. J Rheumatol 1997; 24(suppl 48):46–52.

Sullivan KM, Furst DE. The evolving role of blood and marrow transplantation for the treatment of autoimmune diseases. J Rheumatol 1997; 24(suppl 48):1–4.

Sullivan KM, Siadak M. Stem cell transplantation. In: Johnson FE, Virgo KS, Edge SB, et al., eds. Cancer Patient Follow-Up. St. Louis: Mosby-Yearbook, 1997:490–501.

Sullivan KM, Shulman HM, Storb R, Weiden PL, Witherspoon RP, McDonald GB, Schubert MM, Atkinson K, Thomas ED. Chronic graft-versus-host disease in 52 patients: adverse natural course and successful treatment with combination immunosuppression. Blood 1981; 57:267–276.

Sullivan KM, Storb R, Shulman HM, Shaw C-M, Spence A, Beckham C, Clift RA, Buckner D, Stewart P, Thomas ED. Immediate and delayed neurotoxicity after mechlorethamine preparation for bone marrow transplantation. Ann Intern Med 1982; 27:182–189.

Sullivan KM, Meyers JD, Flournoy N, Storb R, Thomas ED. Early and late interstitial pneumonia following human bone marrow transplantation. Int J Cell Cloning 1986; 4:107–121.

Sullivan KM, Witherspoon RP, Storb R, Weiden P, Flournoy N, Dahlberg S, Deeg JH, Sanders JE, Doney KC, Appelbaum FR, McGuffin R, McDonald GB, Meyers J, Schubert MM, Gauvreau J, Shulman HM, Sale GE, Anasetti C, Loughran TP, Strom S, Nims J, Thomas ED. Prednisone and azathioprine compared with prednisone and placebo for the treatment of chronic graft-versus-host disease: prognostic influence of prolonged thrombocytopenia after allogeneic marrow transplantation. Blood 1988; 72:546–554.

Sullivan KM, Storb R, Buckner CD, Fefer A, Fisher L, Weiden PL, Witherspoon RP, Appelbaum FR, Banaji M, Hansen J, Martin P, Sanders JE, Singer J, Thomas ED. Graft-versus-host disease as adoptive immunotherapy in patients with advanced hematologic neoplasms. N Engl J Med 1989; 320:828–834.

Sullivan KM, Siadak MF, Witherspoon RW. Cyclosporine treatment of chronic graft-versus-host disease following allogeneic bone marrow transplantation. Transplant Proc 1990; 22:1336–1338.

Sullivan KM, Agura E, Anasetti C, Appelbaum F, Badger C, Bearman S, Erickson K, Flowers M, Hansen J, Loughran T, Martin P, Matthews D, Petersdorf E, Radich J, Riddell S, Rovira D, Sanders J, Schuening F, Siadak M, Storb R, Witherspoon R. Chronic graft-versus-host disease and other late complications of bone marrow transplantation. Semin Hematol 1991; 28:250–259.

Sullivan KM, Mori M, Sanders JE, Siadak M, Witherspoon RP, Anasetti C, Appelbaum FR, Bensinger W, Bowden R, Buckner CD, Clark J, Crawford S, Deeg HJ, Doney K, Flowers M, Hansen J, Loughran T, Martin P, McDonald G, Pepe M, Petersen FB, Schuening F, Stewart P, Storb R. Late complications of allogeneic and autologous marrow transplantation (review). Bone Marrow Transplant 1992; 10:127–134.

Sullivan KM. Graft-versus-host disease. In: Forman SJ, Blume KG, Thomas ED, eds. Bone Marrow Transplantation. Boston: Blackwell, 1994:339–362.

Sullivan KM, Storek J, Kopecky KJ, Jocom J, Longton G, Flowers M, Siadak M, Nims J, Witherspoon RP, Anasetti C, Appelbaum F, Bowden RA, Buckner D, Crawford SW, Deeg HJ, Hansen JA, McDonald GB, Sanders JE, Storb R. A controlled trial of long-term administration of intravenous immunoglobulin to prevent late infection and chronic graft-versus-host disease after marrow transplantation: clinical outcome and effect on subsequent immune recovery. Biol Blood Bone Marrow Transplant 1996; 2:44–53.

Syrjala KL, Chapko MK, Vitaliano PP, Cummings C, Sullivan KM. Recovery after allogeneic marrow transplantation: prospective study of predictors of long-term physical and psychosocial functioning. Bone Marrow Transplant 1993; 11:319–327.

Tanner JM, Whitehouse RH. Clinical longitudinal standards for height, weight, weight velocity, and stages of puberty. Arch Dis Child 1976; 51:170–179.

Thompson CB, Sanders JE, Flournoy N, Buckner CD, Thomas ED. The risks of central nervous system relapse and leukoencephalopathy in patients receiving marrow transplants for acute leukemia. Blood 1986; 67:195–199.

Thurston GM, Hayden DL, Burrows P, Clark JI, Taret VG, Kandel J, Courogen M, Peetermans JA, Dowen MS, Miller D, Sullivan KM, Storb R, Stern H, Benedek GB. Quasielastic light scattering study of the living human lens as a function of age. Curr Eye Res 1997; 16:197–207.

Vogelsang GB, Farmer ER, Hess AD, Altamonte V, Beschorner WE, Jabs DA, Corio RL, Levin LS, Colvin OM, Wingard JR, Santos GW. Thalidomide for the treatment of chronic graft-versus-host disease. N Engl J Med 1992; 326:1055–1058.

Walters MC, Patience M, Leisenring W, Eckman JR, Scott JP, Mentzer WC, Davies SC, Ohene-Frempong K, Bernaudin F, Matthews DC, Storb R, Sullivan KM. Bone marrow transplantation for sickle cell disease. N Engl J Med 1996; 335:369–376.

Weiden PL, Sullivan KM, Flournoy N, Storb R, Thomas ED, Seattle Marrow Transplant Team. Anti-leukemic effect of chronic graft-versus-host disease. N Engl J Med 1981; 304:1529–1533.

Wingard JR, Piantadosi S, Vogelsang GB, Farmer ER, Jabs DA, Levin LS, Beschorner WE, Cahill RA, Miller DF, Harrison D, Saral R, Santos GW. Predictors of death from chronic graft-versus-host disease after bone marrow transplantation. Blood 1988; 74:1428–1435.

Wingard JR, Curbow B, Baker F, Piantadosi S. Health, functional status, and employment of adult survivors of bone marrow transplantation. Ann Intern Med 1991; 114:113–118.

Wingard JR, Plotnick LP, Freemer CS, Zahurak M, Piantadosi S, Miller DF, Huibert M, Vriesendorp HM, Yeager AM, Santos GW. Growth in children after bone marrow transplantation: busulfan plus cyclophosphamide versus cyclophosphamide plus total body irradiation. Blood 1992; 79:1068–1073.

Winston DJ, Schiffman G, Wang DC, Feig SA, Lin C-H, Marso EL, Ho WG, Young LS, Gale RP. Pneumococcal infections after human bone marrow transplantation. Ann Intern Med 1979; 91:835–841.

Witherspoon RP, Lum LG, Storb R. Immunologic reconstitution after human marrow grafting. Semin Hematol 1984; 21:2–10.

Witherspoon RP, Fisher LD, Schoch G, Martin P, Sullivan KM, Sanders J, Deeg HJ, Maloney K, Thomas D, Storb R, Thomas ED. Secondary cancers after bone marrow transplantation for leukemia or aplastic anemia. N Engl J Med 1989; 321:784–789.

Witherspoon RP, Storb R, Pepe M, Longton G, Sullivan KM. Cumulative incidence of secondary solid malignant tumors in aplastic anemia patients given marrow grafts after conditioning with chemotherapy alone. Blood 1992; 79:289–292.

25

Prevention of Acute Graft-Versus-Host Disease by Delayed or Selected Lymphocyte Add Back

JOHN BARRETT

National Heart, Lung and Blood Institute, National Institutes of Health, Bethesda, Maryland

DIMITRIOS MAVROUDIS

University General Hospital of Heraklion, Crete, Greece

I. INTRODUCTION

Bone marrow transplants (BMTs) or peripheral blood stem cell transplants confer on the recipient not only donor-derived hematopoietic engraftment but also donor immunological reconstitution. For a successful outcome, engraftment should be prompt, complete, and sustained; leukemia must be eradicated; and immunity against a spectrum of pathogenic microorganisms restored. Tolerance between the donor and the host is a prerequisite for long-term survival. With new approaches, the engraftment barrier can be overcome, even in human leucocyte antigen (HLA)–mismatched situations, by increasing the stem cell dose with granulocyte colony-stimulating factor (G-CSF)–mobilized peripheral blood progenitor cells (1,2) and by increasing the immunosuppressive capacity of the preparative regimen (3,4). After hematopoietic engraftment, immune recovery becomes the key issue. The donor alloresponse to the leukemia—the so-called graft-versus-leukemia (GVL) effect—contributes to the cure of the leukemia (5). On the other hand, the alloresponse also causes graft-versus-host disease (GVHD), delaying immunological reconstitution, predisposing to serious infections, and causing major organ damage and death (6). Since the nature of the immune recovery largely determines the outcome after the transplant, the separation of GVL and GVHD reactions has become an area of intensive research. Table 1 presents some of the new strategies to improve immunological recovery currently under investigation.

Table 1 Novel Approaches for the Prevention of Acute GVHD

Manipulation of cytokines
  use of cytokine antagonists
  induce donor Th2-type CD4+T cells
  delayed add back of donor cells
Manipulation of donor T cells
  costimulatory signal blockade
  insertion of the TK suicide gene
  CD8+ subset depletion
  selective immunodepletion
    immunotoxins against activation markers
    TCR Vβ subset depletion

GVHD, graft-versus-host disease; TK, thymidine kinase; TCR, T-cell receptor.

II. MANIPULATION OF CYTOKINES

A better understanding of the mechanisms underlying acute GVHD has been gained from animal and in vitro studies, which should lead to improved GVHD prevention in clinical practice. Acute GVHD is the result of an alloresponse involving donor cells and cytokines (7). Donor T cells are essential for the initiation of the alloresponse, whereas proinflammatory cytokines, primarily secreted by cells of the monocyte-macrophage lineage, mediate most of the tissue damage (7,8). At the time of transplantation, the chemoradiation used in the conditioning regimen, together with coexisting infections and perhaps the disease itself, stimulate host tissues to produce inflammatory cytokines, in particular interleukin-1 (IL-1) and tumor necrosis factor-α (TNF-α), increasing the immunogenicity of the host tissues. In this cytokine-rich milieu, donor T cells react vigorously to host alloantigens, (major and/or minor histocompatibility antigens), releasing IL-2 and interferon-γ (IFN-γ) in turn activating macrophages and natural killer (NK) cells. These secondary effector cells, once stimulated, produce large quantities of inflammatory cytokines resulting in a "cytokine storm," which amplifies the immune reaction (9). The end result is damage to host tissues, mediated by both activated donor effector cells [cytotoxic T cells (CTLs) and NK cells] and inflammatory cytokines (TNF-α, IL-1, IFN-γ). The cytokines IL-2 and IFN-γ involved in GVHD reactions are part of the spectrum of cytokines produced by Th1 T cells and are critical for the development of acute GVHD (7).

A. Cytokine Antagonists

In human and animal studies, antagonists to IL-2, IL-1, and TNF-α have been used to prevent or treat acute GVHD (10–12). When administered in the peritransplant period, they can modestly reduce or delay acute GVHD (10,13). However, preliminary studies suggest that only a minority of patients with refractory GVHD benefit from this approach (11,13). The addition of an IL-2 receptor antibody to methotrexate and cyclosporine prophylaxis in one study actually reduced leukemia-free survival when compared with methotrexate and cyclosporine alone (14). Since GVHD is the result of several cytokines acting in concert, combinations of cytokine antagonists might be more effective, especially in conjunction with other preventive treatments. It is possible, however, that cytokines causing GVHD also contribute to GVL reactions. Treatment with cytokine antagonists could therefore abolish the GVL effect. Future studies with different combinations of cytokine antagonists given at different time points after transplantation may help discriminate between GVHD and GVL reactivities.

B. Th2-Type Donor Cells

In murine studies, the administration of donor cells with Th2 cytokine phenotype reduces the severity and lethality of experimental GVHD. Such cells have been generated by treating the mice with a combination of IL-2 and IL-4 (15,16) or G-CSF (17). Although successful in animal models, this approach could abrogate GVL and other alloimmune responses mediated by Th1-type cells. In transplants for malignant diseases, where the GVL effect is critical, this Th1–Th2 strategy is therefore problematic and will require refinement to preserve the GVL reaction. Nevertheless, it could be used to prevent acute GVHD in transplants for nonmalignant disorders, providing that such manipulation does not increase the risk of graft rejection.

C. Delayed Add Back of Donor Cells

Based on new understanding of the importance of cytokines in the process of acute GVHD, Johnson and Truitt elegantly showed in murine major histocompatibility complex (MHC)–matched and haplotype-mismatched BMT models that infusion of immunocompetent donor cells delayed until 21 days after transplantation conferred a long-lasting antileukemic effect without causing severe acute GVHD (18,19). In these experiments, alloreactive donor cells behaved differently when infused at different time points posttransplant. The mechanism of the protective effect is not yet defined. The reduced risk from GVHD may be due to avoidance of the cytokine storm or to the emergence of tolerance accompanying the establishment of a donor-derived antigen-presenting system. The concept of delayed lymphocyte add back has now been tested clinically. In a study where Campath-1 antibodies were used for T-cell depletion, donor lymphocytes were infused either starting early after transplant with weekly 1-log increments for up to four doses (days $+ 1, + 6, + 14, + 21$ with $10^4, 10^5, 10^6, 10^7$ T cells/kg recipient weight, respectively) or starting on day 28 and given only to patients without signs of acute GVHD (days $+ 28, + 56, + 84$ infused with $10^5, 10^6, 10^7$ T cells/kg, respectively) (20). In this nonprospective randomized heterogeneous study group of relatively young patients, delayed administration of donor lymphocytes caused clinically significant acute GVHD in 42–53% of patients and was associated with a low probability of leukemia relapse. Unfortunately, owing to patient variability and study design, it is not possible from these data to determine the cell dose and timing critical for the prevention of acute GVHD. Investigating the effect of delayed T-cell add back on the risk of acute GVHD, we treated 42 patients with hematological malignancies at the National Institutes of Health (NIH), using marrow grafts T-cell depleted by elutriation, followed by delayed add back of donor lymphocytes to prevent leukemia relapse (21). Cyclosporine was used for GVHD prophylaxis for a minimum of 6 months after BMT. Twenty-two patients had standard-risk chronic myelogenous leukemia (CML) in chronic or accelerated phase and 20 had high-risk disease: CML in blastic transformation (three patients), acute myelogenous leukemia (AML) in partial remission or myelodysplastic syndrome (MDS) in transformation to AML (nine patients), and multiple myeloma (eight patients). The mean T-cell dose in the bone marrow graft was 2×10^5/kg (range 1.6–3.5). In six patients, elutriation failed to separate T cells from stem cells and the whole product was given as a T-cell–replete graft (group A). Twenty-seven patients were evaluable for development of GVHD before lymphocyte add back (group B). Twenty of these patients received add backs of 2×10^6/kg donor T cells on day 30 and 5×10^7/kg on day 45 (group C). Nine patients received add back of 10^7/kg donor T cells on day 30 only (group D). Eighty percent of patients receiving T-cell–replete transplants (group A) developed grade II or more acute GVHD compared with a 14% risk following the T-depleted transplant and before lymphocyte add back (group B). Add back of 10^7/kg lymphocytes on day 30 resulted in a 100% risk of grade II or more acute GVHD, whereas a further 22% developed acute GVHD > grade I after add backs of 2×10^5/kg and 5×10^7/kg (group C). Of note, no patient in group C developed acute GVHD between days 30 and 45. With a median follow-up of 360 days, 60% of the patients from group C have developed chronic GVHD requiring treatment. The probability of leukemia relapse was 19% for the standard-risk group and 49.5% for the high-risk group. Improved results were achieved in a later study using T-cell–depleted peripheral blood stem cell transplants (PBSCTs) followed by delayed T-cell add back of 1×10^7 and 5×10^7 CD3$^+$ cells/kg, respectively, on days 45 and 100 posttransplant. In 30 patients with hematological malignancies, GVHD grade II–III developed in six patients—two after transplant, two after day 45, and two after day 100. There was a correspondingly low incidence of chronic GVHD, with three patients (30% probability) developing limited disease (22).

Delayed lymphocyte add back has also been investigated in partially mismatched-related transplants (23). Twenty-seven patients with advanced hematological malignancies were transplanted with T-cell–depleted bone marrow grafts from one to three antigen-mismatched–related donors. Starting between days 26 and 74, a cumulative T-cell dose of $0.23–16.5 \times 10^6$/kg was infused to preempt leukemia relapse under low-dose cyclosporine and steroid coverage. The results were compared with a historical group of similar patients treated at the same institution with T-cell–depleted BMT without the delayed addition of donor lymphocytes. A high incidence of acute GVHD was observed in the group receiving lymphocyte add back compared to historical controls (56 vs 11%). When more than 10^6/kg donor T cells were infused, the risk of developing GVHD was higher (88%) with significant GVHD-related mortality. Moreover, development of acute GVHD did not result in more GVL reactivity, since there was no difference in relapse rate between the add back group and historical controls at 18 months posttransplant (56 vs 58%).

Based on our current experience with delayed donor lymphocyte infusions, it thus appears that for HLA-matched sibling pairs, a T-cell dose of 10^6/kg given on day 30 or 10^7/kg given on day 45 under cyclosporine coverage is associated with a low risk of inducing severe acute GVHD and may still confer a GVL effect, especially in CML. However, in the HLA-mismatched setting, despite cyclosporine and steroid protection, administration of even low doses of unmanipulated donor lymphocytes induces severe GVHD.

These results indicate that the degree of donor-recipient matching, timing, and lymphocyte dose infused all determine the incidence and severity of acute GVHD following lymphocyte add back. With this approach, the GVL effect is preserved. Nevertheless, it is clear that no technique using add back of unselected lymphocytes can avoid some degree of acute and chronic GVHD. Further research will be directed toward the complete elimination of GVHD following T-cell–depleted transplants so as to provide a platform for the reconstitution of the immune repertoire using selected lymphocyte add back to avoid GVHD while conserving useful immune function. Improved stem cell selection techniques yielding PBSCTs rich in CD34$^+$ cells and delivering a fixed low dose of CD3$^+$ cells (in the region of 5 × 10^4/kg) facilitate these goals (24).

III. MANIPULATING DONOR T CELLS

As in every primary immune reaction, a functional T-cell response requires two signals: an antigen-specific signal via the T-cell receptor (TCR)/MHC–peptide interaction and a costimulatory signal via CD28/B7 interaction. TCR signaling without costimulation leads to antigen-specific unresponsiveness (25). Although the mechanism is not known, it is clear that the establishment of tolerance avoids the development of GVHD (26). Several in vitro and animal studies have investigated ways of inducing host-specific tolerance to reduce or abrogate GVHD reactions (27,28).

Gene transfer technology has made it possible to transduce donor lymphocytes with a "suicide gene" that makes them a target for pharmacological elimination in vivo. The in vitro insertion of the herpes simplex thymidine kinase gene has been developed for clinical use. This makes it possible to deplete gene-marked T cells in vivo by treating the patient with the antiviral drug ganciclovir should GVHD occur (29,30). This approach could be useful as a "safety net" to abort GVHD reactions in experimental add back studies to treat relapsed leukemia, Epstein-Barr virus (EBV)–lymphoproliferative disease, and cytomegalovirus (CMV) reactivation. It would be particularly applicable in mismatched donor-recipient pairs where the risk from lethal acute GVHD is high. A potential problem with highly efficient elimination of donor lymphocytes is the risk of severe immune deficiency which could increase the chance of leukemic relapse, recurrent infection, or reactivation of viruses leading to CMV disease and EBV lymphoproliferation. At least in transplants for CML, it may be necessary to maintain the GVL effect: the Philadelphia chromosome fusion gene *bcr-abl* is sometimes detectable for several years after BMT in the absence of relapse. This suggests that GVL is not a single immunological hit against the leukemia but rather a long-term process controlling residual disease. Elimination of the GVL suppressor cells could thus lead to leukemia relapse (5).

GVHD and GVL reactions are part of the donor's alloresponse to the host (5,26). Alloresponses to both leukemia and normal cells from the patient can be detected after BMT (31). The cells involved in the GVHD/GVL alloresponse include not only CD4$^+$ and CD8$^+$ T cells but also γδT cells, NK cells, and monocytes (5,32). In the HLA-mismatched setting, primary responders are CD4$^+$ T cells recognizing HLA class II differences and CD8$^+$ T cells recognizing HLA class I differences. In the HLA-matched setting, both CD4$^+$ and CD8$^+$ T cells respond to minor antigen differences (33,34). In rodents, depletion of CD8$^+$ cytotoxic/suppressor subset of T cells is sufficient to reduce or prevent GVHD in some, but not all, donor-recipient strain combinations; identical in major but disparate in minor histocompatibility antigens (35,36). Based on these observations, clinical trials to prevent GVHD using CD8$^+$ T-cell–depleted transplants have been initiated (37–41).

Since the responder cells in the alloimmune reactions between HLA-matched individuals are immunophenotypically diverse, and dependent on minor antigen disparities unique to each particular donor-recipient pair, a potentially superior approach to T-cell subset depletion would be to deplete the donor cells based on their ability to react to selected host cells. In this method, donor lymphocytes are stimulated with irradiated recipient cells in a mixed lymphocyte culture. Alloreacting donor cells express activation markers, including CD25 (high-affinity IL-2 receptor), CD69, or HLA-DR. The alloresponding cells can be eliminated with immunotoxins targeting activation antigens, by fluorescence-activated cell sorting, or using antibody-coated magnetic beads (42–44). The advantage of this approach is that depletion is specific for the population of donor lymphocytes reacting against the selected stimulator. Therefore, donor cells with other reactivities are spared. In the transplant setting, it is hoped this will translate to a selective depletion of only the GVHD-reacting cells and conservation of other beneficial donor immune functions. Several in vitro studies have shown that distinct subsets of donor T cells preferentially react against leukemic and nonleukemic targets in HLA-identical siblings (31,45). Furthermore, a recent multicenter report on the efficacy of donor lymphocyte transfusions used to treat leukemia relapse posttransplant has shown that approximately 25% of the patients responding to this treatment do not develop GVHD; suggesting that GVL and GVHD effector cells may be different (46). Analysis of the TCR Vβ subsets shows that both mixed and lineage-restricted reactivities against leukemic and nonleukemic cells are present in donor-versus-host interactions (47). These observations suggest that the once elusive goal of separating GVHD from favorable donor-derived immunity after BMT may be achieved by selective immunodepletion of the alloresponse.

IV. CLINICAL APPROACHES TO DONOR T-CELL MANIPULATION

A. Costimulatory Signal Blockade

Various antibodies, including anti–B7-1, anti–B7-2, cytotoxic T-lymphocyte–associated antigen-4–immunoglobulin (CTLA4-Ig), and anti–leucocyte fixation antigen-1 (LFA-1), have been used to block the costimulatory signal (27,28,48,49). In murine models of MHC-mismatched donor-recipient pairs, the use of CTLA4-Ig with anti–LFA-1 resulted in donor engraftment with prevention of GVHD-induced lethality and without global immunosuppression (48). In vitro studies have shown that the combined use of anti–B7-1 and anti–B7-2 results in host alloantigen-specific anergy without depletion of donor cells with other specificities (28). This approach to inducing host-specific anergy could be used to prevent acute GVHD in MHC-mismatched transplants. It is, however, unlikely that a significant GVL effect will be retained, since donor cells will most likely become tolerant to the leukemic cells as well as the normal cells of the host. A further concern is the possibility that anergy will eventually be reversed leading to delayed GVHD.

B. Insertion of the Thymidine Kinase Suicide Gene

In order to obtain T cells vulnerable to depletion by ganciclovir, a retroviral vector was used containing the herpes simplex thymidine kinase (TK) gene (29). Administration of ganciclovir to the patient resulted in specific inhibition of alloreactive TK-transduced cells. It was also demonstrated that gene expression was stable in vitro for more than three months. In another study, the TK gene was inserted into HLA-specific CD4+ cytotoxic T-cell clones. These clones retained their specificity, function, and sensitivity to ganciclovir with stable gene expression detected for more than 6 months (30). These studies open the way to clinical trials using genetically engineered T cells for the induction and control of GVHD and GVL alloreactions.

C. CD8+ Subset Depletion

Based on the initial animal data (35,36), human studies began using CD8+ T-cell depletion for the prevention of GVHD (37,38). In the initial study (37), 36 patients with leukemia received bone marrow grafts from HLA-identical siblings and CD8$^+$ T-cell–depleted bone marrow combined with posttransplant cyclosporine. Twenty-eight percent of recipients developed acute GVHD > grade I, which was usually mild and limited to the skin. Four patients failed to engraft, highlighting an important role of CD8$^+$ cells in engraftment. The leukemia relapse rate was only 11% and none of the 13 patients with CML relapsed, suggesting that the GVL effect was retained. In a prospective randomized double-blind study (38), 38 patients with leukemia received bone marrow grafts from their HLA-identical sibling donors, either unmanipulated or CD8$^+$ depleted, with posttransplant cyclosporine. Acute GVHD > grade I developed in 20% of the CD8$^+$-depleted group versus 80% (with five deaths) in the control group. Leukemia relapse was the same in the two groups and graft failure occurred in two patients in the CD8$^+$-depleted group but in none of the controls. Although GVHD prophylaxis was suboptimal for the control group, it seems that CD8$^+$ T-cell depletion in combination with cyclosporine is an effective method to reduce acute GVHD in HLA-identical sibling transplants without losing the GVL effect but at the expense of compromising engraftment in some patients. In another study (39), CD8$^+$ depletion followed by posttransplant cyclosporine effectively prevented acute GVHD in HLA-identical siblings but not in transplants from less well-matched donors. More recently, CD8$^+$-depleted donor lymphocytes have been used successfully to treat CML and multiple myeloma relapsing after allogeneic BMT with a low incidence of acute GVHD (41,50).

D. Selective Immunodepletion

In CML, the majority of circulating T-lymphocytes are not part of the leukemic clone (51,52) and therefore may be used as normal host cells. In a series of CML patients transplanted from HLA-matched siblings (10 patients) or matched unrelated donors (10 patients), donor lymphocytes were stimulated with phytohemagglutinin (PHA)–stimulated lymphoblasts from the patient. The alloreactive cells were then eliminated using a ricin-conjugated anti-CD25 immunotoxin. After depletion, donor lymphocytes lost their capacity to respond to PHA-lymphoblasts (<10% reactivity) but retained (>75%) their reactivity against the CML cells of the patient (53). Using a similar approach in six HLA-identical sibling pairs (54), donor lymphocytes reacting against OKT3/IL-2 expanded lymphoid cells from patients with CML were eliminated using a Pseudomonas exotoxin–based immunotoxin, which targets the high-affinity IL-2 receptor expressed exclusively on activated cells. A sensitive limiting dilution assay for alloreactive helper T-lymphocyte precursor frequencies (HTLPFs) was used to measure alloresponses against normal and leukemic host cells before and after the depletion. Although the HTLPFs against host cells were significantly reduced to a range predicting a low risk for GVHD (55,56), the frequencies against the leukemia cells were largely conserved, suggesting that the GVL effect was retained (57). The importance of donor CD4$^+$ lymphocytes in GVL reactions for CML has been demonstrated not only by the clinical observation that GVL is retained after CD8$^+$ depletion but also by in vitro studies (58), where alloreacting CD4$^+$ cells were shown to exert both cytotoxic and cytokine-mediated antileukemia effects.

The selective immunodepletion technique has also been tested in haplotype-mismatched donor-recipient pairs both in vitro (43) and in animals (42). In 10 haplo-identical pairs, depletion with the Pseudomonas-based anti–IL-2 receptor immunotoxin resulted in about 7.5% residual reactivity against the haploidentical stimulator and 65% against a third party (Table 2) (43). Moreover, the immunotoxin had no adverse effect

Table 2 Selective Immunodepletion of the Haplotype
Alloresponse

Residual response ± standard deviation	
Haploidentical stimulator	Third-party stimulator
14 ± 0.1	49 ± 5
13 ± 0.1	62 ± 2
5 ± 1	87 ± 4
12 ± 4	82 ± 9
1 ± 0.1	51 ± 5
4 ± 2	65 ± 16
8 ± 5	87 ± 11
5 ± 2	62 ± 9
11 ± 9	45 ± 15
3 ± 3	52 ± 7
Mean ± SEM 7.6 ± 1.5	64 ± 5

Stimulator lymphocytes were incubated for 24 h with equal numbers of haplotype-mismatched responder cells. After 24 h, 0.1 mg/
mL anti-Tac(Fv)–PE38 immunotoxin was added and cultures were
incubated a further 24 h. Immunotoxin-treated or immunotoxin-
untreated culture were restimulated with equal numbers of either
the original haploidentical stimulator or a human leucocyte antigen
(HLA)–mismatched third party. Tritiated thymidine uptake was
measured on day 5. Results shown are the percentage of control
tritiated thymidine uptake in cultures not incubated with immunotoxin of 10 different donor-recipient pair combinations. SEM =
standard error of the mean.

on granulocyte-macrophage colony-forming unit (CFU-GM) growth of normal bone marrow cells. When this approach was tested in a murine haploidentical BMT model, it significantly reduced GVHD lethality, prevented graft rejection, and induced specific tolerance for donor cells in chimeras (42). It remains to be seen whether this selective
immunodepletion can effectively prevent the development of acute GVHD in clinical trials
in HLA-matched and HLA-mismatched BMT and whether GVL reactivity and donor immunity are preserved.

V. CONCLUSION

New understanding of the pathogenesis of GVHD and of the basic mechanisms involved
in alloreactions has dramatically changed the way acute GVHD prevention is pursued in
experimental studies. Instead of the global immunosuppression conferred by pharmacological agents and nonselective T-cell–depletion methods, new approaches focus on the induction of specific tolerance, which prevents the development of acute GVHD during the
establishment of donor immunity. It is reasonable to expect that the prevention of GVHD
with improved immunological reconstitution posttransplant and preservation or augmentation of the GVL effect will result in improved outcome for allogeneic BMT in the near
future. The improved ability to control donor immune reconstitution should make bone
marrow stem cell transplants treatment safe even in patients lacking a fully matched related
donor.

REFERENCES

1. Aversa F, Tabilio A, Terenzi A, Velardi A, Falzetti F, Giannoni C, Iacucci R, Zei T, Martelli MP, Gambelunghe C, Rosetti M, Caputo P, Latini P, Ariseti C, Raymondi C, Reisner Y, Martelli M. Successful engraftment of T-cell depleted haploidentical "three-loci" incompatible transplants in leukemia patients by addition of recombinant human granulocyte colony-stimulating factor-mobilized peripheral blood progenitor cells to bone marrow inoculum. Blood 1994; 84:3948–3955.

2. Bensinger W, Clift R, Martin P, Appelbaum F, Demirer T, Gooley T, Lilleby K, Rowley S, Sanders J, Storb R, Buckner CD. Allogeneic peripheral blood stem cell transplantation in patients with advanced hematologic malignancies: a retrospective comparison with marrow transplantation. Blood 1996; 88:2794–2800.

3. Rigden JP, Cornetta K, Srour EF, Hanna M, Broun ER, Hromas R, Baute J, Hilton J, Cox E, Rubin L, Gonin R, Tricot G. Minimizing graft rejection in allogeneic T-cell depleted bone marrow transplantation. Bone Marrow Transplant 1996; 18:913–919.

4. Aversa F, Tabilio A, Velardi A, Cunningham I, Terenzi A, Falzetti F, Ruggeri L, Barbabietola G, Aristei C, Latini P, Reisner Y, Martelli MF. Treatment of high-risk acute leukemia with T-cell–depleted stem cells from related donors with one fully mismatched HLA haplotype. N Engl J Med 1998; 339:1186–1193.

5. Barrett AJ, Malkovska V. Graft-versus-leukemia: understanding and using the alloimmune response to treat haematological malignancies. Br J Haematol 1996; 93:754–761.

6. Ferrara JLM, Deeg JH. Graft-versus-host disease. N Engl J Med 1991; 324:667–674.

7. Krenger W, Ferrara JLM. Graft-versus-host disease and the Th1/Th2 paradigm. Immunol Res 1996; 15:50–73.

8. Antin JH, Ferrara JLM. Cytokine dysregulation and acute graft-versus-host disease. Blood 1992; 80:2964–2968.

9. Neste FP, Price KS, Seemayer TA, Lapp WS. Macrophage priming and lipopolysaccharide-triggered release of tumor necrosis factor-α during graft-versus-host disease. J Exp Med 1992; 175:405–413.

10. Anasetti C, Martin PJ, Storb R, Applebaum FR, Beatty PG, Calori E, Davis J, Doney K, Reichert T, Stewart P, Buckner CD, Thomas ED. Prophylaxis of graft-versus-host disease by administration of the murine anti–IL-2 receptor antibody 2A3. Bone Marrow Transplant 1991; 7:375–381.

11. Herve P, Flesch M, Tiberghien P, Wijdenes J, Racadot E, Bordignon P, Plouvier QE, Stephan JL, Bourdeau H, Holler E, Lioure B, Roche C, Vilmer E, Demeocq F, Kuenz M, Cahn JY. Phase I-II trial of a monoclonal anti-tumor necrosis factor-α antibody for the treatment of refractory severe acute graft-versus-host disease. Blood 1992; 79:3362–3368.

12. Antin JH, Weinstein HJ, Guinan EC, McCarthy P, Bierer BE, Gilliland DG, Parsons SK, Ballen KK, Rimm IJ, Falzarano G. Recombinant human interleukin-1 receptor antagonist in the treatment of steroid-resistant graft-versus-host disease. Blood 1994; 84:1342–1348.

13. Anasetti C, Hansen JA, Waldman TA. Treatment of acute graft-versus-host disease with humanized anti-Tac: an antibody that binds to the interleukin-2 receptor. Blood 1994; 84:1320–1327.

14. Blaise D, Olive D, Michallet M, Marit G, Leblond V, Maraninchi D. Impairment of leukaemia-free survival by addition of interleukin-2 receptor antibody to standard graft-versus-host prophylaxis. Lancet 1995; 345:1144–1146.

15. Fowler DH, Kurasawa K, Husebekk A, Cohen PA, Gress RE. Cells of the Th-2 cytokine phenotype prevent LPS-induced lethality during graft-versus-host reaction. J Immunol 1994; 152:1004–1013.

16. Fowler DH, Kurasawa K, Smith R, Eckhaus MA, Gress RA. Donor CD4-enriched cells of Th-2 cytokine phenotype regulate graft-versus-host disease without impairing allogeneic engraftment in sublethally irradiated mice. Blood 1994; 84:3540–3549.

17. Pan L, Delmonte J, Jalonen CK, Ferrara JLM. Pretreatment of donor mice with granulocyte

colony-stimulating factor polarizes donor T lymphocytes toward type-2 cytokine production and reduces severity of experimental graft-versus-host disease. Blood 1995; 86:4422–4429.

18.   Johnson BD, Drobyski WR, Truitt RL. Delayed infusion of normal donor cells after MHC-matched bone marrow transplantation provides an antileukemia reaction without graft-versus-host disease. Bone Marrow Transplant 1993; 11:329–336.

19.   Johnson BD, Truitt RL. Delayed infusion of immunocompetent donor cells after bone marrow transplantation breaks graft-host tolerance and allows for persistent antileukemic reactivity without severe graft-versus-host disease. Blood 1995; 85:3302–3312.

20.   Naparstek E, Or R, Nagler A, Cividalli G, Engelhard D, Aker M, Gimon Z, Waldmann H, Steinberg SM, Slavin S. T-cell depleted allogeneic bone marrow transplantation for acute leukaemia using Campath-1 antibodies and post-transplant administration of donor's peripheral blood lymphocytes for prevention of relapse. Br J Haematol 1995; 89:506–515.

21.   Barrett AJ, Mavroudis D, Tisdale J, Molldrem J, Dunbar C, Cottler-Fox M, Phang S, Carter C, Okunnieff P, Young NS, Read EJ. T-cell depleted bone marrow transplantation followed by delayed T-cell add-back to prevent severe acute GVHD. Bone Marrow Transplant 1998; 21:543–551.

22.   Barrett AJ, Bahceci E, Childs R, van Rhee F, Dunbar C, Young NS, Carter C, Sing A, Jacobs C, Read EJ. Low incidence of GVHD following T cell depleted peripheral blood stem cell transplant (PBSCT) followed by limited delayed T cell add-back. Blood 1998; 92(suppl 1): 139a.

23.   Godder KT, Abhyankar SH, Lamb LS, Best RG, Geier SS, Pati AR, Gee AP, Henslee-Downey PJ. Donor leukocyte infusion for treatment of graft rejection post partially mismatched related donor bone marrow transplant. Bone Marrow Transplant 1998; 22:111–113.

24.   Read EJ, Vigue FE, Carter CS, Sing A, Jacobs C, Phang S, Barrett AJ. Clinical trial of automated 2-step T cell depletion of peripheral blood progenitor cells for matched related allogeneic transplant. Blood 1998; 92(suppl 1):446a.

25.   Schultze J, Nadler LM, Gribben JG. B7-mediated costimulation and the immune response. Blood Rev 1996; 10:111–127.

26.   Theobald M. Allorecognition and graft-versus-host disease. Bone Marrow Transplant 1995; 15:489–498.

27.   Blazar BR, Taylor PA, Linsley PS, Vallera D. In vivo blockade of CD28/CTLA4: B7/BB1 interaction with CTLA4-Ig reduces lethal murine graft-versus-host disease across the major histocompatibility complex barrier in mice. Blood 1994; 83:3815–3825.

28.   Gribben J, Guinan E, Boussiotis Ke X-Y, Linsley L, Sieff C, Gray GS, Freeman GJ, Nadler LM. Complete blockade of B7 family-mediated costimulation is necessary to induce human alloantigen-specific anergy: a method to ameliorate graft-versus-host disease and extend the donor pool. Blood 1996; 87:4887–4893.

29.   Thiberghien P, Reynolds CW, Keller J, Spence S, Deschaseaux M, Certoux J-M, Contassot E, Murphy WJ, Lyons R, Chiang Y, Herve P, Longo D, Ruscetti FW. Ganciclovir treatment of herpes simplex thymidine kinase-transduced primary T lymphocytes: an approach for specific in vivo donor T-cell depletion after bone marrow transplantation? Blood 1994; 84:1333–1341.

30.   Gallot G, Hallet M, Gaschet J, Moreau JF, Vivien R, Bonneville M, Milpied N, Vie H. Human HLA-specific T-cell clones with stable expression of a suicide gene: a possible tool to drive and control a graft-versus-host-graft-versus-leukemia reaction? Blood 1996; 88:1098–1103.

31.   Hoffman T, Theobald M, Bunjes D, Weiss M, Heimpel H, Heit W. Frequency of bone marrow T cells responding to HLA-identical non-leukemic and leukemic stimulator cells. Bone Marrow Transplant 1993 12:1–8.

32.   Rhoades JL, Cibull ML, Thompson JS, Henslee-Downey PJ, Jennings CD, Sipp HP, Brown SA, Eichhorn TR, Cave ML, Jezek DA. Role of natural killer cells in the pathogenesis of human acute graft-versus-host disease. Transplantation 1993; 56:113–120.

33. Truitt RL, Atasoylu AA. Contribution of CD4+ and CD8+ T cells to graft-versus-host disease and graft-versus-leukemia reactivity after transplantation MHC-compatible bone marrow. Bone Marrow Transplant 1991; 8:51–58.

34. Okunewick J, Kociban D, Machen L, Buffo M. Effect of selective donor T-cell depletion on graft-versus-leukemia reaction in allogeneic marrow transplantation. Transplant Proc 1992; 24:2998–2999.

35. Korngold R, Sprent J. T-cell subsets and graft-versus-host disease. Transplantation 1987; 44: 335–340.

36. Korngold R, Sprent J. Variable capacity of L3T4+ T cells to cause lethal graft-versus-host disease across minor histocompatibility barriers in mice. J Exp Med 1987; 165:52–57.

37. Champlin R, Ho W, Gajewski J, Nimer S, Lee K, Territo M, Winston D, Tricot G, Reichert T. Selective depletion of CD8+ T lymphocytes for prevention of graft-versus-host disease after allogeneic bone marrow transplantation. Blood 1990; 76:418–423.

38. Nimer SD, Giorgi J, Gajewski JL, Ku N, Schiller GJ, Lee K, Territo M, Ho W, Feig S, Selch M, Isacescu V, Reichert TA, Champlin R. Selective depletion of CD8+ cells for prevention of graft-versus-host disease after bone marrow transplantation. Transplantation 1994; 57:82–87.

39. Jansen J, Hanks S, Akard L, Martin M, Thompson J, Chang Q, Ash R, Garrett D, Figg F, English D. Selective T cell depletion with CD8-conjugated magnetic beads in the prevention of graft-versus-host disease after allogeneic bone marrow transplantation. Leukemia 1995; 9: 271–278.

40. Palathumpat V, Dejbakhsh-Jones S, Strober S. The role of purified CD8+ T cells in graft-versus-leukemia activity and engraftment after allogeneic bone marrow transplantation. Transplantation 1995; 60:355–361.

41. Giralt S, Hester J, Huh Y, Hirsch-Ginsberg C, Rondón G, Seong D, Lee M, Gajewski J, Van Besien K, Khouri I, Mehra R, Przepiorka D, Körbling M, Talpaz M, Kantarjian H, Fischer H, Deisseroth A, Champlin R. CD8-depleted donor lymphocyte infusion as treatment for relapsed chronic myelogenous leukemia after allogeneic bone marrow transplantation. Blood 1995; 86: 4337–4343.

42. Cavazzana-Calvo M, Stephan JL, Sarnacki S, Chevret S, Fromont C, de Coene C, Le Deist F, Guy-Grand D, Fischer A. Attenuation of graft-versus-host disease and graft rejection by ex vivo immunotoxin elimination of alloreactive T cells in an H-2 haplotype disparate mouse combination. Blood 1994; 83:288–298.

43. Mavroudis DA, Jiang YZ, Hensel N, Lewalle P, Couriel D, Kreitman R, Pastan I, Barrett AJ. Specific depletion of alloreactivity against haplotype mismatched related individuals by a recombinant immunotoxin: a new approach to graft-versus-host disease prophylaxis in haploidentical bone marrow transplantation. Bone Marrow Transplant 1996; 17:793–799.

44. Rencher SD, Houston JA, Lockey TD, Hurwitz JL. Eliminating graft-versus-host potential from T cell immunotherapeutic populations. Bone Marrow Transplant 1996; 18:415–420.

45. van Lochem E, de Gast B, Goulmy E. In vitro separation of host specific graft-versus-host and graft-versus-leukemia cytotoxic T cell activities. Bone Marrow Transplant 1992; 10:181–183.

46. Kolb HJ, Schattenberg A, Goldman JM, Hertenstein B, Jacobsen N, Arcese W, Ljungman P, Ferrant A, Verdonk L, Niederwieser D, van Rhee F, Mittermuller J, de Witte T, Holler E, Ansari H. Graft-versus-leukemia effect of donor lymphocyte transfusions in marrow grafted patients. Blood 1995; 86:2041–2050.

47. Jiang YZ, Mavroudis D, Hensel N, Barrett AJ. Preferential usage of T cell receptor (TCR) Vβ by allogeneic T cells recognising myeloid leukemia cells: implications for separating GVL from GVHD. Bone Marrow Transplant 1997; 19:899–903.

48. Blazar BR, Taylor PA, Panoskaltsis-Mortari A, Gray GS, Vallera DA. Co-blockade of the LFA1:ICAM and CD28/CTLA4:B7 pathways is a highly effective means of preventing acute

lethal graft-versus-host disease induced by fully major histocompatibility complex-disparate donor grafts. Blood 1995; 85:2607–2618.

49. Blazar BR, Sharpe AH, Taylor PA, Panoskaltsis-Mortari A, Gray GS, Korngold R, Vallera DA. Infusion of anti-B7.1 (CD80) and anti-B7.2 (CD86) monoclonal antibodies inhibits murine graft-versus-host disease lethality in part via direct effects on CD4+ and CD8+ T cells. J Immunol 1996; 157:3250–3259.

50. Alyea EP, Schlossman RL, Canning C, Collins H, Pickett C, Wang Y, Soiffer RJ, Ritz J. CD8-depleted donor lymphocyte infusions mediate graft-versus-multiple myeloma effect. Blood 1996; 88(suppl 1):258a.

51. Jonas D, Lubbert M, Kawasaki ES, Henke M, Bross KJ, Mertelsmann R, Herrmann F. Clonal analysis of bcr-abl rearrangement in T lymphocytes from patients with chronic myelogenous leukemia. Blood 1992; 79:1017–1023.

52. Tsukamoto N, Karasawa M, Maehara T, Okamoto K, Sakai H, Naruse J, Morita K, Tsuchiya J, Omine M. The majority of T lymphocytes are polyclonal during the chronic phase of chronic myelogenous leukemia. Ann Hematol 1996; 72:61–65.

53. Datta AR, Jiang YZ, Guimarães A, Madrigal A, van Rhee F, Barrett AJ. Distinct T-cell populations distinguish chronic myeloid leukemia cells from lymphocytes in the same individual: a model for separating GVHD from GVL reactions. Bone Marrow Transplant 1994; 14:517–524.

54. Mavroudis DA, Jiang YZ, Hensel N, Lewalle P, Couriel D, Kreitman R, Pastan I, Barrett AJ. Selective immunodepletion between HLA matched siblings that reduces the risk for GVHD and preserves reactivity against the leukemia and Epstein-Barr virus. Blood 1996; 88(suppl 1):254a.

55. Theobald M, Nierle T, Bunjes D, Arnold R, Heimpel H. Host-specific interleukin-2-secreting donor T-cell precursors as predictors of acute graft-versus-host disease in bone marrow transplantation between HLA-identical siblings. N Engl J Med 1992; 327:1613–1617.

56. Schwarer AP, Jiang YZ, Brookes PA, Barrett AJ, Batchelor JR, Goldman JM, Lechler RI. Frequency of anti-recipient alloreactive helper T-cell precursors in donor blood and graft-versus-host disease after HLA-identical sibling bone marrow transplantation. Lancet 1993; 341:203–205.

57. Mavroudis DA, Dermime S, Molldrem J, Jiang YZ, Raptis A, van Rhee F, Hensel N, Fellowes V, Eliopoulos G, Barrett AJ. Specific depletion of alloreactive T cells in HLA-identical siblings—a method for separating graft-vs-host and graft-vs-leukaemia reactions. Br J Haematol 1998; 101:565–570.

58. Jiang YZ, Barrett AJ. Cellular and cytokine-mediated effects of CD4-positive lymphocyte lines generated in vitro against chronic myelogenous leukemia. Exp Hematol 1995; 23:1167–1172.

26

Blood Stem Cell Versus Bone Marrow Transplantation
A Critical Appraisal

ANNE KESSINGER

University of Nebraska Medical Center, Omaha, Nebraska

I. INTRODUCTION

Transplantation of hematopoietic stem/progenitor cells is essential for survival if high-dose myelotoxic anticancer therapy has caused permanent marrow ablation or damage severe enough to produce a dangerously prolonged period of neutropenia that cannot be sufficiently shortened with growth factor administration. If the transplanted cells are autologous, one must have already anticipated the necessity for transplant and collected the cells prior to the administration of high-dose therapy. If the cells are to be allogeneic, a suitable donor must have been identified prior to the high-dose therapy. Clinical results from dose-escalation studies have improved the accuracy of predictions that marrow ablation or prolonged marrow suppression will result after a particular high-dose regimen is given, but the variable health of stem cells, especially in patients who have already been treated with myelotoxic agents before high-dose therapy administration, precludes precise predictions.

In the adult, sites from which safe and effective collections of stem/progenitor cells for either allogeneic or autologous transplant can be accomplished are restricted to the pelvic bone marrow and the circulating blood stream. Currently, autologous cells for transplant are more commonly collected from the blood and allogeneic cells are more commonly collected from the marrow. Some controversy exists regarding which source of stem cells is preferred in a specific situation, and this chapter will explore some of the relevant issues in that regard.

II. RELIABLE, SUSTAINED HEMATOPOIETIC RECOVERY

When a patient has received therapy that is truly marrow lethal, reliable, sustained hemato-poietic recovery following transplant becomes an especially critical issue. Allogeneic bone marrow transplantation has been used successfully for decades, and no concerns are currently being raised about the possibility that these marrow graft products may not contain cells capable of restoring sustained hematopoietic function. In the mid 1980s, during the birth of the modern era of blood stem cell transplantation, some hematologists were skeptical that true pluripotent hematopoietic stem cells were present in the circulation, although the existence of circulating progenitors was well accepted. Hematopoietic progenitors in the peripheral blood of humans were first documented with culture assays (1) and later on by the identification of CD34$^+$ cells in human peripheral blood (2). Expression of the CD34 differentiation antigen is limited to hematopoietic precursors, but it does not necessarily distinguish between progenitors and stem cells. When autologous CD34$^+$ cells were positively selected from either marrow or blood stem cell collections (see Section III on CD34$^+$ selection, this volume) and transplanted, reliable recovery of hematopoietic function resulted (3,4). If only progenitors and not pluripotent stem cells were present in a blood stem cell graft product, then patients receiving marrow-ablative therapy and a blood cell transplant would experience hematopoietic recovery followed by marrow aplasia as the transplanted progenitors completed the maturation pathway and the life span of the terminally differentiated blood cells ended. As more experience with clinical blood stem/progenitor cell autografts was gained, and follow-up became longer, the lack of reports of secondary aplasia was reassuring (5) and lessened but did not eliminate the uneasiness, because complete marrow ablation was not thought to be common following high-dose therapy and autografting. As a result, blood stem cell transplants have been described in the literature with a variety of names. Those who believed that pluripotent stem cells were present in the circulation referred to the procedure as a "peripheral stem cell transplantation" or a "peripheral blood stem cell transplantation," whereas others who awaited proof positive that the stem cell circulated used titles such as "peripheral progenitor cell transplantation" or "blood progenitor cell transplantation." The more recent observation that allogeneic blood stem cell transplantation results in long-term hematopoietic function of donor cell origin (6) should now put to rest doubts regarding the sustainability of hematopoiesis following blood stem cell transplants. These studies and observations lead to the conclusion that stem cells collected from marrow or from blood in either the allogeneic or the autologous setting are equally effective at providing long-term hematopoietic recovery following high-dose therapy.

III. RATE OF HEMATOPOIETIC RECOVERY

Because long periods of neutropenia following high-dose therapy are associated with increased morbidity, occasional mortality, and increased medical expense, transplant products which can provide shorter periods of neutropenia as well as anemia and thrombocytopenia should offer clear advantages in certain clinical situations. Prior to the availability of hematopoietic growth factors, transplanted autologous stem/progenitor cells collected during steady-state hematopoiesis from either the marrow or the blood were found to provide equivalent rates of hematopoietic recovery following high-dose chemotherapy (7). However, autografting blood stem cells that were collected while the patient recovered from suppressed myelopoietic function resulting from treatment with conventional doses of myelotoxic chemotherapy was followed by more rapid neutrophil recovery (8). Recovery from chemotherapy-induced cytopenia was shown to be associated with a marked increase in circulating hematopoietic progenitor numbers (9); a phenomena referred to as mobilization.

New horizons were opened regarding the rapidity of marrow recovery following high-dose therapy and transplant when granulocyte-macrophage colony-stimulating factor (GM-CSF) and granulocyte colony-stimulating factor (G-CSF) became available for clinical use. These hematopoietic growth factors were found to be good blood stem/progenitor cell mobilizers when used in conjunction with myelosuppressive chemotherapy or when used alone (10,11). Autografts of $CD34^+$ stem/progenitor cells selected from well-mobilized blood stem/progenitor cell collections produced the same rate of accelerated neutrophil recovery as did unseparated well-mobilized blood cell autografts (4), and growth factor administration following mobilized blood stem/progenitor cell transplants further accelerated circulating neutrophil recovery (12,13). Although retrospective (14,15) and small randomized prospective studies (16) as well as data from registries (17) suggested that autologous bone marrow transplantation with or without administration of growth factor at the time of transplant results in less rapid neutrophil and platelet recovery than similarly administered autologous blood stem/progenitor cell transplantation, a large randomized study reported in 1997 provided confirmation (18). Some investigators, however, have suggested that these comparisons are not appropriate, because transplantation of growth factor–mobilized, or "activated," marrow should be compared to mobilized blood stem/progenitor cell transplantation for speed of hematopoietic recovery (19). Transplanted marrow collected after growth factor stimulation may prove to facilitate hematopoietic recovery as effectively as mobilized blood stem/progenitor cells, but only a limited number of trials have been reported which address this possibility (19,20), and currently growth factor–activated marrow transplants are not commonly performed or reported.

When allogeneic blood cell transplants have been compared retrospectively with allogeneic bone marrow transplants for hematopoietic recovery, some (21–22,23), but not all (24), investigators found an increase in the speed of neutophil recovery, whereas all have reported that more rapid platelet recovery was associated with the blood cell transplants.

These hematopoietic recovery advantages of blood cell as compared with marrow transplants in both the allogeneic and the autologous settings are subject to changes in the future as, for example, new growth factors become available for clinical use. For now, however, if rapid hematopoietic recovery is a paramount consideration for the transplant patient in question, the graft product of choice is blood stem/progenitor cells.

IV. TUMOR CELL CONTAMINATION OF AUTOLOGOUS GRAFT PRODUCTS

Long-term disease-free survival has been described in some patients who received autologous bone marrow transplants that were known to contain occult tumor cells (25,26); demonstrating that reinfusion of small numbers of autologous tumor cells does not invariably result in tumor relapse. However, occult tumor cells in transplanted autologous marrow grafts have also been documented as being contributors to relapse in other patients (27). Although infusion of overt chronic myelogenous leukemic cells collected in blood cell autografts routinely reintroduces the disease (28,29), the metastatic potential of occult tumor cells in infused autologous blood cell products has not been systematically investigated. One study has shown that 35% of patients with low-grade non-Hodgkin's lymphoma had no detectable tumor cells in the blood or bone marrow, as determined with a polymerase chain reaction (PCR) assay for the t(14;18) translocation, after being autografted with PCR-positive blood cell harvests; indicating that reinfused tumor cells collected from the circulation may not be sustained, at least in some instances (30). Differences in the biological characteristics and behavior of circulating occult tumor cells versus those metastatic to marrow seem likely to exist. Nonetheless, and in spite of the lack of concrete evidence to the contrary, the presence of occult tumor cells in a blood stem cell autograft product intuitively has dangerous potential. Interestingly, patients with evidence of occult or overt marrow metastases do not routinely have concomitant occult tumor cells in the circulation (25). The majority of studies involving solid tumors and lymphomas published thus far have reported that unpurged marrow harvests are either more likely to contain occult tumor cells or to contain more occult tumor cells than unpurged blood cell autograft products (31–33).

Taken as a whole, transplantation of autologous blood cell grafts is less likely to reintroduce tumor cells to a patient than transplantation of autologous bone marrow. The in vivo clonogenic potential of circulating tumor cells collected in a blood cell autograft product is not known. Some circumstantial evidence has suggested that mobilized occult lymphoma cells do not contribute to disease relapse if reinfused (34). The risks of occult tumor cells contributing to relapse may vary from one disease to another and from one stage of a disease to another. The development of effective purging techniques for marrow and blood cell autografts in the future, provided occult tumor cells in the blood cell products do have clonogenic potential in vivo, will, however, neutralize any apparent current advantage blood cell autograft products may have.

V. PROMPT IMMUNOLOGICAL RECOVERY FOLLOWING TRANSPLANTATION

Immunological as well as hematological damage results from high-dose therapy administration. Although recovery of hematological function is critical for the patient in the short term, recovery of immunological function following autologous transplantation has important implications for both long-term survival and life quality. Rapid restoration of immunological surveillance may provide antitumor activity against certain tumor cells that may have survived the high-dose therapy. In addition, immune recovery provides protection from infections not associated with neutropenia.

The rate and quality of immunological recovery could be influenced by specific cell populations that can be included in the autograft. An investigation of blood stem cell products demonstrated that GM-CSF not only mobilizes hematopoietic precursors into the circulation but also increases the number of circulating immune cells (35). Significant differences in the immunological profile of cells collected in marrow and blood autograft harvests have been described (36). Specifically, blood stem cell products were found to contain more cells that expressed the CD4, CD8, CD45RO, and CD56 phenotypes than did bone marrow harvests (36,37), although T-cell precursors have been identified in both peripheral blood and bone marrow (38). Blood stem cell harvests were also superior to bone marrow collections with respect to developing effective natural killer activity after culture with interleukin-7 (IL-7), IL-12, or IL-2 plus IL-12 (39). Cellular immune function, including natural killer (NK) and inducible lymphokine-activated killer (LAK) function have been reported to recover more rapidly if autologous blood stem cells rather than autologous marrow are infused following high-dose therapy (36,37), and circulating lymphocytes appear earlier and in greater numbers after blood versus marrow autografting (40).

Although certain immunological parameters do seem to recover more quickly and with greater vigor following blood cell transplants, the important issue is whether this rapid recovery provides any clinical advantage. Not much information is available regarding protection from infection after hematopoietic recovery, although in the pediatric population, the incidence of varicella-zoster infections posttransplant was reported to be similar whether blood or marrow autografts are performed (41).

Whether the antitumor cytotoxic activity found in graft products is valuable is debatable. Although the explanation is very likely to be multifactorial, one retrospective study has suggested that autologous blood stem cell transplantation is associated with longer disease-free survival than autologous bone marrow transplantation (42). Other retrospective studies have not been able to confirm these findings (43).

In regard to immune cytotoxic effector cells, since NK activity and inducible LAK activity are restored more quickly, blood stem cell transplants could theoretically provide some antitumor therapeutic efficacy or autologous graft-versus-tumor effect that marrow autografting could not provide. Mechanisms are reported to exist that might further enhance such an antitumor effect. GM-CSF administration following autologous marrow transplantation has been reported to increase activated killer cell function and possibly diminish the relapse rate for patients with acute myelogenous leukemia (44). This effect might be amplified if blood stem cell infusions were performed. Another study reported that infusion of mafosfamide-purged autologous marrow resulted in faster NK (CD16$^+$) cell regeneration, as measured with chromium release assays, than nonpurged marrow for patients with non-Hodgkin's lymphoma and acute myelogenous leukemia but not for patients with acute lymphoblastic leukemia (45). Perhaps mafosfamide-purged blood stem cells would provide even faster regeneration. However, purging blood stem cell autograft products with positive selection techniques should be approached with some caution and calculation. Selection of CD34$^+$ cells for autografting would exclude infusion of accessory cells such as NK cells, dendritic cells, and LAK cell precursors which may be important in providing or augmenting autologous graft-versus-tumor effects. If these effects are deemed as being desirable, some sort of add back mechanism of important accessory cells could be considered.

Immune therapy following high-dose therapy and transplant as a strategy to improve the long-term disease-free survival of hematopoietic stem cell transplant patients is gaining favor (46,47). Any differences in the effects of immune-modulating agents administered following blood stem cell transplant or marrow transplant, in either the autologous or the allogeneic setting, have not yet been evaluated. The ability to manipulate the immune system may be different after marrow or blood cell transplantation. If differences are found to exist, then the source of the graft product, marrow or blood, will be an important consideration in the management plan of patients who will benefit from immune therapy.

Even less information is available regarding immune reconstitution following marrow-versus-blood stem cell allografting. This is due, in part, to the newness of allogeneic blood stem cell transplantation in the clinical setting. Initial comparative studies have shown that more naive and memory helper T cells are infused with a blood cell than with a marrow allograft, and that allogeneic blood stem cell recipients have higher numbers of circulating naive and memory helper T cells and B cells as well as increased proliferative responses to phytohemagglutinin, pokeweed mitogen, tetanus toxoid, and *Candida* posttransplant (48). CD3$^+$ cell numbers and the CD4/CD8 ratio on day 100 and at 1 year after allogeneic blood cell transplantation were within the normal range and significantly higher than 100 days and 1 year after allogeneic bone marrow transplantation (6). These data at least suggest that immunohematopoietic recovery is different and earlier following alloge-neic blood stem cell transplantation than after allogeneic bone marrow transplantation.

Although blood cell graft products are associated with faster and more complete immune recovery after transplant, the data used to draw these conclusions are based on ex vivo laboratory assays and not clinical outcome. Therefore, the advantages of marrow or blood cell grafts in regard to immune reconstitution following transplant are not obvious. If clinical outcome is shown to correlate with laboratory-measured immune recovery or if immune modulation posttransplant is better after marrow or blood stem cell transplant, the choice of marrow or blood cells will become clearer.

VI. ALLOGENEIC BLOOD STEM CELL AND MARROW TRANSPLANTATION

Allogeneic transplantation of marrow and blood stem cells is discussed in detail in Chapter 21 of this volume. Here, discussion will be limited to comparisons and contrasts between blood stem cell and marrow allogeneic transplantation.

Until very recently, clinical reports of allogeneic blood stem cell transplants were notable by their absence. Autologous blood stem cell transplants gained widespread ac-ceptability in the early 1990s, but several concerns regarding allogeneic transplants de-layed their clinical emergence. These included the lack of definitive information that hema-topoietic stem cells were present in the human circulation, concern that the increased numbers of lymphocytes in the blood stem cell graft product would result in unacceptable incidence and severity of graft-versus-host disease, and the concern that administration of growth factors to normal donors for mobilization purposed could have immediate or delayed untoward consequences. In 1989 (49) and 1993 (50,51), a series of case reports suggested the concerns were possibly unfounded and modest-sized series of such trans-plants are now available at a number of transplant centers. No prospective randomized studies comparing blood to marrow allografting have been published, although one is underway in Europe. A few retrospective comparisons are available which have suggested that allogeneic blood cell transplantation from human leukocyte antigen (HLA)–identical donors is associated with more rapid engraftment (6,21,22), the need for fewer transfusions of red cells and platelets (22), no greater incidence of acute (6,21,22,24) or chronic graft-versus-host disease (22), a shorter hospital stay, and a similar early survival (6). Perhaps, therefore, allogeneic blood stem cell transplants offer some advantages to marrow allo-grafting, but any conclusions drawn at this time are preliminary at best.

VII. CONCLUSION

The source of the graft product plays an interesting role in outcomes of hematopoietic stem cell transplantation. The donor must either undergo multiple aspirations of pelvic bone marrow or multiple, usually two or three, apheresis procedures. Bone marrow har-vesting can be accomplished more quickly than blood stem cell collection, and it is less labor intensive. Blood cell transplants provide more rapid hematopoietic recovery than marrow transplants; thereby reducing costs and in some cases permitting more of the total transplant experience to occur without the need for hospitalization. The effect of the choice of graft product on the outcome of tumor control, if any, is not yet obvious. These issues are and will be considered in future basic, translational, and clinical research ef-forts.

VIII. ADDENDUM

Recent studies have further considered whether the outcomes of cancer patients are influenced by transplantation of blood-derived versus marrow-derived graft products. In the autologous setting, early data suggests that, provided very large numbers of CD34+ cells are infused, outcomes following blood stem cell transplantation may be superior to that seen following bone marrow transplantation (52,53).

In the allogeneic setting, while the randomized trials ongoing in Europe have not been formally reported, a non-randomized trial has suggested better outcomes for patients with chronic myelogenous leukemia in first chronic phase who were allografted with matched blood stem cell vs matched bone marrow products (54).

Many centers are currently investigating methods to engineer blood stem cell grafts to improve outcomes in both the allogeneic and autologous settings, thus potentially providing therapeutic as well as restorative value to the graft procedure.

REFERENCES

1. McCredie KB, Hersh EM, Freireich EJ. Cells capable of colony formation in the peripheral blood of man. Science 1971; 171(968):293–294.
2. Siena S, Bregni M, Brando M, Ravagnani F, Bonadonna G, Gianni AM. Circulation of CD34+ hematopoietic stem cells in the peripheral blood of high-dose cyclophosphamide-treated patients: enhancement by intravenous recombinant human granulocyte macrophage colony-stimulating factor. Blood 1989; 74(6):1905–1914.
3. Gorin N-C, Lopez M, Laporte J-P, Quittet P, Lesage S, Lemoine F, Berenson R, Isnard F, Grande M, Stachowiak J, Labopin M, Fouillard L, Morel P, Jouet J-P, Noel-Walter M-P, Detourmignies L, Aoudjhane M, Bauters F, Najman A, Douay L. Preparation and successful engraftment of purified CD34+ bone marrow progenitor cells in patients with non-Hodgkin's lymphoma. Blood 1995; 85(6):1647–1654.
4. Brugger W, Henschler R, Heimfeld S, Berenson RJ, Mertelsmann R, Kanz L. Positively selected autologous blood CD34+ cells and unseparated peripheral blood progenitor cells mediate identical engraftment after high-dose VP-16, ifosfamide, carboplatin, and epirubicin. Blood 1994; 84(5):1421–1426.
5. Haas R, Witt B, Mohle R, Goldschmidt H, Hohaus S, Fruehauf S, Wannemacher M, Hunstein W. Sustained long-term hematopoiesis after myeloablative therapy with peripheral blood progenitor cell support. Blood 1995; 85(12):3754–3761.
6. Pavletic ZS, Bishop MR, Tarantolo SR, Martin-Algarra S, Bierman PJ, Vose JM, Reed EC, Gross TG, Kollath J, Nasrati K, Jackson JD, Armitage JO, Kessinger A. Hematopoietic recovery after allogeneic blood stem cell transplantation compared to bone marrow transplantation in patients with hematologic malignancies. J Clin Oncol 1997; 15(4):1608–1616.
7. Kessinger A, Armitage JO, Landmark JD, Smith DM and Weisenburger DD. Autologous peripheral hematopoietic stem cell transplantation restores hematopoietic function following marrow ablative therapy. Blood 1988; 71(3):723–727.
8. Juttner CA, To LB, Ho JQK, Bardy PG, Dyson PG, Haylock DN, Kimber RJ. Early lympho-hematopoietic recovery after autografting using peripheral blood stem cells in acute nonlymphoblastic leukemia. Transplant Proc 1988; 20(1):40–42.
9. To LB, Haylock DN, Kimber RJ, Juttner CA. High levels of circulating haemopoietic stem cells in very early remission from acute nonlymphoblastic leukaemia and their collection and cryopreservation. Br J Haematol 1984; 58(3):399–410.
10. Socinski MA, Cannistra SA, Elias A, Antman KH, Schnipper L, Griffin JD. Granulocyte-macrophage colony stimulating factor expands the circulating haemopoietic cell compartment in man. Lancet 1988; 1(8596):1194–1198.

11. Duhrsen U, Villeval JL, Boyd J, Kannourakis G, Morstyn G, Metcalf D. Effects of recombinant human granulocyte colony-stimulating factor on hematopoietic progenitor cells in cancer patients. Blood 1988; 72(6):2074–2081.

12. Klumpp TR, Mangan KF, Goldberg SL, Pearlman ES, Macdonald JS. Granulocyte colony-stimulating factor accelerates neutrophil engraftment following peripheral-blood stem-cell transplantation: a prospective randomized trial. J Clin Oncol 1995; 13(6):1323–1327.

13. Colombat Ph, Delain M, Desbois I, Domenech J, Binet Ch, Tabah I, Langanere JP, Linassier C. Granulocyte-macrophage colony-stimulating factor accelerates hematopoietic recovery after autologous bone marrow or peripheral blood progenitor cell transplantation and high-dose chemotherapy for lymphoma. Bone Marrow Transplant 1996; 18(2):293–299.

14. Reiffers J, Goldman J, Meloni G, Cahn JY, Gratwohl A. Autologous stem cell transplantation in chronic myelogenous leukemia: a retrospective analysis of the European Group for Bone Marrow Transplantation. Bone Marrow Transplant 1994; 14(3):407–410.

15. Harousseau JL, Attal M, Divine M, Milpied N, Marit G, Leblond V, Stoppa AM, Hourhis JH, Caillot D, Boasson M, Abgrall JF, Facon T, Colombat P, Cahn JY, Lamy T, Troussard X, Gratecos N, Pgnon B, Auzanneau G. Comparison of autologous bone marrow transplantation and peripheral blood stem cell transplantation after first remission induction treatment in multiple myeloma. Bone Marrow Transplant 1995; 15(6):963–969.

16. Beyer J, Schwella N, Zingsem J, Strohscheer I, Schwaner I, Oettle H, Serke S, Huhn S, Siegert W. Hematopoietic rescue after high-dose chemotherapy using autologous peripheral-blood progenitor cells or bone marrow: a randomized comparison. J Clin Oncol 1995; 13(6):1328–1335.

17. Harousseau JL, Attal M, Divine M, Marit G, Leblond V, Stoppa A-M, Bourhis J-H, Caillot D, Boasson M, Abgrall J-F, Facon T, Linassier C, Cahn J-Y, Lamy T, Troussard X, Gratecos N, Pignon B, Auzanneau G, Batialle R. Autologous stem cell transplantation after first remission induction treatment in multiple myeloma: a report of the French registry on autologous transplantation in multiple myeloma. Blood 1995; 85(11):3077–3085.

18. Hartmann O, LeCorroller AG, Blaise D, Michon J, Philip I, Norol F, Janvier M, Pico JL, Baranzelli MC, Rubie H, Coze C, Pinna A, Meresse V, Benhamou E. Peripheral blood stem cell and bone marrow transplantation for solid tumors and lymphomas: hematologic recovery and costs. A randomized, controlled trial. Ann Intern Med 1997; 126(8):600–607.

19. Janssen WE, Smilee RC, Elfenbein GJ. A prospective randomized trial comparing blood and marrow-derived stem cells for hematopoietic replacement following high dose chemotherapy. J Hematother 1995; 4(3):139–140.

20. Dicke KA, Hood DL, Arneson M, Fulbright L, DiStefano A, Firstenberg B, Adams J, Blumenschein GR. Effects of short-term in vivo administration of G-CSF on bone marrow prior to harvesting. Exp Hematol 1997; 25(1):34–38.

21. Urbano-Ispizua A, Solano C, Brunet S, Hernandez F, Sanz G, Alegre A, Petit J, Besalduch J, Vivancos P, Diaz MA, Moraleda JM, Carreras E, Ojeda E, de la Rubia J, Benet I, Domingo-Albos A, Garcia-Conde J, Rozman C. for the allo-PBPCT Spanish group. Allogeneic peripheral blood progenitor cell transplantation: analysis of short-term engraftment and acute GVHD incidence in 33 cases. Bone Marrow Transplant 1996; 18(1):35–40.

22. Bensinger WI, Clift R, Martin P, Appelbaum FR, Demirer T, Gooldy T, Lilleby K, Rowley S, Sanders J, Storb R, Buckner CD. Allogeneic peripheral blood stem cell transplantation in patients with advanced hematologic malignancies: a retrospective comparison with marrow transplantation. Blood 1996; 88(7):2794–2800.

23. Pavletic Z, Bishop M, Tarantolo S, Joshi S, Pirruccello S, Reed E, Bierman P, Vose J, Armitage J, Kessinger A. Immunohematopoietic recovery after allogeneic blood stem cell transplantation. Biol Blood Marrow Transplant 1996; 2:153.

24. Korbling M, Przepiorka D, Huh YO, Engel H, van Besien K, Giralt S, Andersson B, Kleine HD, Seong D, Deisseroth AB, Andreeff M, Champlin R. Allogeneic blood stem cell transplantation for refractory leukemia and lymphoma: potential advantage of blood over marrow allografts. Blood 1995; 85(6):1659–1665.

25. Sharp JG, Kessinger A, Mann S, Crouse DA, Armitage JO, Bierman P, Weisenburger DD.

Outcome of high-dose therapy and autologous transplantation in non-Hodgkin's lymphoma based on the presence of tumor in the marrow or infused hematopoietic harvest. J Clin Oncol 1996; 14(1):214–219.

26. Peters SO, Stackschlader M, Hegewisch-Becker S, Lriger W, Wej HJ, Hossfeld DK, Aancer AR. Infusion of tumor-contaminated bone marrow for autologous rescue after high-dose therapy leading to long-term remission in a patient with relapsed Philadelphia chromosome-positive acute lymphoblastic leukemia. Bone Marrow Transplant 1995; 15(5):783–784.

27. Brenner MK, Rill DR, Moen RC, Krance RA, Mirro J, Anderson WF, Ihle JN. Gene marking to trace origin of relapse after autologous bone-marrow transplantation. Lancet 1993; 341(8837):85–86.

28. Haines ME, Goldman JM, Worsley AM, McCarthy DM, Syatt SE, Dowdling C, Kearney L, Th'ng KH, Wareham NJ, Pollock A, Galvin MC, Samson D, Geary CG, Catovsky D, Galton DAG. Chemotherapy and autografting for chronic granulocytic leukaemia in transformation: probable prolongation of survival for some patients. Br J Haematol 1984; 58(4):711–721.

29. Reiffers J, Trouette R, Marit G, Montastruc M, Faberes C, Cony-Makhoul P, David B, Bourdeau MJ, Bilhou-Nabera C, Lacombe F, Feuillatre-Fabre F, Vezon G, Bernard PH., Broustet A. Autologous blood stem cell transplantation for chronic granulocytic leukaemia in transformation: a report of 47 cases. Br J Haematol 1991; 77(3):339–345.

30. Haas R, Moos M, Karcher A, Mohle R, Witt B, Goldschmidt H, Furhauf S, Flentje M, Wannemacher M, Hunstein W. Sequential high-dose therapy with peripheral-blood progenitor-cell support in low-grade non-Hodgkin's lymphoma. J Clin Oncol 1994; 12(8):1685–1692.

31. Shpall EJ, Jones RB. Release of tumor cells from bone marrow. Blood 1994; 83(3):623–625.

32. Ross AA, Cooper BW, Lazarus HM, Mackay W, Moss TJ, Ciobanu N, Tallman MS, Kennedy MJ, Davidson NE, Sweet D, Winter C, Akard L, Jansen J, Copelan E, Meagher RC, Herzig RH, Klumpp TR, Kahn DG, Warner NE. Detection and viability of tumor cells in peripheral blood stem cell collections from breast cancer patients using immunocytochemical and clonogenic assay techniques. Blood 1993; 82(9):2605–2610.

33. Datta YH, Adams PT, Drobyski WR, Ethier SP, Terry VH, Roth MS. Sensitive detection of occult breast cancer by the reverse-transcriptase polymerase chain reaction. J Clin Oncol 1994; 12(3):475–482.

34. Kessinger A, Bierman PJ, Gowles MK, Anderson JR, Armitage JO, Bishop MR, Vose JM. Mobilized versus non-mobilized peripheral stem cell transplantation after high dose therapy for low grade nonHodgkin lymphoma. Cancer Res Ther Control 1998; 5:113–119.

35. Triozzi PL, Tucker F, Benzies T, Balcerzak SP. Antitumor and accessory immune activities of peripheral blood stem cells mobilized with granulocyte-macrophage colony-stimulating factor. Bone Marrow Transplant 1996; 18(1):47–52.

36. Talmadge JE, Reed EC, Kessinger A, Kuszynski CA, Perry GA, Gordy CL, Mills KC, Thomas ML, Pirrucello SJ, Letheby BA, Arneson MA, Jackson JD. Immunologic attributes of cytokine mobilized peripheral blood stem cells and recovery following transplantation. Bone Marrow Transplant 1996; 17(1):101–109.

37. Scheid C, Pettengell R, Ghielmini M, Radford JA, Morgenstern GR, Sterm PL, Crowther D. Time-course of the recovery of cellular immune function after high-dose chemotherapy and peripheral blood progenitor cell transplantation for high-grade non-Hodgkin's lymphoma. Bone Marrow Transplant 1995; 15(6):901–906.

38. Galy AHM, Webb S, Cen D, Murray LJ, Condino J, Negrin RS, Chen BP. Generation of T cells from cytokine-mobilized peripheral blood and adult bone marrow CD34+ cells. Blood 1994; 84:104–110.

39. Wong EK, Eaves C, Klingemann H-G. Comparison of natural killer activity of human bone marrow and blood cels in cultures containing IL-2, IL-7 and IL-12. Bone Marrow Transplant 1996; 18(1):63–71.

40. Henon PhR, Liang H, Beck-Wirth G, Elsenmann JC, Lepers M, Wunder E, Kandel G. Comparison of hematopoietic and immune recovery after autologous bone marrow or blood stem cell transplants. Bone Marrow Transplant 1992; 9(4):285–291.

41. Takaue Y, Okamoto Y, Kawano Y, Suzue T, Abe T, Saito S-I, Sato J, Hirao A, Makimoto A, Kawahito M, Watanabe W, Shimokawa T, Kuroda Y. Regeneration of immunity and varicella-zoster virus infection after high-dose chemotherapy and peripheral blood stem cell autografts in children. Bone Marrow Transplant 1994; 14(2):219–223.

42. Vose JM, Anderson JR, Kessinger A, Bierman PJ, Coccia P, Reed EC, Gordon B, Armitage JO. High-dose chemotherapy and autologous hematopoietic stem cell transplantation for aggressive non-Hodgkin's lymphoma. J Clin Oncol 1993; 11(10):1846–1851.

43. Brunvand MW, Bensinger WI, Soll E, Weaver CH, Rowley SD, Appelbaum FR, Lilleby K, Clift RA, Gooley TA, Press OW, Fefer A, Storb R, Sanders JE, Martin PL, Chauncey T, Maziraz RT, Zuckerman N, Montgomery P, Dorn R, Weiden PL, Demirer T, Holmberg LA, Schiffman K, McSweeney PA, Maloney DG, Buckner CD. High-dose fractionated total-body irradiation, etoposide, and cyclophosphamide for treatment of malignant lymphoma: comparison of autologous bone marrow and peripheral blood stem cells. Bone Marrow Transplant 1996; 18(1):131–141.

44. Richard C, Baro J, Bello-Fernandez J, Hermida G, Calavia J, Olalla I, Alsar MJ, Loyola I, Cuadrado MA, Iriondo A, Conde E, Aubizarreta A. Recombinant human granulocyte-macrophage colony stimulating factor (rhGM-CSF) administration after autologous bone marrow transplantation for acute myeloblastic leukemia enhances activated killer cell function and may diminish leukemic relapse. Bone Marrow Transplant 1995; 15(5):721–726.

45. Almici C, Manoni L, Carlo-Stella C, Garau D, Cottafavi L, Rizzoli V. Natural killer cell regeneration after transplantation with mafosfamide purged autologous bone marrow. Bone Marrow Transplant 1995; 16(1):95–101.

46. Benyunes M, Massumoto C, York A, Higuhi C, Buckner CD, Thompson JA, Petersen FB, Fefer A. Interleukin-2 with or without lymphokine-activated killer cells as consolidative immunotherapy after autologous bone marrow transplantation for acute myelogenous leukemia: a preliminary report. Bone Marrow Transplant 1993; 12(2):159–163.

47. Weisdorf DJ, Anderson PM, Blazar BR, Uckun FM, Kersey JH, Ramsay NKC. Interleukin 2 immediately after autologous bone marrow transplantation for acute lymphoblastic leukemia. Transplant 1993; 55(1):61–66.

48. Ottinger HD, Beelen DW, Scheulen B, Schaefer UW, Growwe-Wilde H. Improved immune reconstitution after allotransplantation of peripheral blood stem cells instead of bone marrow. Blood 1996; 88(7):2775–2779.

49. Kessinger A, Smith DM, Strandjord SE, Landmark JD, Dooley DC, Law P, Coccia PF, Warkentin PI, Weisenburger EE, Armitage JO. Allogeneic transplantation of blood-derived, T-cell depleted hematopoietic stem cells after myeloablative treatment in a patient with acute lymphoblastic leukemia. Bone Marrow Transplant 1989; 4(6):643–646.

50. Russell NH, Hunter A, Rogers S, Hanley J, Anderson D. Peripheral blood stem cells as an alternative to marrow for allogeneic transplantation. Lancet 1993; 341(8858):1482.

51. Dreger P, Suttorp M, Haferlach T, Loffler H, Schmitz N, Schroyens W. Allogeneic granulocyte colony-stimulating factor-mobilized peripheral blood progenitor cells for treatment of engraftment failure after bone marrow transplantation. Blood 1993; 81(5):1404–1407.

52. Verfaillie CM, Bhatia R, Steinbuch M, DeFor T, Hirsch B, Miller JS, Weisdorf D, McGlave PB. Comparative analysis of autografting in chronic myelogenous leukemia: effects of priming regimen and marrow or blood origin of stem cells. Blood 1998; 92:1820–1831.

53. Gorin NC, Labopin M, Pichard P, Sierra J, Trassoni F. For the acute leukemia working party of the European group for Blood and Marrow Transplantation (EBMT). Higher dose of peripheral blood stem cells is critical to improve the outcome of patients over 60 years of age autografted for acute myelocytic leukemia (AML) (abstr). Proc 10th Int Symp Peripheral Blood Stem Cell Transplant, Sept 8, 1999.

54. Elmaagacli AH, Beelen DW, Opalka B, Seeber S, Schaefer UW. The risk of residual molecular and cytogenetic disease in patients with Philadelphia-chromosome positive first chronic phase chronic myelogenous leukemia is reduced after transplantation of allogeneic peripheral blood stem cells compared with bone marrow. Blood 1999; 94:348–389.

27

Autologous Peripheral Blood Stem Cell Collection and Engraftment

STEFAN HOHAUS and **MARIA TERESA VOSO**

Catholic University "S. Cuore," Rome, Italy

SIMONA MARTIN and **RAINER HAAS**

Heinrich Heine University, Düsseldorf, Germany

I. INTRODUCTION

Efficient mobilization and collection of hematopoietic stem cells (HSCs) from peripheral blood are a prerequisite for a successful peripheral blood stem cell (PBSC) transplantation. Provided that a sufficient number of autologous or allogeneic PBSCs are transplanted, the major advantage of PBSCs compared with bone marrow (BM) is the shortened period of severe cytopenia following high-dose therapy (1,2). Bone marrow has therefore been gradually replaced by mobilized peripheral blood (PB) as a source of HSCs. Circulation of progenitor cells capable of forming granulocytic and monocytic colonies was first observed in 1970 (3). The concentration of these colony-forming units (CFUs) was only 1–10% of that observed in BM. In 1976, Richman et al. found that, in patients with solid tumors, the concentration of circulating CFUs increased up to 20-fold over baseline levels during leukocyte recovery after cytotoxic chemotherapy (4). The introduction of hematopoietic growth factors (HGFs) in the late 1980s resulted in a further significant increase of PBSCs when administered either following cytotoxic chemotherapy or during steady-state hematopoiesis.

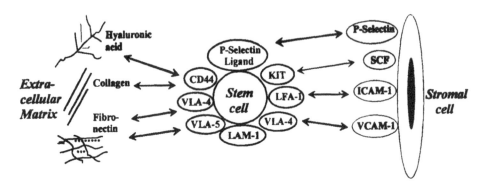

Figure 1 Adhesion molecules on CD34$^+$ cells and their corresponding ligands on stromal cells and extracellular matrix of the bone marrow. ICAM-1, intercellular adhesion molecule-1; LAM-1, leukocyte adhesion molecule-1; LFA-1, leukocyte function antigen-1; VCAM-1, vascular cell adhesion molecule-1; VLA-4, very late antigen-4; SCF, stem cell factor.

II. MECHANISM OF MOBILIZATION AND BIOLOGY OF MOBILIZED PBSCs

The mechanisms of PBSC mobilization still remain elusive. Circulation of HSCs during steady-state conditions suggests that hematopoiesis may be associated with a continuous redistribution of HSCs. Thus, mobilization and egression from BM as well as homing and engraftment after transplantation could be viewed as a migratory circle of HSCs. Egression and redistribution of HSCs prevail when cytotoxic chemotherapy results in empty niches in the marrow while the proliferation of early HSC is stimulated. The stimulatory effect may be partially mediated by growth factors, as high levels of cytokines (e.g., granulocyte-colony stimulating factor, G-CSF) can be measured during chemotherapy-induced cytopenia (5–7). Proliferation-associated release of HSCs from BM therefore appears as a prominent mechanism involved in cytokine-induced PBSC mobilization. The delay of approximately 4 days between administration of hematopoietic growth factors and the appearance of increased numbers of CD34$^+$ cells in the PB argues for a de novo production of PBSC trafficking through the peripheral blood. Cytokines may also contribute to a decrease of binding forces between HSCs and components of the stromal microenvironment which facilitates migration of HSCs into the PB (8). Adhesion molecules are differentially expressed on CD34$^+$ cells residing in the BM (Fig. 1) when compared with circulating HSCs, with higher levels of L-selectin on PB CD34$^+$ cells, and greater levels of α_4-integrin (VLA-4) on BM CD34$^+$ cells (Fig. 2). A decrease in adhesion is the predominant mechanism in the interleukin-8 (IL-8)–related peripheralization of HSCs as a 10- to 100-fold increase of HSCs is observed within 30 min following intravenous injection (9). The importance of changes in adhesive interactions for PBSC mobilization was demonstrated by Papayannopoulou and Nakamoto, who infused anti–VLA-4 antibodies into nonhuman primates (10). VLA-4 is greatly expressed on CD34$^+$ cells and presumably involved in the anchoring of HSCs to endothelial cells of the BM via binding to vascular cell adhesion molecule-1 (VCAM-1). Infusion of anti–VLA-4 antibodies resulted in a rapid up to 200-fold increase of PBSCs over baseline levels.

Cytokine-mobilized PBSCs are different from their counterparts in BM. Circulating HSCs are almost exclusively in the G0/G1 phase of the cell cycle, whereas 30–40% of

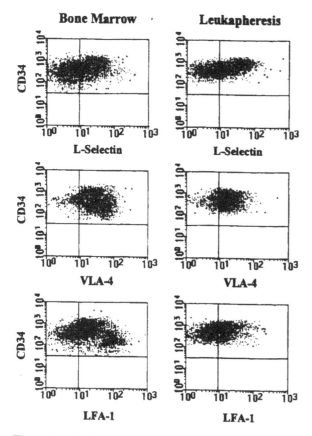

Figure 2 Intraindividual comparison of L-selectin, VLA-4, and LFA-1 coexpression on CD34$^+$ cells from bone marrow (BM) and leukapheresis products (LP) following granulocyte colony-stimulating factor (G-CSF)–supported cytotoxic chemotherapy. Dot plot analysis of BM and LP samples from 10 patients were overlayed. Although blood-derived CD34$^+$ cells express high levels of L-selectin, CD34$^+$ cells from BM contain a particular proportion of cells characterized by strong coexpression of VLA-4 and LFA-1. VLA-4, very late antigen-4; LFA-1, leukocyte function antigen-1.

BM-derived hematopoietic progenitor cells are in S/G2/M-phase (11–13). The expression of differentiation-associated molecules on PBSCs also indicates that a greater proportion of circulating CD34$^+$ cells are early hematopoietic progenitor cells compared with CD34$^+$ cells from bone marrow. In this line, the stem cell–associated antigen Thy1 is expressed on a greater proportion of CD34$^+$ cells from G-CSF–mobilized PB (Fig. 3), whereas expression of c-*kit* and CD45RA, which are found on more mature myeloid and B-cell progenitors, is smaller in comparison with BM-derived CD34$^+$ cells (12,14,15). Culture assays for the determination of long-term culture-initiating cells (LTCICs) and pre–CFU granulocyte-macrophage (GM) corroborated these immunophenotypical findings (16). Some characteristics of PBSCs may depend on the mobilization modality (17). A small proportion of CD34$^+$/CD19$^+$ B-lineage progenitors is typically found postchemotherapy (18–21), while during steady-state hematopoiesis, there is no difference in the proportion of the CD34$^+$/CD19$^+$ cells between BM and PB (20,22).

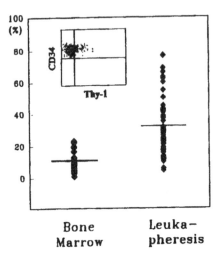

Figure 3 Intraindividual comparison between the proportion of CD34+/Thy1+ cells in bone marrow (BM) samples from 20 cancer patients before the start of cytotoxic chemotherapy and in leukapheresis products (LP) collected during granulocyte colony-stimulating factor (G-CSF)–enhanced marrow recovery. The subset analysis is based on 48 LPs. A threefold greater mean proportion of CD34+/Thy1+ cells was observed in LP products compared with BM: 32.37 ± 2.48% versus 11.05 ± 1.57%. The insert shows a representative two-fluorescence dot plot analysis of an LP product.

III. COLLECTION OF PBSCs USING CYTOKINES

PBSCs for autotransplantations first performed in 1985 were harvested during steady-state hematopoiesis without the use of a particular mobilization regimen (23–26). Up to 10 leukaphereses were required to collect 7–8 × 10⁸ mononuclear cells (MNCs)/kg, containing 8–20 × 10⁴ CFU-GM/kg. Hematological recovery after PBSC-supported high-dose therapy was similar to that observed after bone marrow transplantation (BMT). The time of hematopoietic reconstitution after transplantation and the number of leukaphereses required to harvest a sufficient amount of hematopoietic progenitor cells was significantly reduced when PBSCs were collected postchemotherapy during marrow recovery (27). High-dose cyclophosphamide (4–7 g/m²) induced a 14-fold increase of PB CFU-GM, whereas peak levels were observed 2 days after the white blood cell (WBC) count exceeded 1 × 10⁹/L (27). PBSC collection could be further improved by the introduction of HGF (28,29). When administered alone or following cytotoxic chemotherapy, HGF resulted in a significant increase of circulating progenitor cells. Recombinant human G-CSF and granulocyte-macrophage colony-stimulating factor (GM-CSF) were the first cytokines evaluated for PBSC mobilization, and they are currently the only agents which are approved for autologous PBSC mobilization. The publication of the first studies demonstrating the PBSC-mobilizing effects of these agents in cancer patients dates back to 1988. Socinski et al. (30) found an approximately 18-fold increase of circulating CFU-GM over baseline levels when GM-CSF was administered during steady-state hematopoiesis. GM-CSF administration postchemotherapy resulted in an 62-fold expansion of circulating progenitor cells compared with an 8-fold increase after cytotoxic chemotherapy alone. Duehrsen et al. (31) administered G-CSF during steady-state hematopoiesis (3–5 µg/kg/day) for 4 days and found an up to 100-fold dose-dependent increase of CFU-GM.

The potential of cytokine-mobilized PBSCs to reconstitute hematopoiesis after high-dose therapy was demonstrated first by the addition of PBSCs to BM and later by using PBSCs alone. In 1989, Gianni et al. showed that the addition to bone marrow of PBSCs harvested following GM-CSF–supported cytotoxic chemotherapy resulted in a rapid hematological reconstitution after myeloablative high-dose therapy, with a mean time to achieve 0.5×10^9/L neutrophils and 50×10^9/L platelets of 9.9 and 10.7 days, respectively (29). Our group reported in 1990 on autografting with PBSCs mobilized by GM-CSF administered during steady-state hematopoiesis (32). Complete engraftment following myeloablative chemotherapy was found in five of six patients without additional use of BM or cytokine support posttransplantation. One patient developed relapse of disease with BM involvement interfering with hematological recovery. A first report on the transplantation of G-CSF–mobilized PBSCs was published in 1992. Sheridan et al. harvested PBSCs between days 5 and 7 during steady-state administration of G-CSF (12 µg/kg/day) and reinfused PBSCs with BM after high-dose therapy (33). The time to platelet recovery was significantly shortened in patients who received G-CSF–mobilized PBSCs when compared with a historical group of patients who underwent BMT (15 vs 39 days to achieve platelet counts of greater than 50×10^9/L). In 10 patients with lymphoma, we used cytotoxic chemotherapy and G-CSF (5 µg/kg/day) for PBSC mobilization (18). Following myeloablative therapy, a rapid platelet recovery was observed without additional BM or cytokine support, given that a threshold number of 5×10^6 CD34$^+$ cells/kg bodyweight were autografted (18). Extending this observation to a larger series of 61 patients with lymphoma, the threshold could be refined to 2.5×10^6 CD34$^+$ cells/kg body weight (34). Recently, the results of the first prospective randomized multicenter trial of G-CSF–mobilized autologous PBSC versus autologous marrow transplantation in patients with advanced lymphoma were published (2). The time needed for neutrophil and platelet recovery was significantly shorter in the patients who received PBSCs in comparison with those autografted with BM (11 vs 14 and 16 vs 23 days, respectively). As a consequence, less red blood cells (RBCs) and platelet transfusions were needed in the PBSC group.

We observed greater concentrations of PBSCs following G-CSF–supported chemotherapy than during steady-state administration of G-CSF which was given at the same dose of 5 µg/kg/day (Fig. 4) (20). In an intraindividual comparison, we also observed a seven-fold greater yield of CD34$^+$ cells per leukapheresis (LP). Dose-finding studies were initiated to improve steady-state mobilization (35–37). Several investigators found improved mobilization of PBSCs by increasing the G-CSF dose to 10 µg/kg or even up to 30 µg/kg/day (35–37). Increasing the dose of G-CSF during steady-state might compensate a reduction in the bioavailability of G-CSF which results from G-CSF binding to the largely expanded neutrophils. Similar data for the G-CSF dose during postchemotherapy PBSC collection have not been reported.

Comparing G-CSF with GM-CSF, no difference was found between both cytokines in the ability to mobilize PBSCs. GM-CSF and G-CSF administered at a dose of 5 µg/kg/day during steady-state hematopoiesis increased the number of harvested CFU-GM 33.7- and 35.6-fold over baseline values, respectively (38). In contrast, Lane et al. found greater CD34$^+$ cell counts in normal volunteers on the fifth day of G-CSF treatment when compared with GM-CSF given at the same dose of 10 µg/kg/day (39). Owing to differences in the tolerability of the two cytokines, most centers favor the use of G-CSF over GM-CSF. Adverse reactions to both drugs include bone pain, myalgias, headache, and fatigue (40). At higher doses, fevers, edema, and pericardial and pleural effusions were observed with GM-CSF. Our current standard for PBSC mobilization is to administer a

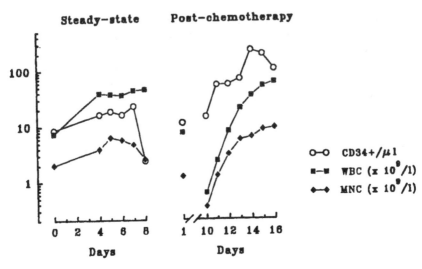

Figure 4 Mean values of CD34⁺ cells, white blood cells (WBCs), and mononuclear cells (MNCs) from seven patients with breast cancer. (a) Granulocyte colony-stimulating factor (G-CSF) during steady-state hematopoiesis was started on day 1. "Day 0" refers to pretreatment values. (b) Treatment with G-CSF after chemotherapy (ifosfamide/epirubicin started on day 1) began on day 3. (O) CD34⁺ cells/μL; (■) WBC (× 10⁹/L); (♦) MNC (× 10⁹/L).

daily dose of 300 μg G-CSF starting 24 h after cytotoxic chemotherapy until the last apheresis has been completed.

In addition to G-CSF and GM-CSF, other cytokines such as IL-3, Pixy 321, and stem cell factor (SCF) have been evaluated in phase I-II studies for their ability to mobilize PBSCs (41–48). The administration of other cytokines with in vitro stimulatory effects on primitive HSCs, such as IL-1 and IL-6, were associated with considerable toxicity, preventing further evaluation. IL-3 and SCF on their own have only modest PBSC-mobilizing effects and were therefore assessed in combination with G-CSF or GM-CSF. We administered IL-3 and GM-CSF sequentially following salvage chemotherapy with high-dose cytosine-arabinoside and mitoxantrone (HAM) in patients with high-grade non-Hodgkin's lymphoma (NHL) (43). IL-3 was given at a dose of 5 μg/kg/day subcutaneously for 6 days followed by GM-CSF at the same dose. Compared to a historical control group who received G-CSF after HAM, no difference was observed in the number of CD34⁺ cells mobilized. The transplantation of IL-3/GM-CSF-mobilized and G-CSF–mobilized PBSCs resulted in a similar median time to recover a neutrophil count of 0.5 × 10⁹/L (14 days vs 14 days) and a platelet count of 20 × 10⁹/L (14 days vs 12 days). Administration of IL-3 (3–5 μg/kg/day) for 4 days before G-CSF (5 μg/kg/day for 7 days) in healthy volunteers similarly did not result in higher peak levels of circulating CD34⁺ cells compared to a treatment with G-CSF alone.

Stem cell factor has recently been shown to induce increased numbers of PBSCs; however, for an efficient mobilization, G-CSF needs to be given at the same time (44,48). Increases in the dose of SCF from 5 to 15 μg/kg/day appeared to be more effective in patients with ovarian cancer when combined with G-CSF (5 μg/kg/day) following 3 g/m² cyclophosphamide (48). Some investigators found a greater clonogenic capacity of PBSCs when IL-3 or SCF was combined with G-CSF, but it is not clear whether this translates into a significant clinical benefit (42,48).

IV. CHEMOTHERAPY REGIMENS FOR MOBILIZATION

Increased numbers of PBSCs were first observed after conventional cytotoxic chemotherapy. Cyclophosphamide as a single agent has been often used as a standard regimen for chemotherapy-induced mobilization. When the dose of cyclophosphamide was increased from 4 to 7 g/m^2 in patients with multiple myeloma (MM), significantly greater levels of circulating $CD34^+$ cells (48 vs 19/μL) were obtained (49). Combinations of cyclophosphamide with etoposide, etoposide and cisplatin or paclitaxel are more cytotoxic and appear to be more effective for PBSC mobilization than cyclophosphamide alone (50). In a study by Demirer et al., the addition of paclitaxel (170 mg/m^2) to cyclophosphamide (4 g/m^2) followed by G-CSF (10 μg/kg/day) resulted in an approximately twofold greater number of $CD34^+$ cells in patients with advanced breast or ovarian cancer when compared with cyclophosphamide (4 g/m^2) alone followed by G-CSF (16 μg/kg/day) (50). Agents that are considered to be stem cell toxic such as carmustine (BCNU), melphalan, and thiotepa are generally thought to be inappropriate for PBSC mobilization. Still, we and other groups have successfully used a combination of dexamethasone, BCNU, etoposide, cytosine-arabinoside, and melphalan (dexaBEAM) for PBSC mobilization in relapsed patients with Hodgkin's disease (51,52).

We therefore usually mobilize PBSCs with a cytotoxic chemotherapy containing drugs which are effective for the tumor in question. This includes dexaBEAM for patients with Hodgkin's disease, high-dose cytosine-arabinoside with mitoxantrone (HAM) for patients with NHL, ifosfamide, epirubicin with or without paclitaxel for patients with breast cancer, and cisplatin, etoposide, and ifosfamide for patients with ovarian and germ cell tumors.

V. FACTORS INFLUENCING MOBILIZATION EFFICIENCY

In patients with solid tumors, an important factor influencing the yield of PBSCs is the amount of previous cytotoxic treatment as well as radiotherapy (53–57). In a group of 61 patients with malignant lymphoma, each cycle of chemotherapy resulted in a decrease of 0.2×10^6 $CD34^+$ cells/kg per LP in nonradiated patients, whereas large-field radiotherapy reduced the collection efficiency by 1.8×10^6/kg $CD34^+$ cells on average (34). In the same line, Tricot et al. reported a correlation between the duration of previous chemotherapy, especially of alkylating agents and the mobilization efficiency in patients with MM (56). In their study, 91% of patients treated for less than 6 months achieved harvests containing more than 5×10^6 $CD34^+$ cells/kg in comparison with 28% of patients who were treated for more than 24 months. In patients with breast cancer, the yield of $CD34^+$ cells harvested after the first cycle of G-CSF–supported chemotherapy with ifosfamide and epirubicin was two-fold smaller compared with the amount collected after the second cycle (57). In other studies, younger age, absence of marrow infiltration, lack of prior radiation, and a low number of previous chemotherapy cycles were factors significantly associated with greater numbers of $CD34^+$ cells obtained following mobilization (58,59).

VI. TIMING OF PBSC HARVESTING

Collection of PBSCs during the peak increase of mobilized PBSCs can help to improve the collection efficiency. During steady-state administration of G-CSF, the $CD34^+$ cell count in PB rises 72 h after the first dose of G-CSF, and peak values are usually observed between the fourth and the sixth day of G-CSF administration. The level of circulating

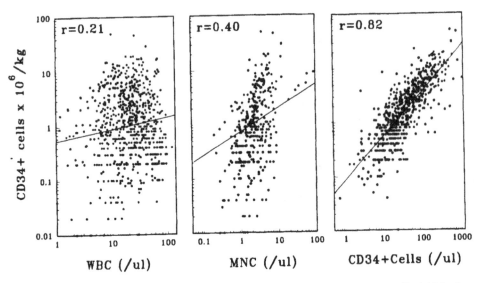

Figure 5 CD34⁺ cells in the peripheral blood. For estimating the progenitor cell yield in the corresponding leukapheresis product, the number of CD34⁺ cells/µL peripheral blood was found to be more reliable than the proportion of CD34⁺ cells to the leukocytes or mononuclear cells (MNCs). The assessment was based on 733 peripheral blood samples and corresponding leukapheresis products from 191 cancer patients. WBCs, white blood cells.

CD34⁺ cells decreases thereafter even though G-CSF administration is continued (60). When administered postchemotherapy, CD34⁺ cells and CFU-GM in PB rise in response to G-CSF and GM-CSF during marrow recovery in parallel to the increase of the WBC counts. PBSC collection may be started as early as the WBC count exceeds 1×10^9 cells/L (27,29). When the cytokine was given only for a certain number of days after chemotherapy, progenitor cell levels increased simultaneously with the increase in WBCs, but peak levels lasted for 1 or 2 days only (28,29). When the administration of G-CSF or GM-CSF was continued until the end of PBSC harvesting, the maximum mobilization effect following cyclophosphamide, epirubicin, 5-fluorouracil, and GM-CSF was consistently observed 2 days after the WBC count had reached more than 2×10^9/L and remained elevated for 4–5 days (61). According to the data of Dreger et al., the optimum mobilization of circulating progenitors after G-CSF–supported dexaBEAM was observed 1–2 days after the WBC count first exceeded 10×10^9/L (59). Pettengell et al. collected a sufficient number of PBSCs by a single LP when they delayed harvesting of PBSCs until a WBC count of $>3 \times 10^9$/L was reached (62). In our experience, patients with high levels of circulating CD34⁺ cells reached their peak level earlier than patients with smaller numbers of circulating CD34⁺ cells. Individual differences in peak levels of CD34⁺ cells and times to reach the peak level make it difficult to predict the optimal time point for PBSC collection. The assessment of PB or BM CD34⁺ cells before mobilization might help to estimate the mobilization ability of a patient (63). Monitoring of CD34⁺ cell counts of PB permits a decision when to start the PBSC collection (18,34,64). In several studies, a good correlation between the number of circulating CD34⁺ cells and the yield of CD34⁺ cells obtained in the leukapheresis product was found (Fig. 5) (34,64–66). In patients with malignant lymphoma, a CD34⁺ cell count of greater than 50/µL in

PB was highly predictable for a yield of more than 2.5×10^6 CD34$^+$/kg in a single regular 10 L LP (34).

We start monitoring CD34$^+$ cells in the PB when the WBC count exceeds 1×10^9/L. If a population of CD34$^+$ cells greater than 20/µL is observed and the WBC count exceeds 5×10^9/L, the first LP will be performed. In some patients, CD34$^+$ cells may not reach 20/µL. In these patients, we start LP after 3 days of CD34$^+$ cell monitoring if the CD34 cell count exceeds 5/µL.

VII. TECHNIQUES OF APHERESIS FOR THE COLLECTION OF PBSCs

Continuous flow centrifugation is mostly used for the concentration of MNCs from PB to harvest PBSCs. Such devices include the CS 3000 (Baxter Healthcare, Deerfield, IL) and the Spectra apheresis system (COBE Laboratories, Lakewood, CO). These devices have a shortened processing time compared with discontinuous-flow separators. Comparisons between different continuous-flow centrifugation devices did not show any significant difference in the collection efficiency for CD34$^+$ cells (67).

For regular LP, 10 L of blood is generally processed at a flow rate between 50 and 70 mL/min. We found that processing of 20 L can significantly increase the yield of CD34$^+$ cells (68). The comparison of 154 large-volume LPs obtained in 88 patients with 838 regular LPs collected from 270 patients showed that the number of CD34$^+$ cells harvested was 2.2-fold greater in the products following large-volume LP (Fig. 6). The greater yield probably results from an increase of CD34$^+$ cells in PB after the processing of 12–16 L of blood. The proportion of leukaphereses sufficient to support one high-dose cycle with more than 2.5×10^6/kg CD34$^+$ cells could be increased to 74% compared with a

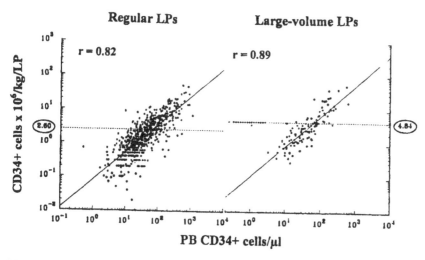

Figure 6   Relationship between the level of circulating CD34$^+$ cells in the peripheral blood (PB) at the day of leukapheresis (LP) and the number of cells/kg body weight contained in the respective product. The close relationship observed was independent whether large-volume or regular LP were performed. Using large-volume LP, the mean number of CD34$^+$ cells harvested/kg body weight was almost twofold greater. The numbers in the circles indicate the mean number of CD34$^+$ cells collected.

proportion of 52% when regular LP were performed (68). Therefore, we now prefer large-volume LP, as 20 L can be processed within 2–3 h given a flow rate of 120–150 mL/min. For this purpose, large-bore double-lumen catheters are needed. The incidence of complications is low when the central catheter is placed just before harvesting and removed after the collection period (69). In a series of 183 patients, the incidence of local infections was 3% and of catheter-related septicemia and thrombosis of the jugular vein 2 and 5%, respectively.

VIII. TUMOR CELLS CONTAMINATING PBSC GRAFTS

Collection of PBSCs from PB in patients with malignant diseases is associated with the potential risk of harvesting tumor cells. It has been shown by gene-marking studies in patients with acute myeloid leukemia and neuroblastoma that reinfused tumor cells can contribute to a relapse of the disease after high-dose therapy (70). Tumor cells may circulate in PB regardless of BM involvement. Contamination of PBSC products by tumor cells has been shown in patients with breast cancer, lymphoma, MM, and leukemia (19,57,71–78). Molecular markers and specific genomic alterations provide the basis for the detection of tumor cells (Table 1).

The PCR can be used as a sensitive method to find translocation-bearing cells as in patients with t(14;18) follicular lymphoma or the t(9;22) in patients with chronic myeloid leukemia. The evaluation of 29 patients with a t(14;18) follicular lymphoma showed that the majority of patients (22 of 29) had PCR-positive PBSC autografts which were harvested during G-CSF–supported recovery postchemotherapy (19). This observation was confirmed in a larger group of 47 patients, as shown in Figure 7.

The design of clone-specific probes for the rearranged immunoglobulin heavy chain and T-cell receptor gene permits a sensitive assessment of tumor cells in patients with MM and other lymphoid malignancies (77,79,80). Several investigators demonstrated that 50–60% of patients with MM have circulating malignant cells at the time of PBSC harvest (77,78).

Most of the solid tumors lack a simple genomic alteration which could be used for monitoring residual tumor cells. Tissue-specific gene expression can help to detect the presence of epithelial cells in PB and LP products. The methods include immunocytological staining and reverse transcription (RT)–PCR for the assessment of protein and messenger RNA expression, respectively (81–84). Still, most investigations use immunocytochemical staining for epithelial antigens such as cytokeratins, which represents the gold standard (85). Brugger et al. found circulating tumor cells during steady-state hematopoiesis in 29% of patients with stage IV breast cancer and in 20% of patients with small cell lung cancer (74). The incidence of circulating tumor cells was greater following G-CSF–supported cytotoxic chemotherapy. Other studies suggest a low risk of mobilizing malignant cells. PBSC collections after cytokine-supported chemotherapy contained fewer tumor cells than BM. The rate of LP products contaminated with tumor cells in patients with breast cancer is between 5 and 20% according to these studies (57,73,76) (Fig. 8).

The biological features of residual tumor cells in PBSC grafts has also been assessed. Ross et al. demonstrated clonogenic tumor cell growth for most specimens from BM and PBSC collections that were immunocytochemically positive (73). Using a semisolid culture assay, Sharp et al. also found malignant clonogenic cells in the PB of patients with Hodgkin's disease and NHL (86). There are ways to reduce the tumor cell contamination of autografts. The time point of PBSC collection could be crucial and ex vivo methods

Table 1 Minimal Residual Disease: Molecular Targets

Tumor	Gene	Abnormality	Frequency (%)	Method
Lymphoma				
B cell	IgH	Rearrangement		PCR
follicular center	BCL2	t(14;18)(q32; q21)	70–90	PCR
mantle cell	BCL1	t(11;14)(q14; q32)	70	PCR
diffuse large cell	BCL6	t(3; ?)(q27; ?)	40	PCR
Burkitt	c-myc	t(8;14)(q24; q32)	100	PCR
T cell	TCR	rearrangement		PCR
anaplastic large cell (CD30⁺)	NPM/ALK	t(2;5)(p23; q35)	80	PCR
Myeloma	IgH	Rearrangement	100	PCR
	CD56/CD38	Aberrant immunophenotype		FACS
Acute Leukemia				
B lymphoid	IgH	Rearrangement		PCR
	bcr/abl	t(19;22)(q34; q11)	90	RT-PCR
	MLL/AF4	t(4;11)(q21; 23)	25–40	RT-PCR
	EZA/PX1	t(1;19)	5	RT-PCR
myeloid M2	AML1/ETO	t(8;21)(q22; q22)	2–3	RT-PCR
M3	PML/RARα	t(15;17)(q22; q11–22)	5–10	RT-PCR
M4E0	CBFβ/MyH11	inv16(p13; q22)	5–10	RT-PCR
M5	MLL/AF9	t(9;11)(p21–22; q23)	5–10	RT-PCR
	CD34/CD56	Aberrant immunophenotype	1–5	FACS
	CD34/CDw65/Telt	Aberrant immunophenotype	20	FACS
Solid tumors of epithelial	CK19	Expression in PB	15	PCR, immunocytochemistry
origin (e.g., breast cancer)	CEA	Expression in PB		PCR
	MUC1	Expression in PB		PCR, immunocytochemistry
	EGF-R	Expression in PB		PCR

PCR, polymerase chain reaction; PB, peripheral blood; RT-PCR, reverse transcriptase-PCR; FACS, fluorescence-activated cell sorter.

PCR technique

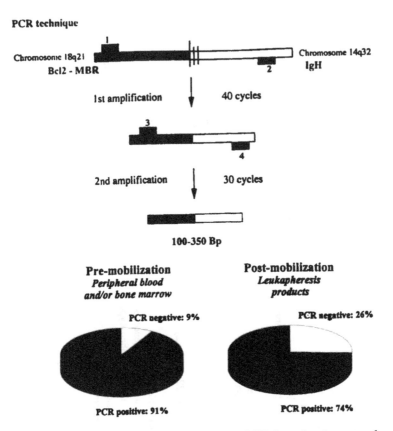

Figure 7 A nested polymerase chain reaction (PCR) is used to detect translocation-bearing cells in patients with t(14;18) follicular lymphoma. Proportions of PCR-positive and PCR-negative samples before the begin of mobilization therapy and PCR status of the leukapheresis products harvested following granulocyte colony-stimulating factor–supported cytotoxic chemotherapy with high-dose cytosine-arabinoside and mitoxantrone in 47 patients bearing the t(14;18) translocation.

for tumor cell depletion such as purging and positive selection of CD34+ cells may be envisaged. We have shown in an intraindividual comparison in patients with high-risk breast cancer that collection of PBSCs resulted in a lower incidence of tumor cell–positive LP products when PBSCs were harvested after the second and not after the first cycle of induction therapy (57). On the other hand, each cycle of chemotherapy is associated with a reduction in the collection efficiency of CD34+ cells. In our patients with breast cancer, the number of CD34+ cells collected per leukapheresis after the second cycle of chemotherapy was half of that obtained after the first cycle (57). The proportion of the CD34+ cells to tumor cells in PB may also vary during the mobilization period.

During GM-CSF–supported recovery following high-dose cyclophosphamide mobilization, Gazitt et al. found maximum levels of CD34+ cells during the first 2 days of LP, whereas the greatest proportion of myeloma cells was observed on days 4 and 6 (77). In contrast, Lemoli et al. observed concomitant mobilization of PBSCs and myeloma cells after high-dose cyclophosphamide with G-CSF support (78). Ex vivo methods to reduce

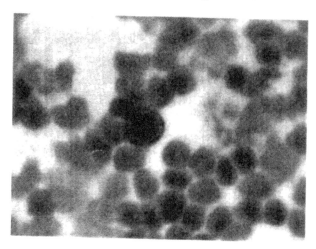

Figure 8 Immunocytochemical staining of leukapheresis–derived mononuclear cells from a patient with breast cancer. A "red" tumor cell is detectable by the alkaline phosphatase antialkaline phosphatase (APAAP) technique, using a cocktail of anticytokeratine 8, 18, 19, antimucine 1, and antihuman epithelial antigen (HEA) antibodies.

contamination of leukapheresis products with tumor cells include purging and selection techniques. CD34$^+$ cell selection results in a 2- to 4-log reduction of breast cancer or myeloma cells (87–92). CD34$^+$ selection is only possible when the tumor cells do not express this antigen. We studied CD34$^+$ cell fractions and their B-lymphoid CD19$^+$ subsets in 14 patients with follicular lymphoma and did not detect t(14;18) translocation-bearing cells in the CD34$^+$ cells of 13 of 14 patients (93). Using an immunomagnetic selection device [Baxter Isolex 300SA (Baxter Immunotherapy, Irvine, CA)] we were able to achieve a 95% purity (median, range 82–92%) of the CD34-selected cells in patients with breast cancer. Later on we also used this technique for patients with low-grade NHL and MM (91) (Fig. 9). The CD34$^+$ cell selection of a single large-volume LP product resulted in numbers sufficient to support at least two cycles of high-dose chemotherapy with an amount of 2.5 × 10^6 CD34$^+$ cells/kg for each course in 62% of the patients.

The significance of infused residual malignant cells for the clinical outcome remains unclear. We studied the bone marrow of 52 patients with breast cancer after high-dose chemotherapy and found isolated tumor cells in 34 patients (65%)(94). Only 12 of 133 autografts contained tumor cells. On the other hand, 71 of bone marrow specimens obtained before high-dose therapy harbored tumor cells. These data argue for a persistence of tumor cells rather than a reinfusion. Contamination of PBSCs by tumor cells might therefore simply reflect the tumor burden in vivo as a prognostic parameter (94).

IX. HEMATOPOIETIC RECONSTITUTION AFTER PBSCT

The time needed for hematopoietic reconstitution primarily depends on the number of stem and progenitor cells reinfused. The relation between the number of CD34$^+$ cells and the speed of marrow recovery appears to be a threshold phenomenon. We found that 2.5 × 10^6 CD34$^+$ cells/kg are sufficient to assure a rapid reconstitution of both granulocytes and platelets (18,34) (Fig. 10). Other groups found threshold numbers between 2 and 5 ×

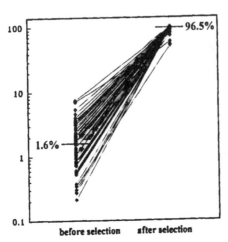

Figure 9 Using the Baxter Isolex 300SA Magnetic Cell Separator System, CD34⁺ cells from leukapheresis products (LP) of 70 patients with low-grade non-Hodgkin's lymphoma, multiple myeloma, and breast cancer were enriched to high purity. The median proportion of CD34⁺ cells in the unseparated LP products was 1.6% (range 0.21–7.41%), whereas a median purity of 96.5% (range 53.24–100%) was achieved in the selected fraction.

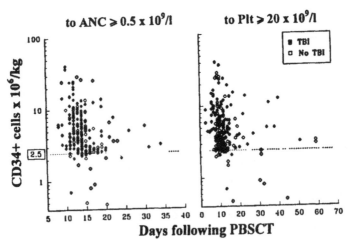

Figure 10 Hematological reconstitution after peripheral blood progenitor cell–supported high-dose therapy in 312 patients with hematological malignancies and solid tumors. The majority of autografts contained more than 2.5 × 10⁶ CD34⁺ cells/kg. There was no significant difference in the speed of hematological reconstitution between patients receiving total body irradiation (TBI, filled diamonds) or not (hollow diamonds). ANC, absolute neutrophil count; PLT, platelets; PBSCT, peripheral blood stem cell transplantation.

10^6 CD34$^+$ cells/kg (54,56,95,96). Differences in this number may be explained by different methods for CD34$^+$ cell assessment and/or different patient selection. Characterization of particular CD34$^+$ cell subsets might help to predict the speed of hematological reconstitution. Dercksen et al. found that the time to neutrophil and platelet recovery correlated better with the number of transplanted CD34$^+$/CD33$^+$ and CD34$^+$/CD41$^+$ cells, respectively, than with the total number of CD34$^+$ cells (21). The investigators also observed that the amount of CD34$^+$ cells coexpressing the adhesion molecule L-selectin correlated better with hematological recovery than with the total CD34$^+$ cell population (97).

Other factors which might influence the kinetics of reconstitution include the underlying diagnosis, purging of the autograft with chemotherapeutic agents, and possibly the type of conditioning regimen. At least one study suggested a higher risk for delayed engraftment after conditioning including busulfan or total body irradiation (TBI) (98). Considering the toxic effect of this regimen on stromal cells, a deficit in the marrow microenvironment to support the proliferation and differentiation of hematopoietic stem and progenitor cells might contribute to a delayed engraftment.

Animal studies show that rapidly dividing progenitor and stem cell clones contribute to hematopoiesis early after transplantation, whereas a smaller number of long-term repopulating clones emerges later for maintenance of long-term hematopoiesis (99,100). It is a matter of speculation whether mobilized cells are capable of sustaining long-term reconstitution or whether long-term hematopoiesis is maintained by small numbers of stem cells surviving TBI-containing regimens. High-dose therapy supported by PBSC transplantation (PBSCT) or BMT is associated with a long-term impairment of the hematopoietic system (98,101,102). More than 6 months after PBSCT, the proportion of CD34$^+$ cells is still significantly smaller than before mobilization. This reduction is most pronounced for the primitive BM progenitor subsets such as the CD34$^+$/DR$^-$ and CD34$^+$/Thyl$^+$ cells. This reduction is not associated with a functional deficit, as PB counts posttransplantation were normal in the majority of patients. The long-term impairment was not related to the amount of CD34$^+$ cells infused (102).

In conclusion, the efficient collection of PBSC and rapid hematological reconstitution after PBSC-supported high-dose therapy has widened the therapeutic options for many patients with malignant diseases. The therapeutic benefits of PBSCT still has to be proven in many conditions.

REFERENCES

1. To LB, Roberts MM, Haylock DN, Dyson PG, Branford AL, Thorp D, Ho JQ, Dart GW, Horvath N, Davy ML, Juttner CA. Comparison of haematological recovery times and supportive care requirements of autologous recovery phase peripheral blood stem cell transplants, autologous bone marrow transplants and allogeneic bone marrow transplants. Bone Marrow Transplant 1992; 9:277–284.

2. Schmitz N, Linch DC, Dreger P, Goldstone AH, Boogaerts MA, Ferrant A, Demuynck HM, Link H, Zander A, Barge A. Randomised trial of filgrastim-mobilised peripheral blood progenitor cell transplantation versus autologous bone-marrow transplantation in lymphoma patients. Lancet 1996; 347:353–357.

3. McCredie KB, Hersh EM, Freireich EJ. Cells capable of colony formation in the peripheral blood of man. Science 1970; 171:293–294.

4. Richman CM, Weine RS, Yankee RA. Increase in circulating stem cells following chemotherapy in man. Blood 1976; 47:1031–1039.

5. Haas R, Gericke G, Witt B, Cayeux S, Hunstein W. Increased serum levels of granulocyte

colony-stimulating factor after autologous bone marrow or blood stem cell transplantation. Exp Hematol 1993; 21:109–113.

6. Cairo MS, Suen Y, Sender L, Gillan ER, Ho W, Plunkett JM, van de Ven C. Circulating granulocyte colony-stimulating factor (G-CSF) levels after allogeneic and autologous bone marrow transplantation: endogenous G-CSF production correlates with myeloid engraftment. Blood 1992; 79:1869–1873.

7. Shimazaki C, Uchiyama H, Fujita N, Araki S, Sudo Y, Yamagata N, Ashihara E, Goto H, Inaba T, Haruyama H. Serum levels of endogenous and exogenous granulocyte colony-stimulating factor after autologous blood stem cell transplantation. Exp Hematol 1995; 23:1497–1502.

8. van der Loo JC, Ploemacher RE. Marrow- and spleen-seeding efficiencies of all murine hematopoietic stem cell subsets are decreased by preincubation with hematopoietic growth factors. Blood 1995; 85:2598–2606.

9. Laterveer L, Lindley IJ, Heemskerk DP, Camps JA, Pauwels EK, Willemze R, Fibbe WE. Rapid mobilization of hematopoietic progenitor cells in rhesus monkeys by single intravenous injection of interleukin-8. Blood 1996; 87:781–788.

10. Papayannopoulou T, Nakamoto B. Peripheralization of hemopoietic progenitors in primates treated with anti–VLA-4 integrin. Proc Natl Acad Sci USA 1993; 90:9374–9378.

11. Roberts AW, Metcalf D. Noncycling state of peripheral blood progenitor cells mobilized by granulocyte colony-stimulating factor and other cytokines. Blood 1995; 86:1600–1605.

12. Donahue RE, Kirby MR, Metzger ME, Agricola BA, Sellers SE, Cullis HM. Peripheral blood CD34$^+$ cells differ from bone marrow CD34$^+$ cells in Thy-1 expression and cell cycle status in nonhuman primates mobilized or not mobilized with granulocyte colony-stimulating factor and/or stem cell factor. Blood 1996; 87:1644–1653.

13. Rutella S, Rumi C, Teofili L, Etuk B, Ortu-La Barbera E, Leone G. RhG-CSF–mobilized peripheral blood haemopoietic progenitors reside in G0/G1 phase of cell cycle independently of the expression of myeloid antigens. Br J Haematol 1996; 93:737–738.

14. Möhle R, Haas R, and Hunstein W. Expression of adhesion molecules and c-kit on CD34$^+$ hematopoietic progenitor cells: comparison of cytokine-mobilized blood stem cells with normal bone marrow and peripheral blood. J Hematother 1993; 2:483–489.

15. Haas R, Möhle R, Pförsich M, Fruehauf S, Witt B, Goldschmidt H, Hunstein W. Blood-derived autografts collected during granulocyte colony-stimulating factor–enhanced recovery are enriched with early Thy-1+ hematopoietic progenitor cells. Blood 1995; 85: 1936–43.

16. Tarella C, Benedetti G, Caracciolo D, Castellino C, Cherasco C, Bondesan P, Omede P, Ruggieri D, Gianni AM, Pileri A. Both early and committed haemopoietic progenitors are more frequent in peripheral blood than in bone marrow during mobilization induced by high-dose chemotherapy + G-CSF. Br J Haematol 1995; 91:535–543.

17. To LB, Haylock DN, Dowse T, Simmons PJ, Trimboli S, Ashman LK, Juttner CA. A comparative study of the phenotype and proliferative capacity of peripheral blood (PB) CD34$^+$ cells mobilized by four different protocols and those of steady-phase PB and bone marrow CD34$^+$ cells. Blood 1994; 84:2930–2939.

18. Hohaus S, Goldschmidt H, Ehrhardt R, Haas R. Successful autografting following myeloablative conditioning therapy with blood stem cells mobilized by chemotherapy plus rhG-CSF. Exp Hematol 1993; 21:508–514.

19. Haas R, Moos M, Karcher A, Möhle R, Witt B, Goldschmidt H, Fruehauf S, Flentje M, Wannenmacher M, Hunstein W. Sequential high-dose therapy with peripheral-blood progenitor-cell support in low-grade non-Hodgkin's lymphoma. J Clin Oncol 1994; 12:1685–1692.

20. Möhle R, Pförsich M, Fruehauf S, Witt B, Krämer A, Haas R. Filgrastim postchemotherapy mobilizes more CD34$^+$ cells with a different antigenic profile compared with use during steady-state hematopoiesis. Bone Marrow Transplant 1994; 14:827–832.

21. Dercksen MW, Rodenhuis S, Dirkson MK, Schaasberg WP, Baars JW, van der Wall E,

Slaper Cortenbach IC, Pinedo HM, Von dem Borne AE, van der Schoot CE. Subsets of CD34$^+$ cells and rapid hematopoietic recovery after peripheral-blood stem-cell transplantation. J Clin Oncol 1995; 13:1922–1932.

22. Bender JG, Unverzagt KL, Walker DE, Lee W, Van Epps DE, Smith DH, Stewart CC, To LB. Identification and comparison of CD34-positive cells and their subpopulations from normal peripheral blood and bone marrow using multicolor flow cytometry. Blood 1991; 77:2591–2596.

23. Körbling M, Dörken B, Ho AD, Pezzutto A, Hunstein W, Fliedner TM. Autologous transplantation of blood derived hemopoietic stem cells after myeloablative therapy in a patient with Burkitt's lymphoma. Blood 1986; 67:529–532.

24. Reiffers J, Bernard P, David B, Vezon G, Sarrat A, Marit G, Moulinier J, Broustet A. Successful autologous transplantation with peripheral blood hematopoietic cells in a patient with acute leukemia. Exp Hematol 1986; 14:312–315.

25. Kessinger A, Armitage JO, Landmark JD, Weisenburger DD. Reconstitution of human hematopoietic function with autologous cryopreserved circulating stem cells. Exp Hematol 1986; 14:192–196.

26. To LB, Dyson PB, Juttner CA. Cell dose effect in circulating stem-cell autografting. Lancet 1986; 16:404–405.

27. To LB, Shepperd M, Haylock DN, Dyson PG, Charles P, Thorp DL, Dale BM, Dart GW, Roberts MM, Sage RE, Juttner CA. Single high doses of cyclophosphamide enable the collection of high numbers of hemopoietic stem cells from the peripheral blood. Exp Hematol 1990; 18:442–447.

28. Siena S, Bregni M, Brando B, Ravagnani F, Bonadonna G, Gianni AM. Circulation of CD34$^+$ hematopoietic stem cells in the peripheral blood of high-dose cyclophosphamide-treated patients: enhancement by intravenous recombinant human granulocyte-macrophage colony-stimulating factor. Blood 1989; 74:1905–1914.

29. Gianni AM, Siena S, Bregni M, Tarella C, Stern AC, Pileri A, Bonadonna G. Granulocyte-macrophage colony-stimulating factor to harvest circulating haemopoietic stem cells for auto-transplantation. Lancet 1989; 2:580–585.

30. Socinski MA, Cannistra SA, Elias A, Antman KH, Schnipper L, Griffin JD. Granulocyte-macrophage colony stimulating factor expands the circulating hematopoietic progenitor cell compartment in man. Lancet 1988; 1:1194–1198.

31. Dührsen U, Villeval JL, Boyd J, Kannourakis G, Morstyn G, Metcalf D. Effects of recombinant human granulocyte colony-stimulating factor on hematopoietic progenitor cells in cancer patients. Blood 1988; 72:2074–2081.

32. Haas R, Ho AD, Bredthauer U, Cayeux S, Egerer G, Knauf W, Hunstein W. Successful autologous transplantation of blood stem cells mobilized with recombinant human granulocyte-macrophage colony-stimulating factor. Exp Hematol 1990; 18:94–98.

33. Sheridan WP, Begley CG, Juttner CA. Effect of peripheral-blood progenitor cells mobilised by filgrastim (G-CSF) on platelet recovery after high-dose chemotherapy. Lancet 1992; 339:640–694.

34. Haas R, Möhle R, Frühauf S, Goldschmidt H, Witt B, Flentje M, Wannenmacher M, Hunstein W. Patient characteristics associated with successful mobilizing and autografting of peripheral blood progenitor cells in malignant lymphoma. Blood 1994; 83:3787–3794.

35. Grigg AP, Roberts AW, Raunow H, Houghton S, Layton JE, Boyd AW, McGrath KM, Maher D. Optimizing dose and scheduling of filgrastim (granulocyte colony-stimulating factor) for mobilization and collection of peripheral blood progenitor cells in normal volunteers. Blood 1995; 86:4437–4445.

36. Höglund M, Smedmyr B, Simonsson B, Totterman T, Bengtsson M. Dose-dependent mobilisation of haematopoietic progenitor cells in healthy volunteers receiving glycosylated rHuG-CSF. Bone Marrow Transplant 1996; 18:19–27.

37. Zeller W, Gutensohn K, Stockschlader M, Dierlamm J, Kroger N, Koehne G, Hummel K,

Kabisch H, Weh HJ, Kuhnl P, Hossfeld DK, Zander AR. Increase of mobilized CD34-positive peripheral blood progenitor cells in patients with Hodgkin's disease, non-Hodgkin's lymphoma, and cancer of the testis. Bone Marrow Transplant 1996; 17:709–713.

38. Winter JN, Lazarus HM, Rademaker A, Villa M, Mangan C, Tallman M, Jahnke L, Gordon L, Newman S, Byrd K, Cooper BW, Horvath N, Crum E, Stadtmauer EA, Conklin E, Bauman A, Martin J, Goolsby C, Gerson SL, Bender J, O'Gorman M. Phase I/II study of combined granulocyte colony-stimulating factor and granulocyte-macrophage colony-stimulating factor administration for the mobilization of hematopoietic progenitor cells. J Clin Oncol 1996; 14:277–286.

39. Lane TA, Law P, Maruyama M, Young D, Burgess J, Mullen M, Mealiffe M, Terstappen LWMM, Hardwick A, Moubayed M, Oldham F, Corringham RET, Ho AD. Harvesting and enrichment of hematopoietic progenitor cells mobilized into the peripheral blood of normal donors by granulocyte-macrophage colony-stimulating factor (GM-CSF) or G-CSF: potential role in allogeneic marrow transplantation. Blood 1995; 85:275–282.

40. Hohaus S, Martin H, Wassmann B, Egerer G, Haus U, Färber L, Burger KJ, Goldschmidt H, Hoelzer D, Haas R. Recombinant human granulocyte and granulocyte-macrophage colony-stimulating factor (G-CSF and GM-CSF) administered following cytotoxic chemotherapy have a similar ability to mobilize peripheral blood stem cells. Bone Marrow Transplant 1998; 22:625–630.

41. Andrews RG, Bensinger WI, Knitter GH, Bartelmez SH, Longin K, Bernstein ID, Appelbaum FR, Zsebo KM. The ligand for c-kit, stem cell factor, stimulates the circulation of cells that engraft lethally irradiated baboons. Blood 1992; 80:2715–2720.

42. Brugger W, Bross K, Frisch J, Dern P, Weber B, Mertelsmann R, Kanz L. Mobilization of peripheral blood progenitor cells by sequential administration of interleukin-3 and granulo-cyte-macrophage colony-stimulating factor following polychemotherapy with etoposide, ifosfamide, and cisplatin. Blood 1992; 79:1193–1200.

43. Haas R, Ehrhardt R, Witt B, Goldschmidt H, Hohaus S, Pförsich M, Ehrlich H, Färber L, Hunstein W. Autografting with peripheral blood stem cells mobilized by sequential interleu-kin-3/granulocyte-macrophage colony-stimulating factor following high-dose chemotherapy in non-Hodgkin's lymphoma. Bone Marrow Transplant 1993; 12:643–649.

44. Moskowitz CH, Stiff P, Gordon MS, McNiece I, Ho AD, Costa JJ, Broun ER, Bayer RA, Wyres M, Hill J, Jelaca-Maxwell K, Nichols CR, Brown SL, Nimer SD, Gabrilove J. Recombinant methionyl human stem cell factor and filgrastim for peripheral blood progenitor cell mobilization and transplantation in non-Hodgkin's lymphoma patients—results of a phase I/II trial. Blood 1997; 89:3136–3147.

45. Geissler K, Peschel C, Niederwieser D, Goldschmitt J, Hladik F, Fritz A, Ohler L, Bettelheim P, Huber C, Lechner K. Effect of interleukin-3 pretreatment on granulocyte/macrophage colony-stimulating factor induced mobilization of circulating haemopoietic progenitor cells. Br J Haematol 1995; 91:299–305.

46. Huhn RD, Yurkow EJ, Tushinski R, Clarke L, Sturgill MG, Hoffman R, Sheay W, Cody R, Philipp C, Resta D, George M. Recombinant human interleukin-3 (rhIL-3) enhances the mobilization of peripheral blood progenitor cells by recombinant human granulocyte colony-stimulating factor (rhG-CSF) in normal volunteers. Exp Hematol 1996; 24:839–847.

47. Roman-Unfer S, Bitran JD, Garrison L, Proeschel C, Hanauer S, Schroeder L, Johnson L, Klein L, Martinec J. A phase II study of cyclophosphamide followed by PIXY321 as a means of mobilizing peripheral blood hematopoietic progenitor cells. Exp Hematol 1996; 24:823–828.

48. Weaver A, Slowley C, Woll PJ, et al. A randomized comparison of progenitor cell mobilization using chemotherapy plus stem cell factor (r-metHuSCF) and filgrastim (r-methHuG-CSF) or chemotherapy plus filgrastim (abstr). Proc Am Soc Clin Oncol 1996; 15:269.

49. Goldschmidt H, Hegenbart U, Haas R, Hunstein W. Mobilization of peripheral blood pro-genitor cells with high-dose cyclophosphamide (4 or 7 g/m^2) and granulocyte colony-

stimulating factor in patients with multiple myeloma. Bone Marrow Transplant 1996; 17: 691–697.

50. Demirer T, Rowley S, Buckner CD, Appelbaum FR, Lilleby K, Storb R, Schiffman K, Bensinger WI. Peripheral blood stem cell (PBSC) collections after Taxol®, cyclophosphamide and recombinant human granulocyte-colony stimulating factor (rhG-CSF). J Clin Oncol 1995; 13:1714–1719.

51. Haas R, Hohaus S, Egerer G, Ehrhardt R, Witt B, Hunstein W. Recombinant human granulocyte-macrophage colony-stimulating factor (rhGM-CSF) subsequent to chemotherapy improves collection of blood stem cells for autografting in patients not eligible for bone marrow harvest. Bone Marrow Transplant 1992; 9:459–465.

52. Dreger P, Marquardt P, Haferlach T, Jacobs S, Mulverstedt T, Eckstein V, Suttorp M, Löffler H, Müller-Ruchholtz W, Schmitz N. Effective mobilization of peripheral blood progenitor cells with Dexa-BEAM and G-CSF–timing of harvesting and composition of the leukapheresis product. Br J Cancer 1993; 68:950–957.

53. Menichella G, Pierelli L, Foddai ML, Paoloni A, Vittori M, Serafini R, Benedetti-Panici P, Scambia G, Baiocchi G, Greggi S, Bizzi B. Autologous blood stem cell harvesting and transplantation in patients with advanced ovarian cancer. Br J Haematol 1991; 79:444–450.

54. Bensinger W, Appelbaum F, Rowley S, Storb R, Sanders J, Lilleby K, Gooley T, Demirer T, Schiffman K, Weaver C. Factors that influence collection and engraftment of autologous peripheral-blood stem cells. J Clin Oncol 1995; 13:2547–2555.

55. Dreger P, Kloss M, Petersen B, Haferlach T, Löffler H, Loeffler M, Schmitz N. Autologous progenitor cell transplantation: prior exposure to stem cell–toxic drugs determines yield and engraftment of peripheral blood progenitor cells but not of bone marrow grafts. Blood 1995; 86:3970–3978.

56. Tricot G, Jagannath S, Vesole D, Nelson J, Tindle S, Miller L, Cheson B, Crowley J, Barlogie B. Peripheral blood stem cell transplants for multiple myeloma: identification of favorable variables for rapid engraftment in 225 patients. Blood 1995; 85:588–596.

57. Haas R, Schmid H, Hahn U, Hohaus S, Goldschmidt H, Murea S, Kaufmann M, Wannenmacher M, Wallwiener D, Bastert G, Hunstein W. Tandem high-dose therapy with ifosfamide, epirubicin, carboplatin and peripheral blood stem cell support is an effective adjuvant treatment for high-risk primary breast cancer. Eur J Cancer 1997; 33:372–378.

58. Bensinger WI, Longin K, Appelbaum F, Rowley S, Weaver C, Lilleby K, Gooley T, Lynch M, Higano T, Klarnet J. Peripheral blood stem cells (PBSCs) collected after recombinant granulocyte colony stimulating factor (rhG-CSF): An analysis of factors correlating with the tempo of engraftment after transplantation. Br J Haematol 1994; 87:825–831.

59. Dreger P, Haferlach T, Eckstein V, Jacobs S, Suttorp M, Löffler H, Müller-Ruchholtz W, Schmitz N. G-CSF-mobilized peripheral blood progenitor cells for allogeneic transplantation: safety, kinetics of mobilization, and composition of the graft. Br J Haematol 1994; 87:609–613.

60. Sekhsaria S, Fleisher TA, Vowells S, Brown M, Miller J, Gordon I, Blaese RM, Dunbar CE, Leitman S, Malech HL. Granulocyte colony-stimulating factor recruitment of CD34+ progenitors to peripheral blood: impaired mobilization in chronic granulomatous disease and adenosine deaminase–deficient severe combined immunodeficiency disease patients. Blood 1996; 88:1104–1112.

61. Ho AD, Glück S, Germond C, Sinoff C, Dietz G, Maruyama M, Corringham RE. Optimal timing for collections of blood progenitor cells following induction chemotherapy and granulocyte-macrophage colony-stimulating factor for autologous transplantation in advanced breast cancer. Leukemia 1993; 7:1738–1744.

62. Pettengell R, Morgenstern GR, Woll PJ, Chang J, Rowlands M, Young R, Radford JA, Scarffe JH, Testa NG, Crowther D. Peripheral blood progenitor cell transplantation in lymphoma and leukemia using a single apheresis. Blood 1993; 82:3770–3777.

63. Fruehauf S, Haas R, Conradt C, Murea S, Witt B, Möhle R, Hunstein W. Peripheral blood

progenitor cell (PBSC) counts during steady-state hematopoiesis allow to estimate the yield of mobilized PBPC after filgrastim (R-metHuG-CSF)-supported cytotoxic chemotherapy. Blood 1995; 85:2619–2626.

64. Siena S, Bregni M, Brando B, Belli N, Ravagnani F, Gandola L, Stern AC, Lansdorp PM, Bonadonna G, Gianni AM. Flow cytometry for clinical estimation of circulating hematopoietic progenitors for autologous transplantation in cancer patients. Blood 1991; 77:400–409.

65. Passos-Coelho JL, Braine HG, Davis JM, Huelskamp AM, Schepers KG, Ohly K, Clarke B, Wright SK, Noga SJ, Davidson NE, Kennedy M. Predictive factors for peripheral-blood progenitor-cell collections using a single large-volume leukapheresis after cyclophosphamide and granulocyte-macrophage colony-stimulating factor mobilization. J Clin Oncol 1995; 13: 705–714.

66. Möhle R, Murea S, Pförsich M, Witt B, Haas R. Estimation of the progenitor cell yield in leukapheresis products by previous measurement of CD34$^+$ cells in the peripheral blood. Vox Sang 1996; 71:90–96.

67. Menichella G, Pierelli L, Vittori M, Serafini R, Foddai ML, Rossi PL, Leone G, Sica S, Scambia G, Benedetti-Panici L, Bizzi B. Five-year experience in PBSC collection: results of the Catholic University of Rome. Int J Artif Organs 1993; 16(suppl 5):39–44.

68. Murea S, Goldschmidt H, Hahn U, Pförsich M, Moos M, Haas R. Successful collection and transplantation of peripheral blood stem cells in cancer patients using large-volume leukapheresis. J Clin Apheresis 1996; 11:185–194.

69. Hahn U, Goldschmidt H, Salwender H, Haas R, Hunstein W. Large-bore central venous catheters for the collection of peripheral blood stem cells. J Clin Apheresis 1995; 10:12–16.

70. Brenner MK, Rill DR, Moen RC, Krance RA, Mirro J Jr, Anderson WF, Ihle JN. Gene-marking to trace origin of relapse after autologous bone marrow transplantation. Lancet 1993; 341:85–86.

71. Maurer J, Janssen JW, Thiel E, van Denderen J, Ludwig WD, Aydemir U, Heinze B, Fonatsch C, Harbott J, Reiter A. Detection of chimeric BCR-ABL genes in acute lymphoblastic leukaemia by the polymerase chain reaction. Lancet 1991; 337:1055–1058.

72. Gribben JG, Neuberg D, Freedman AS, Gimmi CD, Pesek KW, Barber M, Saporito L, Woo SD, Coral F, Spector N, Nadler L. Detection by polymerase chain reaction of residual cells with the bcl-2 translocation is associated with increased risk of relapse after autologous bone marrow transplantation for B-cell lymphoma. Blood 1993; 81:3449–3457.

73. Ross AA, Cooper BW, Lazarus HM, Mackay W, Moss TJ, Ciobanu N, Tallman MS, Kennedy MJ, Davidson NE, Sweet D. Detection and viability of tumor cells in peripheral blood stem cell collections from breast cancer patients using immunocytochemical and clonogenic assay techniques. Blood 1993; 82:2605–2610.

74. Brugger W, Henschler R, Heimfeld S, Berenson RJ, Mertelsmann R, Kanz L. Mobilization of tumor cells and hematopoietic progenitor cells into peripheral blood of patients with solid tumors. Blood 1994; 83:636–640.

75. Lin F, Goldman JM, Cross NC. A comparison of the sensitivity of blood and bone marrow for the detection of minimal residual disease in chronic myeloid leukemia. Br J Haematol 1994; 86:683–685.

76. Passos-Coelho JL, Ross AA, Moss TJ, Davis JM, Huelskamp AM, Noga SJ, Davidson NE, Kennedy MJ. Absence of breast cancer cells in a single-day peripheral blood progenitor cell collection after priming with cyclophosphamide and granulocyte-macrophage colony-stimulating factor. Blood 1995; 85:1138–1143.

77. Gazitt Y, Tian E, Barlogie B, Reading CL, Vesole DH, Jagannath S, Schnell J, Hoffman R, Tricot G. Differential mobilization of myeloma cells and normal hematopoietic stem cells in multiple myeloma after treatment with cyclophosphamide and granulocyte-macrophage colony-stimulating factor. Blood 1996; 87:805–811.

78. Lemoli RM, Rosti G, Visani G, Gherlinzoni F, Miggiano MC, Fortuna A, Zinzani P, Tura

S. Concomitant mobilization of plasma cells and hematopoietic progenitors in peripheral blood of multiple myeloma patients: positive selection and transplantation of enriched CD34$^+$ cells to remove circulating tumor cells. Blood 1996; 87:1625–1634.

79. Ouspenskaia MV, Johnston DA, Roberts WM, Estrov Z, Zipf TF. Accurate quantitation of residual B-precursor acute lymphoblastic leukemia by limiting dilution and a PCR-based detection system: a description of the method and the principles involved. Leukemia 1995; 9:321–328.

80. Henry JM, Sykes PJ, Brisco MJ, To LB, Juttner CA, Morley AA. Comparison of myeloma cell contamination of bone marrow and peripheral blood stem cell harvests. Br J Haematol 1996; 92:614–619.

81. Cote RJ, Rosen PP, Lesser ML, Old LJ, Osborne MP. Prediction of early relapse in patients with operable breast cancer by detection of occult bone marrow micrometastases. J Clin Oncol 1991; 9:1749–1756.

82. Diel IJ, Kaufmann M, Goerner R, Costa SD, Kaul S, Bastert G. Detection of tumor cells in bone marrow of patients with primary breast cancer: a prognostic factor for distant metastasis. J Clin Oncol 1992; 10:1534–1539.

83. Datta YH, Adams PT, Drobyski WR, Ethier SP, Terry VH, Roth MS. Sensitive detection of occult breast cancer by the reverse-transcriptase polymerase chain reaction. J Clin Oncol 1994; 12:475–482.

84. Fields KK, Elfenbein GJ, Trudeau WL, Perkins JB, Janssen WE, Moscinski LC. Clinical significance of bone marrow metastases as detected using the polymerase chain reaction in patients with breast cancer undergoing high-dose chemotherapy and autologous bone marrow transplantation. J Clin Oncol 1996; 14:1868–1876.

85. Pantel K, Schlimok G, Angstwurm M, Weckermann D, Schmaus W, Gath H, Passlick B, Izbicki JR, Riethmuller G. Methodological analysis of immunocytochemical screening for disseminated epithelial tumor cells in bone marrow. J Hematother 1994; 3:165–183.

86. Sharp JG, Joshi SS, Armitage JO, Bierman P, Coccia PF, Harrington DS, Kessinger A, Crouse DA, Mann SL, Weisenburger DD. Significance of detection of occult non-Hodgkin's lymphoma in histologically uninvolved bone marrow by a culture technique. Blood 1992; 79:1074–1080.

87. Berenson RJ, Bensinger WI, Hill RS, Andrews RG, Garcia-Lopez J, Kalamasz DF, Still BJ, Spitzer G, Buckner CD, Bernstein ID, Thomas ED. Engraftment after infusion of CD34+ marrow cells in patients with breast cancer or neuroblastoma. Blood 1991; 77:1717–1722.

88. Shpall EJ, Jones RB, Bearman SI, Franklin WA, Archer PG, Curiel T, Bitter M, Claman HN, Stemmer SM, Purdy M, Myers SE, Hami L, Taffs S, Heimfeld S, Hallagan J, Berenson RJ. Transplantation of enriched CD34-positive autologous marrow into breast cancer patients following high-dose chemotherapy: Influence of CD34-positive peripheral-blood progenitors and growth factors on engraftment. J Clin Oncol 1994; 12:28–36.

89. Gorin NC, Lopez M, Laporte JP, Quittet P, Lemoine F, Berenson RJ, Isnard F, Grande M, Stachowiak J, Labopin M, Fouillard L, Morel P, Jouet JP, Noel-Walter MP, Detourmignies L, Aoudjhane M, Bauters F, Najman A, Douay L. Preparation and successful engraftment of purified CD34+ bone marrow progenitor cells in patients with non-Hodgkin's lymphoma. Blood 1995; 85:1647–1654.

90. Mahé B, Milpied N, Hermouet S, Robillard N, Moreau P, Letortorec S, Rapp MJ, Bataille R, Harousseau JL. G-CSF alone mobilises sufficient peripheral blood CD34+ cells for positive selection in newly diagnosed patients with myeloma and lymphoma. Br J Hematol 1996; 92:263–268.

91. Hohaus S, Pförsich M, Murea S, Abdallah A, Lin YS, Funk L, Voso MT, Kaul S, Schmid H, Wallwiener D, Haas R. Immunomagnetic selection of CD34+ peripheral blood stem cells for autografting in patients with breast cancer. Br J Haematol 1997; 97:881–888.

92. Mapara MY, Körner LJ, Hildebrandt M, Bargou R, Krahl D, Reichardt P, Dörken B. Monitoring of tumor cell purging after highly efficient immunomagnetic selection of CD34+ cells

from leukapheresis products in breast cancer patients: comparison of immunocytochemical tumor cell staining and reverse transcriptase-polymerase chain reaction. Blood 1997; 89: 337–344.

93. Voso MT, Hohaus S, Moos M, and Haas R. Lack of t(14;18) PCR-positive cells in highly purified CD34$^+$ cells and their CD19 subsets in patients with follicular lymphoma. Blood 1997; 89:3763–3768.

94. Hohaus S, Funk L, Martin S, Schlenk RF, Abdallah A, Hahn U, Egerer G, Goldschmidt H, Schneeweiß A, Fersis N, Kaul S, Wallwiener D, Bastert G, Haas R. Stage III and oestrogen receptor negativity are associated with poor prognosis after adjuvant high-dose therapy in high-risk breast cancer. Br J Cancer 1999; 79:1500–1507.

95. Bender JG, To LB, Williams S, Schwartzberg LS. Defining a therapeutic dose of peripheral blood stem cells. J Hematother 1992; 1:329–341.

96. Schwartzberg L, Birch R, Blanco R, Wittlin F, Muscato J, Tauer K, Hazelton B, West W. Rapid ans sustained hematopoietic reconstitution by peripheral blood stem cell infusion alone following high-dose chemotherapy. Bone Marrow Transplant 1993; 11:369–374.

97. Dercksen MW, Gerritsen WR, Rodenhuis S, Dirkson MK, Slaper-Cortenbach IC, Schaasberg WP, Pinedo HM, von dem Borne AE, van der Schoot CE. Expression of adhesion molecules on CD34+ cells: CD34$^+$ L-selectin$^+$ cells predicts a rapid platelet recovery after peripheral blood stem cell transplantation. Blood 1995; 85:3313–3319.

98. Domenech J, Linassier C, Gihana E, Dayan A, Truglio D, Bout M, Petitdidier C, Delain M, Petit A, Bremond JL. Prolonged impairment of hematopoiesis after high-dose therapy followed by autologous bone marrow transplantation. Blood 1995; 85:3320–3327.

99. Jordan CT, Lemischka IR. Clonal and systemic analysis of long-term hematopoiesis in the mouse. Genes and Dev 1990; 2:220–232.

100. Keller G, Snodgrass R. Life span of multipotential hematopoietic stem cells in vivo. J Exp Med. 1990; 171:1407–1418.

101. Haas R, Witt B, Möhle R, Goldschmidt H, Hohaus S, Fruehauf S, Wannenmacher M, Hunstein W. Sustained long-term hematopoiesis after myeloablative therapy with peripheral blood progenitor cell support. Blood 1995; 85:3754–3761.

102. Voso MT, Murea S, Goldschmidt H, Hohaus S, Haas R. High-dose chemotherapy with PBSC support results in a significant reduction of the haematopoietic progenitor cell compartment. Br J Haematol 1996; 94:757–763.

28

Stem Cell Transplantation for Hodgkin's Disease

RAM KANCHERLA and TAUSEEF AHMED

New York Medical College, Valhalla, New York

I. INTRODUCTION

Therapy for Hodgkin's disease has evolved over the past few decades. This malignancy affects 7500 people in the United States yearly. The majority can be cured with radiation and/or combination chemotherapy. However, without appropriate salvage measures, a significant number will die of the disease. Strategies to identify this subgroup and therapeutic plans to best treat them have been the focus of considerable work in recent years. Long-term follow-up results of the MOPP [mechlorethamine, Oncovin (vincristine), procarbazine, prednisone] regimen at the National Cancer Institute (NCI) showed 82% survival at 5 years for patients achieving complete remission (CR) (1). However, none of those who failed to achieve CR survived beyond 5 years. With the use of combination regimens, including MOPP, ABVD (doxorubicin, bleomycin, vincristine, dacarbazine), MOPP alternating with ABVD, hybrid MOPP/ABV (without dacarbazine), and Ch1VPP (chlorambucil, vinblastine, procarbazine, prednisone) regimens, CR can be achieved in 75–90% of patients with advanced disease. Thirty percent of the patients ultimately fail conventional therapy. The prognosis for these patients is extremely poor.

Conventional salvage chemotherapy or radiation can improve long-term survival only in a minority of patients. Longo et al. reported data on 107 patients relapsing after having achieved CR out of 439 patients treated with first-line combination chemotherapy between 1964 and 1990 at the NCI (2). Half the relapses occurred within the first year of achieving remission and 82% within 3 years. The estimated 20-year survival of relapsed patients is 17%. Other studies report a CR in 13–67% of relapsed or refractory patients and a remission duration of 5–47 months. A 34% CR rate is reported with the MINE regimen (mitoguazone, ifosfamide, vinorelbine, etoposide) in 100 patients (3). DHAP (dexamethasone, cytarabine, cisplatin) produced 11% CR in 37 patients (4), HOPE-Bleo (doxorubicin, vincristine, prednisone, etoposide, bleomycin) 59% in 44 patients (5), and mini-BEAM (carmustine, etoposide, cytarabine, melphalan) 32% in 44 patients (6). We tried ACES (cytarabine, carboplatin, etoposide, methylprednisolone) in 20 patients with non-Hodgkin's lymphoma (NHL) and 13 with Hodgkin's disease. The CR rate was 12% (7). The variation in the results of the more recent studies is probably a consequence of the wide heterogeneity in the characteristics of their patient populations and their relatively small size.

II. HIGH-DOSE TREATMENT AND AUTOLOGOUS BONE MARROW TRANSPLANTATION

High-dose treatment with autologous bone marrow rescue is a viable option for patients with relapsed disease. Appelbaum first reported successful engraftment of cryopreserved autologous bone marrow in patients with malignant lymphoma (8). Following this, many investigators used high-dose chemotherapy and radiotherapy to overcome chemoresistance. Most of the initial studies used autologous bone marrow as a source for stem cells, but the use of peripheral blood has increased markedly in recent years.

Several investigators report that high-dose chemotherapy and/or radiotherapy and autologous bone marrow transplantation (ABMT) can produce long-term disease-free survival in 25–50% of patients with relapsed and refractory disease. A variety of conditioning regimens with different agents, doses, and schedules have been used. Table 1 shows some of the common conditioning regimens, and Table 2 summarizes the results of the various studies.

The efficacy of high-dose cyclophosphamide, carmustine, and etoposide (CBV) followed by ABMT was reported in 30 patients with relapsed Hodgkin's disease (9). At the time of transplantation, 23 patients had progressive disease while receiving salvage chemotherapy. The investigators used cyclophosphamide 6 g/m^2 over 4 days, carmustine 300 mg/m^2 as a single dose, and etoposide 600–900 mg/m^2 divided over six doses given every 12 h. Of the 30 patients, 15 achieved a complete remission and 10 a partial response, whereas 5 had no response. Three patients developed carmustine-induced pulmonary toxicity. A larger follow-up of this trial with 128 patients from both the M.D. Anderson Cancer Center and the University of Nebraska Medical Center was published (10). Of these, 65 (51%) achieved CR after ABMT. Overall survival at 4 years is estimated at 45%, with 25% surviving without progression of disease.

With intensive CBV at different high dosages followed by ABMT in 128 patients with advanced or refractory disease, a CR rate of 52% was reported, with 24% of the patients remaining in CR at a minimal follow-up of 3 years (11).

In a dose-escalation study of CBV with ABMT in 30 patients with refractory and relapsed Hodgkin's disease and 28 patients with intermediate- and high-grade NHL, the maximal tolerated dose (MTD) was 7200 mg/in^2 for cyclophosphamide, 450 mg/in^2 for carmustine, and 2000 mg/in^2 for etoposide (12). Interstitial pneumonia developed in 5 of 18 patients receiving 600 mg/in^2 of carmustine. Treatment-related mortality was 5% at levels up to the MTD and 22% at higher doses. Fourteen of the 30 patients remain free from progression at a median follow-up of 265 days. There is no difference in either complete or total response rates in the various dose levels.

High-dose BEAM (carmustine, etoposide, cytarabine, melphalan) was used with ABMT in 155 poor-risk patients (13). The actuarial overall and progression-free survival at 5 years was 55% and 50%, respectively. Procedure-related mortality was 10%. Eleven

Table 1 Conditioning Regimens for Autotransplant in Hodgkin's Disease

CBV (9)
   cyclophosphamide 1.5/m²/day, days-6 to -3
   etoposide 100–150 mg/m² q12h, days-6 to -4
   carmustine 300 mg/m² day-6
CBV (augmented) (15)
   cyclophosphamide 1.8 g/m²/day, days-7 to -4
   etoposide 400 mg/m² q12h, days-7 to -5
   carmustine 600 mg/m² day-3
CBV ± cisplatin (29)
   etoposide 2.4 g/m² (over 34 h) day-7
   cyclophosphamide 1800 mg/m²/day, days-6 to -3
   carmustine 500 mg/m², day-2
   ± cisplatin 50 mg/m² day, days-7 to -5
BEAM (13)
   carmustine 300 mg/m² day-6
   etoposide 100–200 mg/m² day, days-5 to -2
   cytarabine 100–200 mg/m² q12h, days-5 to -2
   melphalan 140 mg/m² iv, day-1
Cy-TBI (17)
   cyclophosphamide 60 mg/kg/day, days-5 and -4
   total body irradiation 1000–1400 cGY
Cy-VP/TBI or BCNU (30)
   total body irradiation 1200 cGY in six fractions, days-8 to -5
   or
   carmustine 150 mg/m² day, days-6 to -4
   etoposide 60 mg/m² day-4
   cyclophosphamide 100 mg/kg day-2
Cy-VP-TLI (18)
   total lymphoid irradiation 20.04 Gy over 4 days, 1.67 Gy fraction (3 times a
     day) days -11 to -7
   etoposide 250 mg/m²/day, days -6 to -4
   cyclophosphamide 60 mg/kg/day, days-3 and -2
MBE (58)
   carmustine 300–600 mg/m² day-5
   melphalan 80–140 mg/m² day-4
   etoposide 100 mg/m²/day, days-5 to -3
Melphalan–etoposide (59)
   etoposide 60 mg/kg day-4
   melphalan 160 mg iv day-3
Bu-Cy or Cy-TBI (21)
   busulfan 1 mg/kg po qid. for 4 days
   then cyclophosphamide 50 mg/kg/day for 4 days
   or
   cyclophosphamide 50 mg/kg/day for 4 days
   then total body irradiation 1200–1440 cGY divided over 4 days
BEC-2 (16)
   carmustine 400 mg/m² day-5
   etoposide 1800 mg/m² day-5
   cyclophosphamide 2500 mg/m²day, days-5 and -4
TMJ (16)
   thioteopa 250 mg/m²/day, days-7 to -5
   mitoxantrone 40 mg/m² day-7
   carboplatin 330 mg/m²/day, days-7 to -5
EC (16)
   etoposide 600 mg/m²/day, days-8 to -6
   cyclophosphamide 2.5 g/m²/day, days-6 to -4
   ± total body irradiation 10 Gy in five fractions, days-3 to -1

Table 2 Autologous Bone Marrow Transplant for Hodgkin's Disease: Regimens and Results

Regimen (references)[a]	No. of patients	Disease-free survival (%)	Survival (%)	Median follow-up (months)	Procedure-related mortality (%)
CBV (9)	30	31 (at 3–44 months)	63	NA	NA
CBV (10)	128	25 (4-yr actuarial)	45	48	7
CBV (60)	62	38 (3-yr actuarial)	45	45	0
CBV dose escalation (12)	30	50 (1-yr actuarial)	70	9	17
CBV augmented (15)	56	47 (5-yr actuarial)	NA	41	21
CBV ± cisplatin (29)	58 (all relapsed)	64 (2-yr actuarial)	72	27	7
BEAM (13)	155	50 (5-yr actuarial)	55	NA	10
Cy-TBI (17)	26	<25 (4-yr actuarial)	35	44	23
Cy-VP (47)	85	58 (2-yr actuarial)	75	25	13
TBI or BCNU Cy-VP-TLI (18)	47	53 (3-yr actuarial)	NA	40	17
MBE (58)	89	41 (5-yr actuarial)	41	43	22
Melphalan—etoposide (59)	73	40 (4-yr actuarial)	NA	30	10
Bu-Cy or Cy-TBI (21)	50 / 28	30 (3-yr actuarial)	NA	26	34
BACE (61)	37	38 (at 38–79 mo.)	38	61	NA
Etoposide—melphalan (62)	48	>50 (45-mo. actuarial)	>50	45	NA
Sequential chemoradiotherapy (63)	25	48 (6-yr actuarial)	NA	72	0
CTEB (20)	20	38 (2-yr actuarial)	38	22	15
CVB (11)	128	NA	NA	32	8
Sequential ABMT (16)	122	37 (3-yr actuarial)	48	48	16

[a] See text for definitions of abbreviations.

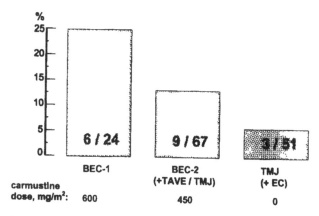

Figure 1 Incidence of lethal or potentially lethal lung toxicity of two conditioning regimens with different carmustine doses and a carmustine-free conditioning in three consecutive autologous bone marrow transplant studies. BEC, carmustine, etoposide, cyclophosphamide ; TMJ, thiotepa, mitoxantrone, carboplatin; EC, etoposide, cyclophosphamide.

(7%) patients had interstitial pneumonitis. Of 155 patients, 78 were chemoresistant and 33 were in chemosensitive relapse. Forty-four patients had untested relapse.

In 1989, we reported 23 advanced Hodgkin's disease patients treated with myeloablative chemotherapy using carmustine 450–600 mg/in², etoposide 1500–2000 mg/in², and cyclophosphamide 120 mg/kg followed by ABMT (14). Nineteen patients had disease refractory to previous chemotherapy. Ten patients (43%) achieved a complete remission with the study regimen. Median duration of response was only 6 months. Ten patients (43%) had evidence of pulmonary dysfunction and three died as a result of interstitial pneumonia.

An augmented CBV regimen with cyclophosphamide 7200 mg/in², carmustine 600 mg/in², and etoposide 2400 mg/in² was used in 56 patients, 80% of whom achieved CR; 21% had a toxic death due to sepsis or interstitial pneumonia (15).

Thus, although dose-intensive therapy with high-dose carmustine, etoposide, and cyclophosphamide can be beneficial for a subset of patients, not all can be effectively salvaged and there is a price to pay for such therapy. Specifically, escalating the dose of carmustine leads to an increase in toxicity and therapy-related fatality (Fig. 1). This led us and others to evaluate regimens without carmustine (16). The solid line in Figure 2 shows the actuarial survival probability of 47 patients with sensitive relapse treated with the TMJ (thiotepa, mitoxantrone, carboplatin) conditioning regimen at New York Medical College.

Since radiotherapy is clearly useful in patients with Hodgkin's disease, dose-intensive combination therapy and irradiation have also been evaluated by several groups. Phillips et al. used cyclophosphamide and total body irradiation (TBI) followed by ABMT in 26 patients with progressive Hodgkin's disease (17). Selected patients also received involved field radiotherapy. Eight patients were in untreated relapse. Six patients (23%) died of treatment-related toxicity and three of idiopathic interstitial pneumonitis, whereas seven (27%) remain continuously progression free for a median of 3.8 years. The efficacy of high-dose cyclophosphamide, etoposide, and accelerated hyperfractionated total lymphoid irradiation (TLI) was reported in 47 patients with refractory or relapsed disease

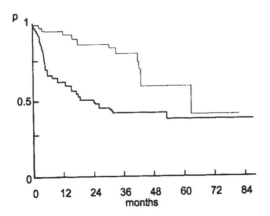

Figure 2   Actuarial survival from autologous bone marrow transplant of patients with sensitive (dotted line) and refractory disease (solid line) (at the start of treatment) in the New York Medical College sequential transplant studies.

(18). Involved field boost radiation to all areas of residual or recurrent disease was given following reinduction chemotherapy. Twenty-six patients (55%) responded to chemotherapy and 21 (45%) are resistant. Eight patients died of treatment-related toxicity. Of these, five died of pulmonary decompensation with clinical and radiological manifestations suggestive of alveolar hemorrhage. Twenty-five patients (53%) were alive and disease-free at a median follow-up of 40 months. In the only randomized comparison between high-dose chemotherapy followed by ABMT and conventional dose salvage therapy, with 20 patients in each arm (BEAM + ABMT vs mini-BEAM), the 3-year actuarial event-free survival was 53% in the BEAM and 10% in the mini-BEAM group (19). The trial was closed early because of poor recruitment.

A.   Disease Status at Transplantation

One of the reasons for the differences in survival estimates of patients in different high-dose chemotherapy/ABMT studies is the heterogeneity of the patients with respect to their disease status prior to the procedure; that is, first CR, failure to achieve CR with induction chemotherapy ("primary refractory"), chemosensitive relapse, and chemoresistant relapse. A source of difficulty in comparing different studies is the variable definition of previous response. Some accept relapse within a year of standard induction therapy as evidence of resistance. Others define responsiveness as any response according to traditional criteria. However, such responsiveness is not necessarily clinically relevant. Patients who fail to achieve a CR with initial chemotherapy are likely to have a poor outlook. In addition, patients with Hodgkin's disease may have persistent radiographic abnormalities after therapy that represent fibrosis. Here, lack of progression of disease may or may not be clinically relevant. The criteria used at New York Medical College/Arlin Cancer Institute are outlined in Table 3.

> *Primary refractory disease*: Even though long-term survival in primary refractory patients is somewhat better with high-dose chemotherapy and stem cell transplantation when compared to conventional measures, it remains significantly lower than that of relapsed patients. In the study reported by Yahalom, disease-

Table 3 New York Medical College Criteria to
Define Previous Tumor Response

Sensitive Relapse:
Standard-dose treatment prior to autologous bone
  marrow transplant achieves complete or near-
  complete elimination of clinically detectable disease
  in relapsed patient.
Refractory relapse:
Relapsed patient still has significant amount of tumor
  at the end of standard-dose therapy.
Primary refractory disease:
Patient never achieved complete response.

---

free survival at 40 months was 33% for primary refractory disease as compared
to 79% for relapsed patients (18). Five-year progression-free survival for primary
refractory patients on the high-dose BEAM protocol was 33% as opposed to 70%
for patients in the third or later relapse (13).

Sensitive versus resistant disease: Several studies of ABMT showed that progression-free survival for patients with chemosensitive relapse is superior to that of
patients with chemoresistant relapse. Median progression-free survival in one
study using CBV was 6 months for resistant relapse patients (20). The study by
Jones et al. showed about 50% disease-free survival for patients with sensitive
relapse, whereas none of the resistant relapse patients were disease free at 14
months (21). In the BEAM protocol, progression-free survival at 5 years for chemosensitive and chemoresistant patients was 52% and 32%, respectively (13).
Only 4 of 16 patients with chemoresistant relapse versus 25 of 35 patients with
sensitive relapse in a study reported by Carella et al. had a CR to the different
CBV regimens (11).

To improve the outcome of primary refractory and chemoresistant relapsed patients, at
New York Medical College we employed a sequential transplant approach. We gave BEC-
2 (carmustine, etoposide, cyclophosphamide) for the first transplant and TAVE (thiotepa,
cytarabine, vinblastine) or TMJ (thiotepa, mitoxantrone, carboplatin) for the second transplant in the first study. TMJ was given for the first and EC (etoposide, cyclophosphamide ± TBI) for the second transplant in the second study. Currently, the conditioning
regimen for the first transplant consists of the TMJ regimen and the second of ICE (ifosfamide, carboplatin, etoposide). Patients with sensitive relapse received a single high-dose
chemotherapy treatment with ABMT, whereas those with primary refractory disease or
chemoresistant relapse were offered a second course, provided they had not progressed
after the first transplant and their physiological functions had recovered sufficiently. Some
investigators give conventional chemotherapy to debulk tumor prior to dose-intensive therapy and ABMT. We used conventional dose chemotherapy to test the tumor sensitivity,
which determined whether one or two cycles of dose-intensive therapy would be administered. Of the 122 patients, 39 were with sensitive and 83 resistant relapse (42 primary
refractory and 41 refractory relapse). After a median follow-up of 4 years, the survival
of patients with sensitive relapse was superior to patients with refractory relapse or primary
refractory disease (see Fig. 2). However, when compared to patients with sensitive relapse,

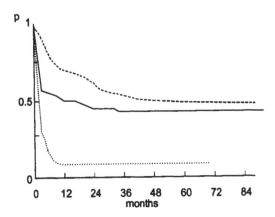

Figure 3 Life table curve of progression-free survival of patients with sensitive disease (dotted line), patients with refractory disease who received two sequential transplants (solid line), and patients with refractory disease who had one transplant only (dashed line).

those with refractory disease receiving both cycles of dose-intensive therapy had almost identical progression-free survival (Fig. 3). It is conceivable that this could reflect a genuine alteration in the biology of the disease by the second transplant. However, the first ABMT is likely to select for second ABMT patients with a prognosis better than that of refractory patients in general. Half the partial responders after the first ABMT converted into complete responders with the second course, and all of them are still alive without relapse except in one case of fatal pulmonary toxicity. Thus, the first ABMT can identify those patients with refractory disease who are likely to benefit from a second cycle. Whether sequential transplantation should be used in sensitive relapse is a question worth pondering. With improved supportive measures, multicycle dose-intensive regimens are feasible and could be beneficial.

Transplant in first CR: Among 993 autotransplants performed between 1989 and 1995 for Hodgkin's disease and reported to the Autologous Blood and Marrow Transplant Registry (ABMTR), the 3-year probability of survival was 86% for 49 patients transplanted in first remission, 60% for 463 transplanted in first relapse, 76% for 224 transplanted in second or subsequent remission, and 49% for 257 patients never in remission (22). Similar outcomes at first CR were reported in different studies (23,24). Even though excellent results were seen in first remission, this approach is not automatically justifiable in all patients. Initial conventional chemotherapy and/or radiotherapy is curative for the majority of them. Moreover, the cost in terms of drug toxicity and monetary expenditure can be prohibitively high. Identification of patients at high risk for relapse at the time of initial diagnosis is of paramount importance.

Straus et al. reported that patients presenting initially with two or more unfavorable factors (i.e., low hemoglobin, high LDH, age >45 years, inguinal lymph node involvement, mediastinal mass wider than 45% of the thoracic diameters, and bone marrow involvement) are at high risk for relapse (25). Investigators from Scotland and the Newcastle Lymphoma Group developed a numerical prognostic index based on hemoglobin, absolute lymphocyte count, stage, and age (26). Their model correctly identifies poor-risk patients, including some in stages I and II.

Hodgkin's disease patients reported to the European Bone Marrow Transplantation (EBMT) registry with early ABMT were evaluated (27). The overall and disease-free survival for patients who were in first CR prior to ABMT is 76 + 8% and 70 ± 8%, respectively, at 7 years. Similar results were reported for patients in partial remission (PR) prior to ABMT. These results compare favorably with conventional chemotherapy or combined modality treatment. Randomized trials are ongoing, and longer follow-up of these trials is needed to substantiate such an approach (28).

III. PROGNOSTIC FACTORS FOR ABMT

The prognostic factors which influence survival in relapsed patients before undergoing standard-dose chemotherapy include the length of initial relapse-free interval, initial disease stage, B symptoms at relapse, age, sex, and performance status. Table 4 lists prognostic characteristics reported as independently significant for patients with recurrent or refractory disease at the time of ABMT.

Prognosis is generally dependent on both the disease and its therapy. Factors identified as significant at the time of standard-dose salvage will thus be different from those most often noted at ABMT; that is, performance status, disease status at ABMT, number of prior chemotherapy regimens, bulk of disease, and extranodal involvement. Initial remission duration (greater or less than 1 year) is reported as an independently significant factor in one publication only (29). Nademanee et al. reported 51% disease-free survival in patients with an initial remission <12 months (30). Patients who had received more than two chemotherapy regimens had a poorer disease-free survival and were at increased risk for transplant-related mortality, possibly because of increased drug resistance and cumulative organ toxicity from cytotoxic agents. Patients with refractory disease have a poor survival and higher transplant-related mortality than those with sensitive disease, as noted by both us and others.

Prior bleomycin lung toxicity is reported as the only independently significant factor in a multivariate analysis of 30 patients who received CBV and cisplatin followed by ABMT after failing to achieve a CR with combination chemotherapy (31). On the other hand, multivariate analysis of 56 patients with relapsed disease who underwent a similar high-dose chemotherapy with ABMT indicate that an initial remission of less than 12 months, B symptoms at relapse, and extranodal disease at relapse are poor prognostic factors (29). Differences in the factors identified as independently significant reflect not only the wide heterogeneity of the study populations but also the characteristics included in the analysis, their number, the number of study patients and of those with completed follow-up, and finally the method of analysis.

An analysis of 150 patients with sensitive or refractory Hodgkin's disease who underwent ABMT at New York Medical College identified response to prior salvage treatment, age, prior radiation, and initial stage as the main prognostic features. Prior irradiation and early stage at diagnosis were adverse factors. The reason for the negative impact of these characteristics is unclear. It may possibly be due to referral bias; that is, the fact that most patients with early disease are cured with initial treatment and those with truly resistant disease are preferentially referred for therapy of relapse. It is also conceivable that early irradiation modifies the biology of the disease. The real reason could be best

Table 4 Independent Prognostic Factors for Autologous Bone Marrow Transplant in Hodgkin's Disease

Investigator year (reference)	Regimen[a]	Most significant factors
Jagannath et al., 1989 (20)	CBV	Failed prior therapies >2
		Performance status
Vose et al., 1990 (64)	CBV	Failed prior therapies >2
		Disease bulk > 10 cm
Reece et al., 1994 (29)	CBV ± cisplatin	B symptoms at relapse
		Extranodal disease at relapse
		Remission duration >1 year
Chopra et al., 1993 (13)	BEAM	Tumor bulk >10 cm
		Prior treatment regimens >2
		Patient's sex
		Relapse status
Ahmed et al., 1997 (16)	Double transplants	Previous response
		Prior radiation
		Age
Phillips et al., 1989 (17)	Cy-TBI	Performance status
		Duration of disease
Crump et al., 1993 (59)	Melphalan, etoposide	Disease status at transplant
		(no evidence vs bulky disease)
Nademanee et al., 1995 (30)	Cy-VP-TBI	Prior chemotherapy regimens >3
	Cy-VP-BCNU	
Jones et al., 1990 (21)	Bu-CY	Previous response status
	Cy-VP-TLI	Original response to chemotherapy
		(relapsed vs primary refractory)
Yahalom et al., 1993	Cy-VP-TLI	Original response to chemotherapy
		(relapsed vs primary refractory)
Seymour et al., 1994 (62)	Melphalan, etoposide	Disease status at transplant
		Liver involvement
Carella et al., 1991 (11)	CVB	Performance status
		Disease status at transplant
Burns et al., 1995 (60)	CBV	B symptoms
Horning et al., 1997 (65)	Cy-Vp-TBI	B symptoms at relapse
	CBV	Disseminated lung or marrow disease at relapse
	Cy-VP-CCNU	> Minimal disease at transplant

[a] See text for definitions of abbreviations.

discerned by including in the analysis the true denominator of patients with early-stage Hodgkin's disease.

IV. ALLOGENEIC BONE MARROW TRANSPLANTATION

The theoretical advantages of allogeneic BMT (alloBMT) are the avoidance of tumor cell infusion and a possible graft-versus-Hodgkin's disease effect, both of which might reduce the probability of relapse after BMT (32). Most alloBMT studies included only few patients with Hodgkin's disease. No prospective randomized trial is available. A nonrandomized study showed a similar event-free survival rate and a 17% decrease in the relapse rate for 21 allogenic bone marrow recipients compared with 28 autologous bone marrow recipients (21). Analysis of patients with Hodgkin's disease who underwent marrow transplantation at the Fred Hutchinson Cancer Research Center in Seattle revealed a lower relapse rate of human leukocyte antigen (HLA)–identical sibling transplants compared to autologous transplants (45 vs 75% 5-year actuarial estimate) (33). The differences in 5-year event-free survival (26 vs 14%) and nonrelapse mortality rates (53 vs 43%) were not statistically significant. There was no association between acute graft-versus-host disease (GVHD) and relapse. Frequency of relapse at previously uninvolved sites was similar between autologous and allogeneic recipients. These investigators felt that, since there is no evidence that reinfusion of autologous tumor cells leads to the higher relapse rate among autologous recipients, graft-versus-tumor effects following alloBMT is the most logical explanation for the lower relapse rate in HLA-identical sibling transplant patients.

Forty-five patients who underwent alloBMT for Hodgkin's disease reported to the EBMT registry were compared to 45 patients who had received ABMT and were matched for sex and age at transplantation, stage at diagnosis, bone marrow involvement at diagnosis and transplantation, year of transplantation, disease status at transplantation, time from diagnosis to transplantation, and conditioning regimen with or without TBI (34). The 4-year actuarial probability of survival and progression-free survival were 25 and 15% for alloBMT and 37 and 24% for ABMT. No difference in relapse was seen in this analysis as opposed to the Seattle experience. In patients with sensitive relapse, the 4-year survival probability was 30% after alloBMT and 64% after ABMT, but transplant-related mortality from alloBMT was substantially higher. A graft-versus-Hodgkin's effect is associated with grade II or worse acute GVHD, but its positive effect on relapse is largely offset by its toxicity.

Another analysis of 100 patients who received HLA-identical sibling BMT reported to the International Bone Marrow Transplant Registry (IBMTR) revealed the 3-year probability of survival and disease-free survival rates of 21 and 15%, respectively (35). Because of these contradictory results and the lack of donor availability for the majority of Hodgkin's disease patients, alloBMT is markedly restricted in its use.

V. SUPPORTIVE CARE

In recent years, improved supportive care techniques have lead to shorter hospital stays and lowered peritransplant morbidity/mortality. Also in recent years, peripheral blood stem cells (PBSCs) have been used clinically in humans (36). PBSCs collected in the unperturbed (steady) state were clinically effective in restoring hematopoiesis after dose-intensive therapy. They were initially used in patients with fibrotic inaspirable marrow, marrow involvement by disease, or inadequate marrow collection. The advantages of using PBSCs are avoidance of general anesthesia, collection in an outpatient setting, less risk of tumor contamination of the product, and ability to collect enough stem cells even in patients who have received pelvic radiation. The disadvantages are the necessity of a central catheter placement and catheter-related infections. Kessinger et al. reported on CBV followed by PBSC transplantation in 56 relapsed patients with marrow abnormalities (either hypocellularity or tumor involvement) (37). Neither chemotherapy nor hematopoietic growth factors were used to mobilize stem cells. Median time to recovery to 0.5×10^9/L granulocytes was 30 days. Median time to independence from red cell and platelet transfusions were 22 and 25 days, respectively. The actuarial event-free survival at 3 years was 37%, which was at least as good as that reported for relapsed Hodgkin's disease patients treated with CBV and ABMT. In our own experience, marrow involvement was not associated with shorter survival. There are as yet no comparative randomized studies of marrow versus PBSC transplant. The general opinion is that patients receiving PBSCs show less morbidity. Mobilization with chemotherapy and hematopoietic growth factors, that is, recombinant granulocyte-macrophage colony-stimulating factor (GM-CSF) and granulocyte colony-stimulating factor (G-CSF), reduced the number of apheresis procedures required per patient for adequate PBSC collection. A randomized trial comparing filgrastim (recombinant G-CSF)–mobilized PBSC transplant with ABMT as hematopoietic stem cell support in lymphoma patients showed that filgrastim-mobilized PBSCs significantly reduced the number of platelet transfusions, the time to platelet and neutrophil recovery, and led to earlier discharge from the hospital (38). Mobilization of stem cells with chemotherapy and cytokines needs fewer apheresis procedures. However, chemomobilization has greater morbidity (39). Thus, combining chemotherapy and cytokine mobilization is perhaps best reserved for patients with inadequate CD34$^+$ cell yield following cytokine mobilization alone or for those in whom the mobilization regimen is intended as cytoreductive therapy preliminary to high-dose treatment.

Cytokines have likewise reduced peritransplant morbidity. In a randomized multicenter study of recombinant G-CSF in 54 patients with Hodgkin's disease or NHL undergoing ABMT, patients were randomized to receive 10 or 30 µg/kg/dose of G-CSF or no growth factor (40). The duration of neutropenia was reduced from 27 days in the control group to 11 and 13 days in the G-CSF groups. Fewer days of febrile neutropenia were observed in the G-CSF groups (5 and 6 days) than in the controls (10 days). No significant effects of G-CSF on the number of days with fever, the use of intravenous antibiotics, and hospitalization were detected. Another phase III study showed the efficacy of recombinant GM-CSF in reducing the duration of neutropenia after ABMT for lymphoid malignancies (41). Median follow-up of 36 months demonstrated the middle-term safety of GM-CSF. No apparent deleterious effects on bone marrow function were observed. Moreover, disease-free survival and overall survival were similar on both treatment arms. A randomized study of erythropoietin and G-CSF versus placebo and G-CSF for patients with Hodgkin's disease and non-Hodgkin's lymphoma undergoing ABMT did not show a reduction in the total number of red blood cell and platelet transfusions with the combination of G-CSF and erythropoietin (42).

Initial phase I-II studies with recombinant interleukin-3 used with either GM-CSF or G-CSF are interesting (43,44). New cytokines in future clinical use may lead to even faster count recovery. It is unclear whether cytokines currently in use provide a significant improvement over PBSC support alone. Cytokine combinations used ex vivo might expand the stem cell pool for transplantation (45,46). They might help obviate the need for multiple apheresis and allow for repetitive cycles of dose intensive therapy. However, a greater understanding of the biology of ex vivo expansion and its precise utility is necessary before recommending it for general use.

VI. THERAPY AFTER RELAPSE FOLLOWING BMT

Most relapses occur in the first year following ABMT, mainly in previous disease sites, especially when involved field radiation treatment was not given (47). In relapsing patients, median time to relapse is less than year. Varterasian et al. (1995) reported on 26 patients who relapsed after ABMT or PSCT at Wayne State University (48). Median time from BMT to disease progression was 6 months and median survival 11 months for this cohort. Twenty-one of 26 relapses occurred in the first year. Six patients survived longer than 2 years after progression. Only three patients (12%) relapsed after 3 years posttransplant. Most patients received treatment after progression. These treatments included involved field radiation therapy, steroids, interferon, chemotherapy, or second ABMT. On multivariate analysis, only time from ABMT to progression was significantly correlated to postprogression survival.

Allogeneic transplantation is perhaps best reserved for patients who develop myelodysplastic syndromes. The high morbidity and mortality of alloBMT compared with ABMT obviously favors dose-intensive therapy and ABMT. The use of donor lymphocyte infusions (DLIs) may in fact afford a graft-versus-Hodgkin's disease effect without the toxicity of drugs such as busulfan, which has not been demonstrated to have activity in Hodgkin's disease, or of TBI, which has inadequate direct therapeutic benefit. The use of DLI, however, may be complicated by GVHD and pancytopenia. Its true efficacy is as yet unclear, but it probably warrants further study.

Three of six patients achieved a CR with yttrium-90–labeled antibodies (49). A more recent update of the same group included 44 patients (50). In five of these patients, polyclonal antiferritin failed to target the tumor. Thirty-nine patients received intravenous ^{90}Y-labeled antiferritin and ABMT. Ten patients achieved CR, 10 had PR, 2 were stable, and 17 had progressive disease. No patient produced antiantibodies, probably because of immunosuppression from Hodgkin's disease. The investigators speculate that the responses to this low-dose protein (2–5 mg) were due to radiation rather than the immunological effects of the antibody, and high-dose treatment with ABMT may not be required for tumor response.

Twelve patients were treated with ^{90}Y-labeled antiferritin and dose-intensive therapy (CBV) followed by ABMT (51). Four patients had procedure-related mortality. Four patients are alive more than 2 years following transplantation and three are free from disease progression. The 1-year progression-free survival is estimated at 21%. Yttrium-labeled antiferritin therapy is probably most useful in patients with minimal disease. Further studies combining antibodies and high-dose chemotherapy and also exploring antibody dose escalation are needed.

To improve survival after BMT, several investigators used different agents and methods to enhance the antitumor immune response. Interleukin (IL) with or without lymphokine-activated killer (LAK) cells was used post-BMT in both Hodgkin's disease and NHL (52). Actuarial probability of relapse at 4 years is 54%. One of the five Hodgkin's disease patients relapsed and another died in relapse at a median follow-up of 37 months. The other three patients were in continued CR. Further trials seem to be warranted. The use of IL-1 post-BMT may increase cytolytic function, but its impact on decreasing relapse rates is undetermined (53).

Interferon-α (IFN-α) was administered to 32 patients with lymphoma, 11 of whom had Hodgkin's disease (54). Six of these patients had refractory relapse. Patients were first given high-dose chemotherapy (CCV) followed by ABMT/PBSCT. IFN-α was started at 1×10^6 U/in^2 with escalating doses monthly following engraftment. The 36-month probability of survival and relapse-free survival was 42% and 14%, respectively, at a median follow-up of 18 months. There is a significant difference in overall survival estimates between the IFN-α group and the untreated group. Only three Hodgkin's disease patients received IFN-α in this study. These patients were able to tolerate IFN-α. Efficacy cannot be determined because of the small numbers. A randomized trial is needed to evaluate the role of IFN-α posttransplantation.

A complete response was observed in a patient with Hodgkin's disease in relapse after ABMT treated with interleukin-fusion toxin (DAB486 IL-2) (55). This targeting agent may have a role in the treatment of IL-2–expressing hematological malignancies like Hodgkin's disease, which needs to be studied further.

VII. LONG-TERM COMPLICATIONS

After a follow-up of 5 years, many investigators observed an increased incidence of myelo-dysplasia (MDS) and/or acute myelogenous leukemia (AML) in patients who underwent ABMT/PBSCT. Miller et al. reviewed 206 patients who underwent ABMT for Hodgkin's disease and NHL, of whom 9 developed MDS or secondary acute leukemia with 34 months median follow-up after BMT (56). In vitro bone marrow purging had no effect on the incidence of MDS, but projected MDS incidence is higher in patients who received PBSCs. All patients received radiation before the diagnosis of MDS. Darrington et al. reviewed patients with Hodgkin's lymphoma or NHL who underwent autologous stem cell transplantation at the University of Nebraska Medical Center (57). Twelve patients developed MDS or AML at a median follow-up of 44 months following ABMT/PBSCT. Age >40 years at transplant and TBI-containing conditioning were risk factors for developing MDS or AML in this group. Such a difference between TBI and a non–TBI-containing regimen was not reported in a prognostic factor analysis of 85 patients (30). The investigators felt that prior exposure to alkylating agents may be the most likely cause of MDS in these patients.

The incidence of other long-term complications of high-dose therapy in relapsed or refractory Hodgkin's disease is insufficiently reported. In particular, other secondary malignancies and cardiac, pulmonary, and endocrine chronic toxicity could be expected following ABMT. However, the follow-up of most reported studies might be too short for a definitive evaluation of these complications.

VIII. FUTURE DIRECTIONS

Future high-dose therapy with ABMT is now well established as a salvage treatment for recurrent Hodgkin's disease. The use of high-dose carmustine can be complicated by interstitial pneumonitis. Our experience shows that regimens without carmustine are associated with a high response and disease-free survival. Sequential ABMT for patients with refractory disease results in a progression-free survival equal to that of patients with sensitive disease receiving a single transplant. Transplant for high-risk Hodgkin's disease as part of initial therapy is a viable option, although results of the randomized study are not in as yet. Improvement in supportive care techniques has led to low mortality and reduced morbidity. The availability of PBSCs, the potential for ex vivo expansion, and cytokine support, among other advances, can facilitate the administration of multiple cycles of dose-intensive therapy. Methods such as immune modulation, DLI, and newer salvage regimens and dose-intensive regimens hold a potential for a better outcome for patients with high-risk relapsed or refractory Hodgkin's disease.

ACKNOWLEDGMENTS

The authors want to thank Paula Martin and Elsbeth Sofia for their accurate and efficient assistance in preparing the manuscript.

REFERENCES

1. DeVita VT, Simon RM, Hubbard SM, Young RC, Berard CW, Moxley JH, Frei E, Carbone PP, Canellos GP. Curability of advanced Hodgkin's disease with chemotherapy. Ann Intern Med 1980; 92:587–595.
2. Longo DL, Duffey PL, Young RC, Hubbard SM, Ihde DC, Glatstein E, Phares JC, Jaffe ES, Urba WJ, Devita VT. Conventional-dose salvage combination chemotherapy in patients relapsing with Hodgkin's disease after combination chemotherapy: the low probability for cure. J Clin Oncol 1992; 10:210–218.
3. Ferme C, Bastion Y, Lepage E, Berger F, Brice P, Morel P, Gabarre J, Nedellec G, Raman O, Cheron N. The MINE regimen as intensive salvage chemotherapy for relapsed and refractory Hodgkin's disease. Ann Oncol 1995; 6:543–549.
4. Brandwein JM, Callum J, Sutcliffe SB, Keating A. Evaluation of cytoreductive therapy prior to high dose treatment with autologous bone marrow transplantation in relapsed and refractory Hodgkin's disease. Bone Marrow Transplant 1990; 5:99–103.
5. Perren TJ, Selby PJ, Milan S, Meldrum M, McElwain TJ. Etoposide and adriamycin containing combination chemotherapy (HOPE-Bleo) for relapsed Hodgkin's disease. Br J Cancer 1990; 61:919–923.
6. Colwill R, Crump M, Couture F, Danish R, Stewart AK, Sutton DMC, Scott JG, Sutcliffe SB, Brandwein JM, Keating A. Mini-BEAM as salvage therapy for relapsed or refractory Hodgkin's disease before intensive therapy and autologous bone marrow transplantation. J Clin Oncol 1995; 13:396–402.
7. Ahmed T, Cook P, Feldman E, Coombe N, Puccio C, Mittelman A, Chun H, Coleman M, Helson L. Phase I-II trial of high dose ara-C, carboplatinum, etoposide and steroids in patients with refractory or relapsed lymphomas. Leukemia 1994; 8:531–534.
8. Appelbaum FR, Herzig GP, Ziegler JL, Graw RG, Levine ASS, Deisseroth AB. Successful engraftment of cryopreserved autologous bone marrow in patients with malignant lymphoma. Blood 1978; 52:85–95.
9. Jagannath S, Dicke KA, Armitage JO, Cabanillas F, Horwit LJ, Vellekoop L, Zander AR, Spitzer G. High-dose cyclophosphamide, carmustine, and etoposide and autologous bone marrow transplantation for relapsed Hodgkin's disease. Ann Intern Med 1986; 104:163–168.
10. Bierman PJ, Bagin PG, Jagannath S, Vost JM, Spitzer G, Kessinger A, Dickie KA, Armitage JO. High dose chemotherapy followed by autologous hematopoietic rescue in Hodgkin's disease: long term follow-up in 128 patients. Ann Oncol 1993; 4:767–773.
11. Carella A, Carlier P, Congiu A, Occhini D, Meloni G, Anselmo AP, Mandelli F, Mazza P, Tura S, Mangoni L. Nine years' experience with ABMT in 128 patients with Hodgkin's disease: an Italian study group report. Leukemia 1991; 5(suppl):1:68–71.
12. Wheeler C, Antin JH, Churchill WH, Come SE, Smith BR, Bubley GJ, Rosenthal DS, Rappaport JM, Ault KA, Schnipper LR, Eder JP. Cyclophosphamide, carmustine, and etoposide with autologous bone marrow transplantation in refractory Hodgkin's disease and non-Hodgkin's lymphoma: a dose-finding study. J Clin Oncol 1990; 8:648–656.
13. Chopra R, McMillan AK, Linch DC, Yuklea S, Tsaghipour G, Zpeascrce R, Patterson KG, Goldstone AH. The place of high-dose BEAM therapy and autologous bone marrow transplantation in poor-risk Hodgkin's disease. A single-center eight year study of 155 patients. Blood 1993; 81:1137–1145.
14. Ahmed T, Ciavarella D, Feldman E, Ascensao J, Hussain F, Engelking C, Gingrich S, Mittel

man A, Coleman M, Arlin Z. High-dose, potentially myeloablative chemotherapy and autologous bone marrow transplantation for patients with advanced Hodgkin's disease. Leukemia 1989; 3:19–22.

15. Reece D, Barnett MJ, Connors J, Fairey RN, Geer JP, Herzig GP, Herzig RH, Kingemann HG, O'Reilly SE, Shepherd JO, Spinelli JJ, Voss NJ, Wolff SN, Phillips G. Intensive chemotherapy with cyclophosphamide, BCNU and etoposide followed by autologous bone marrow transplantation for relapsed Hodgkin's disease. J Clin Oncol 1991; 9:1871–1879.

16. Ahmed T, Lake DE, Beer M, Feldman EJ, Preti RA, Seiter K, Helson K, Mittelman A, Kancherla R, Ascensao J, Akhtar T, Cook P, Goldberg R, Coleman M. Single and double autotransplants for relapsing/refractory Hodgkin's disease: results of two consecutive trials. Bone Marrow Transplant 1997; 19:449–454.

17. Phillips GL, Wolff SN, Herzig RH, Lazarus HM, Fay JW, Lin HS, Sinha DC, Glasgow GP, Griffith RC, Lamb CW, Herzig GP. Treatment of progressive Hodgkin's disease with intensive chemoradiotherapy and autologous bone marrow transplantation. Blood 1989; 7: 2086–2092.

18. Yahalom J, Gulati SC, Toia M, Maslak P, McCarron EG, O'Brien JP, Portlock CS, Straus DJ, Phillips J, Fuks Z. Accelerated hyperfractionated total-lymphoid irradiation, high-dose chemotherapy and autologous bone marrow transplantation for refractory and relapsing patients with Hodgkin's disease J Clin Oncol 1993; 11:1062–1070.

19. Kessinger A, Bierman PJ, Vose JM, Armitage JO. High-dose cyclophosphamide, carmustine, and etoposide followed by autologous peripheral stem cell transplantation for patients with relapsed Hodgkin's disease. Blood 1991; 77:2322–2325.

20. Jagannath S, Armitage JO, Dicke KA, Tucker SL, Velasquez WS, Smith K, Vaughan WP, Kessinger A, Horwitz LJ, Hagemeister FB, McLaughlin P, Cabanillas F, Spitzer G. Prognostic factors for response and survival after high-dose cyclophosphamide, carmustine and etoposide with autologous bone marrow transplantation for relapsed Hodgkin's disease J Clin Oncol 1989; 7:179–185.

21. Jones RJ, Piantadosi S, Mann RB, Ambinder RF, Seifter EJ, Vriensendrop HM, Abeloff MD, Bruns WH, May WS, Rowley SD, Vogelsang GB, Wagner JE, Wiley JM, Wingard JR, Yeager AM, Saral R, Santos GW. High-dose cytotoxic therapy and bone marrow transplantation for relapsed Hodgkin's disease. J Clin Oncol 1990; 8:527–537.

22. Rowlings PA. 1996 Summary slides show current use and outcome of blood and marrow transplantation. ABMTR Newsletter 1996; 3:6–12.

23. Carella AM, Carlier P, Congiu A, Occhini D, Nati S, Santini G, Pieluigi D, Giordano D, Bacigalupo A, Damasio E. Autologous bone marrow transplantation as adjuvant treatment for high risk Hodgkin's disease in first complete remission after MOPP/ABVD protocol. Bone Marrow Transplant 1991b; 8:99–103.

24. Fleury J, Legros M, Colombat P, Cure H, Travade P, Tortochaux J, Dionet C, Chollet P, Linassier C, Lamagnere JP, Blaise D, Viens P, Maraninchi D, Plagne R. High-dose therapy and autologous bone marrow transplantation in first complete or partial remission for poor prognosis Hodgkin's disease. Leuk Lymphoma 1996; 20:259–266.

25. Straus DJ, Gaynor JJ, Myers J, Merke DP, Caravelli J, Chapman D, Yahalom J, Clarkson BD. Prognostic factors among 185 adults with newly diagnosed advanced Hodgkin's disease treated with alternating potentially noncross-resistant chemotherapy and intermediate-dose radiation. J Clin Oncol 1990; 8:1173–1186.

26. Proctor SJ, Taylor P, Mackie MJ, Donnan P, Boys R, Lennard A, Prescott RJ. A numerical prognostic index for clinical use in identification of poor-risk patients with Hodgkin's disease at diagnosis. The Scotland and Newcastle Lymphoma Group (SNLG) Therapy Working Party. Leuk Lymphoma 1992; 7(suppl):17–20.

27. Moreau P, Fleury J, Bouabdallah R, Colombat AP, Brice P, Lioure D, Voillat L, Sandoun A, Francois S, Lamy T, Casasnovas O, Linassier C, Legros M, Milpied N, Bastion Y, Biron P, Andre M, Divine M, Ferme C, Jovet JP, Harousseau JL. Early intensive therapy with autolo-

gous stem cell transplantation (ASCT) in high-risk Hodgkin's disease. Report of 158 cases from the French Registry. Blood 1996; 88:486a.

28. Federico M, Clo V, Carella AM. High-dose therapy with autologous stem cell transplantation vs conventional therapy for patients with advanced Hodgkin's disease responding to first-line therapy: analysis of clinical characteristics of 51 patients enrolled in the HD01 protocol. EBMT/ANZLG/Intergroup HD01 trial. Leukemia 1996; 10:69–71.

29. Reece DE, Connors JM, Spinelli JJ, Barnett MJ, Fairey RN, Klingemann HG, Nantel SH, O'Reilly S, Shepherd JD, Sutherland HJ, Voss N, Chan KW, Phillips GL. Intensive therapy with cyclophosphamide, carmustine, etoposide ± cisplatin, and autologous bone marrow transplantation for Hodgkin's disease in first relapse after combination chemotherapy. Blood 1994; 83:1193–1199.

30. Nademanee A, O'Donnell MR, Snyder DS, Schmidt GM, Parker PM, Stein AS, Smith EP, Molina A, Stepan DE, Somlo G, Margolin KA, Sniecinski I, Dagis AC, Niland J, Pezner R, Forman SJ. High-dose chemotherapy with or without total body irradiation followed by autologous bone marrow and/or peripheral blood stem cell transplantation for patients with relapsed and refractory Hodgkin's disease: Results in 85 patients with analysis of prognostic factors. Blood 1995; 85:1381–1390.

31. Reece DE, Barnett MJ, Shepherd JD, Hogge DE, Klasa RJ, Nantel SH, Sutherland HJ, Klingemann HG, Fairey RN, Voss NJ, Connors JM, O'Reilley SE, Spineilli JJ, Philips GL. High-dose cyclophosphamide, carmustine (BCNU), and etoposide (VP16-213) with or without cisplatin (CBV ± P) and autologous transplantation for patients with Hodgkin's disease who fail to enter a complete remission after combination chemotherapy. Blood 1995; 86:451–456.

32. Jones RJ, Ambinder RF, Piantadosi S, Santos GW. Evidence of a graft-versus-lymphoma effect associated with allogenic bone marrow transplantation. Blood 1991; 77:649–663.

33. Anderson JE, Litzow MR, Appelbaum FR, Schoch G, Fisher LD, Buckner CD, Petersen FB, Crawford SW, Press OW, Sanders JE, Bensinger WI, Martin PJ, Storb R, Sullivan KM, Hansen JA, Thomas ED. Allogeneic, syngeneic, and autologous marrow transplantation for Hodgkin's disease: The 21-year Seattle experience. J Clin Oncol 1993; 11:2342–2350.

34. Milpied N, Fielding AK, Pearce RM, Ernst P, Goldstone AH. Allogeneic bone marrow transplant is not better than autologous transplant for patients with relapsed Hodgkin's disease. European Group for Blood and Bone Marrow Transplantation. J Clin Oncol 1996; 14:1291–1296.

35. Gajewski JL, Phillips GL, Sobocinski KA, Armitage JO, Gale RP, Champlin RE, Herzig RH, Hurd DD, Jagannagh S, Klein JP, Lazarus HM, McCarthy PL, Pasvolvsky S, Petersen FB, Rowlings PA. Bone marrow transplants from HLA-identical siblings in advanced Hodgkin's disease. J Clin Oncol 1996; 14:572–578.

36. Ahmed T, Wuest D, Ciavarella D. Peripheral blood stem cell mobilization by cytokines. J Clin Apheresis 1992; 7:129–131.

37. Kessinger A, Bierman PJ, Vose JM, Armitage JO. High-dose cyclophosphamide, carmustine and etoposide followed by autologous peripheral stem cell transplantation for patients with relapsed Hodgkin's disease. Blood 1991; 77:2322–2325.

38. Schmitz N, Linch DC, Dreger P, Goldstone AH, Boogaerts MA, Ferrant A, Demuynck HM, Link H, Zasnder AS, Barge AS, Borkett K. Randomised trial of filgrastim-mobilized peripheral blood progenitor cell transplantation versus autologous bone-marrow transplantation in lymphoma patients. Lancet 1996; 347:353–357.

39. Goldberg SL, Mangan KF, Klumpff TR. Complications of peripheral blood stem cell harvesting: review of 554 PBSC leukaphereses. J Hematothera 1995; 4:85–90.

40. Schmitz N, Dreger P, Zander AR, Ehinger G, Wandt H, Fauser AA, Holb HJ, Zumsprekel A, Martin A, Hecht T. Results of a randomised, controlled, multicentre study of recombinant human granulocyte colony-stimulating factor (filgrastim) in patients with Hodgkin's disease and non-Hodgkin's lymphoma undergoing autologous bone marrow transplantation. Bone Marrow Transplant 1995; 15:261–266.

41. Rabinowe SN, Neuberg D, Bierman PJ, Vose JM, Nemunaitis J, Singer JW, Freedman AS, Demetri G, Onetto N. Long-term follow-up of a phase III study of recombinant human granulocyte-macrophage colony-stimulating factor after autologous bone marrow transplantation for lymphoid malignancies. Blood 1993; 81:1903–1908.

42. Chao NJ, Schriber JR, Long GD, Negrin RS, Castolico M, Brown BW, Miller LL, Blume KG. A randomized study of erythropoietin and granulocyte colony-stimulating factor (G-CSF) versus placebo and G-CSF for patients with Hodgkin's and non-Hodgkin's lymphoma undergoing autologous bone marrow transplantation. Blood 1994; 83:2823–2828.

43. Fay JW, Lazarus H, Herzig R, Saez R, Stevens DA, Collins JRH, Pineiro LA, Cooper BW, Dicesare J, Campion M, Felser JM, Herzig G, Bernstein H. Sequential administration of recombinant human interleukin-3 and granulocyte-macrophage colony-stimulating factor after autologous bone marrow transplantation for malignant lymphoma: a phase I/II multicenter study. Blood 1994; 84:2151–2157.

44. Vose JM, Bierman PJ, Weisenburger DD, Armitage JO. The importance of early autologous bone marrow transplantation (ABMT) in the management of patients (pts) with Hodgkin's disease (HD). Proc Am Soc Clin Oncol 1990; 9:256a.

45. Henschler R, Brugger W, Luft T, Frey T, Mertelsmann R, Kanz L. Maintenance of transplantation potential in ex vivo expanded CD34+ selected human peripheral blood progenitor cells. Blood 1996; 84:2988–2903.

46. Bertolini F, Soligo D, Lazzari L, Corsini C, Servida F, Sirchia G. The effect of interleukin-12 in ex-vivo expansion of human haemopoietic progenitors. Br J Haematol 1995; 90:935–938.

47. Mundt AJ, Sibley G, Williams S, Hallahan D, Nautiyal J, Weischselbaum RR. Patterns of failure following high-dose chemotherapy and autologous bone marrow transplantation with involved field radiotherapy for relapsed/refractory Hodgkin's disease. Int J Radiat Oncol Biol Phys 1995; 33:261–270.

48. Varterasian M, Ratanatharathorn V, Uberti JP, Karnes C, Abella E, Momin F, Kasten-Sportes C, Al-Katib A, Lum L, Heilbrun L, Sensenbrenner LL. Clinical course and outcome of patients with Hodgkin's disease who progress after autologous transplantation. Leuk Lymphoma 1995; 20:59–65.

49. Vriesendorp HM, Herpst JM, Leichner PK, Klein JL, Order SE. Polyclonal ^{90}yttrium labeled antiferritin for refractory Hodgkin's disease. Int J Radiat Oncol Biol Phys 1989; 17:815–821.

50. Herpst JM, Klein PK, Quadri SM, Vriesendorp HM. Survival of patients with resistant Hodgkin's disease after polyclonal yttrium 90–labeled antiferritin treatment. J Clin Oncol 1995; 13:2394–2400.

51. Bierman PJ, Vose JM, Leichner PK, Quadri SM, Armitage JO, Klein JL, Abrams RA, Dicke KA, Vriesendrop HM. Yttrium 90–labeled antiferritin followed by high dose chemotherapy and autologous bone marrow transplantation for poor-prognosis Hodgkin's disease. J Clin Oncol 1993; 11:698–703.

52. Benyunes MC, Higuchi C, York A, Lindgren C, Thompson JA, Buckner CD, Fefer A. Immunotherapy with interleukin 2 with or without lymphokine-activated killer cells after autologous bone marrow transplantation for malignant lymphoma: a feasibility trial. Bone Marrow Transplant. 1995; 16:282–288.

53. Katsanis E, Weisdorf E, Xu Z, Dancisak BB, Halet ML, Blazar BR. Infusions of interleukin-alfa after autologous transplantation for Hodgkin's disease and non-Hodgkin's lymphoma induce effector cells with antilymphoma cytolytic activity. J Clin Immunol 1994; 14:205–211.

54. Schenkein DP, Dixon P, Desforges JF, Berkman OE, Erban JK, Ascensao JL, Miller KB. Phase I/II study of cyclophosphamide, carboplatin, and etoposide and autologous hematopoietic stem-cell transplantation with posttransplant interferon alfa-2b for patients with lymphoma and Hodgkin's disease. J Clin Oncol 1994; 12:2423–2431.

55. Tepler I, Schwartz G, Parker K, Charette J, Kadin ME, Woodworth TG, Schnipper LE. Phase I trial of an interleukin-2 fusion toxin (DAB486IL-2) in hematologic malignancies: complete

response in a patient with Hodgkin's disease refractory to chemotherapy. Cancer 1994; 73: 1276–1285.

56. Miller JS, Arthur DC, Litz CE, Neglia JP, Miller WJ, Weisdorf DJ. Myelodysplastic syndrome after autologous bone marrow transplantation: an additional late complication of curative cancer therapy. Blood 1994; 83:780–786.

57. Darrington DL, Vose JM, Anderson JR, Bierman PJ, Bishop MR, Chan WC, Morris ME, Reed C, Sanger WAG, Tarantolo SR. Incidence and characterization of secondary myelodysplastic syndrome and acute myelogenous leukemia following high-dose chemoradiotherapy and autologous stem-cell transplantation for lymphoid malignancies. J Clin Oncol 1994; 12:2527–2534.

58. O'Brien ME, Milan S, Cunningham D, Jones AL, Nicolson M, Selby P, Hickish T, Hill M, Gore ME, Viner C. High-dose chemotherapy and autologous bone marrow transplant in relapsed Hodgkin's disease—a pragmatic prognostic index. Br J Cancer 1996; 73:1271–1277.

59. Crump M, Smith AM, Brandwein J, Couture F, Sherret H, Sutton D, Scott JG, McCrae J, Murray C, Pantalony D, Sutcliffe SB, Keating A. High-dose etoposide and melphalan, and autologous bone marrow transplantation for patients with advanced Hodgkin's disease: importance of disease status at transplant. J Clin Oncol 1993; 11:704–711.

60. Burns LJ, Daniels KA, McGlave PB, Miller WJ, Ramsay NKC, Kersey JH, Weisdorf DJ. Autologous stem cell transplantation for refractory and relapsed Hodgkin's disease: factors predictive of prolonged survival. Bone Marrow Transplant. 1995; 16:13–18.

61. Snyder MJ, Johnson DB, Daly MB, Giguere JK, Hasrman GH, Harden EA, Johnson RA, Leff RS, Mercier RJ, Messerschmidt GL. Carmustine, Ara C, cyclophosphamide and etoposide with autologous bone marrow transplantation in relapsed or refractory lymphoma: a dose-finding study. Bone Marrow Transplant. 1994; 14:595–600.

62. Seymour LK, Dansey RD, Bezwoda WR. Single high-dose etoposide and melphalan with non-cryopreserved autologous marrow rescue as primary therapy for relapsed, refractory and poor-prognosis Hodgkin's disease. Br J Cancer 1994; 70:526–530.

63. Gianni AM, Siena S, Bregni M, Lombardi F, Gandola L, Di-Nicola M, Magni M, Peccatori F, Valagussa P, Bonadonna G. High-dose sequential chemo-radiotherapy with peripheral blood progenitor cell support for relapsed or refractory Hodgkin's disease—a 6-year update. Ann Oncol 1993; 4:889–891.

64. Vose JM, Anderson JE, Bierman PJ, Appelbaum FR, Anderson JR, Garrison L, Lebsack ME, Armitago JO. Phase ITT trial of PIXY321 to enhance engraftment following autologous bone marrow transplantation for lymphoid malignancy. J Clin Oncol 1996 14:520–526.

65. Horning SJ, Chao NJ, Negrin RS, Hoppe RT, Kwak LW, Long GD, Stallbaum B, O'Connor P, Blume KG. High-dose therapy and autologous hematopoietic progenitor cell transplantation for recurrent or refractory Hodgkin's disease: analysis of the Stanford University results and prognostic indices. Blood 1997; 89:801–813.

29

Stem Cell Transplantation for Multiple Myeloma—10 Years Later

DAVID S. SIEGEL, SEAH H. LIM, GUIDO TRICOT, K.R. DESIKAN,
A. FASSAS, JAYESH MEHTA, SEEMA SINGHAL, ELIAS ANAISSIE,
SUNDAR JAGANNATH, and BARTHEL BARLOGIE

University of Arkansas for Medical Sciences, Little Rock, Arkansas

I. INTRODUCTION

Multiple myeloma (MM) is the most aggressive member in the spectrum of diseases called plasma cell dyscrasias. It is characterized by the accumulation of large numbers of clonal, transformed plasma cells. Patients suffer from the consequences of (1) local tumor infiltration and destruction; (2) abnormal cytokine production with anemia, hypercalcemia, bone destruction, and suppression of normal immunoglobulin production; (3) monoclonal immunoglobulin production which can be associated with deposition diseases (light chain cast nephropathy, amyloid, light chain deposition disease), hyperviscosity, coagulopathies, and occasionally autoimmune phenomena; and (4) renal failure. In the United States, multiple myeloma occurs with a frequency of approximately 1% of all malignancies and 10% of all hematological malignancies. The median age at diagnosis is between 65 and 70 years (1).

A. Treatment with Standard-Dose Chemotherapy

Three decades ago, the combination of melphalan and prednisone (MP) was first introduced for the treatment of patients with multiple myeloma (2). The subsequent 30 years of experience have shown MP to provide symptomatic relief and short-term disease control in approximately 50% of patients (3). This regimen has remained the mainstay of myeloma therapy (4).

There have been clinical trials involving many thousands of patients comparing

MP to combination chemotherapy. Investigators added cyclophosphamide and vincristine (VMCP), among other agents, to MP (5). The dose intensity of corticosteroids was examined. VAD chemotherapy introduced by Barlogie and his colleagues at the M.D. Anderson Cancer Center utilized vincristine, doxorubicin, and high-dose dexamethasone, a potent inducer of apoptosis in plasma cells (6). These studies established that adding other agents and increasing the dose of glucocorticosteroids could significantly improve the rapidity and degree of response. Although combinations such as VAD and VMCP produced a significantly higher response rate, they did not lead to any significant survival advantage over the original MP. Median survival remained less than 3 years, and <5% of patients were alive 10 years after diagnosis (7–9).

The most important conclusion resulting from this generation of studies was that, although a marginal increase in dose intensity does result in improved response rates, this has not translated into a substantially improved outcome. However, a meta-analysis that included most of the large-scale, standard-dose, clinical trials done prior to the 1990s demonstrated a survival advantage for patients receiving greater dose intensity of corticosteroids and alkylating agents (10). A subsequent study conducted by the Southwest Oncology Group (SWOG) and involved over 500 patients confirmed a modest survival advantage in those receiving higher doses of glucocorticoids (11), but the difference in mean survival was marginal. The low-dose corticosteroid arm had a median overall survival (OS) of 31 months, the two higher dose corticosteroid arms had median OS of 35 and 40 months.

The other important concept was the establishment of prognostic factors relevant to the outcome of patients with multiple myeloma. The most important of these have been β_2-microglobulin (β_2M) as an indicator of tumor mass and renal function, C-reactive protein (CRP) as a surrogate marker of interleukin-6 (IL-6) activity, and a plasma cell labeling index (PCLI) as a measurement of the proliferative capacity (4,12–16). Using standard chemotherapy, patients with low β_2M (<6 g/L) and a low PCLI (<2%) were shown to have a median survival of 71 months, those with only a single favorable variable had a median survival of 40 months, whereas the median survival was only 16 months in the absence of any favorable variables (4). Similarly, using the combination of β_2M (<6 mg/L) and CRP (<6 mg/L), median survival was 54 months for the good-risk group (low β_2M *and* CRP), 27 months for the intermediate-risk group (low β_2M *or* CRP), and only 6 months for those in the high-risk group (neither low β_2M *nor* low CRP) (12).

B. Dose Escalation for MM

One of the seminal observations made by McElwain and colleagues was that high-dose intravenous melphalan at 140 mg/m^2 (MEL140), without growth factor or stem cell support, induced complete responses in MM patients with high-risk and advanced drug refractory disease (17). This report was followed by a series of studies using high-dose melphalan without stem cell support in patients with both newly diagnosed and refractory disease (18–21). One hundred and thirty-eight patients were included in these studies. Treatment-related mortality was approximately 15%. This treatment was associated with prolonged neutropenia of 25–30 days and thrombocytopenia of 30–35 days (Table 1). For patients treated with refractory disease, the complete remission (CR) rate was only about 10%; the median event-free survival (EFS) and OS rates were correspondingly disappointing at 5 and 8 months, respectively. In contrast, 35% of previously untreated patients achieved CR, with an EFS and OS of 17 and 45 months, respectively. Most remarkably, 5% of

Table 1 High-Dose Melphalan Without Autotransplants

Type of Diseases	N	%ED	%CR	%≥PR	EFS	OS
Refractory						
Vesole et al. (21)	47	19	6	40	5	7
Selby et al. (20)	15	13	13	66	6	10
Newly Diagnosed						
Cunningham et al. (18)	63	14	32	82	18	47
Lokhorst et al. (19)	13	15	46	85	16	41+

ED, early death; CR, complete remission; PR, partial remission; EFS, event-free survival; OS, overall survival.

patients in these studies remained in CR for 5 years after high-dose therapy with no further treatment.

The addition of growth factor support to the original MEL140 regimen substantially decreased the duration of aplasia associated with high-dose melphalan (22,23). Despite this, the duration of neutropenia (granulocytes <500/µL) was approximately 25 days and of thrombocytopenia (platelets <50,000/µL) was approximately 35 days.

II. AUTOTRANSPLANT FOR MM

The significant morbidity and mortality associated with the prolonged aplasia in earlier studies with high-dose melphalan led to the next generation of therapies using stem cell support and further escalation of dose intensity. The first published efforts utilized MEL140 with autologous bone marrow stem cell support (24). The duration of cytopenia was decreased to 2–3 weeks and the morbidity associated with chemotherapy correspondingly improved. Peripheral blood stem cells, initially collected in steady state (25), followed by peripheral blood stem cells mobilized with high-dose chemotherapy and hematopoietic growth factors (26), and finally peripheral blood stem cells collected with growth factor alone (27), reduced the duration of aplasia to less than 1 week and the transplant-related mortality to less than 5% (28–31). This treatment-related mortality rate is not significantly different from the 2–10% seen in most standard-dose chemotherapy trials (32–34).

The improved safety profile associated with stem cell support led to trials in previously untreated MM patients and to further dose escalation. The first truly myeloablative conditioning regimens utilized in the autotransplant setting added total body irradiation (TBI) to the original MEL140 (35). In other studies, the dose of melphalan was pushed to 200 mg/m² (MEL200) (21). The results of some of the larger studies can be seen in Table 2. Many critical observations came out of these studies: (1) CR rates and EFS were significantly higher than those observed with conventional therapy in the untreated population, proving the dose-response concept in myeloma (35,36); and (2) in patients with refractory disease, there was a significantly higher EFS (37 vs 17 months) and OS (43 vs 21 months) in patients with primary refractory disease or relapsed disease (21). Subsequently the concept of tandem autotransplants was introduced, using two cycles of MEL200 (21,30). An analysis of the data from the University of Arkansas showed an improvement in EFS and OS as the dose intensity was increased from nonmyeloablative doses of melphalan to a single transplant with MEL200 and subsequently to tandem transplants (Fig. 1) without any increase in transplant-related mortality.

Table 2 Autotransplants in Multiple Myeloma

Type of disease	Type of transplant	N	%ED	%CR	EFS (mos)	OS (mos)	AGC >0.5 × 10⁹/L (days)	Plt >50 × 10⁹/L (days)
Refractory								
Vesole et al. (21)	ABMT	21	24	10	8	16	23	34
Vesole et al. (21)	PBSC	67	1	12	21	43+	14	18
Newly Diagnosed								
Cunningham et al. (36)	ABMT	53	2	75	20+	54+	19	24[b]
Harousseau et al.[a] (37)	ABMT/PBSC	133	4	27	33	46	17	23[c]

ED, early death; CR, complete remission; EFS, event-free survival; OS, overall survival; AGC, absolute granulocyte count; Plt, platelet; ABMT, autologous bone marrow transplant; PBSC, peripheral blood stem cell.
[a] Patients were initially treated with standard chemotherapy or high dose melphalan.
[b] Days to recover platelets ≥ 25 × 10⁹/L.
[c] Days to recover platelets ≥ 25 × 10⁹/L.

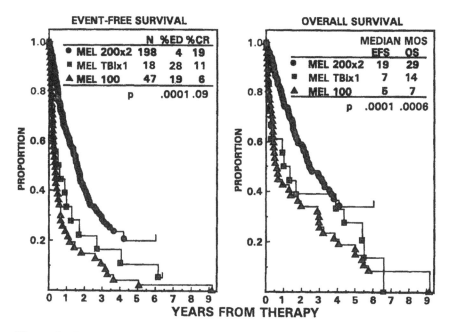

Figure 1 Improved outcome in refractory myeloma with greater dose intensity. Note that treatment-related mortality within 60 days is only 4% with double transplants. Marked prolongation in EFS and OS was observed as regimen intensity increased from melphalan 100 mg/m² (MEL100) to melphalan 140 mg/m² + TBI 850 cGy (MEL/TBI ×1) to two cycles of high-dose therapy with melphalan 200 mg/m² (MEL200 × 2).

These studies clearly established that high-dose therapy could overcome drug resistance in patients relapsing after or refractory to standard dose therapy and could produce significantly higher CR rates in newly diagnosed patients. What still remained to be answered was whether the higher CR rates in newly diagnosed patients translated into improved disease-free and overall survival. In the French Myeloma Intergroup (IFM) study (37), patients initially received 4 months of VMCP alternating with VBAP chemotherapy. Patients were then randomized to autotransplantation using MEL140 plus low-dose TBI (800 cGy) versus eight additional cycles of VMCP/VBAP. This study showed significant advantage for patients who received myeloablative consolidation. EFS and OS at 5 years were 28 and 52%, respectively, for the high-dose group and 10 and 12% for the conventional arm. Although further phase III work is ongoing, and much needs to be learned about the timing of high-dose therapy, its advantage finally appears to be clearly established.

The largest autologous experience in newly diagnosed MM patients has been obtained at the University of Arkansas. The Total Therapy program that started in 1990 employed tandem transplantation for newly diagnosed MM patients. Eligibility criteria stipulated that patients be under the age of 70 years, had received no or at the most one cycle of standard therapy, and that they have adequate pulmonary and cardiac function. Patients with renal failure were eligible but were dropped from the study if their creatinine did not improve to ≤ 2 mg/dL by the time they were scheduled to receive high-dose cyclophosphamide (HDCTX) for peripheral blood stem cell (PBSC) mobilization. Patients

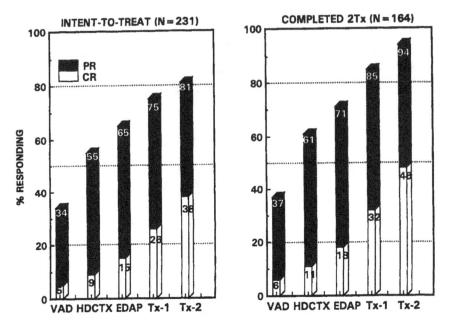

Figure 2   Marked increase in the incidence of partial remission (PR) and complete remission (CR) as patients proceed through the different phases of Total Therapy, consisting of remission induction with mutually non–cross-resistant regimens (VAD; high-dose cyclophosphamide, HDCTX; etoposide-dexamethasone-ara-C-cisplatin, EDAP) and two transplants.

initially received three cycles of VAD (6) chemotherapy. This was chosen because of its well-established high rate and speed of response without inflicting hematopoietic stem cell damage. Patients then proceeded to receive HDCTX (6 g/m^2) with granulocyte-macrophage colony-stimulating factor (GM-CSF) support for PBSC mobilization. Subsequent to adequate stem cell collection, patients received one cycle of etoposide, dexamethasone, cytarabine, and cisplatin (EDAP) (38) targeting the more immature, plasmablastic compartment that probably exists in all MM patients even at diagnosis (39). After this induction phase with non–cross-resistant active agents, patients received tandem transplants using MEL200 as the conditioning regimen. These transplants were administered 3–6 months apart in order to limit toxicity. Patients who did not achieve and maintain at least a partial response (PR) after their first transplant received a second transplant with MEL-TBI or MEL-CTX. On completion of tandem transplant, maintenance therapy with interferon-α was offered to all patients. Two hundred and thirty-one patients were enrolled in this study. Despite the rigorous nature of the treatment program, 84% completed one transplant and 71% completed both. Of the 164 patients who completed two transplants, the PR and CR rates were 94 and 48% respectively. For all patients entered in the study, these rates were 81 and 38% (Fig. 2). Median EFS and OS for the patients in the study were 43 and 62 months with a median duration of CR of 54 months (Fig. 3). A pair-mate analysis of previously untreated patients enrolled in this study comparing them to a group of patients treated on Southwest Oncology Group conventional dose chemotherapy trials demonstrated dramatically and statistically significant EFS and OS advantages for patients receiving Total Therapy (40).

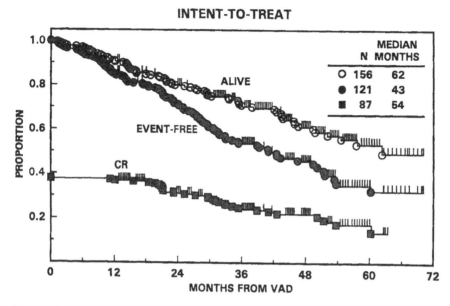

Figure 3 Kaplan-Meier plots of event-free and overall survival as well as CR duration for patients receiving Total Therapy.

III. PROGNOSTIC FACTORS IN AUTOTRANSPLANTATION

A. Mobilization Phase

There has been a highly significant correlation between the number of CD34$^+$ cells infused and prompt recovery of both granulocytes and platelets. The Arkansas data showed no difference in patients receiving PBSCs alone versus those receiving PBSCs and autologous marrow (41). The median time to granulocyte ($>0.5 \times 10^9$/L) and platelet ($>50 \times 10^9$/L) recovery was comparable following first and second transplant. The length of standard alkylating agent therapy prior to stem cell collection had a highly significant prognostic value. Patients with a longer prior exposure to standard-dose alkylating agents showed significantly delayed engraftment. This was true even in patients with ≤6 months of treatment. The "threshold" dose of CD34$^+$ cells required for prompt hematopoietic recovery was ≥2 $\times$ 10^6/kg and ≥5 $\times$ 10^6/kg in patients with ≤24 months and >24 months of prior therapy, respectively. Adequate numbers of CD34$^+$ cells could be collected in the vast majority of patients with ≤24 months of prior therapy (91%), whereas only 28% of patients >24 months of prior therapy had threshold numbers of cells collected.

Since many MM patients still present for PBSC mobilization after having been heavily pretreated, the need for high-dose chemotherapy as part of the mobilization regimen is a significant issue. High-dose cyclophosphamide therapy is associated with significant morbidity owing to prolonged aplasia and has only modest antimyeloma activity in heavily pretreated patients. We have examined the need for high-dose cyclophosphamide in mobilization in a randomized study of 44 patients (42). Half of the patients received G-CSF alone and half CTX plus G-CSF for mobilization. Although the number of CD34$^+$ cells recovered were significantly higher in the HDCTX arm, engraftment kinetics and toxicities posttransplant were similar.

Table 3 Patient Characteristics
(N = 427)

Parameter	%
Age > 50 years	53
CRP > 4.0 mg/L	48
Stage III at diagnosis	48
> 12 Months of prior therapy	47
β_2-microglobin > 2.5 mg/L	45
Refractory disease	39
IgA isotype	18
Creatinine > 2.0 mg/dL	5

Attempts to optimize PBSC collection in this heavily pretreated population have included a randomized trial of G-CSF alone versus G-CSF plus recombinant human stem cell factor (SCF). Preliminary result (43) has shown significantly better stem cell recoveries in the arm receiving SCF plus G-CSF. The median total CD34$^+$ cells/kg recovered was 3.2×10^6 in the G-CSF arm versus 7.0×10^6 in the G-CSF plus SCF arm. Whether this will result in differences in engraftment kinetics remains to be seen.

B. Pretransplant Characteristics

We have recently analyzed 427 patients (all with at least 1 year of follow-up and treated in Arkansas) to identify prognostic variables for patients undergoing tandem transplants. The characteristics for this population are summarized in Table 3. Multivariate analysis identified the absence of "unfavourable cytogenetics" (any translocation and/or abnormalities of 11q or 13q (44,45), low β_2M ($\leq$ 2.5 mg/L), less than 1 year of prior therapy, and low CRP ($\leq$ 4 mg/L) as independent prognosticators predicting improved EFS and OS (Table 4). An increased risk of early death was significantly higher in patients with elevated LDH (8 vs 2%), in patients with primary refractory myeloma (5 vs 1%) and in patients over the age of 50 years (4 vs 1%) (46).

Table 4 Multivariate Analysis (N = 542) with Cytogenetics

EFS	P	OS	P
No "unfavorable" karyotype	.0001	No "unfavorable" karyotype	.0001
$\leq$ 12 mos. of prior therapy	.0001	β_2-microglobin $\leq$ 2.5 mg/L	.0001
β_2-microglobin $\leq$ 2.5 mg/L	.0001	Sensitive disease	.0002
CRP $\leq$ 4.0 mg/L	.0009	CRP $\leq$ 4.0 mg/L	.003
LDH $\leq$ 190 U/L	.005	LDH $\leq$ 190 U/L	.004
Sensitive disease	.01	$\leq$ 12 mos. of prior therapy	.02
Stage <III at diagnosis	.04	Non-IgA isotype	.2
Non-IgA isotype	.07	Albumin > 3.5 g%	.3

EFS, event-free survival; OS, overall survival.

IV. HIGH-DOSE THERAPY IN PATIENTS WITH RENAL FAILURE AND ADVANCED AGE

Most clinical trials for MM have not included patients over the age of 65 years or with creatinine levels over 2 mg/dL. Pharmacokinetic studies have demonstrated a similar melphalan clearance for patients with and without normal renal function (47). We have recently reviewed our pilot experience utilizing high-dose melphalan in 23 patients with a creatinine >2 mg/dL at the time of the first transplant (48). Seven of these patients were hemodialysis dependent. Pair-mate analysis showed that early mortality, engraftment kinetics, and response rates were equivalent in the two populations. Ten of the 23 patients treated had improvement in their creatinine to ≤ 1.2 mg/dL. Patients with renal insufficiency did experience more severe and longer lasting mucositis, febrile episodes, and anorexia.

A recent pair-mate analysis of patients treated with high-dose melphalan over the age of 65 years (the oldest patient was 83 years of age) showed that the regimen was well tolerated. The quantity of CD34$^+$ cells/kg mobilized and the engraftment kinetics posttransplantation were similar and that EFS and OS were identical (49,50).

V. TUMOR CELL CONTAMINATION OF THE GRAFT

One of the most obvious issues in autologous transplantation for MM is whether tumor cell contamination of the graft is relevant for relapse. Most of the early studies with high-dose therapy for MM, particularly those carried out in relapsed and refractory patients, did not yield clinical complete remissions in more than a small fraction of patients. In this situation, the tumor load remaining in the body after transplant is at least 10^9 clonal cells. Therefore, most relapses were not related to the 10^7 or 10^8 tumor cells reinfused with most grafts but to the insensitivity of endogenous tumor cells to the myeloablative regimen. With the increased aggressiveness with which myeloma is now approached, that is, tandem transplants and transplantation as part of the initial treatment plan, clinical CRs can be achieved in close to half of newly diagnosed patients. In this situation, potential contamination of the graft becomes a much more critical issue.

There has been substantial data showing that PBSCs mobilized with either high-dose chemotherapy and/or hematopoietic growth factors are contaminated with cells clonally related to the myelomatous plasma cells. These cells have been identified morphologically (51,52), by immunoglobulin gene fingerprinting (53–55), and by polymerase chain reaction (PCR) for patient-specific sequences in the immunoglobulin hypervariable regions (56–58). The percentage of circulating clonal cells has varied between <0.01 and >10.0%; being between 0.1 and 1.0% clonal cells in most patients. Since 2–5 × 10^{10} PBSCs are usually infused per transplant, most patients will be receiving between 10^7 and 10^8 clonal cells, so that they may conceivably be a cause of posttransplant relapse.

The fact that a fraction of MM patients undergoing syngeneic transplants will be long-term disease-free survivors (59–61) implies that some patients have disease sensitive enough to be eradicated by currently available conditioning regimens. If this is the case, then purging of the graft may increase the chance of cure and/or prolong remission in a minority of MM patients who have exceptionally chemosensitive disease.

There are two basic approaches to minimize tumor cell contamination of the graft. The first is negative selection. One method to remove contaminating tumor cells is to expose the graft to chemotherapy ex vivo. The activated cyclophosphamide analog 4-hydroperoxycyclophosphamide (4-HC) has been used for this purpose but has resulted in a substantial delay in hematopoietic recovery (62). The other major negative selection approach has been the use of monoclonal antibodies directed at cell surface markers found on the malignant population. At the Dana-Farber Cancer Center, Boston, MA, a cocktail of monoclonal antibodies has been used to purge the marrow autografts (63,64). This cocktail is composed of antibodies against CALLA (CD10), PCA-1, and CD20. Patients were only eligible for this regimen if marrow plasmacytosis could be reduced to <10% by standard chemotherapy. Eleven of 36 patients treated in this fashion remained in continuous CR at 16 months posttransplant. Engraftment was somewhat delayed with median recovery of granulocytes to $>0.5 \times 10^9$/L and platelets to $>20 \times 10^9$/L at 21 and 23 days, respectively.

The second purging strategy emphasizes positive selection of hematopoietic stem cells. The more widely utilized technology is based on the immobilization of monoclonal antibodies to a solid matrix. A number of such strategies have been developed. These have included immobilization of cells via biotinylated anti-CD34 monoclonal antibody and passage through avidin-conjugated columns, the anti-CD34 monoclonal antibody being conjugated to either immunomagnetic beads or to tissue culture flasks. Schiller and colleagues (65) reported on 37 MM patients transplanted with CD34$^+$ cells collected using the biotin/avidin column. Using PCR to detect patient-specific hypervariable region sequences, five of eight with detectable contamination in the product prior to processing were purged to undetectable levels. Overall, a greater than 2.7- to 4.5-log reduction in the number of contaminating clonal cells was achieved. Median time to platelet ($>20 \times 10^9$/L) and neutrophil ($>0.5 \times 10^9$/L) was 12 days.

An alternative strategy utilized in Arkansas is based on high-speed cell sorting (66). PBSC products were subjected to clinical-scale high-speed cell sorting for CD34$^+$Thy$^+$Lin$^-$ phenotype. PCR for hypervariable region determinants sensitive to 1 in 10^5 cells has shown that grafts can consistently be purged to negativity. With approximately 10 patients having received such a product, trilineage hematopoiesis was successfully demonstrated, although somewhat delayed.

VI. POSTTRANSPLANT RELAPSE

Salvage chemotherapy after high-dose therapy is often felt to be futile. Physicians and patients alike often perceive transplantation as the final intervention. We have recently examined the outcome in patients with recurrent or progressive disease postautotransplant. One hundred and five of these patients relapsed after a single transplant and 91 after tandem transplants. Of the total 196 patients, 49 proceeded directly with high-dose therapy and transplantation and 147 received standard chemotherapy as initial therapy. The transplant-related mortality was 10%. CRs were achieved in 8% of patients. Overall, postsalvage EFS and OS were 8 and 14 months, respectively. Multivariate analysis showed that EFS and OS were significantly longer in patients with transplant as primary salvage and with a presalvage β_2M $\leq$ 2.5 mg/L. For the 25 of 196 patients with both favorable features, the CR rate was 32% and EFS/OS were 64+/64+ months. When patients with one (n = 105) and two (n = 91) prior transplants were examined separately, primary transplant and low β_2M were found to be the most important features. EFS and OS were substantially longer in the group with these two favorable variables (EFS of 64+ vs 9 months, P = .0001 and OS of 64+ vs 11 months, P = .0001) (67). For patients who relapsed after tandem transplant, late relapse (>12 months) and low β_2M at relapse predicted for better survival with EFS of 8 versus 5 months ($P = .05$) and OS of 15 versus 9 months ($P = .0003$).

The combination of dexamethasone, cyclophosphamide, etoposide,and cis-platinum (DCEP) has become our routine standard dose chemotherapy regimen for posttransplant relapses. A recent review (68) of 51 such patients treated with this combination has demonstrated a CR rate of 10% and PR (>75% reduction in paraprotein and resolution of marrow plasmacytosis) rate of 41%. There were only two (4%) treatment-related deaths. Thus, patients who relapse following transplant should not a priori be excluded from further therapy. Patients relapsing after single transplants can often be salvaged with further high-dose therapy, especially if they have a low β_2M at relapse. It should therefore be part of the initial stem cell collection plan to have enough stem cells for at least three transplants. In those selected patients who relapse after tandem transplant, further therapy can be expected to salvage a significant proportion, although response duration is limited in the majority of these patients.

VII. MDS/AML POSTAUTOTRANSPLANT

One of the major concerns in long-term survivors of alkylating agent–based standard chemotherapy is the development of myelodysplastic syndrome (MDS) and acute myelogenous leukemia (AML). Most of the relevant data come from experience with lymphoma treatment (69). This is perhaps an even more important concern in myeloma, where most standard therapies are based on very protracted use of the most stem cell–damaging alkylating agents such as melphalan and BCNU. However, since high-dose melphalan with or without TBI is the most widely used conditioning regimen for autologous transplantation in myeloma, it is possible that the preparative regimen with alkylating agents itself may be leukemogenic. To answer this question, the Arkansas group has compared the incidence of these disorders in a group of 71 patients enrolled in the Total Therapy program, which limits alkylating agent use prior to mobilization, with 117 patients who had undergone extensive conventional therapy prior to mobilization. Seven cases of MDS occurred in the group having received extensive prior therapy and none occurred in the Total Therapy group. This implies that prolonged standard-dose alkylating agent use rather than the myeloablative conditioning chemotherapy is primarily responsible for secondary MDS/AML in this population of patient (70).

VIII. CONCLUSION

We do not yet understand why MM remains resistant to all know treatment modalities. Is it because of complex genetic changes? Cytogenetic abnormalities are noted in >90% of patients at diagnosis and *ras* mutations are seen in 40% of patients. Alternatively, is chemoresistance an inherent characteristic of plasma cells and their precursors related to their stage of differentiation? This notion may be supported by observation in patients undergoing myeloablative or near myeloablative chemotherapy for disease such as acute leukemia. In such scenario, the predominant cell type in the aplastic marrow is often the plasma cell. In spite of these limitations, we do understand from the history of dose-escalation studies that "more is better." This has been proven in randomized trials and in single-arm studies related to historical controls. There is enough confidence in these findings that the Intergroup Study currently being conducted in the United States (SWOG 93-21) has chosen to address a different question. Following induction therapy, all patients have PBSCs collected and are then randomized to consolidation with standard-dose therapy or high-dose therapy (MEL/TBI) with PBSC support. Patients who relapse on the standard-dose therapy arm are then salvaged with an autotransplant, using the same MEL/TBI. Thus, the question that will hopefully be answered is not whether stem cell transplantation is appropriate in MM, but whether early (consolidative) or late (salvage) transplants are more advantageous.

Other ongoing studies will answer whether tandem transplantation offers significant advantage over single transplants (IFM Study). Numerous ongoing studies at many institutions, including our own, are aimed at answering whether tumor cell contamination of the grafts contributes significantly to relapse. All of these questions are of vital importance and the general approach to transplantation in myeloma will change as these questions are answered.

Although these basic questions are being answered, we have chosen to focus on posttransplant manipulations on a risk-based approach. The identification of cytogenetics, pretransplant $\beta_2 M$, and duration of prior therapy as the major predictors of posttransplant outcome allows us to stratify patients into different risk groups. Patients with only favorable variables are good risk, whereas those with only two such features would be considered intermediate risk, and those with one or no favorable variables are considered highest risk. Because good-risk patients can be expected to have EFS and OS of approximately 4 years and greater than 6 years, respectively, we do not feel that interventions likely to subject these patients to high risk of morbidity and/or mortality are justified. We have therefore chosen this population for immune modulation–based approaches posttransplant with vaccines using autologous myeloma idiotype.

The first study is being undertaken in collaboration with Larry Kwak, MD, PhD, at the National Cancer Institute (NCI) and involves the generation of a vaccine by conjugation of idiotypic protein to the immunostimulatory carrier protein, keyhole limpet hemocyanin (KLH). Patients are then vaccinated around the time of their second tandem transplant. Idiotypic protein is unique to the clonal plasma cell and its precursor populations. The presence of T-cell subsets reactive to myeloma idiotype has been clearly demonstrated in myeloma patients, as has been the ability of Id to elicit/augment idiotype-specific T-cell responsiveness by vaccination of patients with monoclonal gammopathies or myeloma (71–75). The magnitude of this T-cell reactivity has been inversely correlated with tumor load and tumor progression (73,74). The low-risk patient population will be vaccinated at the point of minimal residual disease. The generation of T-cell clones reactive to this small remaining malignant cell population may result in the elimination of this population by cytotoxic cells or alternatively reassert the control mechanisms that prevent or retard proliferation of the clonal population. The second vaccine approach involves the pulsing of autologous dendritic cells with idiotypic protein and/or tumor lysate. Dendritic cells, which represent the most efficient of the professional antigen-presenting cells, are cultured from the PBSC collection product. On loading with the appropriate antigenic materials, these cells can then be reintroduced into the patient to elicit maximal immune responsiveness. Early results on seven patients reported by Lim and his colleagues (76,77) using this approach demonstrated the ability to elicit idiotype-specific immune responses. In one patient, there was an associated and persistent 25% drop of circulating idiotype and in another, a transient response was observed. Alternatively, antigen-loaded dendritic cells can be used to generate reactive T cells ex vivo which can be returned to the patient. A further extrapolation of this approach is to clone DNA encoding hypervariable region or other sequences unique to tumor populations. Proteins encoded by these sequences are then translated in situ following plasmid vaccination (78–80). Results obtained in a murine model of myeloma has demonstrated the ability of this genetic strategy of targeting idiotype to prevent the development of transplantable myeloma (81).

Intermediate-risk patients have a significantly worse outcome with an EFS and OS of 28 months and 47 months, respectively. These patients have been targeted for more aggressive interventions. Based on the excellent results with patients relapsing after autotransplant, we have chosen these patients for inclusion on a study testing the role of maintenance DCEP chemotherapy. Patients will receive four cycles of this regimen on completion of the second transplant.

Poor-risk patient have an EFS and OS of less than 12 months. Patients with an available sibling donor will proceed with an allogeneic transplantation. Graft-versus-myeloma (GVM) activity is now clearly established (82,83), and efforts are being directed at separating this activity from graft-versus-host disease (GVHD) complications. Most patients will receive T-cell–depleted transplants with the intention to give back T cells to those patients with persistent disease. Currently, a protocol involving "gene therapy" is ongoing. Donor mononuclear cells are transduced with a suicide gene, the herpes simplex thymidine kinase (TK), prior to infusion into the patients. This allows the donor cells to be eliminated with subsequent administrating of ganciclovir and enables GVHD complications to be minimized (84).

For patients ineligible for allotransplantation, other strategies directed at harnessing GVM activity is being developed. Patients are receiving infusions of haploidentical peripheral blood mononuclear cells at the time of PBSC rescue with their second autotransplant. During the period of maximal immunosuppression following the transplant conditioning regimen, these cells are expected to persist; but as the patient's graft recovers, these cells are expected to be eliminated. During this window between infusion and elimination, these cells can be expected to exert some GVM activity on neoplastic cells that have survived the conditioning regimen.

We have also extended stem cell transplantation in MM to patients previously considered to the ineligible. They include heavily pretreated patients, in whom new mobilization strategies are helping us achieve adequate PBSC collections for the safe conduct of autotransplants. Patients with renal insufficiency are now being transplanted routinely, often with substantial improvements in their renal function. Finally, the elderly, who comprise the bulk of myeloma patients, have not only been transplanted safely but with excellent results comparable to those seen in younger patients.

Multiple myeloma continues to represent a dilemma both as a clinical entity and as a basic scientific question. The last decade has led to new insights into the biology of myeloma, as well as to tangible advances in its treatment. Nonetheless, relapses after both autologous and allogeneic transplants remain a serious concern. Although efforts to "push the edges to the envelope" with cytotoxic agents continue and have proven worthwhile, myeloma is a disease in which the interplay of the immune system may play a dominant role. The observation by Massaia and colleagues (85,86) that there are large numbers of plasma cell–reactive T cells in patients with myeloma is encouraging. An extension of this observation is that the magnitude of disease in patients with plasma cells dyscrasias is inversely proportional to the number of idiotype-reactive T cells (74). Another exciting observation is that soluble Fc receptor γIII, produced by CD8$^+$ T cells and natural killer (NK) cells in patients with myeloma, is capable of binding to surface immunoglobulin on human myeloma cells with subsequent suppression of tumor cell growth and immunoglobulin production (87). It thus appears that a cure for this disease is attainable. Based on carefully selected clinical trials and with the help of the basic science community, we can hope to realize this goal in the foreseeable future.

REFERENCES

1. Niesvyzky R, Siegel D, Michaeli J. Biology and treatment of multiple myeloma. Blood Rev 1993; 7:24–33.
2. Alexanian R, Haut A, Khan AU, Lane M, McKelvey EM, Migliore PJ, Stuckey WJ Jr, Wilson HE. Treatment for multiple myeloma. Combination chemotherapy with different melphalan dose regimens. JAMA 1969; 208:1680–1685.
3. Boccadoro M, Pileri A. Standard chemotherapy for myelomatosis: an area of great controversy. Hematol/Oncol Clin North Am 1992; 6:371–382.
4. Greipp PR, Lust JA, O'Fallon W, Katzmann J, Witz T, Kyle R. Plasma cell labeling index and β_2-microglobulin predict survival independent of thymidine kinase and C-reactive protein in multiple myeloma. Blood 1993; 81:3382–3387.
5. Alexanian R, Haut A, Khan A. Combination therapy for multiple myeloma. Cancer 1977; 49: 2765–2771.
6. Barlogie B, Smith L, Alexanian R. Effective treatment of advanced multiple myeloma refractory to alkylating agents. N Engl J Med 1984; 310:1353–1356.
7. Barlogie B, Alexanian R, Jagannath S. Plasma cell dyscrasias. JAMA 1992; 268:2946–2951.
8. Kyle R. Long-term survival in multiple myeloma. N Engl J Med 1983; 308:314.
9. Tsuchiya J, Murakami H, Kanoh T, Kosaka M, Sezaki T, Mikuni C, Kawato M, Takagi T, Towawa A, Isobe T, Suzuki K, Immamura Y, Takatsuki K. Ten-year survival and prognostic factors in multiple myeloma. Br J Haematol 1994; 87:832–834.
10. Gregory W, Richard M, Malpas J. Combination chemotherapy versus melphalan and prednisolone in the treatment of multiple myeloma: an overview of published trials. J Clin Oncol 1992; 10:334–342.
11. Salmon S, Crowley J, Grogan T, Finley P, Pugh R, Barlogie B. Combination chemotherapy, glucocorticoids and interferon alpha in the treatment of multiple myeloma: a Southwest Oncology Group Study. J Clin Oncol 1994; 12:2405–2414.
12. Bataille R, Boccadoro M, Klein B, Durie B, Pileri A. C-reactive protein and β_2 microglobulin produce a simple and powerful myeloma staging system. Blood 1992; 80:733–737.
13. Durie B, Stock-Novack D, Salmon S, Finley P, Beckford J, Crowley J, Coltman C. Prognostic value of β2 microglobulin in myeloma: a Southwest Oncology Group Study. Blood 1990; 75: 823–830.
14. Ffrench M, Ffrench P, Remy F, Chapuiscellier C, Wolowiec D, Ville D, Bryon PA. Plasma cell proliferation in monoclonal gammopathy—relations to other biologic variables—diagnostic and prognostic significance. Am J Med 1995; 98:60–66.
15. Latreille J, Barlogie B, Johnston D, Drewinko B, Alexanian R. Ploidy and proliferative characteristics in monoclonal gammopathies. Blood 1982; 59:43–51.
16. San Miguel JF, Garciasanz R, Gonzalez M, Moro MJ, Hernandez JM, Ortega F, Borrego D, Carnero M, Casanova F, Jimenez R, Portero JA, Orfao A. A new staging system for multiple myeloma based on the number of S-phase plasma cells. Blood 1995; 85:448–455.
17. McElwain T, Powles R. High dose intravenous melphalan for plasma cell leukemia and myeloma. Lancet 1983; 2:822–824.
18. Cunningham D, Paz-Ares L, Gore M, Malpas J, Hickish T, Nicolson M, Meldrum M, Viner C, Milan S, Selby P, Normal A, Raymond J, Powles R. High dose melphalan for multiple myeloma: Long term follow-up data. J Clin Oncol 1994; 12:764–768.
19. Lokhorst H, Meuwissen O, Verdonck L, Dekker A. High-risk multiple myeloma treated with high dose melphalan. J Clin Oncol 1992; 10:47–51.
20. Selby P, McElwain T, Nandi AC, Perren TJ, Powles RL, Tillyer CR, Osborne RJ, Slevin ML,

Malpas JS. Multiple myeloma treated with high dose intravenous melphalan. Br J Haematol 1987; 66:55–62.

21. Vesole D, Barlogie B, Jagannath S, Cheson B, Tricot G, Alexanian R, Crowley J. High dose therapy for refractory multiple myeloma: improved prognosis with better supportive care and double transplants. Blood 1994; 84:950–956.

22. Barlogie B, Jagannath S, Dixon D, Cheson B, Smallwood L, Hendrickson A, Purvis J, Bonnem E, Alexanian R. High-dose melphalan and granulocyte-macrophage colony-stimulating factor for refractory multiple myeloma. Blood 1990; 76:677–680.

23. Moreau P, Fiere D, Bezwoda W, Facon T, Attal M, Laporte J, Colombat P, Haak H, Moncon-duit M, Lockhorst H, Girault D, Harousseau J. Prospective randomized placebo-controlled study of granulocyte-macrophage colony stimulating factor without stem-cell transplantation after high dose melphalan in patients with multiple myeloma. J Clin Oncol 1997; 15:660–666.

24. Barlogie B, Hall R, Zander A, Dicke K, Alexanian R. High dose melphalan with autologous bone marrow transplantation for multiple myeloma. Blood 1986; 67:1298–1301.

25. Ventura G, Barlogie B, Hester J, Yau J, LeMaistre C, Wallerstein R, Spinola J, Dicke K, Horwitz L, Alexanian R. High dose cyclophosphamide, BCNU and VP-16 with autologous stem cell support for refractory multiple myeloma. Bone Marrow Transplant 1990; 5:265–268.

26. Gianni A, Siena S, Bregni M, Tarella C, Stern A, Pileri A, Bonadonna G. Granulocyte-macro-phage colony-stimulating factor to harvest circulating hematopoietic stem cells for autotrans-plantation. Lancet 1989; 2:580–585.

27. Bensinger W, Singer J, Appelbaum F, Lilleby K, Longin K, Rowley S, Clarke E, Clift R, Hansen J, Shields T, Storb R, Weaver C, Weiden P, Buckner C. Autologous transplantation with peripheral blood mononuclear cells collected after administration of recombinant granulo-cyte-colony stimulating factor. Blood 1993; 81:3158–3163.

28. Bjorkstrand B, Ljungman P, Bird JM, Samson D, Brandt L, Alegre A, Auzanneau G, Blade J, Brunet S, Carlson K, Cavo M, Ferrant A, Gravett P, Delaurenzi A, Prentice HG, Proctor S, Remes K, Troussard X, Verdonck LF, Williams C, Gahrton G. Autologous stem-cell trans-plantation in multiple myeloma—results of the European Group for Bone Marrow Trans-plantation. Stem Cells 1995; 13:140–146.

29. Jagannath S, Tricot G, Vesole D, Desikan K, Munshi N, Siegel D, Crowley J, Bracy D, Mattox S, Nauke S, Barlogie B. Total therapy (TT) with tandem autotransplants (2TX) for 231 newly diagnosed patients with multiple myeloma (MM). Blood 1996; 88:685a.

30. Jagannath S, Vesole D, Glenn L, Crowley J, Barlogie B. Low risk intensive therapy for multi-ple myeloma with combined autologous and blood stem cell support. Blood 1992; 80:1666–1672.

31. Vesole DH, Tricot G, Jagannath S, Desikan KR, Siegel D, Bracy D, Miller L, Cheson B, Crowley J, Barlogie B. Autotransplants in multiple myeloma—what have we learned. Blood 1996; 88:838–847.

32. Blade J, Lopez-Guillermo A, Bosch F, Cervantes F, Reverter J-C, Montserrat E, Rozman C. Impact of response to treatment on survival in multiple myeloma: results in a series of 243 patients. Br J Haematol 1994; 88:117–121.

33. Boccadoro M, Marmont F, Tibalto M, Avvisati G, Andriani A, Barburi T, Cantonetti M, Cara-ternuto M, Camotti B, Dammacoco F, Frieri R, Gallamini A, Gallone G, Giavongrossi P, Grignani F, Lauta V, Lberati M, Musto P, Neretto G, Petrucci M, Resegotti L, Pileri A, Mande-lli F. Multiple myeloma: VMCP/VBAP alternating combination therapy is not superior to melphalan and prednisolone even in high risk patients. J Clin Oncol 1991; 9:444–448.

34. Cooper M, Dear K, McIntyre O, Ozer H, Ellerton J, Canellos G, Bernhardt B, Duggan D, Faraghen D, Schiffer C. A randomized trial comparing melphalan/prednisolone with or with-out interferon alpha-2β in newly diagnosed patients with multiple myeloma. J Clin Oncol 1993; 11:155–160.

35. Barlogie B, Alexanian R, Dicke K, Zagars G, Spitzer G, Jagannath S, Horowitz L. High dose

chemoradiotherapy and autologous bone marrow transplantation for resistant multiple myeloma. Blood 1987; 70:869–872.

35a. Cunningham D, Paz-Ayes L, Milan S, Powles R, Nicolson M, Hickish T, Selby P, Treleaven J, Viner C, Malpas J *et al.* High-dose melphalan and autologous bone marrow transplantation as consolidation in previously untreated myeloma. J Clin Oncol 1994; 12:759–763.

35b. Harousseau JL, Attal M, Divine M, Marit G, Leblond V, Stoppa AM, Bourhis JH, Caillot D, Boasson M, Abgrall JF, *et al.* Autologous stem cell transplantation after first remission induction treatment in multiple myeloma: a report of the French Registry for autologous transplantation in multiple myeloma. Blood 1995; 85:3077–3085.

36. Vesole D, Jagannath S, Tricot G, Miller L, Cheson B, Bracy D, Barlogie B. 400 autotransplants (AT) for multiple myeloma (MM). Blood 1994; 84:535a.

37. Attal M, Harousseau J-L, Stoppa A-M, Sotto J-J, Fuzibet J-G, Rossi J-F, Casassus P, Maisonneuve H, Facon T, Ifrah N, Payen C, Bataille R. A prospective randomized trial of autologous bone marrow transplant and chemotherapy in multiple myeloma. N Engl J Med 1996; 335: 91–97.

38. Barlogie B, Alexanian R, Cabanillas F. Etoposide, dexamethasone, cytarabine and cisplatin in vincristine, doxorubicin and dexamethasone refractory myeloma. J Clin Oncol 1989; 7:1514–1517.

39. Greipp P, Raymond N, Kyle R, O'Fallon W. Multiple myeloma: significance of the plasmablastic subtype in morphological classification. Blood 1985; 65:305–310.

40. Barlogie B, Jagannath S, Vesole D, Naucke S, Cheson B, Mattox S, Bracy D, Salmon S, Jacobson J, Crowley C, Tricot G. Superiority of tandem autologous transplantation over standard therapy for previously untreated multiple myeloma. Blood 1997; 89:789–793.

41. Tricot G, Jagannath S, Vesole D, Nelson J, Tindle S, Miller L, Cheson B, Crowley J, Barlogie B. Peripheral blood stem cell transplants for multiple myeloma—identification of favorable variables for rapid engraftment in 225 patients. Blood 1995; 85:588–596.

42. Desikan K, Jagannath S, Siegel D, Munshi N, Bracy D, Barlogie B, Tricot G. Post-transplant engraftment kinetics and toxicities in multiple myeloma patients are comparable following mobilization of PBSC with G-CSF with or without high dose cyclophosphamide. Blood 1996; 88:2703a.

43. Tricot G, Jagannath S, Desikan K, Siegel D, Munshi N, Olson E, Wyres M, Parker W, Barlogie B. Superior mobilization of peripheral blood progenitor cells with r-metHuSCF (SCF) and r-metHuG-CSF (filgastim) in heavily pretreated multiple myeloma patients. Blood 1996; 88: 1540a.

44. Tricot G, Sawyer J, Jagannath S, Desikan K, Siegel D, Vesole D, Naucke S, Mattox S, Bracy D, Munshi N, Barlogie B. The unique role of cytogenetics in the prognosis of patients with multiple myeloma receiving high dose therapy and autotransplants. J Clin Oncol. 1997; 15: 2659–2666.

45. Tricot G, Barlogie B, Jagannath S, Bracy D, Mattox S, Vesole DH, Naucke S, Sawyer JR. Poor prognosis in multiple myeloma is associated only with partial or complete deletions of chromosome 13 or abnormalities involving 11q and not with other karyotype abnormalities. Blood 1995; 86:4250–4256.

46. Siegel D, Dhodapkar M, Tricot G, Jagannath S, Vesole D, Flick J, Desikan K, Vaught L, Barlogie B. Prognostic factors identifying myeloma-related mortality within 6 months (Mrm-6m) after autotransplantation (At) in multiple myeloma (MM). Blood 1995; 86:819a.

47. Tricot G, Alberts D, Johnson C, Roe D, Dorr R, Vesole D, Jagannath S, Meyers R, Barlogie B. Safety of autotransplants with high dose melphalan in renal failure: a pharmacokinetic and toxicity study. Clin Cancer Res. 1996; 2:947–952.

48. Jagannath S, Barlogie B, Vesole D, Bracy D, Mattox S, Tricot G. Autotransplants (AT) can be performed safely in multiple myeloma (MM) patients with renal insufficiency. Blood 1995; 86:809a.

49. Vesole DH, Jagannath S, Tricot G, Siegel D, Desikan KR, Vaught L, Barlogie B. Efficacy and safety of high dose therapy with autotransplantation (AT) in multiple myeloma (MM) patients over age 60. Blood 1995; 86:812a.

50. Siegel DS, Desikan KR, Mehta J, Singhal S, Fassas A, Munshi N, Anaissie E, Naucke S, Ayers D, Spoon D, Vesole G, Tricot G, Barlogie B. Age is not a prognostic variable with autotransplants for multiple myeloma. Blood 1999; 1:51–54.

51. Vora A, Toh C, Peel J, Greaves M. Use of granulocyte colony-stimulating factor (G-CSF) for mobilizing peripheral blood stem cells: risk of mobilizing clonal myeloma cells in patients with bone marrow infiltration. Br J Haematol 1994; 86:180–182.

52. Witzig TE, Gertz MA, Pineda AA, Kyle RA, Greipp PR. Detection of monoclonal plasma-cells in the peripheral blood stem cell harvests of patients with multiple myeloma. Br J Haematol. 1995; 89:640–642.

53. Bird J, Bloxham D, Russell N, Samson D, Apperley J. Detection of clonally rearranged cells in PBSC harvests in multiple myeloma by immunoglobulin gene fingerprinting. Blood 1993; 82:265a.

54. Bird JM, Wilmore HP, Samson D. Detection of cells with clone-specific immunoglobulin gene rearrangements in the peripheral blood of myeloma patients using immunoglobulin gene fingerprinting. Eur J Haematol 1996; 56:259–261.

55. Dreyfus F, Ribrag V, Leblond V, Ravaud P, Melle J, Quarre MC, Pillier C, Boccaccio C, Varet B. Detection of malignant B-cells in peripheral blood stem cell collections after chemo-therapy in patients with multiple myeloma. Bone Marrow Transplant 1995; 15:707–711.

56. Belch AR, Bergsagel PL, Szczepek A, Lansdorp P, Pilarki LM. CD34+ B-cells in the blood of patients with multiple myeloma express clonotypic IgH sequences. Blood 1994; 84:385a.

57. Gazitt Y, Reading CC, Hoffman R, Wickrema A, Vesole DH, Jagannath S, Condino J, Lee B, Barlogie B, Tricot G. Purified CD34(+) Lin(−)Thy(+) stem cells do not contain clonal myeloma cells. Blood 1995; 86:381–389.

58. Vescio R, Hong C, Cao J, Kim A, Schiller GJ, Lichtenstein A, Berenson J. The hematopoeitic stem cell antigen CD34 is not expressed on the majority of malignant cells in multiple my-eloma. Blood 1994; 84:3283–3290.

59. Fefer A, Cheever M, Greenberg P. Identical-twin (syngeneic) marrow transplantation for he-matologic cancers. J Natl Cancer Inst 1986; 76:1269–1273.

60. Durie BGM, Gale RP, Horowitz MM. Allogeneic and twin transplants for multiple myeloma—an IBMTR analysis. Blood 1994; 84:202a.

61. Bensinger W, Demirer T, Buckner C, Appelbaum F, Storb R, Lilleby K, Weiden P, Bluming A, Fefer A. Syngeneic marrow transplant in patients with multiple myeloma. Bone Marrow Transplant 1996; 18:527–531.

62. Reece DE, Barnett MJ, Connors JM, Klingemann HG, O'Reilly SE, Shepherd JD, Sutherland HJ, Phillips GL. Treatment of multiple myeloma with intensive chemotherapy followed by autologous BMT using marrow purged with 4-hydroperoxycyclophosphamide. Bone Marrow Transplant 1993; 11:139–146.

63. Anderson K, Barut B, Ritz J, Freedman A, Takvorian T, Rabinowe S, Soiffer R, Heflin L, Coral F, Dear K, Mauch P, Nadler L. Monoclonal antibody-purged autologous bone marrow transplant for multiple myeloma. Blood 1991; 77:712–720.

64. Seiden M, Schlossman R, Andersen J, Freeman A, Robertson K, Soiffer R, Freedman A, Mauch P, Ritz J, Nadler L, Anderson K. Monoclonal antibody-purged bone marrow trans-plantation therapy for multiple myeloma. Leuk Lymphoma 1995; 17:87–93.

65. Schiller G, Vescio R, Freytes C, Spitzer G, Sahebi F, Lee M, Wu CH, Cao J, Lee JC, Hong CH, Lichtenstein A, Lill M, Hall J, Berenson R, Berenson J. Transplantation of CD34(+) peripheral blood progenitor cells after high dose chemotherapy for patients with advanced multiple myeloma. Blood 1995; 86:390–397.

66. Tricot G, Gazitt Y, Jagannath S, Vesole D, Reading C, Juttner C, Hoffman R, Barlogie B. CD34+Thy+Lin- peripheral blood stem cells (PBSC) effect timely trilineage engraftment in multiple myeloma (MM). Blood 1995; 86:1160a.

67. Tricot G, Jagannath S, Desikan K, Munshi N, Siegel D, Bracy D, Barlogie B. Salvage trans-plants for early relapse after a single autotransplant are effective and improve outcome. Blood 1996; 88:513a.

68. Munshi N, Desikan K, Jagannath S, Siegel D, Bracy D, Tricot G, Barlogie B. Dexamethasone, cyclophosphamide, etoposide and cis-platinum (DCEP), an effective regimen for relapse after high-dose chemotherapy and autologous transplant. Blood 1996; 88:2331a.

69. Shulman N. Therapy related second malignancies. Hematol/Oncol Clin North Am 1993; 7: 325–335.

70. Govindarajan R, Jagannath S, Flick J, Vesole D, Sawyer J, Barlogie B, Tricot G. Preceding standard therapy is the likely cause of MDS after autotransplantation for multiple myeloma. Br J Haematol 1996; 95:349–353.

71. Bergenbrant S, Yi Q, Osterborg A, Bjorkholm M, Osby E, Mellstedt H. Modulation of antiidiotypic immune response by immunization with autologous M-component protein in multiple myeloma patients. Br J Haematol 1996; 92:840–846.

72. Yi Q, Bergenbrant S, Osterborg A, Osby E, Ostman R, Bjorkholm M, Holm G, Lefvert AK. T-cell stimulation induced by idiotypes on monoclonal immunoglobulins in patients with monoclonal gammopathies. Scand J Immunol 1993; 38:529–534.

73. Yi Q, Osterborg A. Idiotype-specific T-cells in multiple myeloma—targets for an immunotherapeutic intervention. Med Oncol 1996; 13:1–7.

74. Yi Q, Osterborg A, Bergenbrant S, Mellstedt H, Holm G, Lefvert AK. Idiotype-reactive T-cell subsets and tumor load in monoclonal gammopathies. Blood 1995; 86:3043–3049.

75. Wen YJ, Ling M, Lim SH. Immunogenicity and cross-reactivity with idiotypic IgA of VH CDR3 peptide in multiple myeloma. Br J Haematol 1998; 100:464–468.

76. Wen YJ, Ling M, Bailey-Wood R, Lim SH. Idiotypic protein-pulsed adherent peripheral blood mononuclear cell-derived dendritic cells prime immune system in multiple myeloma. Clin Cancer Res 1998; 4:957–962.

77. Lim SH, Bailey-Wood R. Id-pulsed dendritic cell vaccination in multiple myeloma. Blood 1998; 10:108a.

78. Hawkins R, Winter G, Hamblin T, Stevenson F, Russel S. A genetic approach to idiotype vaccination. J Immunother 1993; 14:273–278.

79. Hawkins R, Zhu D, Ovecka M, Winter G, Hamblin T, Long A, Stevenson F. Idiotypic vaccination against human B-cell lymphoma. Rescue of variable region gene sequences from biopsy material for assembly of single-chain Fv personal vaccines. Blood 1994; 83:3279–3288.

80. Stevenson F, Zhu D, King C, Ashworth L, Kumar S, Hawkins R. Idiotypic DNA vaccines against B-cell lymphoma. Immunol Rev 1995; 145:211–228.

81. King CA, Spellerberg MB, Zhu D, Rice J, Sahota SS, Thompsett AR, Hamblin TJ, Radl J, Stevenson FK. DNA vaccines with single-chain Fv fused to fragment C of tetanus toxin induce protective immunity against lymphoma and myeloma. Nature Med 1998; 4:1281–1286.

82. Tricot G, Vesole DH, Jagannath S, Hilton J, Munshi N, Barlogie B. Graft-versus-myeloma effect—proof of principle. Blood 1996; 87:1196–1198.

83. Verdonck L, Lockhorst H, Dekker A, Nieuwenhuis H, Petersen E. Graft-versus-myeloma effect in two cases. Lancet 1996; 447:800–801.

84. Munshi N, Govindarajan R, Drake R, Ding L, Iyer R, Saylors R, Kornbluth J, Marcus S, Chiang Y, Ennist D, Kwak L, Tricot B, Barlogie B. Thymidine kinase gene-transduced human lymphocytes can be highly purified, remain fully functional and are killed efficiently with ganciclovir. Blood 1997; 89:1334–1340.

85. Massaia M, Bianchi A, Attisano C, Peola S, Redoglia V, Dianzani U, Pileri A. Detection of hyperreactive T cells in multiple myeloma by multivalent cross-linking of the CD3/TCR complex. Blood 1991; 78:1770–1780.

86. Massaia M, Attisano C, Peola S, Montacchini L, Omede P, Corradini P, Ferrero D, Boccadoro M, Bianchi A, Pileri A. Rapid generation of antiplasma cell activity in the bone marrow of myeloma patients by CD3-activated T cells. Blood 1993; 82:1787–1797.

87. Hoover RG, Lary G, Page R, Travis P, Owens R, Flick J, Kornbluth J, Barlogie B. Autoregulatory circuits in myeloma—tumor-cell cytotoxicity mediated by soluble CD16. J Clin Invest 1995; 95:241–247.

30

High-Dose Therapy for Primary and Metastatic Breast Cancer

GARY SPITZER

Cancer Centers of the Carolinas, Greenville, South Carolina

KENNETH MEEHAN

Georgetown University Medical Center, Washington, D.C.

DOUGLAS ADKINS

Washington University School of Medicine, St. Louis, Missouri

I. INTRODUCTION

The utilization of high-dose chemotherapy to treat early and late metastatic and high-risk early-stage breast cancer will be discussed in this chapter. There is some enlargement on the new interest in immediate high-dose therapy, repetitive cycles of therapy, sequential high-dose therapy, and the addition of immunotherapy. The significance of marrow contamination in breast cancer, its detection, and approaches to remove tumor cells are described. The patterns and biology of hematopoietic recovery following high-dose chemotherapy and new approaches to modify and shorten the hematopoietic toxicity following high-dose therapy with recombinant growth factors and peripheral blood cells is described in other chapters in this text.

II. HIGH-DOSE THERAPY STUDIES IN REFRACTORY BREAST CANCER

Early studies demonstrated that single-agent high-dose chemotherapy administered to patients with refractory metastatic breast cancer resulted in higher objective response rates when compared with cytotoxic agents used at "standard doses" (1–5). However, complete remissions (CRs) were uncommon (<10%), remission durations were short (3–4 months), and survival was unaltered. High-dose combination chemotherapy, initially with combinations of alkylating agents (but more recently with combinations including mitoxantrone, carboplatin, etoposide, ifosfamide, and thiotepa), have demonstrated higher overall response rates in patients with refractory metastatic breast cancer (60–80%) and a higher percentage of CRs (3–13). Although CRs are seldom durable in refractory patients, these encouraging results have formed the basis of incorporating multiple agents in the treatment of less heavily pretreated patients.

However, it is highly likely that patients referred for first-generation single-agent studies had more advanced disease that had often progressed on therapy than those treated with multiple agent therapy. Alternatively, this may explain the lower response rates and CR rates observed with single agents used alone.

One alternative to using alkylating agents alone in the combination is to incorporate mitoxantrone, a deoxyribonucleic acid (DNA) intercalator, with a better toxicity profile for dose escalation than doxorubicin (Adriamycin). In our studies (10,13), the majority of patients developed progressive disease while receiving Adriamycin, but a proportion were responsive to alternative conventional therapy. CRs were predominately achieved in patients with minimal or less tumor bulk whose disease responded to alternative salvage therapy. Fields and coworkers (14,15), using similar combinations but at higher doses, have described impressive CR rates with a small percentage of disease-free survivors (DFSs) after 1 year. However, overall the results in breast cancer patients with multiple relapses are poor. This lack of impact in patients experiencing multiple relapses suggests that the dose response of metastatic breast cancer is shallow and drug resistance more prevalent than observed in the treatment of hematological malignancies.

Reevaluating the comparative activity of combination versus single-agent chemotherapy at maximally tolerated doses may help to realize methods to improve the results achieved thus far in early-stage disease, but is unlikely to benefit the long-term outcome in patients with advanced disease. Tumor burden is, generally, inversely correlated with response rate and length of survival, and drug-resistant clones of cells would limit the effectiveness of therapy. Thus, the maximum benefit of chemotherapy (including high-dose chemotherapy) would be anticipated in patients with minimal residual disease which is responsive to therapy.

III. HIGH-DOSE INTENSIFICATION THERAPY STUDIES IN HORMONE REFRACTORY METASTATIC BREAST CANCER

In the most recent generation of clinical studies utilizing high-dose chemotherapy, a "standard dose" combination chemotherapy induction regimen is administered to the point of maximal response followed by the administration of high-dose chemotherapy as "consolidation" treatment (intensification) in responsive and sometimes stable patients (8,12,16–22). Standard-dose therapy has usually included an anthracycline combined with antimetabolites and/or alkylating agents. Because of the extensive use of Adriamycin as adjuvant therapy, the recent addition of paclitaxel (Taxol), either alone or in combination with other agents, is being increasingly used as induction therapy. Intensification has incorporated combinations of alkylating agents frequently combined with cisplatin or carboplatin, combinations extensively discussed under refractory disease and conditioning regimens and variations of our *double* high-dose CVP [cyclophosphamide, etoposide (VP-16) and cisplatin] combination.

The uncertain natural history of the subgroup of patients entered into these trials and the magnitude of the selection of patients offered marrow or stem cell transplantation has resulted in controversy. The patients enrolled in metastatic disease trials have generally not been treated previously with chemotherapy for metastatic disease and in earlier trials were either estrogen receptor negative (ER⁻) or hormone refractory. The median survival of patients with ER⁻ tumors approximates, at best, 15–18 months (23). Maximal 3-year progression-free and overall survival is 10%.

Recent publications reviewing the natural history of stage IV breast cancer provide a better impression of the outcome and durability of response in these patients. Experience at the M.D. Anderson Cancer Center with standard Adriamycin-containing combination chemotherapy programs in 1424 patients with metastatic breast cancer (ER⁻ and ER⁺) has been reviewed (24). The median disease-free interval was 19 (range 0–36) months. The majority of patients were of good performance status and the median number of metastatic sites was two. Two hundred and twenty-two (16%) of these patients achieved a complete remission (CR) with FAC (fluorouracil, Adriamycin, and cyclophosphamide). The median duration of CR was 24 months (8% disease free at 2 years); however, 5 years after initiation of therapy, only 12% of the CR patients remain in remission. Therefore, even among those patients achieving a CR with conventional therapy, very few are long-term disease-free survival (DFS). In Cancer and Leukemia Group B (CALGB) studies, the median duration of response of 400 patients younger than age 55 years with metastatic breast cancer was 8 months, and the median survival was 19 months. Improved survival rates were seen in women with ER⁺ tumors (median survival 2.5 years) who achieved CR with standard therapy (median 2.8 years) or had a small volume of local disease (median >4 years). However, only an approximate 2% are disease free at 36 months (25). The M.D. Anderson experience was also analyzed by a different approach, subdividing their database into high-dose chemotherapy candidates (HDCs) and noncandidates. HDCs included patients of less than 60 years of age, with an excellent performance status, normal end organ function, and radiation therapy to less than two sites. Despite including patients with hormone-responsive disease and patients with no prior history of adjuvant therapy, only 18.8% of the patients were alive at 5 years. The proportion of patients disease free is not stated (26).

With this historical perspective, we can appreciate the outcome of high-dose therapy approaches. High-dose therapy intensification strategies in metastatic disease has matured to the point that several studies now have significant median follow-up (8,12,16,17,19, 22,27,28). The CR rates achieved with this strategy (47–70%) are higher than those using other approaches. Up to 50% of patients with measurable disease following induction therapy are converted to CR, and up to 20–30% of patients remain in CR for periods exceeding 24 months. Unpublished data from the Autologous Blood and Marrow Transplant Registry of North America demonstrate a 3-year probability of DFS in stable or progressive disease patients after chemotherapy of 7%, and for those patients in partial remission (PR) or CR, 13 and 32%, respectively. Registry data must be interpreted with caution because of the marked heterogeneity in patient selection. Controversy centers around the probability that patient selection alone could account for the 15% increment in long-term survival. Our studies of high-dose therapy demonstrate that patients with minimal disease (one or two metastatic sites only) and without liver involvement are the patients who experience prolonged DFS (29). When analyzed separately, these patients have a projected DFS of 40%. Patients with metastases only to the lung have an impressive 60% projected survival. Patients with more extensive disease will require different strategies of high-dose therapy or other novel approaches. Others have confirmed the correlation of tumor bulk and disease site to outcome and identified the importance of the disease-free interval (DFI) and prior adjuvant therapy, particularly with Adriamycin (30). These studies suggest that factors predicting improved outcome with conventional therapy are the same for dose-intensive therapy.

Because the minority of patients with stage IV disease will benefit from high-dose therapy, patient and/or tumor features which could predict a favorable outcome with a high-dose approach could restrict this therapy to those patients most likely to benefit. Other patients should be entered on developmental or palliative approaches.

IV. TIMING OF HIGH-DOSE THERAPY FOR METASTATIC DISEASE

Most young patients now considered for high-dose therapy have received prior adjuvant chemotherapy. This consideration brings into question the classic approach to metastatic disease, an introductory three to four cycles of chemotherapy followed by high-dose therapy in those patients demonstrating responsive disease. Recent data and theoretical arguments suggest an advantage to the alternative approach of an immediate cycle or cycles of high-dose therapy without exposure of patients to potentially ineffective therapy. This would be logical given their relapse following adjuvant therapy and the probable element of some drug resistance to conventional therapy doses. Some studies report a shorter than expected continuous long-term CR after high-dose therapy in patients who had received prior Adriamycin chemotherapy (29,30). The administration of chemotherapy prior to dose-intensive therapy may increase the toxicity and decrease the stem cell yield. Peters and colleagues (31) reported an inferior outcome in patients receiving high-dose STAMP 1 (cyclophosphamide, carmustin, cisplatin) chemotherapy immediately after Adriamycin, 5-fluorouracil, and methotrexate (AFM) induction of CR of recurrent disease compared to patients who were later treated with STAMP 1 following relapse from AFM. The explanation is unclear, but it raises concerns regarding the use of high-dose therapy with stem cell support immediately following conventional doses of therapy in patients with metastatic disease. Possible explanations could include the temporary induction of drug resistance with induction therapy and the enhanced therapy-related mortality. In addition, several clinical trials suggest no additional benefit when therapy is initiated prior to high-dose therapy. In an early study of a small group of patients with recurrent disease, patients received only one cycle of STAMP 1 without initial induction chemotherapy with no apparent change in the proportion of long-term DFS (32). Bezwoda and coworkers (33) randomized patients to receive cyclophosphamide for mobilization of stem cells followed by two cycles of high-dose therapy (cyclophosphamide 2.4 G/m^2, mitoxantrone 35–45 mg/m^2, and etoposide 2500 mg/m^2). The second group of patients received modest doses of chemotherapy (cyclophosphamide 600 mg/m^2, mitoxantrone 12 mg/m^2, and vincristine 1.4 mg/m^2). The high-dose regimen produced superior survival and DFS. Despite the short follow-up, this is the first published randomized study, and it demonstrates equivalent, if not superior, median response duration (80 weeks) to other studies of high-dose therapy in metastatic disease. This is intriguing, since the patients were not selected based on responsiveness of disease to chemotherapy and dose escalation was lower when compared to many other high-dose therapy studies.

However, Bezwoda's study (33) has been heavily criticized. It is argued that the response rate and survival are less than that expected of conventional therapy. The CR rate was only 4%, the PR rate 49%, and the response duration 34 weeks in the conventional chemotherapy arm. These outcomes were modestly inferior to the results observed with the same combination in an earlier trial (34). This criticism is not entirely valid, since this was a prospective randomized study and patient demographics of the two arms are equivalent. Many results of conventional therapy reported in contemporary literature document equivalent response rates, duration of response, and survival to that realized in the low-dose arm. A possible explanation for inferior outcomes with time and equivalent therapy is increasing exposure to aggressive adjuvant therapy. A large French study recently documented the influence of prior adjuvant therapy in patients exposed to CMF (cyclophosphamide, methotrexate, 5-fluorouracil) or Adriamycin-containing adjuvant chemotherapy with response rates of only 43–44% (35). Overall survival was also effected by prior adjuvant therapy and response duration was equivalent, as reported in the control arm of this study. A second criticism of Bezwoda's study (33) is the suggestion that the difference between the arms may be related to long-term tamoxifen use for responsive patients, which is an outcome in this patient group which has never been demonstrated. If this is valid, then hormonal effects must be dramatic given the response rate of 95 versus 53% in the conventional therapy arm. Nevertheless, for a variable period of time, 42% more patients received tamoxifen therapy in the high-dose therapy arm. However, considering only 27% of the patients were ER$^+$ and 20% unknown in the high-dose arm compared with 38 and 27%, respectively, in the low-dose group, the probable maximum percentage of patients that may have benefited from hormonal maintenance in this young group of women is approximately 25%, hardly a percentage to effect the median. Assuming this argument is valid, tamoxifen maintenance in responding stage IV patients (many premenopausal) is beneficial. All these arguments are suspect given the fact that this is a randomized trial (evidence 1 data) which must provide strong evidence for a dose response for recurrent disease. A recent update of this study reported that, in the high-dose arm, the 20% of the patients who were alive and in CR at greater than 150 weeks remain (nine patients) in CR for greater than 5 years (36).

Dose-intensive chemotherapy of repetitive cycles of submaximal high-dose therapy without preceding induction therapy for metastatic disease is an approach we and others are investigating. We are currently investigating three to four cycles of Taxol (250 mg/m^2 over 24 h) followed by carboplatin with an area under the curve (AUC) of 16 (37). Hopefully, this strategy will be associated with superior outcome and lesser mortality and morbidity.

V. CONDITIONING REGIMENS

Most conditioning regimens have used combinations of alkylating agents, sometimes with other classes of chemotherapeutic agents. The optimal agents should demonstrate a steep dose-response curve and have hematopoietic toxicity as the predominant toxicity.

Many chemotherapy combinations and sometimes the same combinations at different doses and schedules have been examined for the treatment of metastatic breast cancer. The total dose is somewhat a reflection of the individual investigator's tolerance of toxicity and mortality. For example, Elias and Fields examined the high-dose ICE regimen (ifosfamide, carboplatin, and etoposide), yet reached different conclusions concerning the maximum tolerated dose (MTD). Elias recommended ifosfamide 16 g/m^2, carboplatin 1.8 g/m^2, and etoposide 1.2 g/m^2; all drugs were given over 3 days (38). In contrast, the MTD derived by Fields and colleagues (14,15,39,40) with drugs given over 6 days realized higher doses of ifosfamide and etoposide, 20.1 g/m² and 3 g/m², respectively. Mortality was a little higher (6 vs 4%) and grades 3 and 4 gastrointestinal and liver toxicity increased.

A number of combination chemotherapy regimens include mitoxantrone with the hope that this drug would enable dose escalation (better than Adriamycin) with less toxicity. Fields' group has determined a MTD of 90 mg/m² and 1200 mg/m² of mitoxantrone and thiotepa, respectively, when used together (14,40). Delayed engraftment was observed with marrow infusion separated by only 2–3 days after completion of mitoxantrone infusion. At these doses, mortality in advanced refractory breast cancer patients was elevated at 20% with a similar mortality rate when doses were modified slightly and paclitaxel added (see below). DFS may be improved with the addition of paclitaxel, but these are sequential studies and interpretation is fraught with difficulty. These doses are larger when compared to our earlier reported studies when recommended doses were only 60 mg/m² and 900 mg/m² of mitoxantrone and thiotepa, respectively (13). However, a second cycle was frequently administered at this dose in responding patients who experienced acceptable first-cycle toxicity.

Other combinations that have been investigated include cyclophosphamide (6 g/m²), thiotepa (600 mg/m²), and mitoxantrone (40 mg/m²) (CTM) (41), or a combination with little mortality in minimally pretreated patients of cyclophosphamide 120 mg/kg, mitoxantrone 45 mg/m², and melphalan 140 mg/m² (CMA) (42). Because of the activity of paclitaxel in the treatment of breast cancer, several investigators have incorporated this drug into the preparative program. Researchers at the University of Colorado investigated the addition of paclitaxel up to 775 mg/m² as a 24-h infusion on day 7 as a replacement for the carmustine (BCNU) in STAMP 1 (cyclophosphamide, BCNU, and cisplatin). Major toxicity observed with the addition of paclitaxel included a reversible neurotoxicity. Ongoing studies include BCNU with lower doses of paclitaxel (43). Investigators at the University of South Florida are evaluating the addition of paclitaxel (at doses of 120–360 mg/m² administered over 72 h) to mitoxantrone (75 mg/m²) and thiotepa (900 mg/m²) (40).

VI. SEQUENTIAL HIGH-DOSE CHEMOTHERAPY

The most effective cytoreductive therapy or approach to high-dose therapy is yet to be determined. In an attempt to increase dose intensity, some investigators have administered sequential cycles of high-dose therapy to improve DFS in patients with stage IV disease. An increasing number of studies are exploring this concept.

Our focus has been to develop high-dose regimens which can be administered repetitively to patients with metastatic breast cancer or other tumor types (44). This strategy was developed in part because of the concern that the dose response of most human solid tumors would not be steep enough to warrant expectations that a single cycle of high-dose therapy would achieve results significantly different in advanced stages from those of standard chemotherapy. Tandem or repetitive high-dose therapy cycles also offered a potential means of circumventing kinetic resistance related to the presence of a proportion of G0 cells in a tumor population. Theoretically, the first course of therapy may recruit cells into the cell cycle. Although we were concerned that drug delivery to the center of tumor masses might be problematic, the potential for tumor reduction during the first cycle of chemotherapy might enhance the effects of subsequent cycles.

Our reports have tested identical high doses of chemotherapeutic agents administered in tandem within a short period of time and reported the MTDs that were feasible using such an approach. We defined MTD as that dose which did not produce grade III or IV extramedullary toxic effects (cardiovascular, pulmonary, hepatic, neurological, and vasculitis).

We evaluated cyclophosphamide, etoposide, and cisplatinum (CVP). The long-term outcome of this combination administered in repetitive cycles appears at least equivalent to high-dose single cycles of combinations of alkylating agents (16–18,29,44).

Subsequent studies included a different but hopefully non–cross-resistant mitoxantrone-based combination of agents in the second cycle. This concept was investigated in patients with adverse prognostic features (liver involvement, short DFI, multiple metastatic sites) to do well with CVP alone. Patients received CVP as the initial cycle and mitoxantrone, etoposide, and thiotepa (MVT) in the second cycle (10). The number of patients converting to a CR after developing a PR with CVP alone was small. This suggests the ability to achieve CR with a single high-dose therapy cycle in patients with adverse features may not be enhanced significantly by this approach. This strategy needs to be evaluated in patients with chemosensitive disease. Ayash and coworkers (45) investigated an initial intensification in women with chemosensitive disease with melphalan at doses of 140–180 mg/m^2 supported with peripheral blood stem cells (PBSCs) and a second cycle of high-dose cyclophosphamide, thiotepa, and carboplatin (CTCb). Owing to excessive liver toxicity, the intervals between cycles had to be increased from 28 days to 35 days. Median follow-up of this group is short (less than 2 years), but progression-free survival is continuously falling and may be inferior to the results obtained by these investigators in prior studies with a single cycle of CTCb (46). The investigators discuss many hypotheses for the poor outcome and the less than anticipated effect in patients intensified in CR. Since this is a small series, conclusions cannot be made without randomized trials because of the invariable patient differences between trials.

These investigators subsequently examined repetitive cycles of CTCb at 0.25 dose of the usual CTCb for four cycles with peripheral blood progenitor cells (PBPCs) and granulocyte colony-stimulating factors (G-CSF) support. PBPCs were collected during each of four induction cycles of low-dose CTCb. Of 18 patients initiating therapy, 12 completed all four cycles, but two patients were removed because of progressive disease, one patient refused further therapy, and three patients were removed because of dose-limiting hematological toxicity. Twenty-six percent of the cycles were associated with febrile neutropenia. The total duration of neutropenia, thrombocytopenia, and platelet transfusion requirements were greater than that experienced with the fourfold higher single cycle. In the few evaluable stage IV patients, no CRs were obtained. Repetitive cycles of CTCb at this dose and schedule are associated with significant morbidity, no greater dose intensity, and no improvement in the CR rate (47).

Crown and coworkers have published an interesting series of trials (48–53). They usually started therapy by mobilizing stem cells with high doses of cyclophosphamide, but recently incorporated paclitaxol, usually followed by four cycles of single-agent high-dose alkylating agents, such as carboplatin, thiotepa, and melphalan or combinations of these drugs with cyclophosphamide. Cycles were usually repeated earlier than day 21, and dose intensity delivered has been impressive, approximately 465 mg/m^2/week of carboplatin administered as the MTD. Toxicities appeared to be cumulative, with delayed hematopoietic recovery and a higher frequency of neutropenic fever in later cycles. Doses were frequently modified because of cumulative toxicity. These investigators clearly showed a disturbing increase in the frequency of serious toxicities with a third cycle near full doses. Some patients receiving thiotepa in later cycles experienced fatal pneumonitis, suggesting cumulative doses of certain alkylating agents may reach a threshold for serious nonhematological toxicity. The cumulative hematological toxicity is similar to what others have reported using multiple cycles of high-dose cyclophosphamide, thiotepa, and carboplatin (47). The antitumor activity of this approach is uncertain. Most of the sequential cycles in the studies by Crown have used single agents, unlike the combination therapy used by Bezwoda (33) or the paclitaxel/carboplatin combination explored by our group (37). Given the positive results of two consecutive high-dose therapy cycles as initial therapy for metastatic disease and the ability to administer sequential cycles with PBPC support, further exciting trials comparing variations of multiple high-dose therapy cycles consisting of single drugs or combinations will likely be initiated. However, careful attention needs to be paid to the potential cumulative toxicity of this approach. Prudent selection of agents without overlapping cumulative toxicity and careful choices of total doses of individual agents will be required.

VII. AUTOLOGOUS GRAFT-VERSUS-HOST DISEASE AND OTHER CONCEPTS IN IMMUNOTHERAPY

Further innovative strategies, besides new combinations of high doses or scheduling of sequences, to improve the modest gains in stage IV disease are under investigation. One approach is the induction of an autologous graft-versus-host disease (GVHD) by a short course of cyclosporine therapy after infusion of autologous stem cells. This approach was initiated in lymphoma and leukemia and was recently explored in breast cancer (54,55). Autologous GVHD was first described in a murine transplant model where it is thought that cyclosporine facilitates the development of autoreactive T cells directed against class II targets on tumor cells (56). The development of these autoreactive T cells confers tumor immunity against a variety of tumor cell lines. A significantly frequency of clinical and histological GVHD was induced in patients with stage IV breast cancer who received high-dose therapy, stem cell support, and a short course (28 days) of cyclosporine after stem cell infusion (57). To enhance the expression of class II molecules on tumor cells, interferon-γ has been added to cyclosporine posttransplant. Ongoing phase III studies of this strategy are in progress and should provide definitive insight into this approach (58).

Others (59,60) have investigated interleukin-2 (IL-2) activation of autologous PBSCs followed by parental IL-2 administration beginning the day of transplant. This in vitro activation method generates enhanced tumor-directed cytotoxicity in vivo after stem cell infusion. Hematopoietic recovery does not appear to be effected, and the majority of patients develop skin changes consistent with GVHD.

A recent case report described a temporary CR in a breast cancer patient with stage IV liver disease and the development of tumor-specific cytotoxic lymphocytes after allogeneic transplantation (61). Another report describes 10 patients with metastatic breast cancer that involved the liver or bone marrow that were treated with high-dose chemotherapy and allogeneic PBPC transplantation. The median age was 42 years (range 29–55). The conditioning regimen was cyclophosphamide (6000 mg/m^2), carmustine (BCNU 450 mg/m^2), and thiotepa (720 mg/m^2) (CBT regimen). Patients received GVHD prophylaxis using cyclosporine- or tacrolimus-based regimens. Three patients developed grade 2 or greater acute GVHD and four chronic GVHD. After transplantation, one patient was in CR, five achieved a PR, and four had stable disease. In two patients, metastatic liver lesions regressed in association with skin GVHD after withdrawal of immunosuppressive therapies. The median progression-free survival duration was still only 238 days in this poor-risk group of patients. The regression of tumor associated with GVHD was concluded as being suggestive of clinical evidence that graft-versus-tumor effects against breast cancer (62). There is still only limited experience in breast cancer patients receiving an allogeneic transplantation owing to the high mortality and morbidity associated with the procedure and the uncertainty of the importance of donor lymphoid populations and allogeneic GVHD in this setting. Well-designed studies in young patients are anxiously awaited. Unpublished studies are in progress using cord blood cells in the hope that GVH disease may be less and a GVHD effect maintained.

Other immunotherapy approaches include the use of IL-2 with G-CSF for stem cell mobilization, incubation of stem cells with IL-2 for periods ranging from 1 day to a week or greater, and posttransplant immunotherapy using IL-2, sometimes in combination with interferon (60). These studies have been phase I/II studies that have demonstrated no compromise of engraftment and acceptable toxicity. The effectiveness of this approach will need to be evaluated further, hopefully in randomized trials.

VIII. TUMOR CONTAMINATION AND PURGING

Various methods have detected micrometastatic disease in the bone marrow of patients with early and late disease, suggesting that reinfusion of tumor cells could be responsible for the recurrence following autologous marrow infusion (62–66). Various techniques exist to identify malignant breast cancer cells, including immunochemistry, multicolor immunofluorescence of epithelial antigens and cytokeratins, and molecular detection for epithelial specific messenger ribonucleic acid (mRNA). The significance of finding tumor cells in infused blood or bone marrow in late- or early-stage breast cancer is still unknown. The potential contribution of these cells to recurrence is argued from the negative prognostic importance of marrow tumor cell detection in stage I and II disease and the ability to demonstrate clonogenic cells from positive samples (63,65,67). The significance of the predictive failure (in most studies) is generally increased with the detection of positive cells by immunohistochemistry. However, in both lymphatic and subtypes of myeloid leukemia, the molecular detection of minimal residual disease in marrow, particularly at levels corresponding to one cell in less than 10^{-3} is not always associated with relapse. Both semiquantitative and serial measurements are more predictive (65,68,69). The maximal sensitivity for morphological detection of tumor cells is 0.1% or less. Therefore, if 10^{11} marrow cells were collected and infused, up to 10^7 tumor cells may be contaminating the marrow inoculum. Owing to the greater number of cells infused with PBSCs, despite the lower level of tumor contamination, a similar number of malignant cells could be infused. These reasons stress the need for extensive research into tumor cell detection, isolation, and removal.

Tumor cell contamination is higher in more advanced stage disease and lower in peripheral blood regardless of the mobilization method. There is a direct correlation between blood and marrow contamination. There are conflicting conclusions regarding the incidence of tumor cell contamination utilizing different methods of mobilization (65,67,70,71). Studies utilizing polymerase chain reaction (PCR) detection of cytokeratins suggest a greater sensitivity (1×10^7 vs 1×10^6) when compared to immunochemistry and a greater frequency of abnormal results in both early and late disease compared to immunohistochemistry. There is a surprisingly positive detection rate in marrow of approximately 60% in patients with stage II disease compared with immunochemistry detection rates of approximately 20–30%. However, there is an inferior outcome only in stage IV disease patients (not stage II) receiving marrow products which are positive by PCR for tumor cells (65,72,73). However, some patients infused with marrow containing tumor cells detected by PCR remain disease free for extended periods of time (72). Vredenburgh and colleagues (74) used immunohistochemistry and noticed no prognostic importance in their earlier reports to marrow or blood contamination and outcome after high-dose therapy in patients with stage II or stage IV disease. Longer follow-up by these same investigators suggests an inferior outcome in patients with stage II disease receiving marrow positive for tumor cells (Vredenburgh, unpublished data). The method of detection of minimal residual disease may therefore have differing prognostic value after high-dose therapy.

Some investigators consider that tumor cell contamination has been proven to be a significant source of therapeutic failure because of the detection of genetically marked infused tumor cells at relapse in leukemia and neuroblastoma after autologous marrow infusion (75,76). As a result, phase II studies continue in an attempt to remove tumor cells by either positive selection using CD34 isolation or elimination of tumor cells by drugs or monoclonal antibodies ex vivo (77,78).

Some studies indirectly suggest the importance of tumor cell contamination. Shpall noted that 13 patients transplanted with negative grafts as determined immunohistochemically after CD34 concentration experienced a DFS of 45% compared to 13% in 34 patients with residual detected tumor cells after CD34 isolation (79). A multivariate analysis determined residual tumor cells was an important prognostic variable as was treatment on a phase II rather than phase I trial. Other covariates, such as bulk of disease and response to induction therapy, and risk factors most likely to correlate with the degree of tumor contamination of pheresis products, are not mentioned as prognostic factors (79). These results contrast with earlier attempts in a phase I study at removing tumor cells ex vivo with chemotherapy by the same investigators (80). It was anticipated that further tumor cell removal might be achievable with the addition of monoclonal antibodies (81,82); however, 7 of 11 relapses occurred in CR patients at a median follow-up of only 10 months. This suggests that this approach may not prevent relapse.

The confusing results addressing tumor cell contamination of stem cell products and relapse could be interpreted in a number of ways. The detection of single cells or minimal disease by immunochemistry or PCR may be a reflection of tumor burden, and only if this disease bulk is truly minimal (as may be the case with a positive PCR assay) will the reinfused product be a significant contribution to relapse. Otherwise, the residual volume of disease at the time of transplantation is unlikely to be totally removed by high-dose therapy. A second, not exclusive, explanation is that the majority of these cells do not possess in vivo clonogenic potential, and the number of clonogenic cells varies and shows poor correlation with present tests for tumor detection. If there is poor correlation of the number of cells detected by these assays and tumor cells responsible for tumor regrowth, then correlations will be difficult in small studies. A study utilizing CVP therapy questions the significance of tumor cell contamination as an important factor contributing to relapse. In this study, patients were randomized to high dose chemotherapy with autologous bone marrow transplantation (ABMT) or ABMT only if markedly delayed hematopoietic recovery, neutrophil recovery beyond 28 days after therapy. Long-term DFS was equivalent in both arms and was not compromised by marrow infusion (83). It is unfortunate that a formal trial has not been designed to resolve the importance of removing or reducing tumor cells in the graft.

IX. PATIENTS WITH HIGH-RISK PRIMARY BREAST CANCER

Results from pilot studies in patients with stages II and IIIA breast cancer with extensive nodal involvement are encouraging. The projected DFS of 65–75% at 5 years (21,84,85) compared to, at best, 45% or less with adjuvant therapy (86) suggests that this difference in outcome may not be explained by selection alone. A number of investigators urge caution when interpreting these results because of possible selection of patients. Patients receiving high-dose therapy are usually subjected to extensive staging [e.g., evaluation with computed tomographic (CT) scans, bilateral bone marrow biopsies] prior to entry on the study. The patients entered on these studies have routinely received local irradiation of high technical quality; a modality which in recent randomized studies has been shown to prolong survival (87,88). Patients with estrogen receptor–positive tumors have also received long-term tamoxifen maintenance therapy. The extensive staging evaluation and the additional therapeutic modalities were not used in the historical comparisons. These potentially confounding variables make it difficult to evaluate the true increase in survival garnished by high-dose therapy approaches (89).

Two recently reported studies raise concern regarding the efficacy of a single cycle of high chemotherapy as a final consolidation for high-risk breast cancer. In the first study, 97 women younger than 60 years, who were high risk by extensive axillary nodal metastases (tumor-positive infraclavicular lymph node biopsy), received three courses of neoadjuvant chemotherapy (FE120C). This regimen consisted of cyclophosphamide 500 mg/m^2, epirubicin 120 mg/m^2, and 5-fluorouracil 500 mg/m^2 once weekly for 3 weeks. After surgery, stable patients or those who responded to chemotherapy were randomly assigned conventional therapy [fourth course of FE120C followed by radiation therapy and 2 years of tamoxifen (40 patients)] or high-dose therapy [identical treatment but an additional high-dose regimen and peripheral blood progenitor cell (PBPC) support after the fourth FE120C course (41 patients)]. The high-dose regimen was similar to that used by most and consisted of cyclophosphamide 6 g/m^2, thiotepa 480 mg/m^2, and carboplatin 1600 mg/m^2. With a median follow-up of 49 (range 21–76) months, the 4-year overall and relapse-free survivals for all 97 patients were 75 and 54%, respectively. By intention to treat analyses, there was no significant difference in survival between the two groups (90).

Another small study of different design also failed to show any benefit but greater short-term toxicity. Fluorouracil, Adriamycin, and cyclophosphamide were administered for eight cycles and then patients were randomized to two cycles of CVP followed by ABMT or no further chemotherapy. Seventy-eight patients were registered with a median follow-up of 53 months. The 4-year DFS was 55% and 48% (conventional vs ABMT) by intention to treat analysis. There was similarly no difference in survival, but again there was greater short-term toxicity (91).

Both these studies could be criticized because of the very small number of patients, but these results would suggest that the impact of high-dose therapy if positive in larger randomized studies would be modest at best. Large randomized studies were presented at the May 1999 meeting of the American Association of Clinical Oncology. Studies involving consolidation with high dose were not positive, but suffered from inadequate follow-up. Dr. Bezwoda reported remarkably positive approach with two cycles of high dose therapy alone. Recent audit of this data has not confirmed these results and will be reported. Even if the studies are negative, this may not negate the therapeutic benefit of such an approach. The increment and timing of dose intensity may be flawed and early high-dose repetitive cycles may be a more effective approach (92).

Prognostic factors predicting the outcome after high-dose therapy in stage II disease have not been extensively studied. One small study reported an inferior outcome after high-dose therapy and stem cell support in patients whose tumor demonstrated high expression of Her2/neu (c-erbB2) (93). These results contradict the dose-response effect observed in patients with node-positive disease treated with CAF (cyclophosphamide, Adriamycin, 5-fluorouracil), which showed an increased response to greater total drug administered to patients with c-erbB2–expressing tumors (94). Other studies suggest that tumors expressing high levels of c-erbB2 have a worse prognosis when treated with CMF (cyclophosphamide, methotrexate, 5-fluorouracil) adjuvant therapy (95) or are more responsive to anthracycline combinations. A recent study suggests that ER$^-$ tumors have a worse outcome than ER$^+$ tumors (96).

The long term analysis of prospective randomized trials are eagerly awaited to confirm this effect and to enable a better understanding of true differences in survival, toxicities, and quality of life between the two approaches. An intergroup trial, coordinated by the Eastern Cooperative Oncology Group (ECOG), is currently comparing six cycles of CAF with the same induction followed by a single cycle of high-dose cyclophosphamide and thiotepa and stem cell support. Another study, coordinated by the CALGB, compares four cycles of CAF followed by randomization to either very high-dose cyclophosphamide, carmustine, and cisplatin (STAMP 1) with stem cell support or to these agents at a lower dose without hematopoietic support.

X. PATIENTS WITH FOUR TO NINE POSITIVE LYMPH NODES

The natural history of women with four to nine positive lymph nodes has improved modestly with the introduction of adjuvant therapy, approximating a DFS of 50–60% at 5 years and 40–50% at 10 years (97). It is hoped that if dose intensity results in improved survival in patients with more advanced early and late disease, dose intensity may further enhance the outcome in this patient group where development of drug resistance may be minimal. A CALGB study evaluating three different doses and schedules of CAF for node-positive disease showed a significant improvement in overall survival and DFS with greater total dose and a trend for improvement when this greater dose was delivered at an increased dose rate (98).

A number of pilot studies of dose-intensive therapy for women with lesser nodal involvement have been reported. Bearman (98) used STAMP 1, reducing the BCNU dose to 450 mg/m^2, in an attempt to reduce pulmonary toxicity. There were no treatment-related deaths but a 25% incidence of pulmonary toxicity. The actual progression-free and overall survival with a short median follow-up (277 days) were 88 and 94%, respectively (97). A number of randomized studies using different designs have been initiated comparing variations of treatment without stem cell support with that of induction therapy followed by intensification requiring stem cell support. One design compares an alternating high-dose single agent with growth factor support to a second group receiving four cycles of induction therapy with Adriamycin combined with cyclophosphamide followed by either STAMP I or STAMP V intensification. Another design is comparing an Adriamycin induction followed by randomization to CMF or stem cell collection with cyclophosphamide followed by STAMP V.

XI. INFLAMMATORY BREAST CANCER

Inflammatory breast cancer is an uncommon variant of breast cancer with a variable natural history dependent on the extent of breast and nodal involvement and the response to neoadjuvant therapy. Owing to these factors and the small numbers of patients reported in any one series, it is difficult to evaluate the impact of high-dose therapy with stem cell support.

One recent historical comparison to conventional therapy suggests no difference (99), but other recent larger reports suggest an encouraging 40–50% DFS at 4–5 years (100). Without a randomized study, and the elimination of selection, it is difficult to estimate the impact of high-dose therapy in this aggressive disease.

XII. CONCLUSION AND FUTURE DIRECTIONS

Dose-intensive therapies for early- and late-stage breast cancer have evolved significantly over the years. As described by other investigators, the advances in supportive care and improved experience in managing these patients has significantly reduced morbidity and mortality. No longer is this therapy confined to academic centers, as it can be safely performed by well-trained community physicians. However, the quantitative benefits of this procedure (increases in DFS, overall survival, and quality of life) are difficult to discern accurately. There is a great need for patients to be registered in randomized studies to assess these outcomes accurately. Furthermore, our approach to the delivery of dose-intensive therapy is undergoing rapid change, concentrating on sequential cycles of therapy (with similar or dissimilar drugs) at submaximal dose with PBSC support. This approach may deliver more dose intensity than single aggressive cycles of high-dose therapy and cause less mortality and morbidity.

These are exciting times with many hypotheses to be tested. Possibilities include sequential cycles of therapy, immunomodulation of the graft and posttransplant immune therapy, tumor cell removal and detection, better patient selection, and early disease treatment. Hopefully, patients will participate in these trials and insurance carriers will support these clinical efforts so that these important issues can be addressed. It is unfortunate that as this chapter was going to press, it seems that some of the enthusiasm for immediate administration of high-dose therapy may have been misguided. We await the results of detailed audit of these data. However, we should be patient and wait for long term follow-up of several American and European randomized studies in high-risk disease. It is quite possible that with sufficient follow-up, three years or greater, modest but important benefits will be realized.

REFERENCES

1. Tannir N, Spitzer G, Schell F, Legha S, Zander A, Blumenschein G. Phase II study high-dose amacrine (AMSA) and autologous bone marrow transplantation in patients with refractory metastatic breast cancer. Cancer Treat Rep 1983; 67:599–600.
2. Tannir N, Spitzer G, Dicke KA, DiStefano A, Blumenschein G. Phase II study of high-dose mitomycin with autologous bone marrow transplantation in refractory metastatic breast cancer. Cancer Treat Rep 1984; 68:805–806.
3. Eder JP, Antman K, Peters WP, Henner WD, Elias AD, Shea T, Schryber S, Andersen J, Come S, Schnipper L. High-dose combination alkylating agent chemotherapy with autologous bone marrow support for metastatic breast cancer. J Clin Oncol 1986; 4:1592–1597.
4. Peters WP, Eder JP, Henner WD, Schryber S, Wilmore D, Finberg R, et al. High-dose combination alkylating agents with autologous bone marrow support: a phase I trial. J Clin Oncol 1986; 4:646–654.
5. Antman K, Eder JP, Elias A, Ayash L, Shea TC, Weissman L, Critchlow J, Schryber SM, Begg C, Teicher BA. High-dose thiotepa alone and in combination regimens with bone marrow support. Semin Oncol 1990; 17:33–38.
6. Ayash LJ, Elias AD, Wheeler C, Reich E, Schwartz G, Mazanet R, Tepler I, Warren D,

Lynch C, Gonin R. Double dose-intensive chemotherapy with autologous marrow and periph-eral-blood progenitor-cell support for metastatic breast cancer: a feasibility study. J Clin Oncol 1994; 12:37–44.

7. Williams SF, Mick R, Desser R, Golick J, Beschorner J, Bitran JD. High-dose consolidation therapy with autologous stem cell rescue in stage IV breast cancer. J Clin Oncol 1989; 7: 1824–1830.

8. Peters WP. High-dose chemotherapy and autologous bone marrow support for breast cancer. Important Adv Oncol 1991; 135–150.

9. Eder JP, Elias A, Shea TC, Schryber SM, Teicher BA, Hunt M, Burke J, Siegel R, Schnipper LE, Frei E. A phase I-II study of cyclophosphamide, thiotepa, and carboplatin with autolo-gous bone marrow transplantation in solid tumor patients. J Clin Oncol 1990; 8:1239–1245.

10. Wallerstein RJ, Spitzer G, Dunphy F, Huan S, Hortobagyi G, Yau J, Buzdar A, Holmes F, Theriault R, Ewer M. A phase II study of mitoxantrone, etoposide, and thiotepa with autolo-gous marrow support for patients with relapsed breast cancer. J Clin Oncol 1990; 8:1782–1788.

11. Elias AD, Ayash LJ, Eder JP, Wheeler C, Deary J, Weissman L, Hunt M, Critchlow J, Schnip-per L, Frei E. Escalating doses of carboplatin with high-dose ifosfamide using autologous bone marrow as support: a phase I study. J Cancer Res Clin Oncol 1991; 117(suppl 4):S208–S213.

12. Antman K, Ayash LJ, Elias AD, Wheeler C, Hunt M, Eder JP, Teicher BA, Critchlow J, Bibbo J, Schnipper LE. A phase II study of high-dose cyclophosphamide, thiotepa, and car-boplatin with autologous marrow support in women with measurable advanced breast cancer responding to standard-dose therapy (see Comments). J Clin Oncol 1992; 10:102–110.

13. Bowers C, Adkins D, Dunphy FR, Harrison B, Lemaistre CF, Spitzer G. Dose escalation of mitoxantrone given with thiotepa and autologous bone marrow transplantation for metastatic breast cancer. Bone Marrow Transplant 1993; 12:525–530.

14. Fields KK, Elfenbein GJ, Perkins JB, Hiemenz JW, Janssen WE, Zorsky PE, Ballester OF, Kronish LE, Foody MC. Two novel high-dose treatment regimens for metastatic breast can-cer—ifosfamide, carboplatin, plus etoposide and mitoxantrone plus thiotepa: outcomes and toxicities. Semin Oncol 1993; 20:59–66.

15. Fields KK, Efenbein GJ, Perkins JB, Janssen WE, Ballester OF, Hiemenz JW, Zorksy PE, Kronish LE, Foody MC. High-dose ifosfamide/carboplatin/etoposide: maximum tolerable doses, toxicities, and hematopoietic recovery after autologous stem cell infusion. Semin On-col 1994; 21(suppl 12):86–92.

16. Dunphy FR, Spitzer G. Long-term complete remission of stage IV breast cancer after high-dose chemotherapy and autologous bone marrow transplantation. Am J Clin Oncol 1990; 13:364–366.

17. Dunphy FR, Spitzer G, Buzdar AU, Hortobagyi GN, Horwitz LJ, Yau JC, Spinolo JA, Jagan-nath S, Holmes F, Wallerstein RO. Treatment of estrogen receptor-negative or hormonally refractory breast cancer with double high-dose chemotherapy intensification and bone mar-row support. J Clin Oncol 1990; 8:1207–1216.

18. Dunphy FR, Spitzer G. Use of very-high-dose chemotherapy with autologous bone marrow transplantation in treatment of breast cancer (Letter, Comment). J Natl Cancer Inst 1992; 84:128–129.

19. Williams SF, Gilewski T, Mick R, Bitran JD. High-dose consolidation therapy with autolo-gous stem-cell rescue in stage IV breast cancer: follow up report. J Clin Oncol 1992; 10: 1743–1747.

20. Antman K, Ayash LJ, Elias AD, Wheeler C, Schwartz G, Mazanet R, Tepler I, Schnipper LE, Frei E. High-dose cyclophosphamide, thiotepa, and carboplatin with autologous marrow support in women with measurable advanced breast cancer responding to standard-dose ther-apy: analysis by age. J Natl Cancer Inst Monogr 1994; 91–94.

21. Peters WP, Ross M, Vredenburg JJ, Meisenberg B, Marks LB, Winer E, Kurtzberg J, Jones R, Shpall EJ, Wu K, Rosner G, Gilbert C, Mathias B, Coniglo D, Petros W, Henderson IC, Norton L, Weiss RB, Budmann DR, Hurd D. High-dose chemotherapy and autologous bone marrow support as consolidation after standard dose adjuvant therapy for high-risk primary breast cancer. J Clin Oncol 1993; 11:1132–1143.

22. Antman K, Rowlings P, Vaughan WP, Pelz CJ, Fay J, Fields KK, Freytes CO, Gale RP, Hillner BE, Holland HK, Kennedy MJ, Klein JP, Lazarus HM, McCarthy PL, Saez R, Spitzer G, Stadtmauer EA, Williams SF, Wolff S, Sobocinski KA, Armitage JO, Horowitz MM. High-dose chemotherapy with autologous hematopoietic stem-cell support for breast cancer in North America. J Clin Oncol 1997; 15:1870–1879.

23. Livingston R, Schulman S. Combination chemotherapy and systemic irradiation for poor prognosis breast cancer. Cancer 1987; 59:1249–1254.

24. Greenberg PA, Hortobagyi GN, Smith TL, Ziegler LD, Frye DK, Buzdar AU. Long term follow-up of patients with complete remission following combination chemotherapy for metastatic breast cancer. J Clin Oncol 1996; 14:2197–2205.

25. Mick R, Begg CB, Antman KH, Korzun AH, Frei E. Diverse prognosis in metastatic breast cancer: who should be offered alternative initial therapies? Breast Cancer Res Treat 1989; 13:33–38.

26. Rahman Z, Frye D, Buzdar AU, Hortobagyi GN. A retrospective analysis to evaluate the impact of selection process for high-dose chemotherapy (HDCT) on the outcome of patients (PT) with metastatic breast cancer (MBC) (Abstr). Proc Am Soc Clin Oncol 1995; 13(suppl): 95.

27. Kennedy MJ, Beveridge RA, Rowley SD, Gordon GB, Abeloff MD, Davidson NE. High-dose chemotherapy with reinfusion of purged autologous bone marrow following dose-intense induction as initial therapy for metastatic breast cancer (see Comments). J Natl Cancer Inst 1991; 83:920–926.

28. Kennedy MJ. High-dose chemotherapy of breast cancer: is the question answered? J Clin Oncol 1995; 13:2477–2479.

29. Dunphy FR, Spitzer G, Fornoff JE, Yau JC, Huan SD, Dicke KA, Buzdar AU, Hortobagyi GN. Factors predicting long-term survival for metastatic breast cancer patients treated with high-dose chemotherapy and bone marrow support. Cancer 1994; 73:2157–2167.

30. Ayash LJ, Wheeler C, Fairclough D, Schwartz G, Reich E, Warren D, Schnipper L, Antman K, Frei E, Elias AD. Prognostic factors for prolonged progression-free survival with high-dose chemotherapy with autologous stem-cell support for advanced breast cancer. J Clin Oncol 1995; 13:2043–2049.

31. Peters WP, Jones R, Vredenburg JJ, Shpall EJ, Hussein A, Elkordy M, Rubin P, Ross M, Berry D. A large prospective randomized trial of high-dose combination alkylating agents (CPB) with autologous cellular support (ABMS) as consolidation for patients with metastatic breast cancer achieving complete remission after intensive doxorubicin-based induction (AFM). Breast Cancer Res Treat 1996; 37(suppl):35.

32. Peters WP, Shpall EJ, Jones RB, Olsen GA, Bast RC, Gockerman JP, Moore JO. High-dose combination alkylating agents with bone marrow support as initial treatment for metastatic breast cancer. J Clin Oncol 1988; 6:1368–1376.

33. Bezwoda WR, Seymour L, Dansey RD. High-dose chemotherapy with hematopoietic rescue as primary treatment for metastatic breast cancer: a randomized trial. J Clin Oncol 1995; 13: 2483–2489.

34. Bezwoda WR, Dansey RD, Seymour L. First line chemotherapy of advanced breast cancer with mitoxantrone, cyclophosphamide and vincristine. Oncology 1989; 46:208–211.

35. Venturini M, Bruzzi P, Mastro LD, Garrone O, Bertelli G, Guelti M, Pastorino S, Rasso R, Sertoli R. Effect of adjuvant chemotherapy with or without anthracyclines on the activity and efficacy of first-line cyclophosphamide, epidoxorubicin, and fluorouracil in patients with metastatic breast cancer. J Clin Oncol 1996; 14:764–773.

36. Bezwoda WR. Primary high dose therapy for metastatic breast cancer: update and analysis of prognostic factors (Abstr). Proc Am Soc Clin Oncol 1998; 17(suppl 1):115.

37. Ford C, Spitzer G, Reilly W, Adkins D. A phase II study of repetitive cycles of dose intense carboplatin plus Taxol chemotherapy and peripheral blood stem cells in metastatic breast cancer. Semin Oncol 1997; 24(suppl 17):S17–S24.

38. Elias AD, Ayash LJ, Wheeler C, Schwartz G, Tepler I, Gonin R, McCauley M, Mazanet R, Schnipper L, Frei E. Phase I study of high-dose ifosfamide, carboplatin and etoposide with autologous hematopoietic stem cell support. Bone Marrow Transplant 1995; 15:373–379.

39. Fields KK, Perkins JP, Hiemenz JW, Zorsky PE, Janssen WE, Kronish LE, Machak MC, Elfenbein GJ. Intensive dose ifosfamide, carboplatin, and etoposide followed by autologous stem cell rescue: results of a phase I/II study in breast cancer patients. Surg Oncol 1993; 2: 87–95.

40. Fields KK, Perkins JB, Partyka S, Efenbein GJ. High-dose therapy for the treatment of breast cancer: evaluation of effect of regimen on outcome. Bone Marrow Transplant 1996; 18(suppl 1):30–33.

41. Zander AR, Kruger W, Kroger N, Dumon L, Konigmann M, Berdel WE, Gieseking F, Schafer-Eckart K, Mobus V, Frickhofen N, Wandt H, Illiger HJ, Metzner B, Kolbe K, Wormann B, Trumper L, Huber C, Hossfeld DK, Maass H, Jonat W, for the German GABG-4/eh-93-Studt. High dose mitoxantrone with thiotepa, cyclophosphamide and autologous stem cell rescue for high risk stage II and stage III breast cancer. Bone Marrow Transplant 1996; 18(suppl 1):S24–S25.

42. Gisselbrecht C, Extra JM, Lotz JP, Devaux Y, Janvier M, Peny AM, Guillevin L, Bremond D, Delain M, HErbrecht R, Lepage E, Maraninchi D. Cyclophosphamide/mitoxantrone/melphalan (CMA) regimen prior to autologous bone marrow transplantation (ABMT) in metastatic breast cancer. Bone Marrow Transplant 1996; 18:857–863.

43. Stemmer SM, Cagnoni PJ, Shpall EJ, Bearman SI, Matthes S, Dufton C, Day T, Taffs S, Hami L, Martinez C, Purdy MH, Arron J, Jones RB. High-dose paclitaxel, cyclophosphamide, and cisplatin with autologous hematopoietic progenitor-cell support: a phase I trial. J Clin Oncol 1996; 1:1463–1472.

44. Spitzer G, Champlin R, Scong D, Dunphy FR, Velasquez WS, Petruska C, Bowers C, Broun G, McIntrye W, Niemeyer R, Adkins D. Repetitive high-dose therapy: tolerance and outcome in stage IV breast cancer. In: Dicke KA, Keating A, eds. Autologous Marrow and Blood Transplantation: Proceedings of the Seventh International Symposium. TX: The Cancer Treatment Research and Educational Institute, 95:195–206.

45. Ayash LJ, Elias AD, Wheeler C, Reich E, Schwartz G, Mazanet R, Tepler I, Warren D, Lynch C, Gonin R. Double dose-intensive chemotherapy with autologous marrow and peripheral-blood progenitor-cell support for metastatic breast cancer: a feasibility study. J Clin Oncol 1994; 12:37–44.

46. Ayash LJ, Elias AD, Schwartz G, Wheeler C, Ibrahim J, Reich E, Warren D, Lynch C, Richardson P, Schnipper LE, Frei E, Antman K. Double dose-intensive therapy chemotherapy with autologous stem-cell support for metastatic breast cancer: no improvement in progression-free survival by the sequence of high-dose melphalan followed by cyclophosphamide, thiotepa, and carboplatin. J Clin Oncol 1996; 14:2984–2992.

47. Shapiro CL, Ayash L, Webb IJ, Gelman R, Keating J, Williams L, Demetri G, Clark P, Elias A, Duggan D, Hayes D, Hurd D, Henderson IC. Repetitive cycles of cyclophosphamide, thiotepa, and carboplatin intensification with peripheral-blood progenitor cells and filgrastin in advanced breast cancer patients. J Clin Oncol 1997; 15:674–683.

48. Crown J, Wassherheit C, Hakes T, Fennelly D, Reich L, Moore M, Schneider J, Curtin J, Rubin SC, Reichman B. Rapid delivery of multiple high-dose chemotherapy courses with granulocyte colony-stimulating factor and peripheral blood–derived hematopoietic progenitor cells (Letter). J Natl Cancer Inst 1992; 84:1935–1936.

49. Crown J, Kritz A, Vahdat L, Reich L, Moore M, Hamilton N, Schneider J, Harrison M,

Gilewski T, Hudis C. Rapid administration of multiple cycles of high-dose myelosuppressive chemotherapy in patients with metastatic breast cancer. J Clin Oncol 1993; 11:1144–1149.

50. Crown J, Vahdat L, Raptis G. Rapid cycled courses of high-dose chemotherapy supported by filgastrin and peripheral blood stem cells in patients with metastatic breast cancer. Proc Am Soc Clin Oncol 1994; 13:110.

51. Crown J, Vahdat L, Fennelly D, Francis P, Wasserheit C, Hudis C, Kritz A, Schneider J, Hamilton N, Gilewski T. High-intensity chemotherapy with hematopoietic support in breast cancer (Review). Ann NY Acad Sci 1993; 698:378–388.

52. Fennelly D, Vahdat L, Schneider J, Reich L, Hamilton N, Hakes T, Raptis G, Wasserheit C, Kritz A, Gulati S. High-intensity chemotherapy with peripheral blood progenitor cell support (Review). Semin Oncol 1994; 21(suppl 12):S21–S25.

53. Fennelly D, Wasserheit C, Schneider J, Hakes T, Reich L, Curtin J, Yau TJ, Markman M, Norton L, Crown J. Simultaneous dose escalation and schedule intensification of carboplatin-based chemotherapy using peripheral blood progenitor cells and filgastrin: a phase I trial. Cancer Res 1994; 54:6137–6142.

54. Jones RJ, Vogelsang GB, Hess AD, Farmer ER, Mann RB, Geller RB, Piantadosi S, Santos GW. Induction of graft-versus-host disease after autologous bone marrow transplantation. Lancet 1989; 1:754–757.

55. Kennedy MJ, Jones RJ. Autologous graft-versus-host disease: immunotherapy of breast cancer after bone marrow transplantation (Review). Breast Cancer Res Treat 1993; 26(suppl): S31–S40.

56. Glazier A, Tutschka PJ, Farmer ER, Santos GW. Graft-versus-host disease in cyclosporin A–treated rats after syngeneic and autologous bone marrow reconstitution. J Exp Med 1983; 158:1–8.

57. Kennedy MJ, Vogelsang GB, Beveridge RA, Farmer ER, Altomonte V, Huelskamp AM, Davidson NE. Phase I trial of intravenous cyclosporine to induce graft-versus-host disease in women undergoing autologous bone marrow transplantation for breast cancer. J Clin Oncol 1993; 11:478–484.

58. Kennedy MJ, Vogelsang GB, Jones RJ, Farmer ER, Hess AD, Altomonte V, Huelskamp AM, Davidson NE. Phase I trial of interferon gamma to potentiate cyclosporine-induced graft-versus-host disease in women undergoing autologous bone marrow transplantation for breast cancer. J Clin Oncol 1994; 12:249–257.

59. Meehan KB, Verma UN, Cahill R, Frankel SR, Areman EA, Sacher R, Foelber R, Rajagopal C, Gehan EA, Lippman ME, Mazumder A. Interleukin-2–activated hematopoietic stem cell transplantation for breast cancer: investigation of dose level with clinical correlates. Bone Marrow Transplant 1997; 20:643–652.

60. Meehan KB, Verma UN, Frankel SR, Rajagopal R, Cahill R, Arun-Killic B, Jensen M, Oquendo C, Mazumder A. Immunotherapy with IL-2 and alpha interferon after PBSC transplantation for women with breast cancer (Abstr). Proc Am Soc Clin Oncol 1997; 16(suppl): 94.

61. Eibl B, Schwaighofer H, Nachbaur D, Marth C, Gachter A, Knapp R, Bock G, Gassner C, Schiller L, Petersen F, Niederwieser D. Evidence for a graft-versus-tumor effect in a patient treated with marrow ablative chemotherapy and allogeneic bone marrow transplantation for breast cancer. Blood 1996; 88:1501–1508.

62. Ueno NT, Rondon G, Mirza NQ, Geisler DK, Anderlini P, Giralt SA, Andersson BS, Claxton DF, Gajewski JL, Khouri IF, Korbling M, Mehra RC, Przepiorka D, Rahman Z, Samuels BI, van Besien K, Hortobagyi GN, Champlin RE. Allogeneic peripheral-blood progenitor-cell transplantation for poor-risk patients with metastatic breast cancer. J Clin Oncol 1998; 16:986–993.

63. Cote RJ, Rosen PP, Lesser ML, Old LJ, Osborne MP. Prediction of early relapse in patients with operable breast cancer by detection of occult bone marrow micrometastases. J Clin Oncol 1991; 9:1749–1756.

64. Pantel K, Braun S, Passlick B, Schlimok G. Minimal residual epithelial cancer: diagnostic approaches and prognostic relevance. Prog Histochem Cytochem 1996; 30:1–60.

65. Dwenger A, Lindemann A, Mertelsmann R. Minimal residual disease: detection, clinical relevance, and treatment strategies. J Hematother 1996; 5:537–548.

66. Sharp JG. Micrometastases and transplantation. J Hematother 1996; 5:519–524.

67. Ross AA, Cooper BW, Lazarus HM, Mackay W, Moss TJ, Ciobanu N, Tallman MS, Kennedy MJ, Davidson NE, Sweet D. Detection and viability of tumor cells in peripheral blood stem cell collections from breast cancer patients using immunocytochemical and clonogenic assay techniques. Blood 1993; 82:2605–2610.

68. Brisco MJ, Condon J, Hughes E, Neoh SH, Sykes PJ, Seshadri R, Toogood I, Waters K, Tauro G, Ekert H. Outcome prediction in childhood acute lymphoblastic leukaemia by molecular quantification of residual disease at the end of induction. Lancet 1994; 343:196–200.

69. Kusec R, Laczika K, Knobl P, Friedl J, Greinix H, Kahls P, Linkesch W, Schwarzinger I, Mitterbauer G, Purtscher B. AML1/ETO fusion MRNA can be detected in remission blood samples of all patients with T(8;21) acute myeloid leukemia after chemotherapy or autologous bone marrow transplantation. Leukemia 1994; 8:735–739.

70. Brugger W, Bross KJ, Glatt M, Weber F, Mertelsmann R, Kanz L. Mobilization of tumor cells and hematopoietic progenitor cells into the peripheral blood of patients with solid tumors. Blood 1994; 83:636–640.

71. Precore AL, Lazarus H, Cooper B, Copelan E, Herzig R, Meagher R, Kennedy MJ, Akard L, Jansen J, Isaacs R, Jennis A, Moss TJ. The incidence of breast cancer cell contamination in peripheral blood stem cell (PBSC) collections in relation to the mobilization regimen. Blood 1996; 88(suppl 1):408.

72. Fields KK, Elfenbein GJ, Trudeau WL, Perkins JB, Janssen WE, Moscinski LC. Clinical significance of bone marrow metastases as detected using the polymerase chain reaction in patients with breast cancer undergoing high-dose chemotherapy and autologous bone marrow transplantation. J Clin Oncol 1996; 14:1868–1876.

73. Kruger WH, Stockschalder M, Hennings S, Aschenbrenner M, Gruther M, Gutensohn K, Lobliger C, Gieseking F, Jonat W, Zander AR. Detection of cancer cells in peripheral blood stem cells of women with breast cancer by RT-PCR and cell culture. Bone Marrow Transplant 1996; 18(suppl 1):18–20.

74. Vredenburgh JJ, Peters WP, Rosner G, DeSombre K, Johnston WW, Kamel A, Wu K, Bast RC. Detection of tumor cells in the bone marrow of stage IV breast cancer patients receiving high-dose chemotherapy: the role of induction chemotherapy. Bone Marrow Transplant 1995; 16:815–821.

75. Brenner MK, Rill DR, Moen RC, Krance RA, Mirro JJ, Anderson WF, Ihle JN. Gene-marking to trace origin of relapse after autologous bone-marrow transplantation. Lancet 1993; 341:85–86.

76. Rill DR, Santana VM, Roberts WM, Nilson T, Bowman LC, Krance RA, Heslop HE, Moen RC, Ihle JN, Brenner MK. Direct demonstration that autologous bone marrow transplantation for solid tumors can return a multiplicity of tumorigenic cells. Blood 1994; 84:380–383.

77. Shpall EJ, Stemmer SM, Bearman SI, Myers S, Purdy M, Jones RB. New strategies in marrow purging for breast cancer patients receiving high-dose chemotherapy with autologous bone marrow transplantation. Breast Cancer Res Treat 1993; 26(suppl):S19–S23.

78. Shpall EJ, Jones RB, Bearman SI, Franklin WA, Archer PG, Curiel T, Bitter M, Claman HN, Stemmer SM, Purdy M. Transplantation of enriched CD34-positive autologous marrow into breast cancer patients following high-dose chemotherapy: influence of CD34-positive peripheral-blood progenitors and growth factors on engraftment. J Clin Oncol 1994; 12:28–36.

79. Cagnoni PJ, Nieto Y, Shpall EJ, Bearman SI, Baron AE, Ross M, Mahtes S, Dunbar SE, Jones R. High-dose chemotherapy with autologous hematopoietic progenitor-cell support as part of combined modality therapy with inflammatory breast cancer. J Clin Oncol 1998; 16:16661–1668.

80. Shpall EJ, Jones RB, Bast RC Jr, Rosner GL, Vandermark R, Ross M, Affronti ML, Johnston C, Eggleston S, Tepperburg M. 4-Hydroperoxycyclophosphamide purging of breast cancer from the mononuclear cell fraction of bone marrow in patients receiving high-dose chemotherapy and autologous marrow support: a phase I trial. J Clin Oncol 1991; 9:85–93.

81. Shpall EJ, Bast RC Jr, Joines WT, Jones RB, Anderson I, Johnston C, Eggleston S, Tepperberg M, Edwards S, Peters WP. Immunomagnetic purging of breast cancer from bone marrow for autologous transplantation. Bone Marrow Transplant 1991; 7:145–151.

82. O'Briant KC, Shpall EJ, Houston LL, Peters WP, Bast RC Jr. Elimination of clonogenic breast cancer cells from human bone marrow. A comparison of immunotoxin treatment with chemoimmunoseparation using 4-hydroperoxycyclophosphamide, monoclonal antibodies, and magnetic microspheres. Cancer 1991; 68:1272–1278.

83. Seong D, Mehra R, Anderson B, Giralt S, Van Biesen K, Khouri I, Deisseroth A, Champlin R. Autologous bone marrow infusion does not contribute to relapse following high-dose tandem chemotherapy for recurrent or metastatic breast cancer (Abstr). Proc Am Soc Clin Oncol 1995; 14(suppl 1):210.

84. Gianni A, Sienna S, Bregni M, Di Nicola S, Orefice F, Cusumano B, Salvadori B, Luini A, Greco M, Zucali R, Rilke F, Zambeti M, Valagussa P, Bonadona G. Efficiency, toxicity and applicability of high-dose sequential chemotherapy as adjuvant treatment in operable breast cancer with 10 or more involved axillary nodes: five year results. J Clin Oncol 1997; 15: 2312–2321.

85. Hurd DD, Peters WP. Randomized, comparative study of high-dose (with autologous bone marrow support) versus low-dose cyclophosphamide, cisplatin, and carmustine as consolidation to adjuvant cyclophosphamide, doxorubicin, and fluorouracil for patients with operable stage II or III breast cancer involving 10 or more axillary lymph nodes (CALGB Protocol 9082). Cancer and leukemia Group B. J Natl Cancer Inst Monogr 1995; 19:41–44.

86. Bonadona G, Zambetta M, Valagussa P. Sequential of alternating doxorubicin and CMF regimens in breast cancer with more than three positive nodes. JAMA 1995; 273:542.

87. Overgaard M, Hansen PS, Overgaard J, Rose C, Andersson M, Bach F, Kjaer M, Gadeberg CC, Mouridsen HT, Jensen MB, Zedeler K. Postoperative radiotherapy in high-risk premenopausal women with breast cancer who receive adjuvant chemotherapy. Danish Breast Cancer Cooperative Group 82b Trial. N Engl J Med 1997; 337:949–955.

88. Ragaz J, Jackson SM, Plenderleith IH, Wilson K, Basco V, Knowling M, Worth A, Spinelli J, Ng V. Can adjuvant radiotherapy improve the overall survival of breast cancer in the presence of adjuvant chemotherapy? 10 year analysis of the British Columbia Randomized Trial (Abstr). Proc Am Soc Clin Oncol 1993; 12:60a.

89. Crump M, Goss PE, Prince M, Girouard C. Outcome of extensive evaluation before adjuvant therapy in women with breast cancer and 10 or more positive axillary lymph nodes. J Clin Oncol 1996; 14:66–69.

90. Rodenhuis S, Richel DJ, van der Wall E, Schornagel JH, Baars JW, Koning CC, Peterse JL, Borger JH, Nooijen WJ, Bakx R, Dalesio O, Rutgers E. Randomised trial of high-dose chemotherapy and haemopoietic progenitor-cell support in operable breast cancer with extensive axillary lymph-node involvement. Lancet 1998; 352:515–521.

91. Hortobagyi G, Buzdar AU, Champlin R, Gajewski J, Holmes F, Booser D, Valero V, Thieriault RL. Lack of efficacy of adjuvant high-dose (HD) tandem combination chemotherapy (CT) for high-risk primary breast cancer (HRPBC)—a randomized trial (Abstr). Proc Am Soc Clin Oncol 1998; 17(suppl):123.

92. Basser RL, To B, Collins JP, Begley CG, Keefe D, Cebon J, Bashford J, Durrant S, Szer J, Kotasek D, Juttner CA, Russell I, Maher DW, Olver I, Sheridan WP, Fox RM, Green MD. Multicycle high-dose chemotherapy and filgastin-mobilized peripheral blood progenitor cells in women with high-risk stage II or III breast cancer: five-year follow-up. J Clin Oncol 1999; 17:82–92.

93. Bitran JD, Samuels B, Trujillo Y, Klein L, Schroeder L, Martinec J. Her2/neu overexpression is associated with treatment failure in women with high-risk stage II and IIIa breast cancer

(>10 involved lymph nodes) treated with high-dose chemotherapy and autologous hemato-poietic progenitor cell support following standard-dose adjuvant chemotherapy. Clin Cancer Res 1996; 2:1509–1513.

94. Muss HR, Thor AD, Berry DA, Kuth T, Liu ET, Koerner F, Cirrincione CT, Budman DR, Woods WC, Barcos MD, Henderson CI. C-Erb-2 Expression and response to adjuvant ther-apy in women with node-positive early breast cancer. N Engl J Med 1994; 330:1260–1266.

95. Gusterson BA, Gelber RD, Goldhirsch A, Price KN, Save-Soderborgh J, Anbazhagan R, Styles J, Rudenstam CM, Golouh R, Reed R. Prognostic importance of C-ErbB-2 expression in breast cancer. International (Ludwig) Breast Cancer Study Group (see Comments). J Clin Oncol 1992; 10:1049–1056.

96. Schwartzberg LS, Birch R, West WH, Tauer KW, Wittlin F, Leff R, Campos L, Rymer W, Carter P, Mangum M, Greco FA, Hainsworth J, Raefsky E, Blanco R, Buckner CD, Weaver CH. Sequential treatment including high-dose chemotherapy with peripheral blood stem cell support in patients with high-risk stage II–III breast cancer: outpatient administration in com-munity cancer centers. Am J Clin Oncol 1998; 21:523–531.

97. Wood WC, Budman DR, Korzun AH, Cooper MR, Younger J, Hart RD, Moore A, Ellerton JA, Norton L, Ferree CR. Dose and dose intensity of adjuvant chemotherapy for stage II, node-positive breast carcinoma (see Comments). (Published Erratum Appears in N Engl J Med 1994 Jul 14; 331(2):139.) N Engl J Med 1994; 330:1253–1259.

98. Bearman SI, Overmoyer BA, Bolwell BJ, Taylor CW, Shpall EJ, Cagnoni PJ, Mechling BE, Ronk B, Baron AE, Purdy MH, Ross M, Jones RB. High-dose chemotherapy with autologous peripheral blood progenitor cell support for primary breast cancer in patients with 4–9 in-volved axillary lymph nodes. Bone Marrow Transplant 1997; 20:931–937.

99. Huelskamp AM, Abeloff MD, Armstrong DK, Fetting JH, Gordon G, Davidson NE, Kennedy MJ. High-dose consolidation chemotherapy for stage IIIB breast cancer in remission: inter-mediate follow-up and comparison with intensively treated historical controls. Proc Am Soc Clin Oncol 1995; 14:98.

100. Pnatier P, Morvan F, Espie M, Devaux Y, Cure H, Lotz JP, HErbrecht R, Peny AM, Maolleau JP, Bremond D, Gisselbrecht C. High-dose therapy with autologous bone marrow transplanta-tion (ABMT) as consolidation after standard dose chemotherapy and locoregional treatment for inflammatory breast Cancer (Abstr). Proc Am Soc Clin Oncol 1995; 14:117a.

31

Gene Therapy Using Hematopoietic Stem Cells

DONALD B. KOHN, GAY M. CROOKS, and JAN A. NOLTA

Children's Hospital Los Angeles and University of Southern California School of Medicine, Los Angeles, California

I. INTRODUCTION

The treatment of congenital diseases of blood cells by gene replacement has been a major focus of gene therapy research for more than the past decade (1,2). Any of the congenital diseases affecting the production or function of hematopoietic and lymphoid cells which can be treated by allogeneic bone marrow transplantation (BMT) should be amenable to treatment by gene insertion into pluripotent hematopoietic stem cells (HSCs). HSCs would be the ideal target for clinical gene therapy of many genetic diseases, because they are long-lived, producing new progenitor cells and mature blood cells for the life of the recipient. Diseases which currently meet these requirements are congenital immune deficiencies, lysosomal storage disorders, leukocyte defects, the hemoglobinopathies, and stem cell defects such as Fanconi's anemia (Table 1). Because gene therapy would involve autologous transplant of a patient's own gene-treated cells, the immunological problems encountered in the allogeneic setting, such as graft rejection or graft-versus-host disease, would not be expected to occur.

The technical challenges for successful gene therapy include (1) cloning of a normal copy of the gene responsible for the disease, (2) inserting the gene into pluripotent HSCs at sufficient frequency to produce large percentages of gene-containing cells, and (3) expressing the new gene in the appropriate mature hematopoietic cells derived from the HSCs at a level which will replace the deficient function. Besides these matters of efficacy, additional considerations must be the relative safety of the treatment as well as the financial cost to the individual patient and to society.

Table 1   Candidate Disorders for Gene Therapy Using
Hematopoietic Stem Cells

Inherited disorders:
1. Congenital immune deficiencies
    Severe combined immunodeficiency (ADA, XSCID, others)
    Wiskott-Aldrich syndrome
    X-linked agammaglobulinemia
2. Lysosomal storage disorders
    Gaucher's disease
    Mucopolysaccharidoses
    Adrenoleukodystrophy
3. Leukocyte defects
    Chronic granulomatous disease
    Chediak-Higashi
    Leukocyte adhesion defect
4. Hemoglobinopathies
    Sickle cell anemia
    Thalassemia
    Hemolytic anemias (G6-PD, RBC skeletal defects)
5. Stem cell defects
    Fanconi's anemia
Neoplastic diseases:
1. Decrease myelosuppressive effects of chemotherapy
Infectious diseases:
1. HIV-1 infection (AIDS)

II. RETROVIRAL VECTORS

The gene-delivery system most widely used for preclinical and clinical gene therapy studies to date has been retroviral vectors based on the Moloney murine leukemia virus (MoMuLV) (3,4). Retroviral vectors are, in effect, self-mobilizing expression plasmids which can become stably integrated into the chromosomes of host target cells. Despite the theoretical potential for insertional oncogenicity, retroviral vectors have been found to be safe in the preclinical and clinical studies performed to date.

    A major limitation to the use of MoMuLV-based retroviral vectors for gene delivery is that the target cells must be actively replicating for the vector to be able to integrate permanently into the chromosomes (5). The majority of HSCs are quiescent, in a resting state or G_0 phase of the cell cycle, so that they must be stimulated to proliferate for effective retrovirus-mediated gene transduction. Despite these limits, MoMuLV-based retroviruses are currently the best available system for clinical applications of gene transfer into stem cells. Certainly, better means of gene transfer would permit more effective application of gene therapy, as discussed below.

III. GENE TRANSDUCTION STUDIES USING MURINE BMT MODELS

A. Gene Transfer

It was shown in the mid-1980s that MoMuLV-based retroviruses are capable of inserting exogenous genes into pluripotent HSCs from the bone marrow of mice (6–8). The transduced HSCs can reconstitute lethally irradiated mice, and the new gene is present in cells of the erythroid, granulocytic, monocytic, and lymphoid lineages. Subsequent improvements have been achieved in the basic gene transfer protocols by adding recombinant hematopoietic growth factors to stimulate proliferation of the marrow HSCs and the use of support matrices of either marrow stromal cell monolayers or the extracellular matrix protein fibronectin. Current methodologies typically permit the majority of *murine* stem cells to be successfully transduced, with nearly every hematopoietic cell in transplanted mice containing the inserted gene (9–11).

B. Gene Expression

The task of achieving appropriate expression of a gene introduced into pluripotent HSCs is formidable. The gene transfer event needs to be into the rare, long-lived HSCs to have an enduring effect. But, the gene expression must occur in specific mature hematopoietic and/or lymphoid cells, produced after multiple rounds of progenitor cell division and extensive cellular differentiation from the blast-like stem cell to the mature cell phenotype. An ideal goal is to have an exogenous gene expressed only in specific cell types, under specific physiological conditions, at a specified level. Such precise control is not currently achievable; most gene vectors have used constitutive promoters, such as those from viruses (the retroviral long-term repeating (LTR), cytomegalovirus (CMV), simian virus 40 (SV40), or cellular housekeeping genes (phosphoglycerate kinase, β-actin), seeking to express the gene within a range which would be beneficial and not harmful.

Many of the initial studies used vectors carrying the bacterial neomycin resistance gene (*neo*) as a readily detectable neutral marker (6,7). Subsequent studies examined transduction of human genes directly relevant to specific genetic disorders, such as adenosine deaminase (ADA—responsible for approximately 20% of the cases of severe combined immunodeficiency, SCID), β-globin, or glucocerebrosidase (GC), defective in Gaucher's disease. Generally, it has been possible to demonstrate that expression of these genes can be achieved in the hematopoietic cells of the mice receiving the gene transfer/BMT at levels which would be expected to be corrective of the genetic defect.

For example, as part of preclinical studies toward gene therapy for Gaucher's disease, we have studied insertion of the human GC gene into mouse bone marrow used to engraft irradiated recipient mice. We demonstrated expression of human GC protein in tissue macrophages after transplant, including Kupffer's cells in the liver, splenic and pulmonary macrophages, and a portion of the central nervous system (CNS) microglia (12). Wolfe and coworkers at the University of Pennsylvania have studied gene transfer and expression in mice deficient for β-glucuronidase (β-GUS), a model of human mucopolysaccharidosis type VII (Sly's disease). They have shown that even low levels of transfer and expression of a normal β-GUS cDNA results in significant correction of disease manifestations, including some of the CNS storage of the mucopolysaccharide substrate (13). The ability of an introduced gene to be expressed in cells migrating into the CNS suggests that these techniques may have some benefit for disorders with neurological components, such as Hurler's disease and acquired immunodeficiency syndrome (AIDS) encephalopathy. More recently, retrovirus-mediated gene transfer has been shown to be capable of correcting manifestations of immune deficiency in gene knockout models of Jak-3 kinase-deficient SCID and chronic granulomatous disease (14,15).

Achieving physiologically appropriate expression of β-globin has been a particularly stubborn problem, with relatively low levels of expression being seen when a transferred human β-globin gene has been controlled by its own promoter elements. A first step toward erythrocyte lineage-specific expression was taken in studies by Dzierzak et al. (16) and others since then (17), in which vectors were developed that expressed human β-globin by using the β-globin promoter and enhancers. In murine studies, the human β-globin gene cassette was inserted into bone marrow stem cells and, subsequently, was present in cells of all hematopoietic and lymphoid lineages after BMT. However, only the erythroid cells expressed the β-globin gene, because only they have the necessary array of *trans*-acting transcriptional factors to transcribe the β-globin gene. Although these control elements are sufficient to achieve lineage-specific expression, the quantitative levels of β-globin produced were very low (e.g., 0.1–1.0% of endogenous levels of murine β-globin).

Attempts have subsequently focused on including in the vector portions of the β-globin locus-control region (LCR), a genetic element which is a master switch to activate globin gene expression in erythroid cells (18). These were initially frustrated by the unexpected adverse affects of these fragments on retroviral vector titer and integrity (19,20). Sequences present in the human β-globin gene function as ribonucleic acid (RNA) splice sites and transcription termination/polyadenylation signals when placed within the RNA genome of retroviral vectors. Recent publications describe work in which extensive modifications of the numerous deleterious elements of the human β-globin gene and LCR sequences led to vectors with more acceptable titers and levels of expression approaching those of endogenous globin (21,22). Possibly, these new β-globin vectors may allow the beginning of clinical trials to treat hemoglobinopathies by gene therapy.

Similar problems have recently been noted with the gene for human MDR-1. Efforts are underway to modify the stem cells from patients with solid tumors to be resistant to common chemotherapeutic agents to decrease the extent of myelosuppression. Although initial studies in mice and human marrow have shown some increased resistance to paclitaxel (Taxol) after insertion of the human MDR-1 cDNA, the effects have been suboptimal (23). Sorrentino et al. (24) have subsequently demonstrated that the human MDR-1 cDNA has cryptic splice donor and splice acceptor sites, causing a fraction of the vectors to carry truncated and useless versions of the gene. Work to modify the responsible sequences may eliminate the splicing problems while maintaining effective drug resistance.

Additionally, we and others have reported that loss of gene expression from retroviral vectors may occur in vivo after gene transfer into murine HSCs, as well as dermal fibroblasts, hepatocytes, and myoblasts, possibly as a result of insertion into ectopic sites in the chromosomes which are not permissive for prolonged gene expression (25–27). Although the MoMuLV LTR can be a strong promoter when used in primary murine BMT recipients, the LTR is often inactive when studied using a green fluorescent protein reporter in peripheral blood cells (28) or by serial transplantation of the marrow into secondary recipient mice (27). This lack of expression significantly correlates with methylation of cytosine residues in the LTR. The late loss of gene expression would prevent an enduring clinical benefit to be obtained in vivo after HSC transduction. It will be necessary to identify other transcriptional control elements (e.g., housekeeping promoters, LCR, hypomethylation signals, scaffold attachment regions, insulators) to achieve the necessary level and duration of gene expression for effective gene therapy.

IV. GENE TRANSDUCTION STUDIES IN LARGE ANIMAL BMT MODELS

The most definitive experimental data demonstrating the limits to effective gene transfer come from studies performed on gene transfer into the bone marrow of large animals.

Data from a number of studies in which retrovirus-transduced marrow was transplanted into canine or simian recipients after cytoablative total body irradiation have until recently not exceeded more than 1–2% stem cell marking (29–31). Yet, in many of these studies, in vitro assays of the transduced marrow demonstrated 15–30% transduction of colony-forming units (CFUs). These findings demonstrate that, although gene transfer into clonogenic progenitors is reasonably effective with current methods, the long-lived reconstituting stem cells remain recalcitrant to transduction. Recently, two groups of investigators have reported results of 1–10% gene marking of the peripheral blood cells in monkeys receiving retrovirally transduced autologous bone marrow by using a combination of modifications of the gene transfer protocol which each modestly improve stem cell transduction or survival during ex vivo manipulation (32,33).

V. GENE TRANSDUCTION STUDIES WITH HUMAN HEMATOPOIETIC STEM CELLS

A. In Vitro Bone Marrow Culture

Many studies have demonstrated that gene transduction of human CD34$^+$ cells is increased by growth with specific recombinant cytokines [interleukin (IL)–1α, IL-3, IL-6, IL-11; leukemia inhibitory factor LIF; c-kit ligand; basic fibroblast growth factor] (34–37). Transduction of CD34$^+$ cells is also enhanced when performed on a marrow stromal cell layer, on a fragment of the matrix protein fibronectin, or by centrifugation of the cells for 1–4 h during exposure to retrovirus, as measured at the level of CFU assays, high-proliferative potential colony-forming cells, or long-term culture-initiating cell assays (38–41).

Unfortunately, there is increasing evidence that these in vitro observations do not predict the effectiveness of gene transfer into the true stem cells which lead to long-term hematopoiesis in vivo after transplantation. The numerical preponderance of committed progenitor cells in marrow obscures the presence and activity of the rare pluripotent stem cells from unfractionated marrow or even CD34$^+$-enriched fractions.

Stem cells are operationally defined by their ability to produce sustained, multilineage hematopoietic cell engraftment after transplant. No in vitro systems have been devised which can measure these activities from human stem cells. The long-term bone marrow culture (LTBMC) systems, originally described by Dexter for murine cells and later adapted for growth of human marrow, produce myelomonocytic and erythroid cells but not lymphoid cells. LTBMCs are viable for only a few months, which is less than the time period required after BMT for hematopoiesis to be derived from pluripotent stem cells. We have consistently found that gene transduction of long-term culture initiating cells (LTCICs), commonly taken as an in vitro counterpart of stem cells, occurs to nearly the same frequency as for the directly clonogenic progenitors (42).

In a more stringent assay of primitive human hematopoietic progenitor cells, we have developed a system for single cell growth from cells bearing the immunophenotype of CD34$^+$, CD38$^-$ (43). A subset of these cells will grow as *extended* long-term culture initiating cells (E-LTCICs) for 3–4 months (producing 10^5–10^7 progeny cells) and are capable of both myeloid and B-lymphoid differentiation (44,45). Although transduction with retroviral vectors may be achieved at reasonably high frequencies into the CD34$^+$/CD38$^-$ cells which form colonies in the first 1–2 months of culture (the standard LTCIC time frame), the E-LTCICs are transduced at low frequencies, typically less than 1–2%. This system will provide a useful in vitro model to test new methods to increase gene transduction.

B. In Vivo Models

One possible approach to studying gene transduction of human HSCs is through the use of animal models which allow human marrow growth in immune-deficient mice or fetal sheep (46,47). Dick and coworkers have demonstrated that the human hematopoietic progenitor cells which engraft over 1–2 months in SCID mice (SCID repopulating cells, SRCs) are very inefficiently transduced by retroviral vectors, providing a model to analyze efforts to improve gene transfer (48).

Our group has developed a model which allows sustained human hematopoiesis in severely immune-deficient mice (*beigelnudelxid*) by cotransplanting gene-transduced CD34$^+$ cells with primary human marrow stromal cells expressing recombinant human IL-3 (41,49). Long-term expression of the IL-3 supports human hematopoietic cell proliferation for at least 12 months. Human progenitors as well as mature myeloid and T-lymphoid cells can be recovered from the mice during this period and will express the genes that had been introduced into the CD34$^+$ cells.

Because MoMuLV-based retroviral vectors integrate into the chromosomal DNA at unique sites for each target cell, the vector can serve as a clonal tag, marking all progeny derived from a single stem cell with the vector present at the same integration site. Using inverse polymerase chain reaction (PCR) to define the retroviral vector integration sites, we have been able to demonstrate that it is possible to transduce human stem cells capable of giving rise to both myeloid cells and T lymphocytes (50). However, the transduction of pluripotent human HSCs by this assessment is a rare event. We are currently using this system to define optimal protocols for gene transfer into the long-lived, pluripotent progenitors present in human marrow, cord blood, and peripheral blood.

VI. CLINICAL TRANSPLANTATION OF TRANSDUCED HUMAN HSCs

Initial clinical gene marking studies have shown the same dichotomy seen in the large animal studies, with relatively efficient gene transfer into clonogenic progenitor cells but minimal transduction of HSCs which function in vivo after transplant of the transduced marrow (51). For example, the group led by Dunbar at the National Institutes of Health (NIH) has transplanted patients with either breast cancer or multiple myeloma using gene marking of a portion of the marrow or peripheral blood progenitor cells (52). The gene-transduction protocol involved culturing the CD34$^+$ cells for 3 days in the presence of growth factors IL-3, IL-6, and SCF with daily addition of vector supernatant. Typically, 10–25% of the CFUs formed in vitro by the marked cells contained the vector. In contrast, only a few patients have shown any detectable circulating blood cells containing vector sequences a few months after transplant.

The most informative clinical results to date have been those obtained by the group of Malcolm Brenner at St. Jude Children's Cancer Research Hospital (53,54). They performed gene marking of the marrow being used for autologous BMT of children with either acute myeloid leukemia (AML) or neuroblastoma. The primary goal of these investigations was to determine if any cells in the transplant inoculum contributed to relapse after transplant; if vector-containing malignant cells are detected in the patient at relapse, then they must have come from the transplanted cells. Indeed, they showed that gene-marked cells *do* contribute a portion of the malignant cells at relapse in patients with AML or neuroblastoma. A similar finding has been reported for adults with chronic myeloid leukemia (CML) undergoing autologous transplants (55). (It remains to be seen whether these data will change the views of those who believe that marrow purging is not necessary in autologous BMT).

The gene transfer protocols which were used for these marking studies were purposefully chosen to cause minimal perturbation of the marrow to allow marking of spontaneously proliferating malignant cells. The marrows were exposed to vector supernatant only once on the day of harvest without the addition of cytokines or stroma. These conditions certainly are suboptimal for gene transfer into CFUs and they observed only 5–10% CFU transduction. Somewhat surprisingly, they achieved a significant level of marking of the normal, nonmalignant hematopoietic cells after reconstitution (56).

One interpretation of these results is that all of the efforts which maximize gene transfer into progenitor cells (such as incubation in recombinant cytokines) have little effect on stem cells. The fraction of stem cells transduced may be determined by the percentage which were spontaneously in cycle at the time of marrow collection; in turn, this may reflect the prior chemotherapy treatment status of the patients. The marrows from the St. Jude's patients were harvested as they were recovering from high-dose chemotherapy, which may be associated with a higher than normal cycling fraction (57). However, when this approach was tried in adults with a variety of other malignancies, minimal gene marking was attained. The relative roles of the specific chemotherapy regimens or the younger ages of the patients in the St. Jude's study on the high extents of gene marking remain to be determined.

The failure to transduce a significant fraction of HSCs which engraft after cytoablative conditioning suggests that effective gene therapy for most hematological disorders may not be possible at the present time. If no combination of currently available cytokines can influence stem cell cycling ex vivo and, if even intensive chemotherapy only increases spontaneous stem cell transduction to a few percentages (58), then correction of a significant percentage of stem cells cannot currently be achieved using retroviral vectors.

VII. NEW APPROACHES TO ACHIEVE MORE EFFECTIVE GENE TRANSFER INTO HUMAN HSCs

Because of the problems currently encountered in effective transduction of human HSCs, a large number of approaches are under investigation to increase the percentages of transduced HSCs (Table 2).

A. Purification of Human HSCs to Facilitate Gene Transduction

One approach to increase gene transfer into human HSCs which has not been fully explored is the application of physical and immunological techniques to isolate populations of cells greatly enriched for stem cell activity. Performing the 30- to 100-fold enrichment afforded by CD34$^+$ cell selection does *not* significantly increase gene transduction of clonogenic progenitors (36). However, there are logistical reasons to eliminate the large numbers of mature cells present in the marrow. Enriching for the target stem cells minimizes the amount of vector supernatant needed to treat a clinical aliquot of marrow (as much as 10^9–10^{11} mononuclear cells). Possibly, further purification of stem cell subsets, such as CD34$^+$/CD38$^-$, CD34$^+$/DR$^-$, or CD34$^+$/lin$^-$/Thy^{lo}, may not only further decrease vector needs, but may also allow increases in the relative multiplicity of infection and/or remove cells producing inhibitory factors which suppress stem cell proliferation.

Table 2 Methods to Achieve High Percentages of Transduced Stem Cells

1. Increase the percentage of stem cells initially transduced
   a. Higher titer retroviral vectors
   b. Alternative retroviral envelopes (GALV, VSV)
   c. Induce cycling of HSCs: cytokines, stroma, LTBMCs
   d. "Present" virus: stroma, fibronectin
   e. Optimize transduction: 32°, centrifuge, phosphate deplete
   f. In vivo transduction
   g. Choice of HSC source
   h. Other gene transfer methods (AAV, lentivirus)
2. Selection for transduced cells
   a. In vitro
      i. Selective drugs (e.g., *neo*, *mdr*)
      ii. Surface antigen (e.g., tNGFR, HSA)
   b. In vivo
      i. Selective drugs (e.g., *mdr*, *dhfr*)
3. Cytoreduction/cytoablation prior to transplant
4. Intrinsic selective advantage to transduced cells

B. MoMuLV-Based Vectors with Alternative Envelopes to Bind to Different Receptors

In addition to the limits to retrovirus-mediated gene transfer imposed by the high fraction of resting stem cells, another barrier may be a relatively low level of appropriate receptor molecules for the amphotropic retroviral envelope protein on the surface of hematopoietic stem cells. Using an indirect immunofluorescence assay for virus binding, we demonstrated that CD34$^+$ cells (and the more primitive CD34$^+$/CD38$^-$cells) isolated directly from human bone marrow showed minimal virus binding (59). Culturing the cells in the presence of recombinant cytokines, such as IL-3 and SCF, led to increased viral binding. Orlic and coworkers have confirmed and extended these findings using RT-PCR to measure expression of the amphotropic envelope receptor in hematopoietic progenitor cell populations (60).

The gene encoding the cellular surface protein which acts as the receptor for the murine leukemia virus amphotropic virus envelope was recently cloned (61). It is a phosphate transport protein, which has been subserved by the virus to act as its receptor. Possibly, greater knowledge of this key molecule may lead to methods to increase viral binding to cells. If binding of amphotropic retroviruses plays a rate-limiting role in gene transfer, then vectors using other receptors more frequently or abundantly present on human stem cells may permit more efficient gene transduction. Two possible approaches have recently been described.

Miller and coworkers (62) reported that the standard MoMuLV-based vectors may be packaged into viral particles in which the envelope protein comes from the gibbon ape leukemia virus (GALV). GALV is a retrovirus which infects primates and its envelope glycoprotein binds to cells through a different receptor than the one used by the murine amphotropic retroviruses. The level of the GALV receptor on human cells appears to be higher than that for MoMuLV amphotropic envelope (60). Some reports have described higher efficiency of gene transfer into human cells with vectors using the GALV envelope than with the amphotropic envelope (63–65). Recently, Kiem and coworkers directly compared the efficiency of gene transfer into primate stem cells by GALV and amphotropic-packaged vectors and found a 3- to 10-fold higher transduction by the GALV-packaged vector (66).

Another potential beneficial approach has been reported by Friedmann and coworkers at the University of California, San Diego. They described the production of MoMuLV-based vectors pseudotyped by the G protein from vesicular stomatitis virus (VSV) (67). The receptor for VSV is highly ubiquitous, possibly being a glycolipid, which allows gene transfer by VSV-pseudotyped vectors into a broad range of cell types from organisms as diverse as mammals and fish (68). Additionally, the VSV-coated viruses are physically more stable than the standard MoMuLV amphotropic envelope-coated vectors, allowing concentration of the viruses to achieve greater titers (in the range of 10^9–10^{10}/mL). Recently, stable cell lines producing VSV-coated vectors have been described (69–71).

It has not been definitively determined whether either the GALV- or VSV-enveloped vectors are more effective than the standard amphotropic-enveloped vectors at gene transfer into human CD34$^+$ cells or more primitive stem cell subsets (72). If the breakdown of the nuclear membrane which occurs during mitosis to allow the MoMuLV genome to integrate into chromosomal DNA is ultimately rate limiting, then pseudotyping with these new envelopes may not significantly increase gene transfer into quiescent pluripotent stem cells.

C. New Vector Systems

Lentiviruses are a subset of retroviruses characterized by a more complex genome and slower growth cycle in host organisms than the simple retroviruses, such as the murine leukemia viruses. Human immunodeficiency virus (HIV)–1, the human acquired immunodeficiency syndrome (AIDS) virus, is included in this class of viruses. Lentiviruses have been demonstrated to be capable of infecting nondividing cells, such as blood monocytes (73). This property may be exploited to produce vectors similarly capable of transducing nondividing cells, such as HSCs. Two recent reports describe initial steps in developing lentivirus-based vectors (74,75) which were shown to be capable of transducing postmitotic cells, such as serum-deprived fibroblasts and neurons. Preliminary data from our group and others indicate that the lentiviral vectors are capable of stably transducing human CD34$^+$/CD38$^-$ E-LTCIC cells under conditions where the MoMuLV-based vectors are ineffective (76). It remains to be determined whether these vectors will efficiently and stably transduce quiescent human HSCs in the transplant setting. Additionally, the use of vectors based on the pathogenic HIV-1 will require extensive characterization to determine their safety before they could be considered for clinical application.

Adenoassociated virus (AAV) is another gene-delivery system with potential advantages over retroviruses for gene therapy (77). Like retroviral vectors, AAVs are able to integrate their genomes into target cell chromosomes. Wild-type AAVs have a strong integration site specificity, although this has not been shown for current AAV-based *vectors* (78). Preliminary studies suggest that AAVs can transfer genes into nonreplicating cells (79), although it has been technically difficult to prove this point stringently, especially with HSCs. The initial studies of AAV-mediated gene transfer into human hematopoietic progenitor cells reported to date have essentially reproduced but not exceeded the results with retroviral vectors (80,81). Stable packaging systems are just being established for AAVs, leading to difficulty producing quantities of virus large enough for clinical studies with consistent high titers and purity. Further work is needed with these newer vector systems before their full advantages and disadvantages compared to MoMuLV-based vectors are known. If these technical barriers can be surmounted, the establishment of vectors which transduce quiescent pluripotent stem cells would represent a quantum advance for gene therapy.

Gene transfer techniques which do not result in chromosomal integration (adenovirus, lipofection, electroporation, particle bombardment) have not been shown to be useful in HSCs, which will undergo multiple rounds of subsequent proliferation. Inclusions of elements which allow efficient episomal replication may surmount the need for integration [e.g., Epstein-Barr virus (EBV) origin of replication], but this approach has not been sufficiently developed to be considered for clinical application in the near future.

D. Alternatives to Bone Marrow for HSCs for Gene Transfer

Alternative sources of stem cells other than bone marrow may be more amenable to gene transduction. Moritz et al. (82) have shown that CD34$^+$ cells in umbilical cord blood are susceptible to retroviral transduction. We have demonstrated that the CD34$^+$/CD38$^-$ from human umbilical cord blood have a modest fraction (4–6%) in active cell cycle compared to essentially no cycling cells in CD34$^+$/CD38$^-$ cells from bone marrow (83).

In the first clinical trial to use umbilical cord blood as the cell source for gene therapy, our group at Children's Hospital Los Angeles performed gene transfer into umbilical cord blood CD34$^+$ cells from three neonates with ADA-deficient SCID in May and June of 1993 (84). Following retrovirus-mediated transfer with a vector containing a normal human ADA cDNA, the cells were given back to each infant as intravenous infusions on day 4 of life, without any prior cytoablative conditioning. Follow-up to over 5 years shows the continued production of gene-containing mononuclear cells and granulocytes, although at levels in the range of 1 cell/10,000 (85).

The persistent production of gene-containing cells demonstrates that long-lived multipotent cells in the umbilical cord blood were successfully transduced and were able to engraft without prior ablative therapy in the recipients to "make space." Decreasing the amount of polyethylene glycol–conjugated adenosine deaminase (PEG-ADA) enzyme replacement therapy has resulted in increases in the percentages of T cells containing the introduced ADA gene. These results confirm the postulated selective survival advantage predicted for genetically corrected T lymphocytes in ADA-deficient patients. The long-term benefits from this low level of gene transfer remain unproven, as the patients continue to receive PEG-ADA, although at reduced dosages. Nevertheless, this study does show that umbilical cord blood can be used for gene therapy in newborns and yield long-term production of gene-containing peripheral blood leukocytes of multiple lineages.

Granulocyte colony-stimulating factor (G-CSF)–mobilized peripheral blood CD34$^+$ cells are also quite susceptible to gene transduction, as measured in assays of the clonogenic progenitors (86,87). However, the presence of a large fraction of proliferating progenitor cells which are susceptible to gene transduction does not indicate whether any long-lived pluripotent stem cells which may be present in the cell populations are also capable of being transduced by retroviral vectors. The ongoing clinical trial by Dunbar's group at the National Heart, Lung and Blood Institute of the NIH is directly addressing this question (52). Patients undergoing treatment for breast cancer or multiple myeloma are simultaneously being given both autologous bone marrow and G-CSF–mobilized peripheral blood cells, with each cell fraction being labeled by different retroviral vectors. Serial measurements of the relative ratio of cells containing either the vector that labeled the bone marrow or the vector that labeled the peripheral blood cells will determine the relative contribution of these two sources to long-term hematopoiesis in this setting.

Recently, studies led by Bodine at the NIH have demonstrated that, following administration of G-CSF and SCF for peripheral blood stem cell (PBSC) mobilization, there are increased numbers of actively cycling stem cells in the *bone marrow* of mice, dogs, and monkeys (88,89). It remains to be determined whether these activated cells in the bone marrow will be transduced, engrafted, and produce gene-containing cells for a sustained time.

VIII. CONCLUSION

As gene therapy advances from an experimental science to clinical applications, a number of new logistical hurdles have developed. Large-scale, high-quality production of a complex biological reagent such as a retroviral vector–containing supernatant is more difficult to perform with the stringent reproducibility mandated by the U.S. Food and Drug Administration (FDA) than is the production of traditional drugs or even recombinant proteins. A new generation of fledgling pharmaceutical companies and the NIH-funded National Gene Vector Laboratories have been established to fill this niche. Bone marrow–directed gene therapy also requires the use of other reagents and devices which are investigational, such as CD34$^+$ cell separation products and new recombinant growth factors. Investigators have encountered reluctance from some of the corporate entities which have developed these materials to provide them for investigational gene therapy trials.

Although the initial trials may not provide cures for their subjects, they are necessary first steps toward achieving that goal. Therefore, the current scientific and logistical limits to effective gene therapy through hematopoietic stem cells will need to be surmounted to allow continued progress in this young field.

REFERENCES

1. Anderson WF. Prospects for human gene therapy. Science 1984; 226:401–409.
2. Wolff JA, Lederberg J. An early history of gene transfer and therapy. Hum Gene Ther 1994; 5:469–480.
3. Miller AD. Retroviral vectors. Curr Topics Microbiol Immunol 1992; 158:1–24.
4. Mulligan RC. The basic science of gene therapy. Science 1993; 260:926–932.
5. Miller DG, Adam MA, Miller AD. Gene transfer by retrovirus vectors occurs only in cells that are actively replicating at the time of infection. Mol Cell Biol 1990; 10:4239–4242.
6. Williams DA, Lemischka IR, Nathan DG, Mulligan RC. Introduction of new genetic material into pluripotent haematopoietic stem cells of the mouse. Nature 1984; 310:476–480.
7. Keller G, Paige C, Gilboa E, Wagner EF. Expression of a foreign gene in myeloid and lymphoid cells derived from multipotent hematopoietic precursors. Nature 1985; 318:149–154.
8. Eglitis MA, Kantoff P, Gilboa E, Anderson WF. Gene expression in mice after high efficiency retroviral-mediated gene transfer. Science 1985; 230:1395–1398.
9. Williams DA. Expression of introduced genetic sequence in hematopoietic cells following retroviral-mediated gene transfer. Hum Gene Ther 1990; 1:229–239.
10. Karlsson S. Treatment of genetic defects in hematopoietic cell functions by gene transfer. Blood 1991; 78:2481–2492.
11. Miller AD. Genetic manipulation of hematopoietic stem cells. In: Forman SJ, Blume KG, Thomas ED, eds. Bone Marrow Transplantation, Cambridge, MA: Blackwell, 1994:72–78.

12. Krall WJ, Challita PM, Perlmutter LS, Skelton DC, Kohn DB. Cells expressing human gluco-cerebrosidase from a retroviral vector repopulate macrophages and central nervous system microglia after murine bone marrow transplantation. Blood 1994; 83:2373–2384.

13. Wolfe JH, Sands MS, Barker JE, Gwynn B, Rowe LB, Vogler CA, Birkenmeier EH. Reversal of pathology in murine mucopolysaccharidosis type VII by somatic cell gene transfer. Nature 1992; 360:749–753.

14. Bunting KD, Sangster MY, Ihle JN, Sorrentino BP. Restoration of lymphocyte function in Janus kinase-3 deficient mice by retroviral-mediated gene transfer. Nature Med 1998; 4:58–64.

15. Mardiney M III, Jackson SH, Spratt SK, Li F, Holland SM, Malech HL. Enhanced host defense after gene transfer in the murine p47^{phox}-deficient model of chronic granulomatous disease. Blood 1997; 89:2268–2275.

16. Dzierzak EA, Papayannopoulou T, Mulligan RC. Lineage-specific expression of a human β-globin gene in murine bone marrow transplant recipients reconstituted with retrovirus-trans-duced stem cells. Nature 1988; 331:35–41.

17. Karlsson S, Bodine DM, Perry L, Papayannopoulou T, Nienhuis AW. Expression of the human β-globin gene following retroviral-mediated transfer into multipotential hematopoietic progen-itors of mice. Proc Natl Acad Sci USA 1988; 85:6062–6066.

18. Townes TM, Behringer RR. Human globin locus activation region (LAR): role in temporal control. Trends Genet 1990; 6:219–223.

19. Novak U, Harris EAS, Forrester W, Groudine M, Gelinas R. High-level β-globin expression after retroviral transfer of locus activation region-containing human β-globin gene derivatives into murine erythroleukemia cells. Proc Natl Acad Sci USA 1990; 87:3386–3390.

20. Chang JC, Liu D, Kan YW. A 36-base-pair sequence of locus control region enhances retrovi-rally transferred human beta-globin gene expression. Proc Natl Acad Sci USA 1992; 89:3107–3110.

21. Leboulch P, Huang GMS, Humphries RK, Oh YH, Eaves CJ, Tuan DYH, London IM. Muta-genesis of retroviral vectors transducing human β-globin gene and β-globin locus control re-gion derivatives results in stable transmission of an active transcriptional structure. EMBO J 1994; 13:3065–3076.

22. Sadelain M, Wang CH, Antoniou M, Grosveld F, Mulligan RC. Generation of a high-titer retroviral vector capable of expressing high levels of the human beta-globin gene. Proc Natl Acad Sci USA 1995; 92:6728–6732.

23. Sorrentino BP, Brandt SJ, Bodine D, Gottesman M, Pastin I, Cline A, Nienhuis AW. Selection of drug-resistant bone marrow cells in vivo after retroviral transfer of human mdr1. Science 1992; 257:99–103.

24. Sorrentino BP, McDonagh KT, Woods D, Orlic D. Expression of retroviral vectors containing the human multidrug resistance 1 cDNA in hematopoietic cells of transplanted mice. Blood 1995; 86:491–501.

25. Palmer TD, Rosman GJ, Osborne WR, Miller AD. Genetically modified skin fibroblasts persist long after transplantation but gradually inactivate introduced genes. Proc Natl Acad Sci USA 1991; 88:1330–1334.

26. Dai Y, Roman M, Naviaux RK, Verma IM. Gene therapy via primary myoblasts: long-term expression of factor IX protein following transplantation in vivo. Proc Natl Acad Sci USA 1992; 89:10892–10895.

27. Challita PM, Kohn DB. Lack of expression from a retroviral vector after transduction of mu-rine hematopoietic stem cells is associated with methylation. Proc Natl Acad Sci USA 1994; 91:2567–2571.

28. Halene S, Wang L, Cooper R, Bockstoce DC, Robbins PB, Kohn DB. Improved expression in hematopoietic and lymphoid cells in mice after transplantation of bone marrow transduced with a modified retroviral vector. Blood 1999; 94:3349–3357.

29. Van Beusechem VW, Kakler A, Meidt PJ, Valerio D. Long-term expression of human adeno-

sine deaminase in rhesus monkeys transplanted with retrovirus-infected bone marrow cells. Proc Natl Acad Sci USA 1992; 79:7640–7644.

30. Bodine DM, Moritz T, Donahue RE, Luskey BD, Kessler SW, Martin DIK, Orkin SH, Nienhuis AW, Williams DA. Long-term in vivo expression of a murine adenosine deaminase gene in rhesus monkey hematopoietic cells of multiple lineages after retroviral mediated gene transfer into CD34+ bone marrow cells. Blood 1993; 82:1975–1980.

31. Kiem HP, Darovsky B, von Kalle C, Goehle S, Stewart D, Graham T, Hackman R, Appelbaum FR, Deeg HJ, Miller AD, Storb R, Schuening FG. Retrovirus-mediated gene transduction into canine peripheral blood repopulating cells. Blood 1994; 83:1467–1473.

32. Kiem H-P, Andrews RG, Morris J, Peterson L, Heyward S, Allen JM, Rasko JEJ, Potter J, Miller AD. Improved gene transfer into baboon marrow repopulating cells using recombinant human fibronectin fragment CH-296 in combination with interleukin-6, stem cell factor, FLT-3 ligand, and megakaryocyte growth and development factor. Blood 1998; 92:1878–1886.

33. Huhn RD, Tisdale JF, Agricola BA, Metzger ME, Donahue RE, Dunbar CE. The effects of alternative transduction cytokine combinations (rhMGDF/rhSCF/rhG-CSF vs rhIL-3/rhIL-6/rhSCF) and of cytokine pre-treatment before non-myeloblastive radiation conditioning on the efficacy of retroviral gene marking of hematopoietic cells in rhesus monkeys. American Society of Gene Therapy, Seattle, May 28–31, 1998:86a.

34. Nolta JA, Kohn DB. Comparison of the effects of growth factors on retroviral vector–mediated gene transfer and the proliferative status of human hematopoietic progenitor cells. Hum Gene Ther 1990; 1:257–268.

35. Fletcher FA, Moore KA, Ashkenazi M, De Vries P, Overbeek PA, Williams DE, Belmont JW. Leukemia inhibitory factor improves survival of retroviral vector-infected hematopoietic stem cells in vitro, allowing efficient long-term expression of vector-encoded human adenosine deaminase in vivo. J Exp Med 1991; 174:837–845.

36. Nolta JA, Crooks GM, Overell RW, Williams DE, Kohn DB. Retroviral vector-mediated gene transfer into primitive human hematopoietic progenitor cells: effects of mast cell growth factor (MGF) combined with other cytokines. Exp Hematol 1992; 20:1065–1071.

37. Dilber MS, Bjorkstrand B, Li KJ, Smith CI, Xanthopoulos KG, Gahrton G. Basic fibroblast growth factor increases retroviral-mediated gene transfer into human hematopoietic peripheral blood progenitor cells. Exp Hematol 1994; 22:1129–1133.

38. Moore KA, Deisseroth AB, Reading CL, Williams DE, Belmont JW. Stromal support enhances cell-free retroviral vector transduction of human bone marrow long-term culture-initiating cells. Blood 1992; 79:1393–1399.

39. Moritz T, Patel VP, Williams DA. Bone marrow extracellular matrix molecules improve gene transfer into human hematopoietic cells via retroviral vectors. J Clin Invest 1994; 93:1451–1457.

40. Bahnson AB, Dunigan JT, Baysal BE, Mohney T, Atchison RW, Nimgaonkar MT, Ball ED, Barranger JA. Centrifugal enhancement of retroviral mediated gene transfer. J Virol 1995; 54:131–143.

41. Nolta JA, Smogorzewska EM, Kohn DB. Analysis of optimal conditions for retroviral-mediated transduction of primitive human hematopoietic cells. Blood 1995; 86:101–110.

42. Wells S, Malik P, Pensiero M, Kohn DB, Nolta JA. The presence of an autologous marrow stromal cell layer increases glucocerebrosidase gene transduction of long term culture initiating cells (LTCIC) from the bone marrow of a patient with Gaucher disease. Gene Ther 1995; 2:512–520.

43. Hao QL, Thiemann FT, Petersen D, Smogorzewska EM, Crooks GM. Extended long-term culture reveals a highly quiescent and primitive human hematopoietic progenitor population. Blood 1996; 88:3306–3313.

44. Rawlings DJ, Quan S, Hao QL, Thiemann FT, Smogorzewska M, Witte ON, Crooks GM. Differentiation of human CD34+CD38− cord blood stem cells into B cell progenitors in vitro. Exp Hematol 1997; 25:66–82.

45. Hao QL, Smogorzewska EM, Barsky LW, Crooks GM. In vitro identification of single CD34$^+$ CD38$^-$ cells with both lymphoid and myeloid potential. Blood 1998; 91:4145–4151.

46. Dick JE, Kamel-Reid S, Murdoch B, Doedens M. Gene transfer into normal human hematopoietic cells using in vitro and in vivo assays. Blood 1991; 78:624–634.

47. Srour EF, Zanjani ED, Cornetta K, Traycoff CM, Flake AW, Hedrick M, Brandt JE, Leemhuis T, Hoffman R. Persistence of human multilineage, self-renewing lymphohematopoietic stem cells in chimeric sheep. Blood 1993; 182:3333–3342.

48. Dick J. Characterization of SCID-repopulating cells (SRC) using retrovirus-mediated gene transfer and expression. Exp Hematol 1996; 24:1019a.

49. Nolta JA, Hanley MB, Kohn DB. Sustained human hematopoiesis in immunodeficient mice by co-transplantation of marrow stroma expressing human IL-3: analysis of gene transduction of long-lived progenitors. Blood 1994; 83:3041–3051.

50. Nolta JA, Dao MA, Wells S, Smogorzewska EM, Kohn DB. Transduction of pluripotent human hematopoietic stem cells demonstrated by clonal analysis after engraftment in immune deficient mice. Proc Natl Acad Sci USA 1996; 93:2414–2419.

51. Kohn DB, Nolta JA, Crooks GM. Clinical trials of gene therapy using hematopoietic stem cells. In: Thomas ED, Blume KG, Forman SJ, eds. Hematopoietic Cell Transplantation, 2nd ed. Boston: Blackwell, 1999:97–102.

52. Dunbar CE, Cottler-Fox M, O'Shaughnessy JA, Doren S, Carter C, Berenson R, Brown S, Moen RC, Greenblatt J, Stewart FM, Leitman SF, Wilson WH, Cowan K, Young NS, Nienhuis AW. Retrovirally marked CD34-enriched peripheral blood and bone marrow cells contribute to long-term engraftment after autologous transplantation. Blood 1995; 85:3048–3057.

53. Brenner MK, Rill DR, Holladay MS, Heslop HE, Moen RC, Buschle M, Krance RA, Santana VM, Anderson WF, Ihle JN. Gene marking to determine whether autologous marrow infusion restores long-term haemopoiesis in cancer patients. Lancet 1993; 342:1134–1137.

54. Rill DR, Santana VM, Roberts WM, Nilson T, Bowman LC, Krance RA, Heslop HE, Moen RC, Ihle JN, Brenner MK. Transplantation for solid tumors: direct demonstration that autologous bone marrow can return a multiplicity of tumorigenic cells. Blood 1994; 84:380–383.

55. Deisseroth AB, Zu Z, Claxton D, Hanania EG, Fu S, Ellerson D, Goldberg L, Thomas M, Janicek K, Anderson WF, Hester J, Korbling M, Durett A, Moen R, Berenson R, Heimfeld S, Hamer J, Calvert L, Tibbits P, Talpaz M, Kantarjian H, Champlin R, Reading C. Genetic marking shows that ph+ cells present in autologous transplants of chronic myelogenous leukemia (CML) contribute to relapse after autologous bone marrow in CML. Blood 1994; 83: 3068–3076.

56. Brenner MK, Rill DR, Moen RC, Krance RA, Mirro J Jr, Anderson WF, Ihle JN. Gene-marking to trace origin of relapse after autologous bone-marrow transplantation. Lancet 1993; 341:85–86.

57. Shah AJ, Smogorzewska EM, Hannum C, Crooks GM. Flt3 ligand induces proliferation of quiescent human bone marrow CD34$^+$CD38$^-$ cells and maintains progenitor cells in vitro. Blood 1996; 87:3563–3570.

58. Barquinero J, Kiem HP, von Kalle C, Darovsky B, Goehle S, Graham T, Seidel K, Storb R, Schuening FC. Myelosuppressive conditioning improves autologous engraftment of genetically marked hematopoietic repopulating cells in dogs. Blood 1995; 85:1195–1201.

59. Crooks GM, Kohn DB. Growth factors increase amphotropic retrovirus binding to human CD34 positive bone marrow progenitor cells. Blood 1993; 82:3290–3297.

60. Orlic D, Girard LJ, Jordan CT, Anderson SM, Cline AP, Bodine DM. The level of mRNA encoding the amphotropic retrovirus receptor in mouse and human hematopoietic stem cells is low and correlates with the efficiency of retrovirus transduction. Proc Natl Acad Sci USA 1996; 93:11097–11102.

61. Miller DG, Edwards RG, Miller AD. Cloning of the cellular receptor for amphotropic murine

retroviruses reveals homology to that for Gibbon ape leukemia virus. Proc Natl Acad Sci USA 1994; 91:78–82.

62. Miller AD, Garcia JV, von Suhr N, Lynch CM, Wilson C, Eiden MV. Construction and properties of retrovirus packaging cells based on Gibbon ape leukemia virus. J Virol 1991; 65:2220–2224.

63. Bunnell BA, Muul LM, Donahue RE, Blaese RM, Morgan RA. High-efficiency retroviral-mediated gene transfer into human and nonhuman primate peripheral blood lymphocytes. Proc Natl Acad Sci USA 1995; 15:7739–7743.

64. Bauer TR Jr, Miller AD, Hickstein DD. Improved transfer of the leukocyte integrin CD18 subunit into hematopoietic cell lines by using retroviral vectors having a gibbon ape leukemia virus envelope. Blood 1995; 86:2379–2387.

65. Porter CD, Collins MK, Tailor CS, Parkar MH, Cosset FL, Weiss RA, Takeuchi Y. Comparison of efficiency of infection of human gene therapy target cells via four different retroviral receptors. Hum Gene Ther 1996; 7:913–919.

66. Kiem HP, Heyward S, Winkler A, Potter J, Allen JM, Miller AD, Andrews RG. Gene transfer into marrow repopulating cells: comparison between amphotropic and gibbon ape leukemia virus pseudotyped retroviral vectors in a competitive repopulation assay in baboons. Blood 1997; 90:4638–4645.

67. Burns JC, Friedmann T, Driever W, Burrascano M, Yee JK. Vesicular stomatitis virus g glycoprotein pseudotyped retroviral vectors: concentration to very high titer and efficient gene transfer into mammalian and non-mammalian cells. Proc Natl Acad Sci USA 1993; 90:8033–8037.

68. Lin S, Gaiano N, Culp P, Burns JC, Friedmann T, Yee JK, Hopkins N. Integration and germ-line transmission of a pseudotyped retroviral vector in zebrafish. Science 1994; 265:666–669.

69. Yang Y, Vanin EF, Whitt MA, Fornerod M, Zwart R, Schneiderman RD, Grosveld G, Nienhuis AW. Inducible high-level production of infectious murine leukemia retroviral vector particles pseudotyped with vesicular stomatitis virus G envelope protein. Hum Gene Ther 1995; 6:1203–1213.

70. Iida A, Chen ST, Friedmann T, Yee JK. Inducible gene expression by retrovirus-mediated transfer of a modified tetracycline-regulated system. J Virol 1996; 70:6054–6059.

71. Ory DS, Neugeboren BA, Mulligan RC. A stable human-derived packaging cell line for production of high titer retrovirus/vesicular stomatitis virus G pseudotypes. Proc Natl Acad Sci USA 1996; 93:11400–11406.

72. Agrawal YP, Agrawal RS, Sinclair AM, Young D, Maruyama M, Levine F, Ho AD. Cell-cycle kinetics and VSV-G pseudotyped retrovirus-mediated gene transfer in blood-derived CD34$^+$ cells. Exp Hematol 1996; 24:738–747.

73. Zack JA, Haislip AM, Krogstad P, Chen IS. Incompletely reverse-transcribed human immunodeficiency virus type I genomes in quiescent cells can function as intermediates in the retroviral life cycle. J Virol 1992; 66:1717–1725.

74. Akkina RS, Walton RM, Chen ML, Li QX, Planelles V, Chen ISY. High-efficiency gene transfer into CD34$^+$ cells with a human immunodeficiency virus type 1–based retroviral vector pseudotyped with vesicular stomatitis virus envelope glycoprotein G. J Virol 1996; 70:2581–2585.

75. Naldini L, Blomer U, Gallay P, Ory D, Mulligan R, Gage FH, Verma IM, Trono D. In vivo gene delivery and stable transduction of nondividing cells by a lentiviral vector. Science 1996; 272:263–267.

76. Case SS, Price MA, Jordan CT, Yu XJ, Wang L, Bauer G, Haas DL, Xu D, Stripecke R, Naldini L, Kohn DB, Crooks GM. Stable transduction of quiescent CD34$^+$/CD38$^-$ human hematopoietic cells by HIV-1 based lentiviral vectors. Proc Natl Acad Sci USA 1999; 96:2988–2993.

77. Muzyczka N. Use of adeno-associated virus as a general transduction vector for mammalian cells. Curr Topics Microbiol Immunol 1992; 158:97–129.

78. Samulski RJ, Zhu X, Xiao X, Brook JD, Housman DE, Epstein N, Hunter LA. Targeted integration of adeno-associated virus (AAV) into human chromosome 19. EMBO J 1992; 10: 3941–3950.

79. Podsakoff G, Wong KK Jr, Chatterjee S. Efficient gene transfer into nondividing cells by adeno-associated virus-based vectors. J Virol 1994; 68:5656–5666.

80. Zhou SZ, Cooper S, Kang LY, Ruggieri L, Heimfeld S, Srivastava A, Broxmeyer HE. Adeno-associated virus 2–mediated high efficiency gene transfer into immature and mature subsets of hematopoietic progenitor cells in human umbilical cord blood. J Exp Med 1994; 179:1867–1875.

81. Fisher-Adams G, Wong KK Jr, Podsakoff G, Forman SJ, Chatterjee S. Integration of adeno-associated virus vectors in CD34⁺ human hematopoietic progenitor cells after transduction. Blood 1996; 88:492–504.

82. Moritz T, Keller DC, Williams DA. Human cord blood cells as targets for gene transfer: potential use in genetic therapies of severe combined immunodeficiency disease. J Exp Med 1993; 178:529–536.

83. Hao QL, Shah AJ, Thiemann FT, Smogorzewska EM, Crooks GM. A functional comparison of CD34⁺CD38⁻ cells in cord blood and bone marrow. Blood 1995; 86:3745–3753.

84. Kohn DB, Weinberg KI, Nolta JA, Heiss LN, Lenarsky C, Crooks GM, Hanley ME, Annett G, Brooks JS, El-Khoureiy A, Lawrence K, Wells S, Shaw K, Moen RC, Bastian J, Williams-Herman DE, Elder M, Wara D, Bowen T, Hershfield MS, Mullen CA, Blaese RM, Parkman R. Engraftment of gene-modified cells from umbilical cord blood in neonates with adenosine deaminase deficiency. Nature Med 1995; 1:1017–1023.

85. Kohn DB, Hershfield MS, Carbonaro D, Shigeoka A, Brooks J, Smogorzewska EM, Barsky LW, Chan R, Burotto F, Annett G, Nolta JA, Crooks G, Kapoor N, Elder M, Wara D, Bowen T, Madsen E, Snyder FF, Bastian J, Muul L, Blaese RM, Weinberg K, Parkman R. T lymphocytes with a normal ADA gene accumulate after transplantation of transduced autologous umbilical cord blood CD34⁺ cells in ADA-deficient SCID neonates. Nature Med 1998; 4: 775–780.

86. Bregni M, Magni M, Siena S, Di Nicola M, Bonadonna G, Gianni AM. Human peripheral blood hematopoietic progenitors are optimal targets of retroviral-mediated gene transfer. Blood 1992; 80:1418–1422.

87. Cassel A, Cottler-Fox M, Doren S, Dunbar CE. Retroviral-mediated gene transfer into CD34-enriched human peripheral blood stem cells. Exp Hematol 1993; 21:585–591.

88. Bodine DM, Seidel NE, Gale MS, Nienhuis AW, Orlic D. Efficient retrovirus transduction of mouse pluripotent blood by treatment with granulocyte colony-stimulating factor and stem cell factor. Blood 1994; 84:1482–1491.

89. Bodine DM, Seidel NE, Orlic D. Bone marrow collected 14 days after in vivo administration of granulocyte colony-stimulating factor and stem cell factor to mice has 10-fold more repopulating ability than untreated bone marrow. Blood 1996; 88:89–97.

32

Gene Therapy for Human Immunodeficiency Virus Infection Using Stem Cell Transplantation

ALAIN GERVAIX

University Hospital of Geneva, Geneva, Switzerland

FLOSSIE WONG-STAAL

University of California, San Diego, La Jolla, California

I. INTRODUCTION

The acquired immunodeficiency syndrome (AIDS) was first recognized in 1981 when unusual clusters of *Pneumocystis carinii* and Kaposi's sarcoma were reported in homosexual men in New York City, Los Angeles, and San Francisco and was further identified in every part of the world. The causative agents of AIDS were isolated 2 years later in France and in the United States (1–3) from the blood of patients and were later shown to be an enveloped RNA virus belonging to the lentivirus subfamily of retroviruses (4). By consensus these agents were named *human immunodeficiency viruses* (HIVs). AIDS is considered one of the most challenging pandemics of the end of this century, and the World Health Organization estimates that between 40 and 100 million individuals may be infected with HIV by year 2000 (5). HIV infection induces a progressive and severe immunodeficiency resulting in multiple infections by opportunistic bacteria, viruses, and parasites (6). Despite the development of antiretroviral drugs that improve the quality of life and the survival time of infected individuals, eradication of all virus-infected cells and cure of infection is not currently feasible and calls for novel therapeutic approaches, such as gene therapy.

II. LIFE CYCLE OF HIV

The HIV virion consists of a core composed of two copies of single-stranded genomic length RNA complexed with several HIV encoded core proteins (7). The cylindrical eccentric core of HIV contains p24 proteins, reverse transcriptase, integrase, and other structural proteins encoded by the HIV *gag* and *pol* genes. This core is surrounded by *env* encoded gp120 and gp41 glycoproteins containing lipidic membranes (Fig. 1). At the time of infection, HIV binds to its principal receptor, the CD4 cell surface protein (8,9), and coreceptors (chemokine receptor family) (10–12) to enter the cell. After viral entry and uncoating, the

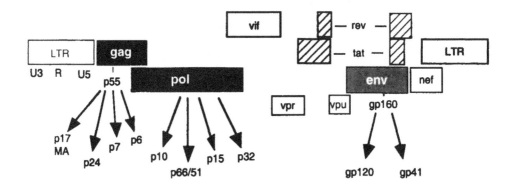

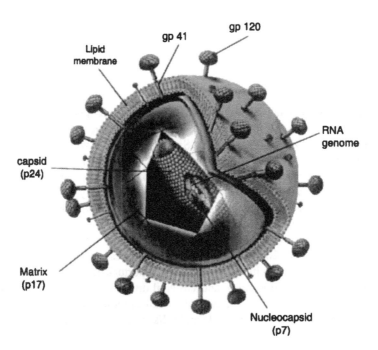

Figure 1   Human immunodeficiency virus (HIV)–1 genome and structure (see text for specific abbreviations).

virion-associated reverse transcriptase characteristic of all retroviruses produces double-stranded proviral deoxyribonucleic acid (DNA) that enters the nucleus and integrates randomly into the host cell's chromosomal DNA. Two viral proteins, matrix (p17MA) and Vpr, have been shown to govern the active transport of the viral preintegration complex through the nucleopores allowing the spread of HIV in such critical targets as terminally differentiated macrophages (13,14).

Once the provirus has been integrated, both cellular and viral factors are necessary to initiate expression of viral genes (15). On activation of the HIV long terminal repeat (LTR), early gene expression is characterized by production of multiply spliced HIV ribonucleic acid (RNA) encoding the nonstructural proteins with regulatory functions, Tat, Rev, Nef, Vif, Vpr, and Vpu. Tat is the most critical of these proteins and acts as a powerful *trans*-activator of viral gene expression and is essential for viral growth (16). *Trans*-activation by Tat requires a specific recognition of this effector protein with a target sequence, TAR, contained in the R region of the virus (17). At the level of transcription, it has been proposed that Tat acts primarily as an antiterminator of RNA elongation, as well as an enhancer of the translational efficiency or stability of the TAR-containing mRNA (18).

Rev is another important *trans*-activator protein which controls the differential expression of viral proteins exclusively at the posttranscriptional level by allowing the accumulation in the cytoplasm of unspliced and singly spliced viral mRNA. The function of Rev is dependent on the presence of a *cis*-acting sequence found within the *env* gene of HIV (19). This RNA sequence, named Rev-responsive element (RRE), forms a complex secondary structure composed of five stem loops among which the second stem loop (SL2) is the most important determinant for Rev responsiveness (20). Rev-RRE interaction results in an efficient extranuclear export of the viral mRNA to the cytoplasm.

The role of Nef in viral replication is still unclear. Recent studies suggest that Nef may function to downregulate CD4 expression and major histocompatibility complex (MHC) class I molecules at the surface of infected cells (21,22). Nef has also been shown to increase the infectivity of viral particles and to enhance the rate of viral replication in vitro (23,24); possibly through the interaction with cellular serine kinases (25). Based on studies in macaques infected with simian immunodeficiency virus (SIV), Nef appears to be important for the maintenance of a high viral burden in vivo (26).

Among the accessory proteins, Vpr is the only one that is incorporated into virions in high copy numbers. Vpr has been shown to arrest infected cells in the G2 phase of the cell cycle, perhaps to prolong their survival, enhancing viral production from these cells (27). This regulatory protein may also serve to facilitate the translocation of the viral genetic material into the cell nucleus, particularly in nondividing cells where nucleic acids must be transported across the intact nuclear membrane (28).

Vif has also been detected in HIV-1 particles (29). Virions produced in the absence of Vif are morphologically defective and are unable to initiate further rounds of replication, suggesting that Vif enhances infectivity (30). These Vif-defective virions can enter target cells normally but subsequently fail to complete reverse transcription of the viral genome (31). Since the activity of the reverse transcriptase is not impaired in these virions, it has been postulated that the Vif defect results in the alteration of the uncoating or the stability of the viral nucleoprotein complex (29).

Vpu has been shown to enhance the release of particles from infected cells and also to mediate the apparent independent function of inducing rapid intracellular degradation of CD4 (32,33). Late viral gene expression results in the increased production of the envelope and core proteins as well as genomic RNAs. Subsequently, HIV genomic RNA is transported to the cell surface and encapsidated into budding viral particles and coated with a plasma membrane containing envelope proteins. The core proteins are then processed by the viral proteases to yield mature virions. Because both Tat and Rev are required during viral replication, they offer the potential for the development of specific strategies against HIV infection.

III. TARGET CELLS FOR GENE THERAPY AGAINST HIV

The main target cells for HIV are monocytes-macrophages, CD4$^+$ T cells, and other cells in the nervous system and gastrointestinal tract (34). Most of them are derived from bone marrow stem cells. Despite conflicting reports, the progenitor/stem cells (CD34$^+$) are not likely infected by HIV (35). After infection, HIV rapidly replicates in target lymph nodes and peripheral blood mononuclear cells (PBMCs) with a high turnover and causes a profound cytopathic effect in CD4$^+$ T cells. This dynamic infectious process results in depletion of helper CD4$^+$ T-cell subset in vivo, in immunological dysfunctions, and subsequently in susceptibility to opportunistic infections (36). Another critical feature of HIV infection is the strain heterogeneity (quasispecies) which occurs in infected individuals with different tissue tropisms. The continuous development of HIV strains with altered epitopes and biological properties contributes to the resistance of HIV to immunological mechanisms and antiretroviral drugs. Since CD4$^+$ cell depletion correlates well with disease development, these cells could be a candidate target for gene therapy.

Several protocols received Recombinant DNA Advisory Committee (RAC) approval to initiate ex vivo gene transfer into CD4$^+$ cells of HIV-infected individuals and reinfusion into the patient. Woffendin et al. (37) have shown that cells transfected with the transdominant mutant protein Rev M10 displayed a survival advantage compared to unprotected cells. However, peripheral blood T cells have a short life span, especially in HIV-infected subjects where a daily turnover of 10^9 infected CD4$^+$ cells and an half-life of 1.6 days have been calculated (38). Finally, the other target cells for HIV such as macrophages will not be protected. In consequence, if CD4$^+$ T-cell–based gene therapy is of value for testing the feasibility and safety of such therapies, the therapeutic benefit will be too limited to use genetically altered CD4$^+$ T cells for gene therapy against HIV.

Because previous studies have shown that primitive hematopoietic stem cells contained in bone marrow and cord blood transplantation were capable of completely and permanently reconstituting all blood lineages and immune functions (39), these cells appear to be suitable for the transfer of exogenous genes interfering with HIV replication; the long-term goal being to reconstitute an immune system with altered HIV target cells resistant to this virus. To consider hematopoietic stem cell gene therapy for HIV infection resulting in therapeutic benefit to the individual, introduction of new genetic material should be efficient in target cells, should have sustained expression over time, and should prevent escape of mutants of HIV. Following these ideas, many efforts have been directed to determine (1) the true hematopoietic stem cells with reconstitutive capabilities using in vivo animal models, (2) the better system for gene transfer and expression into these cells, and (3) the foreign genes to introduce with high and sustained anti-HIV effect.

IV. GENE TRANSFER VECTORS

For a strategy relying on prolonged expression of anti-HIV genes, vectors capable of stable integration into the host genome are required. These vectors ideally should enter the target cells and integrate without affecting cell physiology and developmental capabilities. Three kinds of vectors could satisfy these requirements and include murine retroviral vectors, adeno-associated vectors, and lentiviral vectors.

A. Murine Retroviral Vectors

Murine retroviral vectors are the most commonly used vectors for stable integration into mammalian cells (40). These vectors are likely used for gene therapy because they appear to be safe with cumulative experiences in animals and more recently in human clinical trials (41). Other advantages of such vectors are the ability of large-scale production, the ability to generate deficient virus because the proteins necessary for viral replication can be provided in *trans*, and the ability to accommodate transgenes of up to 7 kb without affecting the packaging efficiency (42). Expression of foreign genes under the control of the retroviral LTR promoter is sustained and has been shown to be expressed for a period greater than 1 year in lymphoblastoid T-cell lines and more importantly in primate hematopoietic cells (43). Using this vector, expression of several anti-HIV genes was shown to be sufficient to inhibit HIV replication in primary human lymphocytes (44) and in macrophages derived from transduced CD34$^+$ (45). However, despite all these promising features, retroviral vectors display two important limitations: (1) The major drawback of murine retroviruses is their inability to infect nondividing cells (46), which considerably limits their use for most hematopoietic stem cell–based gene therapy. High efficiency of transduction (67–100%) of CD34$^+$ cells has been obtained only after stimulation of these cells with growth factors, such as interleukin-3 (IL-3), IL-6, and stem cell factor (47), committing these cells to a more differentiated status. (2) The second disadvantage of retroviruses is their inability to be concentrated to very high titer (>10^8 virions/mL) by ultracentrifugation. Although titers of 10^6 can be achieved, higher titers will be required for in vivo therapeutic approaches. This problem can be overcome by the possibility of replacing the retroviral envelope proteins with the envelope vesicular stomatitis viral glycoproteins (VSV-G) which enable concentrations of the viruses by centrifugation and moreover offer a broader range of target cells to infect (48). However, because of intrinsic toxicity, no stable cell line expressing VSV-G has been established so far. To date, because of all these limitations, only ex vivo (i.e., harvest of cells from a patient, transduction in vitro, and reinfusion to the patient) protocols have been employed for clinical trials.

B. Adenoassociated Vectors

The adenoassociated virus (AAV) is a defective single-stranded DNA human parvovirus. AAV contains at both ends of its genome a 145-base inverted terminal repeated sequence (ITR), which forms T-shaped hairpins serving as viral origins of DNA replication and internal sequences coding for proteins required for replication such as *rep* and *cap* and several *env* genes (49). Although about 80% of the population is seropositive for AAV, this virus has not been found to be associated with any disease in humans.

Used as vector for gene therapy, AAV displays numerous interesting features: (1) The AAV ITR is the only *cis*-element required for the packaging of AAV genome and for integration into the chromosome of host cells (50). Furthermore, AAV DNA has the unique ability to integrate with high-frequency into a defined region of human chromosome 19q13.3-qter in tissue culture (51). This feature could eliminate the potential risk of other vectors for insertional mutagenesis possible with random insertion of DNA either by activating an oncogene or by inactivating a suppressor gene resulting in malignant transformation. The question of whether the Rep proteins, encoded by the *rep* gene which are essential for AAV DNA replication and gene regulation, are required for targeted integration has not be solved satisfactorily. (2) AAV has the ability to infect a wide variety of mammalian cells, including nondividing cells such as hematopoietic stem cells (52,53). (3) AAV particles are very stable and can be concentrated up to 10^{13} particles/mL without losing infectivity. (4) Since the AAV vector (containing no Rep proteins) generates no viral antigens, it is unlikely to be immunogenic.

However, as with the other vectors, AAV also features several disadvantages, including the packaging system and the limited size of the inserted foreign gene. AAV packaging cell lines have been produced following the model of retroviral vector by providing the AAV necessary replication products in *trans*. However, AAV can maintain latency in cells they infect and consequently they do not produce new virions in the absence of helper virus. To date, coinfection with adenovirus is still required for efficient replication (49). Furthermore, low viral titers are obtained from packaging cell lines (10^5–10^6 particles/mL) which survive transiently due to the cytotoxicity of the Rep proteins. Another disadvantage is the limited size (maximum 4.7 kb) of the insert that the vector can withstand.

C. Lentiviral Vectors

The lentiviruses include prototypes HIV-1 and HIV-2 which infect humans. HIV vectors could display multiple advantages for HIV-based gene therapy compared to other vectors (54,55). HIV vectors will target the CD4$^+$ cells, allowing specific transduction of the cells that could be infected by the wild-type HIV virus. Furthermore, if the HIV vector–transduced cells become infected by HIV, it is theoretically possible that the HIV vector could be rescued by the wild-type virus; the latter bringing in *trans* the accessory proteins to package the vector. Through the nuclear targeting properties of both the p17 Gag matrix protein (MA) and the accessory gene Vpr, lentiviruses can penetrate an intact nuclear envelope (14); a property that is not shared by the murine leukemia virus. This ability to infect noncycling cells and postmitotic cells, such as macrophages, is another advantage of HIV vectors, since these cells have been shown to be an important reservoir for HIV.

The unique feature of the lentivirus among other retroviruses to infect noncycling cells is also of consideration for hematopoietic stem cell–based gene therapy (56). However, HIV is not likely to infect CD34$^+$ cells; probably because of the absence of a CD4 receptor at the surface of the cells. To circumvent this limitation, our group and others have replaced the *env* gene of HIV by providing in *trans* the gene encoding for the vesicular stomatitis virus G protein (VSV-G) (56). These pseudotyped vectors have been shown to enter a broad range of mammalian cells including totipotent stem cells and neurons (57). Recent studies from our group demonstrated that, contrary to retroviral vectors, pseudotyped HIV-based vectors could enter and integrate into the genome of CD34$^+$/CD38$^-$ cells without stimulation of the cells with growth factors (58). The majority of these vectors have been obtained by transient cotransfection in cell lines because of the difficulty in establishing a stable cell line expressing high titers of HIV vector. This difficulty is presumably due to the complexity of HIV genetic regulation and because of the toxicity of the HIV and the VSV-G proteins for the packaging cells. Actually, titers of 10^4–10^5 transducing units/mL are achievable with packaging cell lines (56), and even higher titers are seen after ultracentrifugation when pseudotyped with VSV-G. Another concern about the HIV vector is the safety to ensure that competent replicative viruses are not produced by these cell lines.

V. ANTI-HIV GENE THERAPY

Several genetic approaches have been attempted to interfere with HIV (59). Some, based on immunotherapy, expressed HIV proteins in vivo for prophylactic vaccination or for modulation of the immune response (60). Some are based on the expression of host proteins that could interfere with HIV cell entry, such as soluble CD4 receptors (61). All these approaches can be achieved by introducing genetic information into cells that are not mandatory targets for the virus, such as muscle cells. Another approach was to express under drug control a suicide gene (HSV-Tk, diphtheria toxin A) to kill the transduced cells on HIV infection (62,63), but obviously these techniques are not suitable for hematopoietic stem cell gene therapy. Other gene therapy approaches attempt to interfere directly with the HIV life cycle within the target cells. Ribozymes and decoys are two promising gene therapy–based approaches against HIV and are directly applicable to hematopoietic stem cells.

A. Transdominant Mutant Proteins and Anti-HIV RNA Decoys

Because HIV is dependent on interactions between essential viral regulatory proteins (Rev, Tat) and cellular factors, viral genes represent a logical target for gene therapy to inhibit HIV replication. In the Rev protein, a well-conserved leucine-rich domain close to its C-terminus is essential for regulating and stabilizing the nuclear export of unspliced and singly spliced viral messenger RNAs (mRNAs). Two amino acid substitutions at positions 78 (D for L) and 79 (L for E) in this specific region have yielded a mutant protein, Rev M10, that can bind to HIV RRE sequence, multimerize, and prevent the wild-type Rev protein from exporting the mRNA to the cytoplasm (64,65). This defective protein acts as a transdominant inhibitor. Overexpression was shown to inhibit HIV replication in T-cell lines after transient transfection and in primary human CD4$^+$ lymphocytes after transduction with a murine retroviral vector (66). Furthermore, CD4$^+$ cells of HIV-infected individuals transfected with a vector encoding Rev M10 and reinfused into the patient showed survival advantages compared to unprotected cells (37). Similar experiments have been attempted to modify Tat as a transdominant protein (67). Because of the risk that these transdominant proteins could be processed into antigenic peptides resulting in a cytotoxic T-lymphocyte (CTL) response and destruction of altered cells, overexpression of their target RNAs has been used as an alternative. This RNA decoy strategy seeks to sequester viral nucleic acid–binding regulatory proteins through overexpression of their cognate RNA. Sullenger et al. (68) expressed in the lymphoblastoid cell line, CEM, the HIV RRE, and TAR sequences. HIV challenge displayed a dramatic reduction of infectivity in cells expressing the decoys compared to unprotected cells.

B. Ribozymes

Ribozymes are small, catalytic antisense RNAs that bind by the specificity of Watson-Crick base pairing to a substrate RNA and cleave it at specific sites. The cleavage products are rapidly degraded in cells. Based on their secondary structures, ribozymes are designated hammerhead or hairpin (69,70). RNase P, the hepatitis delta virus ribozyme, and the group I introns share the same catalytic properties. Since a ribozyme molecule can cleave many substrate molecules in succession, this provides an advantage over the antisense approach. Ribozyme sequences can be engineered to bind specifically and cleave HIV RNA (71–73). Sarver et al. (74) first showed that ribozymes targeting HIV RNA

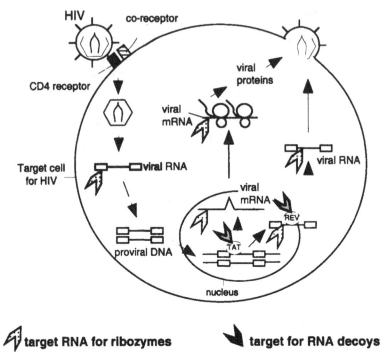

target RNA for ribozymes   **target for RNA decoys**

Figure 2   Schematic representation of the human immunodeficiency virus (HIV) life cycle and the potential targets for ribozyme- and decoy-based gene therapy.

sequences could inhibit HIV replication. Our group has concentrated on hairpin ribozymes targeting multiple substrates in the HIV genome. A ribozyme targeting the U5 region of the HIV 5′ LTR delivered by a murine retrovirus-based vector has been shown to confer protection in T-cell lines (75), in human peripheral blood lymphocytes (PBLs) (44), and in macrophages derived from CD34$^+$ cells challenged with multiple strains of HIV (45,76). An important advantage of ribozymes compared to the other strategies described above on inhibition of viral replication is the theoretical possibility of these molecules having the ability to cleave incoming viral RNA; that is, prior to integration into the host genome as well as de novo synthesized RNA (Fig. 2). In the study of Yamada et al. (77), we showed that expression of the ribozyme decreased 5- to 50-fold the efficiency of the incoming virus to synthesize proviral DNA. However, a point mutation of the target RNA at the cleavage site or to a lesser extent at the binding site can abrogate the catalytic reaction of the ribozyme on its substrate. Because of the exquisite sequence specificity of ribozymes, and to decrease the risk of viral escape by mutation, a combination of different strategies (decoys + ribozymes) has been sought (77). We have engineered a multigene antiviral murine retrovirus-based vector targeting multiple sites in the HIV RNA with different mechanisms of action (ribozyme + RNA decoy) (78). This murine retroviral vector (Fig. 3) has in the 3′ LTR a cassette comprising a ribozyme targeting a very conserved region in the U5 LTR of HIV-1, fused with the stem loop 2 of the RRE, and shown to be an efficient RNA decoy for sequestering the Rev proteins. These antiviral genes are under the control of the housekeeping Pol III tRNA^{val} promoter in an antisense direction. By inserting the cassette in the U3 region of the murine retroviral LTR, this information

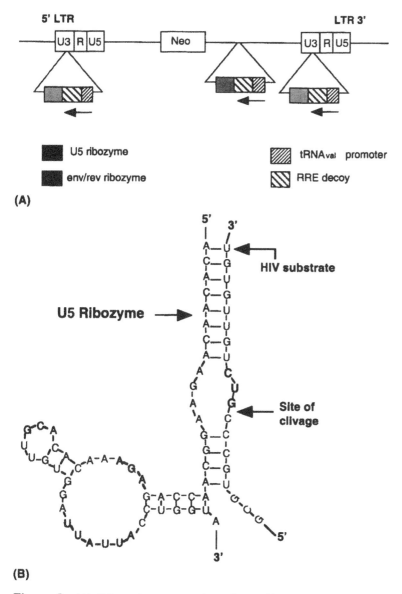

(A)

(B)

Figure 3 (A) Schematic representation of a multigene antihuman immunodeficiency virus (HIV)–1 retroviral vector encoding three ribozyme/decoy fusion molecules driven by a Pol III tRNA^{val} promoter in antisense direction (←). Neo: neomycin resistance gene. (B) The hairpin ribozyme model. This ribozyme targets a specific sequence in the U5 region of HIV-1$_{HXB2}$ long terminal repeat (LTR).

will be copied into the 5′ LTR during the step of reverse transcription at the time of infection of target cells with the vector (79). Furthermore, this vector also contains an internal cassette made of an RRE decoy fused with a ribozyme directed to another sequence (*env/rev*) of the HIV genome. This triple-copy vector displays numerous advantages. (1) Because of the number of cassettes, the expression of the transgenes has been shown to be 100-fold higher than in a single-copy vector. (2) Because of the binding of the RRE decoy to the Rev proteins, the fusion molecule should traffic through the same cellular compartments as HIV, thereby increasing the chance for the ribozymes to encounter its RNA substrate. (3) Fusion of a RRE decoy to the 5' end of hairpin ribozymes has been shown to increase the efficiency of the catalytic activity of the ribozyme (77); possibly by increasing the turnover of the enzyme. Finally, when a T-cell line transduced with different ribozymes expressing vectors was challenged with geographically and philogenetically different strains of HIV (clades A–E), the cells transduced with the multigene antiviral vector resisted HIV infection better than the other transduced cells (78).

VI. AUTOLOGOUS HEMATOPOIETIC STEM CELL TRANSPLANTATION

Isolation and characterization of human hematopoietic progenitor and stem cells represent a long-term challenge due to the low frequency of the cells and lack of markers for positive selection. However, functional studies have shown that the $CD34^+$ surface glycoprotein, found on the surface of 1–4% of human bone marrow cells, is expressed by virtually all hematopoietic progenitors analyzed by in vitro colony assay, long-term culture-initiating cells, and cells with in vivo reconstitutive capacity, but not by mature hematopoietic cells (80,81). Other cell surface phenotypes have been further identified among the $CD34^+$ cells to characterize the most primitive human hematopoietic cell subset such as $CD34^+CD38^-Lin-Thy-1^+$ phenotype (82,83).

Autologous hematopoietic stem cells transplantation with cells transduced with anti-HIV genes could generate multilineage progeny, including peripheral blood cells, lymphoid cells, monocytes-macrophages, and bone marrow–derived dendritic cells, and replace these cell populations that are known to be critical for sustaining HIV replication. However, several questions need to be addressed. (1) Is it possible to mobilize $CD34^+$ cells in HIV-infected individuals? (2) Can these cells be transduced with antiviral genes? (3) Have these cells intact clonogenic capacities? (4) Are the progeny cells resistant to HIV infection? Results from our group (84) and others (85) have shown that after 6 days of daily subcutaneous injection of 10 µg/kg of granulocyte-colony-stimulating factor (G-CSF), between 1.5 and 2.0 million $CD34^+$ cells/kg of body weight were collected after one leukapheresis. The viral burden did not increase significantly during this treatment, as noted by competitive reverse transcriptase assays. In our protocol, part of these cells was subsequently transduced with the multigene antiviral vector (see above) or a control vector after stimulation of the cells with growth factors (IL-3, IL-6, and stem cell factor). Transduction efficiency, assayed by polymerase chain reaction (PCR), varied between 46 and 100% using the clonogenic assay. The capacity of these cells to give rise to progeny CFU-GM and burst-forming units-erythrocyte (BFU-E) was comparable to uninfected subjects. Finally, macrophages derived from $CD34^+$ cells transduced with anti-HIV genes resisted HIV infection. $CD34^+$ cells that had been frozen in liquid nitrogen and then thawed and transduced or first transduced and frozen secondarily displayed a similar testing pattern as the fresh cells (76).

A small number of autologous bone marrow transplantations have been performed in HIV-infected individuals (86,87). Even though the myeloablative conditioning regimen was tolerated, all patients died after a short period of time owing to recurrence of the lymphoma, of AIDS, or of concomitant infections. From this perspective, autologous transplantation of hematopoietic stem cells transduced with anti-HIV gene could be considered in conjunction with antiviral drugs. Recent studies have shown that the combination of inhibitors of HIV reverse transcriptase and protease could substantially decrease the viral load to undetectable levels for several months (88). The better combination could be to cover HIV-infected individuals for several months with a compound of three antiviral drugs to diminish the viral burden. During this period of time, mobilization of hematopoietic stem cells could be obtained by growth factor stimulation, drawn from the patient, transduced with potent anti-HIV vector, and frozen if a myeloablative treatment is needed or directly reinfused to the patient. If these cells can engraft, expand, and sustain anti-HIV gene expression, the progeny cells should benefit from a survival advantage compared to unprotected cells, as suggested by Woffendin et al. (37) with the REV M10 clinical trial.

VII. CONCLUSION

In the last few years, tremendous efforts and progress have been made in improving the understanding of HIV infection and treatment in parallel. Gene therapy technology has also advanced significantly. However, even though in vitro data demonstrated the possibility of transducing hematopoietic stem cells with anti-HIV vectors and conferring resistance to HIV infection in progeny cells, all trials involving more evolved and complex systems as animal (89) or human models (90) have failed to show significant engraftment of genetically altered transfused CD34$^+$ cells and sustained expression of the transgene over time. These actual limitations are perhaps due to the fact that most ex vivo experiments have been performed with murine retrovirus-based vectors and that these vectors require stimulation of the stem cells to integrate stably. However, stimulation of these cells is likely to commit them to differentiate and to lose their pluripotent and self-renewal capacities. Once stable integration in stem cells is achieved and demonstrated by PCR or in situ hybridization, long-term expression of the transgene in vivo will need to be addressed by RNA-based assays to prove that the exogenous promoter is not shut off by the cellular machinery. Finally, challenge with multiple strains of HIV will definitively prove the efficacy of a such therapy. Efficacy in animal models such as immunodeficient mice, reconstituted with human hematopoietic cells, will greatly strengthen the rationale before starting human trials.

REFERENCES

1. Barre-Sinoussi F, Chermann JC, Rey F, Nugeyre MT, Chamaret S, Gruest J, Dauget C, Axler-Blin C, Vezinet-Brun F, Rouzioux C, Rozenbaum W, Montagnier L. Isolation of a T-lymphotrophic retrovirus from a patient at risk for acquired immunodeficiency syndrome (AIDS). Science 1983; 220:868–871.
2. Gallo RC, Salahuddin SZ, Popovic M, Shearer GM, Kaplan M, Haynes BF, Palker TJ, Redfield R, Oleske J, Safai B. Frequent detection and isolation of cytopathic retroviruses (HTLV-3) from patients with AIDS and at high risk for AIDS. Science 1984; 224:500–503.
3. Levy JA, Hoffman AD, Kramer SM. Retroviruses from San Francisco patients with AIDS. Science 1984; 225:840–842.
4. Chiu IM, Yaniv A, Dahlberg C. Nucleotide sequence evidence for relationship of AIDS retrovirus to lentiviruses. Nature 1985; 317:366–368.
5. Mann JM. AIDS the second decade: a global perspective. J Infect Dis 1992; 165:245–250.
6. Schnittman SM, Fauci AS. Human immunodeficiency virus and acquired immunodeficiency syndrome: an update. Adv Intern Med 1994; 39:305–356.
7. Clements JE, Wong-Staal F. Molecular biology of lentiviruses. Virology 1992; 3:137–146.

8. Dalgleish AG, Beverley PC, Clapham PR, Crawford DH, Greaves MF, Weiss RA. The CD4
    (T4) antigen is an essential component of the receptor for the AIDS retrovirus. Nature 1984;
    312:763–767.

9. Klatzmann D, Barre-Sinoussi F, Nugeyre MT, Danquet C, Vilmer E, Griscelli C, Brun-Veziret
    F, Rouzioux C, Gluckman JC, Chermann JC. Selective tropism of lymphadenopathy associated
    virus (LAV) for helper-inducer T lymphocytes. Science 1984; 225:59–63.

10. Deng H, Liu R, Ellmeier W, Choe S, Unutmaz D, Burkhart M, Di Marzio P, Marmon S,
    Sutton RE, Hill CM, Davis CB, Peiper SC, Schall TJ, Littman DR, Landau NR. Identification
    of a major co-receptor for primary isolates of HIV-1. Nature 1996; 381:661–666.

11. Doranz B, Rucker J, Yi Y, Smyth YRJ, Samson M, Peiper SC, Parmentier M, Collman RG,
    Doms RW. A dual-tropic primary HIV-1 isolate that uses fusin and the β-chemokine receptors
    CKR-5, CKR-3, and CKR-2b as fusion cofactors. Cell 1996; 89:1149–1158.

12. Feng Y, Broder CC, Kennedy PE, Berger EA. HIV-1 entry cofactor: functional cloning of a
    seven-transmembrane G protein-coupled receptor. Science 1996; 272:872–877.

13. Von Schwedler U, Kornbluth RS, Trono D. The nuclear localization signal of the matrix pro-
    tein of human immunodeficiency virus type 1 allows the establishment of infection in macro-
    phages and quiescent T lymphocytes. Proc Natl Acad Sci USA 1994; 91:6992–6996.

14. Gallay P, Swingler S, Aiken C, Trono D. HIV-1 infection of nondividing cells: C-terminal
    tyrosine phosphorylation of the viral matrix protein is a key regulator. Cell 1995; 80:379–
    388.

15. Steffy K, Wong-Staal F. Genetic regulation of human immunodeficiency virus. Microbiol Rev
    1991; 55:193–205.

16. Dayton A, Sodroski J, Rosen C, Goh W, Haseltine W. The trans-activator gene of the human
    T-cell lymphotrophic virus type III is required for replication. Cell 1986; 44:941–947.

17. Rosen C, Sodroski J, Haseltine W. The location of cis-acting regulatory sequences in the
    human T-cell lymphotrophic virus type III (HTLV-III) long terminal repeat. Cell 1985; 41:
    313–323.

18. Kao S, Calman P, Luciw P, Peterin B. Antitermination of transcription within the long terminal
    repeat of HIV by tat gene product. Nature 1987; 330:489–493.

19. Malim MH, Tiley L, McCarn D, Rusche J, et al. HIV-1 rev trans-activator acts through a
    structured target sequence to activate nuclear export of unspliced viral mRNA. Nature 1990;
    338:254–257.

20. Lee SW, Gallardo HF, Gilboa E, Smith C. Inhibition of human immunodeficiency virus type
    1 in human T-cells by a potent Rev response element decoy consisting of the 13-nucleotide
    minimal Rev-binding domain. J Virol 1994; 68:8254–8264.

21. Mariani R, Skowronski J. CD4 down-regulation of nef alleles isolated from human immunode-
    ficiency virus type 1-infected individuals. Proc Natl Acad Sci USA 1993; 90:5549–5553.

22. Schwartz O, Marechal V, Le Gall S, Lemonnier F, Heard JM. Endocytosis of major histocom-
    patibility complex class 1 molecules is induced by the HIV-1 Nef protein. Nature Med 1996;
    2:338–342.

23. Miller MD, Warmerdam MT, Gaston I, Green WC, Feinberg MB. The human immunodefi-
    ciency virus-1 nef gene product: a positive factor for viral infection and replication in primary
    lymphocytes and macrophages. J Exp Med 1994; 179:101–113.

24. Spina CA, Kwoh TJ, Chowers MY, Guatelli JC, Richman DD. The importance of nef in
    the induction of human immunodeficiency type 1 replication from primary quiescent CD4
    lymphocytes. J Exp Med 1994; 179:115–123.

25. Sawai ET, Baur A, Struble H, Peterlin BM, Levy JA, Cheng-Mayer C. Human immunodefi-
    ciency virus type 1 Nef associates with a cellular serine kinase in T lymphocytes. Proc Natl
    Acad Sci USA 1994; 91:1539–1543.

26. Kestler HW, Ringler DJ, Mori K, Panicali DL, Sehgal PK, Daniel MD, Desrosiers RC. Impor-
    tance of the nef gene for maintenance of high virus load and for development of AIDS. Cell
    1991; 65:651–662.

27. Jowett JB, Panelles V, Poon B, Shah NP, Chen ML, Chen IS. The human immunodeficiency virus type 1 vpr gene arrests infected T-cells in the G2+ M phase of the cell cycle. J Virol 1995; 69:6304–6313.

28. Heinzinger NK, Bukrinsky MI, Haggerty SA, Ragland AM, Kewalramani V, Lee MA, Gendelman HE, Ratner L, Stevenson M, Emerman M. The Vpr protein of the human immunodeficiency virus type 1 influences nuclear localization of viral nucleic acids in nondividing host cells. Proc Natl Acad Sci USA 1994; 91:7311–7315.

29. Camaur D, Trono, D. Characterization of human immunodeficiency virus type 1 vif particle incorporation. J Virol 1996; 70:6106–6111.

30. Strebel K, Daugherty D, Clouse K, et al. The HIV 'A' (sor) gene product is essential for virus infectivity. Nature 1987; 328:728–731.

31. Sova P, Volsky DJ. Efficiency of viral DNA synthesis during infection of permissive and nonpermissive cells with vif-negative human immunodeficiency virus type 1. J Virol 1993; 67:6322–6326.

32. Klimkait T, Strebel K, Hoggan MD, Martin MA, Orenstein JM. The human immunodeficiency virus type 1–specific protein vpu is required for efficient virus maturation and release. J Virol 1990; 64:621–629.

33. Chen MY, Maldarelli F, Karczewski MK, Willey RL, Strebel K. Human immunodeficiency virus type 1 vpu protein induces degradation of CD4 in vitro: the cytoplasmic domain of CD4 contributes to vpu sensitivity. J Virol 1993; 67:3877–3884.

34. Fauci AS. The human immunodeficiency virus: Infectivity and mechanisms of pathogenesis. Science 1988; 239:617–622.

35. Weichold FK, Zella D, Barabitskaja O, Maciejewski JP, Dunn DE, Sloand E, Young NS. Neither human immunodeficiency virus-1 (HIV-1) nor HIV-2 infects most primitive human hematopoietic stem cells as assessed in long term bone marrow cultures. Blood 1998; 91:907–915.

36. Ho DD, Neumann AU, Perelson AS, Chen W, Leonard JM, Markowitz M. Rapid turnover of plasma virions and CD4 lymphocytes in HIV-1 infection. Nature 1995; 373:123–126.

37. Woffendin C, Ranga U, Yang ZH, Xu L, Nabel GJ. Expression of a protective gene prolongs survival of T cells in human immunodeficiency virus-infected patients. Proc Natl Acad Sci USA 1996; 93:2889–2894.

38. Wei X, Ghosh SK, Taylor ME, Johnson VA, Emini EA, Deutsch P, Lifson JD, Bonhoeffer S, Nowak MA, Hahn BH, Saag MS, Shaw GM. Viral dynamics in human immunodeficiency virus type 1 infection. Nature 1995; 373:117–122.

39. Vormoor J, Lapidot T, Pflumio F, Ridson G, Patterson B, Broxmeyer HE, Dick JE. Immature human cord blood progenitors engraft and proliferate to high levels in severe combined immunodeficient mice. Blood 1994; 83:2489–2497.

40. Fassati A, Dunckley MG, Dickson G. Retroviral vectors. In: Dickson G, ed. Molecular and Cell Biology of Human Gene Therapeutics. London: Chapman & Hall, 1995:1–15.

41. Mulligan RC. The basic science of gene therapy. Science 1993; 260:926–932.

42. Miller AD. Retroviral vectors. Curr Topics Microbiol Immunol 1990; 158:1–24.

43. Van Beusechem B, Kukler A, Heidt P, Valerio D. Long-term expression of human adenosine deaminase in rhesus monkeys transplanted with retrovirus-infected bone-marrow cells. Proc Natl Acad Sci USA 1992; 89:7640–7644.

44. Leavitt MC, Yu M, Yamada O, Kraus G, Looney D, Poeschla E, Wong-Staal F. Transfer of an anti–HIV-1 ribozyme gene into primary human lymphocytes. Hum Gene Ther 1994; 5:1115–1120.

45. Yu M, Leavitt MC, Maruyama M, Yamada O, Young D, Ho AD, Wong-Staal F. Intracellular immunization of human fetal cord blood stem/progenitor cells with a ribozyme against human immunodeficiency virus type 1. Proc Natl Acad Sci USA 1995; 92:699–703.

46. Miller DG, Adam MA, Miller AD. Gene transfer by retroviruses vectors occurs only in cells that are actively replicating at the time of infection. Mol Cell Biol 1990; 10:4239–4242.

47. Lu M, Maruyama M, Zhang N, Levine F, Friedmann T, Ho AD. High efficiency retroviral-mediated gene transduction into CD34+ cells purified from peripheral blood of breast cancer patients primed with chemotherapy and granulocyte-macrophage colony-stimulating factor. Hum Gene Ther 1994; 5:203–208.

48. Friedmann T. Progress towards human gene therapy. Science 1989; 244:1275–1277.

49. Kotin RM. Prospects for the use of adeno-associated virus as a vector for human gene therapy. Hum Gene Ther 1994; 5:793–801.

50. McLaughlin SK, Collis P, Hermonat PL, Muzyczka N. Adeno-associated virus general transduction vectors: analysis of proviral structures. J Virol 1988; 62:1963–1973.

51. Kotin RM, Siniscalco M, Samulski RJ, Zhu X, Hunter L, Laughlin CA, McLaughlin S, Muzyczka N, Rocchi M, Berns KI. Site-specific integration by adeno-associated virus. Proc Natl Acad Sci USA 1990; 87:2211–2215.

52. Muro C, Samulski R, Kaplan D. Gene transfer in human lymphocytes using a vector based on adeno-associated virus. J Immunother 1992; 11:231–237.

53. Zhou SZ, Broxmeyer HE, Cooper S, Harrington MA, Srivastava A. Adeno-associated virus 2-mediated gene transfer in murine hematopoietic progenitor cells. Exp Hematol 1993; 21:928–933.

54. Poznansky M, Lever A, Bergeron L, Haseltine W, Sodroski J. Gene transfer into human lymphocytes by a defective human immunodeficiency virus type 1 vector. J Virol 1991; 65:532–536.

55. Carroll R, Lin JT, Dacquel EJ, Mosca JD, Burke DS, St Louis DC. A human immunodeficiency virus type 1 (HIV-1)–based retroviral vector system utilizing stable HIV-1 packaging cell lines. J Virol 1994; 68:6047–6051.

56. Poeschla E, Corbeau P, Wong-Staal F. Development of HIV vectors for anti-HIV gene therapy. Proc Natl Acad Sci USA 1996; 93:11395–11399.

57. Naldini I, Blomer U, Gage FH, Trono D, Verma IM. Efficient transfer, integration, and sustained long-term expression of the transgene in adult rat brain injected with a lentiviral vector. Proc Natl Acad Sci USA 1996; 93:11382–11388.

58. Poeschla E, Gilbert J, Li X, Huang S, Ho AD, Wong-Staal F. Identification of a human immunodeficiency virus type 2 (HIV-2) encapsidation determinant and transduction of nondividing human cells by HIV-2 based lentivirus vectors. J Virol 1998; 72:6527–6536.

59. Yu M, Poeschla E, Wong-Staal F. Progress towards gene therapy for HIV infection. Gene Ther 1994; 1:13–26.

60. Wang B, Ugen KE, Srikantan V, Weiner DB. Gene inoculation generates immune response against HIV-1. Proc Natl Acad Sci USA 1993; 90:4156–4160.

61. Deen KC, Mc Dougal JS, Inacker R, Folena-Wasserman G, Arthos J, Rosenberg J, Maddon PJ, Axel R, Sweet RW. A soluble form of CD4 (T4) proteins inhibits AIDS virus infection. Nature 1988; 331:82–84.

62. Harrison G, Long C, Curiel T, Maxwell F, Maxwell I. Inhibition of human immunodeficiency virus-1 production resulting from transduction with a retrovirus containing an HIV-regulated diphtheria toxin A gene. Hum Gene Ther 1992; 3:461–469.

63. Caruso M, Klatzman D. Selective killing of CD4+ cells harboring a human immunodeficiency virus inducible suicide gene prevents viral spread in infected cell population. Proc Natl Acad Sci USA 1992; 89:182–186.

64. Malim MH, Bohnlein S, Hauber J, Cullen BR. Functional dissection of the HIV-1 Rev transactivator-derivation of a trans dominant repressor of Rev function. Cell 1989; 58:205–214.

65. Malim MH, Cullen BR. HIV-1 structural gene expression requires the binding of multiple monomers to the viral RRE: implications for HIV-1 latency. Cell 1991; 65:241–248.

66. Malim MH, Freimuth WW, Liu J, Boyle TJ, Lyerly HK, Cullen BR, Nabel JG. Stable expression of transdominant Rev protein in human T-cells inhibits human immunodeficiency virus replication. J Exp Med 1992; 176:1197–1201.

67. Green M, Ishino M, Loewenstein PM. Mutational analysis of HIV-1 Tat minimal domain

peptides: identification of trans-dominant mutants that suppress HIV-LTR driven gene expression. Cell 1989; 58:215–223.

68. Sullenger BA, Gallardo HF, Ungers GE, Gilboa E. Overexpression of TAR sequence renders cells resistant to human immunodeficiency virus replication. Cell 1990; 63:601–608.

69. Hampel A, Tritz R. RNA catalytic properties of the minimum (−)s TRSV sequence. Biochemistry 1989; 28:4929–4933.

70. Cech TR, Uhlenbeck OC. Hammerhead nailed down. Nature 1994; 372:39–40.

71. Lorentzen EU, Wieland U, Kuhn JE, Braun RW. In vitro cleavage of HIV vif RNA by a synthetic ribozyme. Virus Genes 1991; 5:17–23.

72. Yamada O, Kraus G, Leavitt MC, Yu M, Wong-Staal F. Activity and cleavage site specificity of an anti-HIV-1 ribozyme in human T cells. Virology 1994; 205:121–126.

73. Yu M, Poeschla E, Yamada O, Degrandis P, Leavitt MC, Heusch M, Yees JK, Wong-Staal F, Hampel A. In vitro and in vivo characterization of a second functional hairpin ribozyme against HIV-1. Virology 1995; 206:381–386.

74. Sarver N, Cantin EM, Chang PS, Zaia JA, Ladne PA, Stephens DA, Rossi JJ. Ribozyme as potential anti–HIV-1 therapeutic agents. Science 1990; 247:1222–1225.

75. Yu M, Ojwang J, Yamada O, Hampel A, Rappaport J, Looney D, Wong-Staal F. A hairpin ribozyme inhibits expression of diverse strains of human immunodeficiency virus type 1. Proc Natl Acad Sci USA 1993; 90:6340–6344.

76. Gervaix A, Schwartz L, Law P, Looney D, Ho AD, Wong-Staal, F. Gene therapy targeting CD34$^+$ hematopoietic stem cells from peripheral blood of individuals infected with the human immunodeficiency virus type 1. Hum Gene Ther 1997; 8:2229–2238.

77. Yamada O, Kraus G, Luznik L, Yu M, Wong-Staal F. A chimeric human immunodeficiency virus type 1 (HIV-1) minimal Rev response element-ribozyme molecule exhibits dual antiviral function and inhibits cell-cell transmission of HIV-1. J Virol 1996; 70:1596–1601.

78. Gervaix A, Li X, Kraus G, Wong-Staal F. Multigene antiviral vectors inhibit diverse human immunodeficiency virus type 1 clades. J Virol 1997; 71:3048–3053.

79. Hantzopoulos P, Sullenger B, Ungers G, Gilboa E. Improved gene expression upon transfer of the adenosine deaminase minigene outside the transcriptional unit of retroviral vector. Proc Natl Acad Sci USA 1989; 86:3519–3523.

80. Andrews RG, Singer JW, Bernstein ID. Monoclonal antibody 12-8 recognizes a 115-kd molecule present on both unipotent and multipotent hematopoietic colony-forming cells and their precursors. Blood 1986; 67:842–845.

81. Berenson RJ, Andrews RG, Bensinger WI, Kalamasz D, Knitter G, Buckner CD, Bernstein ID. Antigen CD34+ marrow cells engraft lethally irradiated baboons. J Clin Invest 1988; 81: 951–955.

82. Baum CM, Weissmann IL, Tsukamoto AS, Buckle A, Peault B. Isolation of a candidate human hematopoietic stem-cell population. Proc Natl Acad Sci. USA 1992; 89:2804–2808.

83. Henon PR. Peripheral blood stem cell transplantation: past, present and future. Stem Cells 1993; 11:154–172.

84. Law P, Lane TA, Gervaix A, Looney D, Schwartz L, Young D, Ramos S, Wong-Staal F, Recktenwald D, Ho AD. Mobilization of peripheral blood progenitor cells for human immunodeficiency virus-infected individuals. Exp Hematol 1999; 27:147–154.

85. Slobod KS, Bennet TA, Freiden PJ, Kechli AM, Howlett N, Flynn PM, Head DR, Srivastava DK, Boyett JM, Brenner MK, Garcia JV. Mobilization of CD34$^+$ progenitor cells by granulocyte colony-stimulating factor in human immunodeficiency virus type 1–infected adults. Blood 1996; 88:3329–3335.

86. Aboulafia DM, Mitsuyasu RT, Mile SA. Syngeneic bone-marrow transplantation and failure to eradicate HIV. AIDS 1995; 5:344.

87. Saral R, Holland K. Bone marrow transplantation for the acquired immune deficiency syndrome. In: Foreman S, ed. Bone Marrow Transplantation. Boston: Blackwell, 1993:654–664.

88. Gulick R, Mellors J, Havlir D, Eron J. Safety and activity of indinavir (IDV) in combination

with zidovudine (ZDV) and lamivudine (3TC). Abstract. 3rd Conference on Retroviruses and Opportunistic Infections, Washington, DC, 1996.

89. Nolta JA, Smogorzewska EM, Kohn DB. Analysis of optimal conditions for retroviral-mediated transduction of primitive human hematopoietic cells. Blood 1995; 86:101–110.

90. Bordignon C, Notarangelo LD, Nobili N, Ferrari G, Casorati G, Panina P, Mazzolari E, Maggioni D, Rossi C, Servida P, Ugazio AG, Mavilio F. Gene therapy in peripheral blood lymphocytes and bone marrow for ADA-immunodeficient patients. Science 1995; 270:470–475.

33

Autografting Followed by Low-Intensity Conditioning Regimen for Allografting

ANGELO M. CARELLA

Ospedale San Martino, Genoa, Italy

I. INTRODUCTION

Allografting is a well-documented curative therapy for patients with leukemias and other hematological malignancies. Conventional myeloablative regimens for allografting usually involve high-dose chemotherapy alone or in combination with total body irradiation. Such regimens have been considered to be essential for allografting, because they do eliminate from the marrow the host hematopoietic progenitor cells (HPCs) (and therefore they make "space" for the donor HPCs), avoid rejection of these cells, and drastically reduce or eliminate the neoplastic cells of the host (1,2). Recently, it has been demonstrated that the mechanism of tumor cell control is due to the alloreactivity of donor immune cells, and therefore adoptive allogeneic therapy plays a fundamental role mainly in chronic myelogenous leukemia (3), but also in other hematological neoplasias (4). Considering that it is now possible to eradicate high tumor burdens by adoptive allogeneic therapy through donor lymphocyte infusion (DLI) in patients relapsing after high-dose myeloablative approaches, the crucial question is: Is the myeloablation still essential considering that the induction of host-versus-graft tolerance is usually accomplished by successful stable donor cell engraftment?

To reply to this question, two papers have been recently pioneering this new concept in the allografting area (5,6). This new procedure has been called miniallograft; that is, the use of less intensive conditioning regimens. In these regimens, the crucial drug is fludarabine, a purine analog, which is a potent T-cell immunosuppressive agent with no or very low myelotoxicity. The Houston team employed this procedure in patients ineligible for a standard allografting (e.g., advanced age, poor general conditions), whereas the Jerusalem team has included all patients eligible for an allograft. In both groups, a high donor HPC engraftment was achieved in all nonleukemic patients [as confirmed by sensitive polymerase chain reaction (PCR)–based methods]. In many of these patients, donor-versus-host tolerance was not accomplished by grades II–IV acute graft-versus-host disease (GVHD); on the contrary, many of the Jerusalem patients developed chronic GVHD (cGVHD). These preliminary studies, together with other anecdotal reports, appear encouraging (7–9).

In these last months, our team designed a protocol for resistant patients where autografting was combined with subsequent allografting conditioned by an immunosuppressive nonmyeloablative regimen. The idea was to reduce the tumor burden maximally with the eradication of residual cells. Immunosuppression was achieved using fludarabine combined with cyclophosphamide. Fludarabine is a potent immunosuppressive drug that also is able to modulate GVHD. At 30 mg/m^2/day $\times$ 5 days, this drug has already been reported as having a potent immunosuppressive effect allowing engraftment of allogeneic cells with minimal or no toxicity.

II. PATIENTS AND METHODS

Sixteen patients, median age 36 years, were treated. Six patients had primarily refractory (n = 2) or relapsed (n = 4) Hodgkin's disease and two patients had primarily refractory non-Hodgkin's lymphoma. These patients were treated with first- and second-line therapies ± radiotherapy. Two patients had chronic myelogenous leukemia, one in accelerated phase (this patient did not have evidence of the Philadelphia chromosome at diagnosis, but we found a p190 *bcr-abl* gene by the reverse transcriptase PCR) and one in myeloblastic transformation with 70% marrow blasts. They were cytogenetical/molecular resistant to hydroxyurea and interferon-α (5 MU/m^2/die) (10). Four patients had metastatic breast cancer in diffuse metastases in the bone and two patients also in the liver, and two patients had refractory anemia with excess blasts (RAEB). One patient had t(1;3) (p36;q21). The median time from diagnosis to mobilization therapy was 28 months (range 5–49 months). In the first stage of the protocol, autologous peripheral blood stem cells were mobilized from 14 patients: in 12 patients after treatment with cyclophosphamide [3–4 g/m^2 and granulocyte colony-stimulating factor (G-CSF)] and in the two patients with chronic myelogenous leukemia (CML) after the ICE protocol, consisting of idarubicin 8 mg/m^2/d intravenously for 5 days, cytarabine 800 mg/m^2 by 2-hour infusion for 5 days, and etoposide 150 mg/m^2/d by 2-hour infusion for 3 days (blastic phase) or mini-ICE protocol (the same three drugs at the same doses but for 3 days only) (accelerated phase) (11). In preparation for autologous transplant, patients underwent high-dose chemotherapy on protocols appropriate for the underlying disease. Chronic myelogenous leukemia patients received high-dose busulfan 3 mg/kg/day $\times$ 4 days (accelerated phase) or high-dose mitoxantrone (20 mg/m^2/days $\times$ 3 days) with arabinosylcytosine (1000 mg/m^2/day $\times$ 3 days) (blastic phase). Hodgkin's disease and non-Hodgkin's lymphoma (NHL) patients were treated with the BEAM protocol (12): carmustine 300 mg/m^2 iv on day 1, etoposide 200 mg/m^2 iv days 2–5, arabinosylcytosine 200 mg/m^2 bid on days 2–5, and melphalan 140 mg/m^2 iv on day 6. Breast cancer patients received different protocols consisting of cyclophosphamide, mitoxantrone, paraplatin ± taxotere. At a median of 3 weeks after recovery from autografting, all patients with lymphoma and breast cancer were restaged by all available imaging techniques (plain radiographic imaging with computed tomographic scan). Patients who had a >50% reduction in measurable disease were considered to be in partial remission; patients who did not achieve complete or partial remission, or who developed progression of the disease, were considered to have primarily refractory disease. Three patients with Hodgkin's disease and both patients with non-Hodgkin's lymphoma achieved partial remission. The patients with breast cancer achieved bone pain disappearance without modifications of bone or liver localizations and the patients with CML obtained a second chronic phase, but all metaphases were still 100% Philadelphia chromosome positive (blastic phase CML) or *bcr-abl* positive (accelerated phase CML). The patients received fludarabine (Flu) (30 mg/m^2/day on days 1–3) with cyclophosphamide (Cy) (300 mg/m^2/day on days 1–3). GVHD prophylaxis consisted of cyclosporine begun the day before donor stem cell infusion at 1 mg/kg/day by continuous infusion and methotrexate 8 mg/m^2 on days +1, +3, and +5; cyclosporine was continued by intravenous infusion for 12–29 days (median 16 days), after which it was given by oral route at a dosage of 5 mg/kg/daily. The donors were treated with G-CSF at 10 mg/kg bid for 2–4 days and then underwent leukaphereses of stem cells. A median of 3 × 10^6/kg (range 1.3–7.8) donor CD34$^+$ cells were obtained and infused fresh into the patient 48 hs after the conclusion of Flu-Cy therapy. Patient blood samples were serially studied for chimerism.

A. Evaluation of Chimerism

Cytogenetics and DNA polymorphisms by fluorescence-based technology of multiplexed PCR products (STR) on bone marrow cells were used as a marker for chimerism. Allogeneic stem cells have been monitored with this technique, first by multiplex reaction and then by detecting donor/recipient cell population ratios at 10-day interval the first month and 15-day interval in the second and third month after allografting by evaluation of peak areas in singleplexed PCR products of each informative marker.

III. RESULTS

The Flu-Cy protocol was well tolerated with no severe procedure-related toxicity. No patient required platelet or red cell transfusion. Patients were discharged from the hospital 16–28 days (median 19 days) after donor stem cell infusion. There was evidence of 100% donor cell engraftment in nine patients. Severe acute GVHD (aGVHD) was observed in two patients. The first patient was readmitted to the hospital for fever, herpes zoster, and liver grade II aGVHD and successfully treated with acyclovir, high-dose methylprednisolone (125 mg/m^2/day), and continuous infusion (c.i.) cyclosporine (2 mg/kg/day). Soon after, the patient developed evidence of gastrointestinal (GI) tract grade II aGVHD, with a good clinical response to octreotide, methylprednisolone, and cyclosporine. Subsequently, this patient developed cGVHD in the liver combined with extensive and progressive Hodgkin's disease. She died with a complete chimerism 460 days after allografting. The second patient developed GI grade III aGVHD combined with skin grade II. Progressive respiratory failure due to bilateral pneumonia sustained by *Pseudomonas aeruginosa*, *Klebsiella oxytoca*, *Staphylococcus* coagulase negative, *Candida albicans*, and *Aspergillus* was demonstrated by BAL. Specific antibiotic therapy (third-generation cephalosporin and aminoglycosides combined with intravenous vancomycin in continuous infusion) and amphotericin B (subsequently substituted by liposomal derivatives) determined a complete resolution. The patient developed brain hemorrhage and died 120 days later. The autopsy showed *Aspergillus* infection in the brain and confirmed the remission state of the disease.

Limited cGVHD in the skin is now present in the patients with low-grade NHL and accelerated phase CML; both patients are in complete remission after allografting.

A. Disease Response

Two of the Hodgkin's disease (HD) patients, who were in partial remission after autografting, achieved a complete remission: One died of *Aspergillus* infection and brain hemorrhage following, and the second patient is alive in remission 12 months after allografting. Another patient in the third complete remission (CR) after mechlorotamine, vincristine, prednisone, and procarbazine (MOPP) chemotherapy maintains this status after allografting. Of the other three patients, one is alive in partial remission (PR) and he is receiving donor lymphocyte infusion (DLI) (until now without success!); two other patients died of progressive HD or HD and cGVHD. The blastic phase CML patient died of blastic evolution 7 months after allografting. The patient in accelerated phase, who obtained a second chronic phase after autografting, achieved complete disappearance of the *bcr-abl* hybrid transcript, and he is now in complete hematological and molecular remission with 100% donor cells in the marrow on day 330. One patient with RAEB with t(1;3) achieved a complete hematological and cytogenetic remission with 100% donor cells, and she was disease free for 3 months. After that, she relapsed and she was treated with DLI twice. After the second infusion (1×10^6/kg CD3$^+$ cells), she has maintained her hemoglobin level over 9 g/L, and about 30% of diploid cells are present in the marrow. In conclusion, nine patients (56%) are alive with a median follow-up of 252 days (range 62–478 days). Three patients died ≤100 days after miniallograft of lymphoma (two patients) or breast cancer (one patient). Four other patients died over 100 days: one patient of blastic phase CML, two patients of lymphoma, and one patient of lymphoma and cGVHD.

IV. DISCUSSION

Fludarabine, as other purine analogs, has substantial immunosuppressive activity, inducing long-lasting T-cell lymphopenia when used in the treatment of patients with lymphoproliferative disorders and when administered to patients with chronic lymphocytic leukemia as part of their primary therapy before allografting (13). Fludarabine may modulate the host immune system, thereby reducing the severity of the GVHD (14,15); moreover, transfusion-associated GVHD appears to be more frequent in fludarabine-treated patients because of the profound CD4$^+$ and CD8$^+$ T-cell depletion induced by the drug (16).

The efficacy of this drug in combination with other myelosuppressive drugs was recently demonstrated to allow engraftment of human leukocyte antigen (HLA)–matched sibling donor stem cells (5,6). Hepatic toxicity and/or neutropenia was seen in many patients receiving this myelosuppressive/immunosuppressive combination therapy. Five patients died of infections and multiorgan failure in Houston, and four patients died of severe aGVHD in Jerusalem. In addition, in no case was cytogenetic and/or molecular evidence of remission documented. The Flu-Cy protocol employed by our team was free of myelosuppressive drugs but immunosuppressive enough to allow the engraftment of donor cells without potential side effects. No case showed hepatic toxicity, and only one patient with metastatic breast cancer had neutropenia lower than 1×10^9/L for only a few days. Moreover, complete chimerism (100% donor cells) was demonstrated in nine patients.

The second objective of our pilot study was to verify if in these high-risk patients autologous and allogeneic transplantations can be combined in order to harness the reduction of tumor burden following autografting and the immune-mediated effects on minimal residual disease after allografting without high general toxicity and/or procedure-related deaths. We have demonstrated that this approach can be safely pursued in a seriously ill population. No patient experienced procedure-related death, the patients did not require a sterile room, nor did they need a red blood cell or platelet transfusion. They were independent of hyperalimentation, and none of them suffered from mucositis. At a median of 19 days, the patients were discharged from the hospital and followed as outpatients.

Of particular interest are the results achieved in the patients with RAEB with t(1;3) and accelerated phase CML. In the first case, the patient was pretreated with high-dose erythropoietin followed by corticosteroids and chemotherapy without success. In the last months, she was receiving red cell transfusions every week. All metaphases contained t(1;3) (p36;q21). On day 63 after allografting, karyotyping showed only donor cells without evidence of translocations. Reticulocytosis of 12% was showed on day 40 and was followed by an increase in hemoglobin to 12.6 by day 63. No sign of aGVHD was observed. After day +100, the patient relapsed and she was given DLI. After the second infusion of lymphocytes, she showed 30% diploid cells with a stabilization of the hemoglobin value.

The second patient had CML diagnosed in 1996 without evidence of the Philadelphia chromosome but with the p190 *bcr-abl* gene by the RT-PCR. He was treated with hydroxyurea and interferon-alpha (5 MU/m^2/d) for 6 months but RT-PCR remained positive and the white blood cells (WBCs) and platelets increased. In October 1997, the disease was considered to be in accelerated phase with WBCs >100 × 10^9/L and platelets >1200 × 10^9/L. He was treated with the mini-ICE protocol and, while recovering from aplasia, he underwent leukaphereses, which yielded only PCR-positive cells with a *bcr-abl/abl* ratio of 0.1. The patient received autografting but no change in the *bcr-abl/abl* ratio was seen and WBCs and platelets increased. He had a 69-year-old HLA-matched brother, and after the Flu-Cy protocol, mobilized donor hematopoietic stem cells were infused. Granulocytes and platelets never decreased below 1 × 10^9/L and 20 × 10^9/L, respectively. He was discharged on day 14 and followed as an outpatient. Complete chimerism was achieved on day 108 (100% donor cells) with a *bcr-abl/abl* ratio of 0.0008. On day 122, the complete chimerism was confirmed with a *bcr-abl/abl* ratio of 0.0001; on day 330, *bcr-abl* is undetectable and the patient maintains complete chimerism.

V. CONCLUSION

The long-term benefit of this treatment has yet to be determined. The five patients who share normal performance status with disease remission after allografting are reason for cautious optimism. Considering that our patients were all at high-risk, we think that such a sequential procedure can represent a new approach for a large variety of clinical situations with an indication for allografting.

REFERENCES

1. Petersen FB, Bearman SI. Preparative regimens and their toxicity. In: Forman SJ, Blume KG, Thomas ED, eds. Bone Marrow Transplantation. Boston: Blackwell, 1994:79–95.
2. Horowitz MM, Gale RP, Sondel PM, et al. Graft-versus-leukemia reactions after bone marrow transplantation. Blood 1990; 75:555–562.

this book). The c-*kit* antigen is also expressed on this subset of primitive cells, but c-*kit* is expressed on a large percentage of further differentiated cells and is therefore not commonly used in HSC selection strategies (5). There is evidence that the most primitive HSCs in mice may not express CD34 (6), but a cell with this phenotype has not been isolated in humans.

The most commonly used procedure for isolating HSCs is based solely on the selection of cells which are CD34$^+$. Whole blood is incubated with an avidin-conjugated anti-CD34 antibody and subsequently purified by passage over a biotin affinity column (7). Alternate methods using fluorescence-activated cell sorting (FACS) to isolate clinically usable HSCs have been reported (8), and these methods have the benefit of being able to select HSCs based on the expression of multiple surface markers. Some debate exists as to what is the best source of HSCs (be it the bone marrow or peripheral blood in adults or umbilical cord blood from newborns), and it remains to be seen which of these sources contains the most primitive cells with the highest long-term repopulating potential.

III. EX VIVO TRANSDUCTION OF HSCs BY RETROVIRAL VECTORS

After the putative HSCs are selected, they are cultured in vitro prior to the transduction by retroviral vectors. A cocktail of cytokines is commonly added to the culture medium both to keep the cells viable and to prime the cells for transduction (see Chapter 4 of this book by Al-Homsi and Quesenberry for a detailed explanation). Ideally, cytokine addition is intended to help keep the more primitive cells from differentiating, whereas in turn stimulating cell division. The HSCs must be dividing, because all current clinical protocols use murine leukemia virus (MuLV)–based retroviral vectors which require cell division to integrate stably into the host cell deoxyribonucleic acid (DNA) (9). Although there is some controversy as to what constitutes the best mix of cytokines, commonly used cytokines are stem cell factor (SCF), granulocyte colony-stimulating factor (G-CSF), and various members of the interleukin (IL) family (i.e., IL-3, IL-6, IL-11). It has also been demonstrated that the addition of human bone marrow stromal cells to cultures of CD34$^+$ primary cells may help to increase the transduction efficiency of long-term repopulating HSCs (10). However, even with the addition of multiple growth factors to the culture medium, there are several reports which suggest that the most primitive cells (CD34^{bright} and CD34$^+$CD38$^-$) are resistant to transduction by MuLV vectors (11–13).

The retroviral vectors that were used in the first clinical gene therapy trials to transduce human peripheral blood lymphocytes (PBLs) for the treatment of adenosine deaminase deficiency (ADA) contained the amphotropic MuLV envelope (env) protein (1,2). Amphotropic MuLV virus infects a wide range of cell types from different species, including humans. Since these first clinical trials, other groups have used this "standard" retroviral vector to transduce primary CD34$^+$ cells in various gene therapy clinical trials, including the treatment of ADA, chronic granulomatous disease, Fanconi's anemia, Gaucher's disease, chemoprotection (the introduction of the multi–drug-resistance gene), and various cell-marking protocols (for a list of clinical protocols, see *Human Gene Therapy*, 1996, 8, pg 1499–1530). However, it has recently been shown that CD34$^+$ human HSCs express low levels of the receptor PiT-2, recognized by the amphotropic MuLV env protein (14,15), and it was hypothesized that this may be a limiting factor for the transduction of these cells. Pit-2 functions as a sodium-phosphate transporter reviewed by Miller (16), and Kavanaugh and Kabat (17) demonstrated that the surface levels of PiT-2 can be increased by phosphate deprivation. Phosphate starvation of human PBLs has in turn been shown to increase the transduction efficiency by amphotropic MuLV vectors (18), and this is probably due to elevated surface levels of PiT-2. A much more detailed description of ex vivo HSC transduction by retroviral vectors is in Chapter 31.

IV. TRANSDUCTION OF HSCs WITH PSEUDOTYPED MuLV VECTORS

MuLV cores can incorporate various heterologous viral env proteins (pseudotyping), and this property can be used to expand the host range of MuLV retroviral vectors. Several groups have attempted to increase vector transduction efficiency by pseudotyping with an env protein whose receptor is more highly expressed than PiT-2 on the surface of human HSCs (Table 1). For example, the gibbon ape leukemia virus (GALV) receptor, PiT-1 (also a sodium phosphate transporter), is expressed at significantly higher levels than PiT-2 on human hematopoietic cells (19), and many groups have demonstrated higher transduction efficiencies of both human PBLs and CD34$^+$ cells using GALV env pseudotyped vectors (18–20). MuLV can also efficiently incorporate the vesicular stomatitis virus G protein (VSV-G), and packaging cell lines have been generated using this rhabdoviral env protein (21–23). Because the receptor for VSV-G is very widely expressed (24), these

Table 1 Transduction of Primary Human Hematopoietic Cells by Pseudotyped MuLV Retroviral Vectors

Pseudotyping envelope	Cell type	Transduction results	Reference
GALV	TIL	4- to 18-fold higher than amphotropic vector	Lam et al. (19)
	PBL	4- to 12-fold higher than amphotropic vector	
GALV	CFU-GM Marrow	1.7-fold higher than amphotropic vector	
	PBMC	1.7-fold higher than amphotropic vector	
	LTC-IC Marrow	1.5-fold higher than amphotropic vector	Von-Kalle et al. (20)
	PBMC	1.9-fold higher than amphotropic vector	
RD114	PBL	3- to 5-fold higher than amphotropic vector	Porter et al. (20a)
	CD34$^+$	1- to 1.4-fold higher than amphotropic vector	
VSV-G	CD34$^+$	1–2% transduced cells using moi of 10	Agrawal et al. (13)
	CD34$^+$/CD38$^-$	No transduction (mitosis cannot be induced)	
VSV-G	PBL	16–32% transduced cells using moi of 40	Sharma et al. (25)

GALV, gibbon ape leukemia virus; RD114, feline endogenous virus; VSV-G, vesicular stomatitis viral envelope protein; TIL, tumor infiltrating lymphocytes; PBL, peripheral blood lymphocytes; CFU-GM, colony-forming units granulocyte-macrophage; LTC-IC, long term culture initiating cells; PBMC, peripheral blood mononuclear cells; moi, multiplicity of infection.

pseudotyped retroviral vectors have an extremely broad host range, and they have been reported to transduce primary human blood cells with increased efficiency over standard amphotropic vectors (13,25). VSV-G is a single polypeptide, and therefore VSV-G pseudotyped MuLV vectors have the significant advantage of being easily concentrated with little or no loss in transduction ability (26).

As previously mentioned, MuLV retroviral vectors are incapable of transducing nondividing cells. Because the most primitive human HSCs are relatively quiescent, this is potentially a major drawback to the use of MuLV-based vectors in HSC gene therapy. Retroviral vectors based on human immunodeficiency virus (HIV)–1 have been described (27), and these vectors retain the properties of the native virus in that they can transduce nondividing cells both in culture and in vivo (28). Although lentiviral vector systems are still in the developmental stage, these vectors hold considerable promise for use in the transduction of primitive/quiescent pluripotent HSCs. Additionally, HIV cores can be efficiently pseudotyped with various viral env proteins, including MuLV env, and the subsequent discussion of targeted MuLV vectors can be extrapolated to lentiviral systems as well.

V. DEVELOPMENT OF TARGETABLE RETROVIRAL VECTORS FOR IN VIVO GENE TRANSFER

All of the methods described so far for the transduction of human HSCs by retroviral vectors have been ex vivo procedures. Except for several cancer gene therapy trials, all retroviral vector–mediated gene-delivery protocols are currently performed ex vivo. This is for multiple reasons, including (1) the relatively low titer of retroviral vectors, (2) the sensitivity of vectors produced in murine-derived packaging cell lines to lysis by human complement (29), and (3) because the nature of the env protein (e.g., amphotropic, GALV, VSV-G) gives pseudotyped retroviral vectors little cell type specificity. However, there are a number of drawbacks to ex vivo procedures such as (1) the protocols are invasive and labor intensive, (2) there is a limited repertoire of cell types which can be removed and manipulated, and (3) dedifferentiation (or loss of phenotype) of primary cells can occur during ex vivo culture. For these and other reasons, development of a targetable retroviral vector for in vivo use is being pursued.

Retroviral vector targeting is being approached from two general directions: (1) modification of vector binding/entry into target cells and (2) attempts to control the specificity of therapeutic gene expression. We will briefly discuss the advances which have been made in pursuit of cell-specific vector expression, and we will review in more detail efforts attempting to direct the binding of retroviral vectors to specific cell surface molecules.

VI. TARGETING BY TISSUE-SPECIFIC GENE EXPRESSION

After integration of the provirus into the chromosomal DNA, transcription is driven from the retroviral long-terminal repeat (LTR) promoter. Although the MuLV LTR is active in most human cells, expression levels vary depending on the cell type, and they can be low (30,31). Evidence also exists for the silencing of expression from the MuLV LTR over time in vivo (32–34).

These issues led to the design of MuLV vectors with internal heterologous promoters to drive the expression of therapeutic genes. If high-level expression of the inserted gene is desired, strong viral promoters from simian virus (SV40) or cytomegalovirus (CMV) are commonly used. If cell-specific expression of therapeutic genes is to be achieved from a retroviral vector, it must come from an internal promoter, since gene expression from the LTR is fairly constitutive. Insertion of cell-specific promoters into MuLV vectors has been attempted for this reason.

Various hematopoietic cell promoters have been identified which are lineage specific and would appear to be good candidates for use in HSC gene therapy. Several myeloid-specific promoters are known (35–37), and one of these promoters, CD11b, when inserted in a MuLV vector backbone, has resulted in myelomonocytic specific expression of a marker gene in the progeny of transduced primary human CD34$^+$ cells (38). Also, the globin gene locus control region has been placed in a MuLV vector, and expression in erythroid cells was observed (39). Considerable effort is currently being directed toward the understanding of cell-specific gene expression, and these studies will undoubtedly yield more candidate promoters for use in HSC gene therapy.

VII. TARGETING RETROVIRAL VECTORS THROUGH CELL-SPECIFIC BINDING/TRANSDUCTION

As discussed earlier, all retroviral vectors currently used for ex vivo gene therapy have broad cell tropism due to the widespread expression of their receptors. An approach currently being pursued by various groups is to attempt to restrict and/or redirect the vector host range by the addition of cell-specific binding sequences to the viral env protein (40–43). Targeting moieties such as single-chain antibodies (scFv), large ligand sequences, and small peptides have all been used in the construction of such chimeric retroviral env proteins.

Although some degree of success has been achieved in redirecting the tropism of MuLV vectors to specific cell types by this method, transduction efficiencies have been low. The attempts to date are summarized in Table 2. It has become clear from these studies that the modified env protein and the nature of the targeted receptor itself both contribute to the inefficiency of chimeric env-coated vectors.

First, the chimeric env protein must be transported to the plasma membrane and efficiently incorporated into budding viral vector particles. Modification of the env protein by insertion of foreign sequences can result in a chimeric protein which is unstable, and it will not be efficiently incorporated. However, the coexpression of native env protein can sometimes rescue a poorly incorporated chimeric envelope protein (44,45).

Once incorporated into viral particles, the env protein needs both to bind to its cell surface receptor and subsequently catalyze fusion between the viral and cell lipid membranes. Current models for MuLV fusion are based on the influenza env protein, hemagglutinin (HA) (46). On binding to its receptor (sialic acid), HA undergoes a complicated postbinding conformational change triggered by low pH in the endosome. A similar postbinding conformational change has been hypothesized for the MuLV envelope protein, although the "trigger" is not well understood.

Many chimeric env proteins are able to direct vector binding to the targeted cell surface antigen, but the binding does not result in the transduction of the target cell (47–49) (W. F. Anderson, unpublished data). We have demonstrated that some chimeric env proteins are incapable of catalyzing fusion when bound to the targeted antigen (C. A. Benedict and Y. Zhao, unpublished data), and some possible explanations for this are highlighted in Figure 1. Finally, it is also clear that the cell surface antigen itself can play a critical role in the process of targeted vector entry (47). We will review the current status

Table 2 Targeted MuLV Vectors

Targeted antigen (binding moiety)	Insertion site in Mo-MuLV env	Coexpression of wt env	Binding to antigen	Titer (pfu/mL)	Reference
Transferrin receptor (mAb)	X-linking		+	0	Goud et al. (53)
MHCI/MHCII (mAb)	X-linking		+	50–350	Roux et al. (52)
Hapten (scFv)	Between aa 6–7	Yes	+	ND	Russell et al. (54)
EPO-R (epo)	Replacement of aa 18–221	Yes	+	Same as Ampho on K562, HEL cells	Kasahara et al. (44)
EGF-R (egf)	Between aa 6–7	No	+	0[a]	Cosset et al. (47)
LDL-R (scFv)	Between aa 6–7	Yes	+	10^4	Somia et al. (45)
MHCI (scFv)	Between aa 6–7	No	+	3–112[a]	Marin et al. (62)
erbB2/erbB4 (her)	Replacement of aa 18–221	Yes	+	10^3	Han et al. (67)
erbB2/erbB4 (EGF like BD of her)	Between aa 6–7	No	+	0	Schnierle et al. (41)
EGF-R (egf) (Protease activatable)	Between aa −1 and +1 of amphotropic env	No	+	10^4	Nilson et al. (72)
Her2 (scFv or her)	Between aa 6–7	No	+	0[a]	Zhao et al.[b]
CD33 (scFv)	Between aa 6–7	No	+	0[a]	Zhao et al. (43a)
CD34 (scFv)	Between aa 6–7	No	+	0[a]	Benedict et al. (43b)

mAb, monoclonal antibody; aa, amino acid; scFv, single-chain antibody; MHC, major histocompatibility complex; EPO-R, erythropoietin receptor; EGF-R, epidermal growth factor receptor; LDL-R, low-density lipoprotein receptor; her, heregulin; pfu/mL, plaque-forming units/milliliter; BD, binding domain; ND, not determined.

[a]Chimeric env proteins were coexpressed with wild-type env and no difference in titer was observed.

[b]Unpublished data.

A.

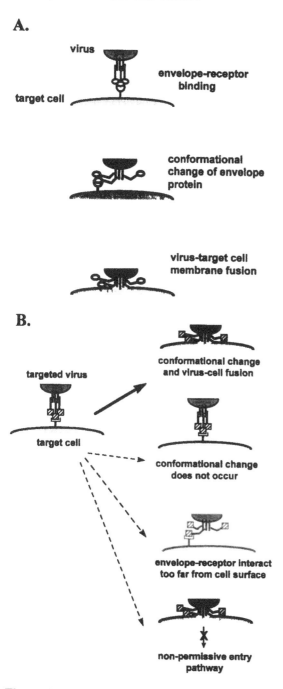

B.

Figure 1 Postbinding conformational changes in the MuLV envelope protein lead to virus-cell fusion. (A) MuLV envelope (env) protein binds to its native receptor, triggering a hypothesized conformational change that leads to fusion between the viral and cellular lipid membranes. (B) Targeted chimeric env proteins must recapitulate this process. Failure to do so may be because (1) binding to the new receptor does not trigger a postbinding conformational change, (2) the envelope/receptor complex is too far from the target cell surface, or (3) the viral core is directed into a nonpermissive entry pathway.

of targeting of MuLV-based retroviral vectors, although successful (albeit low-efficiency) targeting has also been reported for a spleen necrosis virus–based vector (50) and avian leukosis virus–based vector (51) using similar approaches.

VIII. ALTERATION OF MuLV VECTOR TROPISM

Proof that the MuLV vector host range could be expanded was first demonstrated by Roux et al. (52) using an antibody cross-linking approach (Table 2). An ecotropic MuLV (e-MuLV) vector (normally restricted to mouse and rat cells) was precoated with biotinylated anti-env antibody and was bridged to human cells precoated with biotinylated anti–major histocompatability complex (MHC) antibodies via streptavidin. Transduction of the target cells was achieved, although the titers were low (~100 pfu/mL), and it is difficult to imagine how such a strategy could be applied in vivo. Goud et al. (53) used a similar approach to cross link e-MuLV vector to the transferrin receptor expressed on human Hep2 cells. Although the vector was shown to bind to the transferrin receptor and was internalized into the cell, no transduction was seen. Together, these results were the first to suggest that cell surface antigens may differ in their ability to function as viral receptors.

Because "viral-bridging" approaches have been inefficient and would be difficult to perform in vivo, modification of the viral env protein itself has been pursued by various groups (see Table 2). Russell et al. (54) were the first to report the successful presentation of binding moieties on the surface of viral particles by genetic manipulation of the e-MuLV env protein. They displayed an antihapten scFv between amino acids 6 and 7 in the N-terminus of e-MuLV env. The scFv-env protein was expressed in ψ_2 packaging cells which also express the native ecotropic MuLV env protein, and the viral particles produced were coated with both scFv-env and wild-type env protein. Binding of the viral vector to hapten-coated plates through interaction of the displayed scFv was demonstrated. Unfortunately, the question of whether binding through the displayed scFv would lead to transduction could not be addressed owing to difficulties encountered when attempting to coat cells with the hapten molecule.

Although it was not discussed at length by Russell et al. in their initial publication (54), it has become evident that the MuLV env protein is sensitive to the site of insertion of foreign binding moieties. In order for the MuLV env protein to be efficiently incorporated into viral particles it must be (1) translated in the endoplasmic reticulum, (2) oligomerized, (3) glycosylated, (4) cleaved into its mature two-subunit form [gp70 (surface subunit, SU) and p15e (transmembrane subunit, TM)] on transport through the Golgi apparatus, and (5) expressed stably on the surface of the host cell (55). Small modifications of MuLV env such as linker insertions (56) or site-specific mutagenesis (57–59) can result in an env protein which fails to meet one of these five criteria. It is therefore not surprising that the insertion of large binding moieties into MuLV env could result in an env protein which cannot be transported and incorporated into viral particles. A large number of chimeric env constructs have been generated in our laboratory by inserting scFv and ligand sequences into e-MuLV env (C. A. Benedict, unpublished data), and we have yet to identify a site of insertion which is conducive for efficient incorporation of chimeric env into viral particles other than the extreme N-terminus, as reported by Russell et al. (54).

The first success in achieving expanded MuLV vector tropism by genetic modification of the env protein was reported by Kasahara et al. (44). The erythropoietin (epo) ligand coding sequence was inserted into the e-MuLV env protein replacing a large portion of the SU sequences known to be necessary for binding to the native receptor, and it was therefore distinct from the N-terminal scFv fusion construct reported by Russell et al. (54) (see Fig. 2 for different types of chimeric MuLV env constructs). The chimeric epo-env protein was expressed in ψ_2 packaging cells, and a vector-producing cell line was selected which released virus coated with both wild-type and epo-env protein. The resulting vectors were able to transduce human epo receptor (epoR)–expressing HEL and K562 cells, but they did not transduce other human cells which were epoR$^-$.

In this case, coexpression of native MuLV env protein was necessary to allow for incorporation of epo-env (N. Kasahara, unpublished data). Replacement of a large portion of the e-MuLV SU with the epo sequence probably disrupted the structure of the env protein and prevented efficient transport to the cell surface when expressed in the absence of wild-type env. The rescue of incorporation-defective MuLV env mutants by the formation of hetero-oligomers with wild-type env has recently been demonstrated by our laboratory (60), and a similar mechanism for incorporation of the epo-env protein is likely.

It is not clear from the Kasahara et al. (44) study whether the wild-type env protein is contributing to the process of viral entry at a level other than assisting in the incorporation of the epo-env protein into viral particles. The question of whether the epo-env protein can by itself contribute both the binding and the fusion function which are needed for

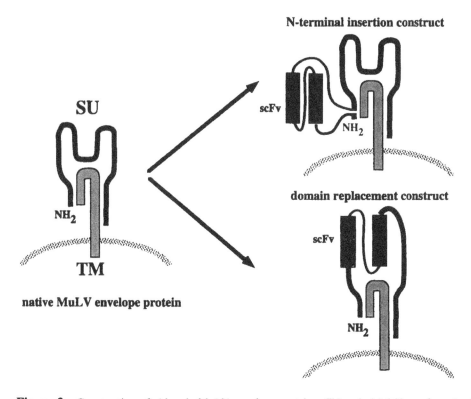

Figure 2   Construction of chimeric MuLV envelope proteins. Chimeric MuLV envelope (env) proteins have been constructed by two general methods: (1) insertion of binding moieties at the extreme N-terminus of SU (e.g., Ref. 54) or (2) replacement of large portions of SU sequences with the targeting ligand (44). Large domain replacements have needed coexpression of wild-type MuLV env protein to allow for incorporation of chimeric env into viral particles. Shown is an insertion of a single-chain antibody molecule into MuLV env.

transduction (see Fig. 1) is difficult to address, since one cannot assay for the function of epo-env protein in the absence of wild-type env owing to its incorporation defect. Interestingly, we have recent data to indicate that a binding competent/fusion defective MuLV env protein can be rescued by coexpression of a binding-defective/fusion-capable env protein (60). This suggests that the binding and fusion functions of MuLV env can be contributed by two different env proteins in the context of a single viral particle. Indeed, other enveloped viruses have evolved strategies where the binding and fusion stages of entry are contributed by two separate proteins. For example, the paramyxoviruses use the HN and F glycoproteins to bind to and then fuse with their target cell, respectively (61).

Even when the problems of transport, processing, and incorporation of chimeric env proteins have been overcome, and the resulting viruses can be shown to bind to their target cells, there are still many examples of such chimeras that do not promote transduction (see Table 2). In particular, the insertion of binding moieties at the N-terminus of e-MuLV env frequently results in targeted vectors with this phenotype (41,47,48) and (W. F. Anderson, unpublished data). However, there are also examples of targeted vectors displaying N-terminal binding moieties which do transduce their target cells (45,62). These differences point to a role for the targeted receptor in determining whether vector entry is successful (see Fig. 2).

IX. RECEPTOR ROLE IN MuLV ENTRY/TRANSDUCTION

Studies targeting MuLV vectors to the transferrin and MHC cell surface molecules (52,53) first suggested that antigen choice may be critical in achieving efficient transduction of cells by engineered MuLV vectors. However, there is little known of the natural MuLV entry pathway into cells and the properties of the receptor that are important for this process.

The receptor for e-MuLV is a cationic amino acid transporter, mCAT-1 (63). e-MuLV entry is sensitive to lysosomotropic agents which inhibit the acidification of endosomes (64,65), suggesting that e-MuLV enters by an endocytic pathway. Notably, e-MuLV titer was reduced by less then two orders of magnitude in these studies, and these effects are cell type dependent, indicating that e-MuLV entry processes may differ from those of typical endocytosed viruses, such as influenza. Therefore, it is possible that e-MuLV may not enter cells via a classic endocytic pathway (66), and in fact may be able to use alternate entry routes. The various cellular entry pathways currently known are summarized in Figure 3A. Determining the entry pathway of e-MuLV following binding to mCAT-1 (Fig. 3B) should enable appropriate cell surface molecules to be chosen as receptors for targeted MuLV vectors.

Work by Cosset et al. (47) has shown that some cell surface antigens are unable to function as viral receptors owing to internalization pathways which result in nonproductive

Figure 3   Possible cellular entry pathways for targeted MuLV vectors. There are several known pathways for molecules to enter cells, and little is known about MuLV entry once bound to its receptor, mCAT-1. Engineered MuLV vectors have been targeted to various cell-surface antigens which enter cells via different pathways, and these pathways are likely to play a role in vector transduction. (A) Known cellular entry pathways. (Adapted from Ref. 78.) (B) Putative entry pathways of cell surface antigens which have been targeted by MuLV vectors.

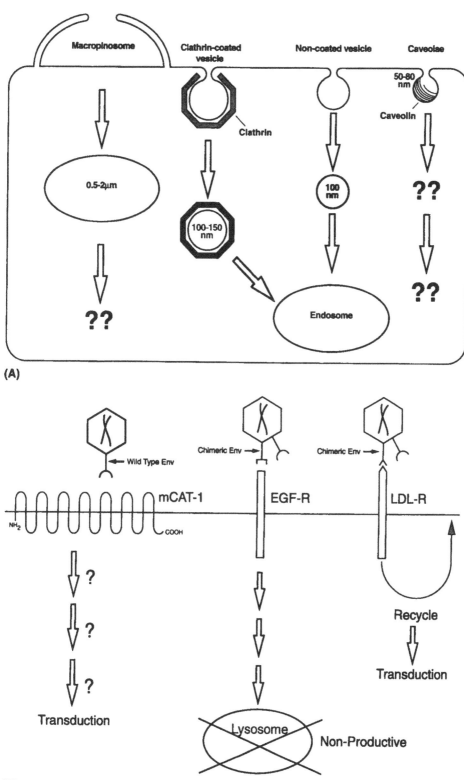

(A)

(B)

viral entry. Vectors coated with e-MuLV env displaying an N-terminal fused epidermal growth factor ligand (EGF-env) could bind efficiently to human cells expressing the EGF receptor (EGF-R) and be internalized into the cells, but internalization did not result in transduction of the target cells (see Table 2). It was suggested that trafficking of EGF-R–bound vector to the lysosomal compartment (see Fig. 3b), as well as deficiencies in the ability of EGF-env to catalyze fusion when bound to EGF-R, were responsible for the lack of transduction. Notably, addition of chloroquine (an inhibitor of endosomal acidification) to the culture medium resulted in low levels of transduction by EGF-env pseudotyped vectors, further supporting the idea that EGF-R–bound vector entered the cell via a nonproductive, lysosomally targeted pathway. Additionally, EGF-env–coated vector particles were still capable of transducing murine NIH-3T3 cells through the binding of mCAT-1, indicating that the EGF-env protein was capable of fusion when the native receptor was used for entry.

Various other cell surface antigens have been targeted by fusing either ligands or scFv molecules to the e-MuLV env protein (see Table 2). Somia et al. (45) reported successful transduction through binding of vector to the human low-density lipoprotein receptor (LDL-R) via an N-terminal fused anti–LDL-R scFv. Titer on LDL-R–expressing HeLa cells was reported to be in the range of 10^4 pfu/mL (the highest titer of targeted MuLV vectors reported to date), and coexpression of the wild-type env protein was required. Interestingly, LDL-R is the only receptor which has been targeted to date that recycles back to the plasma membrane once it has been internalized (see Fig. 3b), and whether this property is responsible for the relatively high titers of LDL-R-targeted vectors should be examined more closely. Marin et al. (62) targeted the MHC class I molecule by N-terminal insertion of an scFv into e-MuLV env which was derived from the same antibody used in the report by Roux et al. (52) (antibody bridging of MuLV vector to the MHCI antigen). Although very low levels of transduction were achieved, the efficiency was no better then the original bridging strategy. Two separate groups have reported attempts to target cells which express the breast cancer antigen erbB2. Han et al. (67) reported transduction of human cancer cell lines expressing erbB2 using a domain-replacement approach similar to that of epo-env (44) in which a large portion of e-MuLV SU was replaced with the extracellular domain of heregulin. Schnierle et al. (49) attempted to target erbB2-expressing cells by fusing the EGF-like binding domain of heregulin between amino acids 6 and 7 of Mo-MuLV env. Although particles pseudotyped with this chimeric env protein were shown to bind to erbB2-expressing cells, no transduction was achieved. We have similarly been able to demonstrate binding to erbB2-expressing human cell lines using either an N-terminal fused anti-erbB2 scFv or the binding domain of heregulin, but transduction was not observed (Y. Zhao, unpublished data).

We have attempted to engineer e-MuLV vectors specifically to transduce human HSCs in our laboratory (C. A. Benedict, unpublished data). We chose to target the CD34 cell surface antigen, since it is believed to be highly expressed on the subset of more primitive human HSCs (4). The ligand for HSC-expressed CD34 is unknown (68), although it is likely that L-selectin is the ligand for CD34 expressed in high endothelial venules in both humans and mice (69). Therefore, we constructed an anti-CD34 scFv to use as the targeting moiety (70) (Fig. 4). We inserted this scFv at multiple sites in e-MuLV SU, but efficient incorporation of the chimeric env protein into viral cores was only achieved when the scFv was fused between amino acids 6 and 7 in the N-terminus of SU. scFv-env coated viral particles were shown to bind to CD34-expressing cells, but transduction of the target cells was not seen.

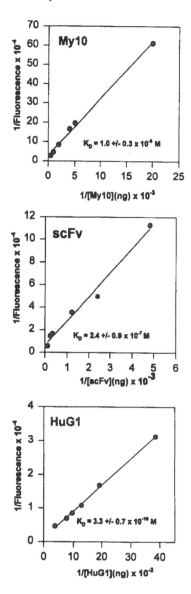

Figure 4 Determination of antibody K_D values by Lineweaver-Burk analysis. CD34 expressing KG-1a cells are the target for all binding experiments presented. (*Top*) Binding of native anti-CD34 antibody My10: (*Center*) Binding of My10-derived anti-CD34 scFv. (*Bottom*) Binding of anti-CD33 antibody, HuG1. (From Ref. 70.)

Recently, a report was published by Fielding et al. (71) describing the addition of sequences encoding for stem cell factor (SCF) to the N-terminus of MuLV SU. Attempts to target specifically hematopoietic cells expressing the Kit receptor were unsuccessful using SCF-env–coated vectors. The reason for the failure of these vectors to promote efficient transduction was identical to that of EGF-env–coated and scFv(CD34)-env–coated vectors; binding to Kit receptors was achieved but blocks in postbinding events prevented gene transfer. Fielding et al. did show that SCF-env vectors could be used to transduce Kit⁻ cells in a mixed population of hematopoietic cells.

X. IMPROVING TARGETED MuLV VECTORS

It is clear from the varied results discussed above that the entry of targeted vectors often does not proceed efficiently when bound to nonnative receptor molecules. Retroviruses have evolved to use specific classes of cellular receptors (16), and attempts to substitute other cell surface molecules for use by targeted vectors in entry has largely been a failure. Therefore, targeted vectors may need to access the natural cellular pathway of viral entry to achieve efficient transduction, while retaining the specificity acquired by the insertion of targeting moieties into the MuLV env protein.

An elegant approach has been reported by Nilson et al. (72) in which the amphotropic (4070A) MuLV env protein was engineered to display a N-terminal binding moiety which is fused to SU by a short linker sequence encoding a protease cleavage site. Binding to the targeted surface antigen (in this case EGF) is achieved by the inserted ligand, protease is added to allow for cleavage of the engineered site, and vector entry then proceeds through the natural amphotropic MuLV receptor, PiT-2. In essence, a concentration of the engineered vector on the surface of the targeted cell occurs via the displayed ligand, and specificity in vector entry is then achieved by spacial proximity to the native viral receptor. This work demonstrates that a vector can be engineered to bind to an antigen (EGF-R) which cannot function as a viral receptor (47), and vector transduction can be rescued via protease cleavage and entry through the natural receptor. Efficiency of the "hand-off" to the native receptor can most likely be optimized further by varying the length of the linker between the displayed binding domain and the remainder of SU (51).

Although the development of protease-activatable MuLV vectors is a significant advance in the field of targetable vector engineering, several issues need to be addressed with regards to in vivo utility. The nonspecific infection of cells through the PiT-2 receptor has to be avoided, and will undoubtedly vary with each different N-terminally displayed ligand. Protease cleavage sites which are readily cleaved by an abundant cell surface protease must be introduced, and these sites should not be cleaved nonspecifically by bloodborne proteases. Finally, the targeted cell must express PiT-2 on its surface to allow for vector entry, and transduction efficiency will probably be proportional to the levels of PiT-2 expression. Because human HSCs express low levels of PiT-2 (14), protease-activatable MuLV vectors may not be optimal for transduction of these cells, and other methods may have to be developed to allow for efficient entry of targeted retroviral vectors into HSCs.

XI. PROSPECTS FOR THE DEVELOPMENT OF INJECTABLE RETROVIRAL VECTORS FOR USE IN HSC GENE THERAPY

Development of a targetable vector for in vivo gene delivery would greatly facilitate the general application of HSC gene therapy procedures. However, injectable retroviral vectors for use in HSC gene therapy need to overcome numerous obstacles to become a reality. Currently, there are a very limited number of known human HSC cell surface markers, which in turn restricts the antigens which can be exploited as receptors by engineered vectors. However, procedures have recently been reported which use phage-displayed peptide libraries to screen surfaces of intact cells, both in culture and in vivo, to identify cell-specific binding peptides (73,74). Application of these methods may prove to be useful in the identification of new markers on the surface of human HSCs, and could result in new targets for engineered retroviral vectors.

Currently, CD34 is one of the very few human HSC markers known, and expression of CD34 on the surface of human endothelial cells (eCD34) (75,76) may further complicate the in vivo utility of this antigen as a target. To avoid transduction of endothelial cells in vivo by a CD34-targeted vector, a binding moiety would have to be developed which specifically recognizes HSC CD34 and not eCD34. Owing to the heavy glycosylation of CD34 (69) and the fact that L-selectin appears to bind to some forms of eCD34 and not to HSC CD34 (68), it is probable that HSC CD34-specific binding moieties could be selected from either peptide or scFv libraries using phage display techniques as well.

Additionally, retroviral vectors used for in vivo gene delivery must avoid lysis by human complement. Lysis of vectors generated in standard murine-derived producer cell lines occurs because of the addition of specific glycosylation epitopes that are recognized by the human immune system (29), but this problem should be solved by the production of vectors in appropriately engineered producer cell lines.

Although all of these issues will need to be dealt with before an injectable vector for use in HSC gene therapy becomes a reality, the outlook is bright. Considerable advances have recently been made in the understanding of why targeted MuLV vectors have not resulted in efficient transduction, and various strategies to circumvent these problems are currently under development. A future targeted retroviral vector will probably contain elements from many of the areas which have been discussed, and the progress being made in the areas of nonviral and alternative viral vector gene-delivery systems will also make an impact on HSC gene therapy.

REFERENCES

1. Blaese RM, Culver KW, Miller AD, Carter CS, Fleisher T, et al. T lymphocyte-directed gene therapy for ADA⁻SCID: Initial trial results after 4 years. Science 1995; 270:475–480.
2. Bordignon C, Notarangelo LD, Nobili N, Ferrari G, Casorati G. Gene therapy in peripheral blood lymphocytes and bone marrow for ADA-immunodeficient patients. Science 1995; 270: 470–475.
3. Kohn DB, Weinberg KI, Nolta JA, Heiss LN, Lenarsky C, et al. Engraftment of gene-modified umbilical cord blood cells in neonates with adenosine deaminase deficiency. Nature Med 1995; 1:1017–1023.
4. Terstapen LWM, Huang S, Safford M, Lansdorp PM, Loken MR. Sequential generations of hematopoietic colonies derived from single nonlineage-committed CD34+CD38− progenitor cells. Blood 1991; 77:1218–1227.
5. Papayannopoulou T, Brice M, Broudy VC, Zsebo KM. Isolation of c-kit receptor expressing cells from bone marrow, peripheral blood, and fetal liver: functional properties and composite antigenic profile. Blood 1991; 78:1403–1412.
6. Osawa M, Hanada K, Hamada H, Nakauchi H. Long-term lymphohematopoietic reconstitution by a single CD34-low/negative hematopoietic stem cell. 1996 Science 273:242–245.
7. Dunbar C, Kohn K. A phase I study: Retroviral vector mediated transfer of the cDNA for human glucocerebrosidase into hematopoietic stem cells of patients with Gaucher disease. Hum Gene Therapy 1996; 7:231–253.
8. Reading C, Sasaki D, Leembuis T, Tichenor E, Chen B et al. Clinical scale purification of CD34+Thy-1+LIN-stem cells from mobilized peripheral blood by high speed fluorescence activated cell sorting for use as an autograft for multiple myeloma patients. Blood 1994; 84(suppl 1):399a.

9. Roe T, Reynolds TC, Yu G, Brown PO. Integration of murine leukemia virus DNA depends on mitosis. EMBO 1993; 12:2099–2108.

10. Nolta JA, Smogorzewska EM, Kohn DB. Analysis of optimal conditions for retroviral-mediated transduction of primitive human hematopoietic cells. Blood 1995; 86:101–110.

11. Hao QL, Thiemann FT, Petersen D, Smogorzewska EM, Crooks GM. Extended long-term culture reveals a highly quiescent and primitive human hematopoietic progenitor population. Blood 1996; 88:3306–3313.

12. Knaan-Shanzer S, Valerio D, Van-Beuschem VW. Cell cycle state, response to hemopoietic growth factors and retroviral vector-mediated transduction of human hemopoietic stem cells. Gene Ther 1996; 3:323–333.

13. Agrawal YP, Agrawal RS, Sinclair AM, Young D, Maruyama M, Levine F, Ho AD. Cell-cycle kinetics and VSV-G pseudotyped retrovirus-mediated gene transfer in blood-derived CD34$^+$ cells. Exp Hematol 1996; 24:734–747.

14. Crooks GM, Kohn DB. Growth factors increase amphotropic retrovirus binding to human CD34+ bone marrow progenitor cells. Blood 1993; 82:3290–3297.

15. Kavanaugh MP, Miller DG, Zhang W, Law W, Kozak SL, Kabat D, Miller AD. Cell-surface receptors for gibbon ape leukemia virus and amphotropic murine retrovirus are inducible sodium-dependent phosphate symporters. Proc Natl Acad Sci USA 1994; 91:7071–7075.

16. Miller DA. Cell-surface receptors for retroviruses and implications for gene transfer. Proc Natl Acad Sci USA 1996; 93:11407–11413.

17. Kavanaugh MP, Kabat D. Identification and characterization of a widely expressed phosphate transporter/retrovirus receptor family. Kidney Int 1996; 49:959–963.

18. Bunnell BA, Muul LM, Donahue RE, Blaese RM, Morgan RA. High-efficiency retroviral-mediated gene transfer into human and nonhuman primate peripheral blood lymphocytes. Proc Natl Acad Sci USA 1995; 92:7739–7743.

19. Lam JS, Reeves ME, Cowherd R, Rosenberg SA, Hwu P. Improved gene transfer into human lymphocytes using retroviruses with the gibbon ape leukemia virus envelope. Hum Gene Therapy 1996; 7:1415–1422.

20. Von-Kalle C, Kiem H-P, Goehle S, Darovsky B, Heimfeld S, Torok-Storb B, Stor R, Schuening, FG. Increased gene transfer into human hematopoietic progenitor cells by extended in vitro exposure to a pseudotyped retroviral vector. Blood 1994; 84:2890–2897.

20a. Porter CD, Collins MK, Tailor CS, Parkar MH, Cosset FL, Weiss RA, Takeuchi Y. Comparison of efficiency of infection of human gene therapy target cells via four different retroviral receptors. Hum Gene Ther 1996; 7:913–919.

21. Yang Y, Vanin EF, Whitt MA, Fornerod M, Zwart R, Schneiderman RD, Grosveld G, Nienhuis AW. Inducible, high-level production of infectious murine leukemia retroviral vector particles pseudotyped with vesicular stomatitis virus G envelope protein. Hum Gene Ther 1995; 6:1203–1213.

22. Ory DS, Neugeboren BA, Mulligan RC. A stable human-derived packaging cell line for production of high titer retrovirus/vesicular stomatitis virus G pseudotypes. Proc Natl Acad Sci USA 1996; 93:11400–11406.

23. Chen ST, Iida A, Guo L, Friedmann T, Yee JK. Generation of packaging cell lines for pseudotyped retroviral vectors of the G protein of vesicular stomatitis virus by using a modified tetracycline inducible system. Proc Natl Acad Sci USA 1996; 93:10057–10062.

24. Schlegel R, Tralka TS, Willingham MC, Pastan I. Inhibition of VSV binding and infectivity by phosphatidylserine: is phosphatidylserine a VSV-binding site? Cell 1983; 32:639–646.

25. Sharma S, Cantwell M, Kipps TJ, Friedmann T. Efficient infection of a human T-cell line and of human primary peripheral blood leukocytes with a pseudotyped retrovirus vector. Proc Natl Acad Sci USA 1996; 93:11842–11847.

26. Yee JK, Friedman T, Burns JC. Generation of high-titer pseudotyped retroviral vectors with very broad host range. Methods Cell Biol 1994; 43:99–112.

27. Shimada T, Fujii H, Mitsuya H, Nienhuis AW. Targeted and highly efficient gene transfer

into CD4+ cells by a recombinant human immunodeficiency virus retroviral vector. J Clin Invest 1991; 83:1043–1047.

28. Naldini L, Blomer U, Gallay P, Ory D, Mulligna R, Gage FH, Verma IM, Trono D. In vivo gene delivery and stable transduction of nondividing cells by a lentiviral vector. Science 1996; 272:263–267.

29. Rother RP, Squinto SP. The alpha-galactosyl epitope: a sugar coating that makes viruses and cells unpalatable. Cell 1996; 86:185–188.

30. Williams D, Orkin SH, Mulligan RC. Retrovirus-mediated transfer of human adenosine deaminase gene sequences into cells in culture and into murine hematopoietic cells in vivo. Proc Natl Acad Sci USA 1986; 83:2566–2570.

31. Couture LA, Mullen CA, Morgan RA. Retroviral vectors containing chimeric promoter/enhancer elements exhibit cell-type-specific gene expression. Hum Gene Ther 1994; 5:667–677.

32. Emerman M, Temin HM. Genes with promoters in retrovirus vectors can be independently suppressed by an epigenetic mechanism. Cell 1984; 39:459–467.

33. Xu L, Yee JK, Wolff JA, Friedmann T. Factors affecting long-term stability of Moloney murine leukemia virus-based vectors. Virology 1989; 171:331–341.

34. Challita P-M, Skelton D, El-Khoueiry A, Yu X-J, Weinberg K, Kohn DB. Multiple modifications in cis elements of the long terminal repeat of retroviral vectors lead to increased expression and decreased DNA methylation in embryonic carcinoma cells. J Virol 1995; 69:748–755.

35. Zhang DE, Hetherington CJ, Gonzalez DA, Chen HM, Tenen DG. Regulation of CD14 expression during monocytic differentiation induced with 1 alpha, 25-dihydroxyvitamin D3. J Immunol 1994; 153:3276–3284.

36. Zhang DE, Hohaus S, Voso MT, Chen HM, Smith LT, Hetherington CJ, Tenen DG. Function of PU.1 (Spi-1), C/EBP, and AML1 in early myelopoiesis: regulation of multiple myeloid CSF receptor promoters. Curr Topics Microbiol Immunol 1996; 211:137–147.

37. Smith LT, Hohaus S, Gonzalez DA, Dziennis SE, Tenen DG. PU.1 (Spi-1) and C/EBP alpha regulate the granulocyte colony-stimulating factor receptor promoter in myeloid cells. Blood 1996; 88:1234–1247.

38. Malik P, Kraff WJ, Yu XJ, Zhou C, Kohn DB. Retroviral-mediated gene expression in human myelomonocytic cells: a comparison of hematopoietic cell promoters to viral promoters. Blood 1995; 86:2993–3005.

39. Sadelain M, Wang CH, Antoniou M, Grosveld F, Mulligan RC. Generation of a high-titer retroviral vector capable of expressing high levels of the human beta-globin gene. Proc Natl Acad Sci USA 1995; 92:6728–6732.

40. Cosset FL, Russell SJ. Review: targeting retrovirus entry. Gene Ther 1996; 3:946–956.

41. Schnierle BS, Groner B. Review: retroviral targeted delivery. Gene Ther 1996; 3:1069–1073.

42. Vile RG, Russell SJ. Review: retroviruses as vectors. Br Med Bull 1995; 51:12–30.

43. Salmons B, Günzburg WH. Review: targeting of retroviral vectors for gene therapy. Hum Gene Ther 1993; 4:129–141.

43a. Zhao Y, Zhu L, Lee S, Li L, Chang E, Soong NW, Dover D, Anderson WF. Identification of the block in targeted retroviral-mediated gene transfer. Proc Natl Acad Sci 1999; 96:4005–4010.

43b. Benedict CA, Tun RY, Rubinstein DB, Guillaume T, Cannon PM, Anderson WF. Targeting retroviral vectors to CD34-expressing cells: binding to CD34 does not catalyze virus-cell infusion. Hum Gene Ther 1999; 10:545–557.

44. Kasahara N, Dozy AM, Kan YW. Tissue-specific targeting of retroviral vectors through ligand-receptor interactions. Science 1994; 266:1373–1376.

45. Somia NV, Zoppé M, Verma IM. Generation of targeted retroviral vectors by using single-chain variable fragment: an approach to in vivo gene delivery. Proc Natl Acad Sci USA 1995; 92:7570–7574.

46. White JM. Membrane fusion. Science 1992; 258:917–924.
47. Cosset FL, Morling FJ, Takeuchi Y, Weiss RA, Collins MKL, Russell S. Retroviral retargeting by envelopes expressing an N-terminal binding domain. J Virol 1995; 69:6314–6322.
48. Ager S, Nilson BHK, Morling FJ, Peng KW, Cosset FL, and Russell SJ. Retroviral display of antibody fragments; interdomain spacing strongly influences vector infectivity. Hum Gene Ther 1996; 7:2157–2164.
49. Schnierle BS, Moritz D, Jeschke M, Groner B. Expression of chimeric envelope proteins in helper cell lines and integration into Moloney murine leukemia virus particles. Gene Ther 1996; 3:334–342.
50. Chu TH, Dornburg R. Toward highly efficient cell-type–specific gene transfer with retroviral vectors displaying single-chain antibodies. J Virol 1997; 71:720–725.
51. Valesesia-Wittmann S, Morling FJ, Nilson BHK, Takeuchi Y, Russell SJ, Cosset F-L. Improvement of retroviral retargeting by using amino acid spacers between an additional binding domain and the N terminus of Moloney murine leukemia virus SU. J Virol 1996; 70:2059–2064.
52. Roux P, Jeanteur P, Piechaczyk M. A versatile and potentially general approach to the targeting of specific cell types by retroviruses: application to the infection of human cells by means of major histocompatibility complex class I and class II antigens by mouse ecotropic murine leukemia virus-derived viruses. Proc Natl Acad Sci USA 1989; 86:9079–9083.
53. Goud B, Legrain P, Buttin G. Antibody-mediated binding of a murine ecotropic Moloney retroviral vector to human cells allows internalization but not the establishment of the proviral state. Virology 1988; 163:251–254.
54. Russell SJ, Hawkins RE, Winter G. Retroviral vectors displaying fuctional antibody fragments. Nucleic Acids Res 1993; 21:1081–1085.
55. Doms RW, Lamb RA, Rose JK, Helenius A. Mini Review: folding and assembly of viral membrane proteins. Virology 1993; 193:545–562.
56. Gray KD, Roth MJ. Mutational analysis of the envelope gene of Moloney murine leukemia virus. J Virol 1993; 67:3489–3496.
57. Bae Y, Kingsman SM, Kingsman AJ. Functional dissection of the Moloney murine leukemia virus envelope protein gp70. J Virol 1997; 71:2092–2097.
58. MacKrell AJ, Soong NW, Curtis CM, Anderson WF. Identification of a subdomain in the Moloney murine leukemia virus envelope protein involved in receptor binding. J Virol 1996; 70:1768–1774.
59. Skov H, Andersen KB. Mutational analysis of Moloney murine leukemia virus surface protein gp70. J Gen Virol 1993; 74:707–714.
60. Zhao Y, Lee S, Anderson WF. Functional interactions between monomers of the retroviral envelope protein complex. J Virol 1997; 71:6967–6972.
61. Lamb RA. Mini Review: Paramyxovirus fusion: a hypothesis for changes. Virology 1993; 197:1–11.
62. Marin M, Noël D, Valsesia-Wittman S, Brockly F, Etienne-Julan M, et al. Targeted infection of human cells via major histocompatibility complex class I molecules by Moloney murine leukemia virus-derived viruses displaying single-chain antibody fragment-envelope fusion proteins. J Virol 1996; 70:2957–2962.
63. Kim JW, Closs EI, Albritton LM, Cunningham JM. Transport of cationic amino acids by the mouse ecotropic retrovirus receptor. Nature 1991; 352:725–730.
64. McClure MO, Sommerfelt MA, Marsh M, Weiss RA. The pH independence of mammalian retrovirus infection. J Gen Virol 1990; 71:767–773.
65. Nussbaum O, Roop A, Anderson WF. Sequences determining the pH dependence of viral entry are distinct from the host range-determining region of the murine ecotropic and amphotropic retrovirus envelope proteins. J Virol 1993; 67:7402–7405.
66. Ragheb JA, Yu H, Hofmann T, Anderson WF. The amphotropic and ecotropic murine leukemia virus envelope TM subunits are equivalent mediators of direct membrane fusion: Implica-

tions for the role of the ecotropic envelope and receptor in syncytium formation and viral entry. J Virol 1995; 69:7205–7215.

67. Han X, Kasahara N, Kan YW. Ligand-directed retroviral targeting of human breast cancer cells. Proc Natl Acad Sci USA 1995; 92:9747–9751.

68. Oxley SM, Sackstein R. Detection of an L-selectin ligand on a hematopoietic progenitor cell line. Blood 1994; 84:3299–3306.

69. Krause DS, Fackler MJ, Civin CI, May WS. Review: CD34: structure, biology, and clinical utility. Blood 1996; 87:1–13.

70. Benedict CA, MacKrell AJ, Anderson WF. Determination of the binding affinity of an anti-CD34 single-chain antibody using a novel, flow cytometry based assay. J Immunol Methods 1997; 201:223–231.

71. Fielding AK, Maurice M, Morling FJ, Cosset FL, Russell SJ. Inverse targeting of retroviral vectors: selective gene transfer in a mixed population of hematopoietic and nonhematopoietic cells. Blood 1998; 91:1802–1809.

72. Nilson BHK, Morling FJ, Cosset FL, Russell SJ. Targeting of retroviral vectors through protease-substrate interactions. Gene Ther 1996; 3:280–286.

73. Pasqualini R, Ruoslahti E. Organ targeting in vivo using phage display peptide libraries. Nature 1996; 380:364–366.

74. Barry MA, Dower WJ, Johnston SA. Toward cell-targeting gene therapy vectors: selection of cell-binding peptides from random peptide-presenting phage libraries. Nature Med 1996; 2:299–305.

75. Fina L, Molgaard HV, Robertson D, Bradley NJ, Monaghan P, Delia D, Sutherland DR, Baker MA, Greaves MF. Expression of the CD34 gene in vascular endothelial cells. Blood 1990; 75:2417–2426.

76. Delia D, Lampugnani MG, Resnati M, Dejana E, Aiello A, Fontanella E, Soligo D, Pierotti MA, Greaves MF. CD34 expression is regulated reciprocally with adhesion molecules in vascular endothelial cells in vitro. Blood 1993; 31:1001–1008.

77. Valsesia-Wittmann S, Drynda A, Deleage G, Aumailley M, Heard J-M, Danos O, Verdier G, Cosset F-L. Modifications in the binding domain of avian retrovirus envelope protein to redirect the host range of retroviral vectors. J Virol 1994; 68:4609–4619.

78. Lamaze C, Schmid SL. The emergence of clathrin-independent pinocytic pathways. Curr Opin Cell Biol 1995; 7:573–580.

Index

Page numbers in italics indicate figures. Page numbers followed by "t" indicate tables.

AAV. *See* Adenoassociated virus
Accessory cells in engraftment, 93–94
Acquired immunodeficiency syndrome, 538, 545, 553
Activin, principal bioactivity, 51
Acute lymphoblastic leukemia, CD34 cells, 243
ADA. *See* Adenosine deaminase
Adenoassociated vectors, 557–558
Adenoassociated virus, 545
Adenosine deaminase, 307
Adenosine deaminase deficiency, 88, 101, 307
Adhesion receptor function, effect of cytokines on, 130, *130*
Adhesion receptors, cell signaling by, 125–136
Adrenoleukodystrophy, 538
Adriamycin, chemotherapy with, 15
AIDS. *See* Acquired immunodeficiency syndrome
Allelic differences, affecting stem cell pool, 115–116
Allogeneic graft engineering, long-term survival, 251–274
Allogeneic transplantation, 403–412

Allografting, low-intensity conditioning regimen for, autografting following by, 569–574
Alopecia, with stem cell transplantation, 423
Alpha-actinin, integrins, 129
Alpha-L-iduronidase-deficient dogs, retrovirus-mediated gene transfer, 184–185
Alpha-thalassemia, 197
Anaplastic large cell, 467
Anastomosis, vascular, 171
Anhidrosis, with stem cell transplantation, 423
Anovulation, 419
Anti-HIV RNA decoys, transdominant mutant proteins and, 559
Antihymocyte serum, 173
Apheresis collection regimens, 334–343
Apheresis collections, timing of, 340–342
Aplastic anemia, 88, 101, 425
Appetite, loss, stem cell transplantation, 424
Arthralgias, stem cell transplantation, 423
Autoimmune disorders, 413
Autoimmune thyroiditis, 100

Autoimmunity, 88, 100
Autologous stem cell transplantation, minimal residual disease, 280
Avascular necrosis, 425

B cell, 467
B lymphocytes, flt3 ligand, 26
B-malignant cells from autografts, immunomagnetic purging of, 293–296, *295*
Bacterial overgrowth, in gut, 424
Bare lymphocyte syndrome, 197
Basophils, 141
Baxter Isolex 300SA Magnetic Cell Separator System, 470
Beta-globin deficiency, 307
Beta-thalassemia, 307
Beta-thalassemia major, 197
Beta-thalassemic mouse model, 200–201
BFU-E. *See* Burst-forming unit-erythroid
Bile displacement therapy, 423
Biology, thrombopoietin, 1–22
Blood cell lineages, hematopoietic stem cell commitment to, 1
Blood progenitor cells, mobilization into peripheral blood, 13–14
Blood stem cell. *See* Hematopoietic stem cell
BMT. *See* Bone marrow transplantation
Bone disease, 414
  with, 425
Bone marrow, flt3, 26
Bone marrow chimerism, 100–101
  diseases potentially treatable with, 88
Bone marrow transplantation, 254
Bone marrow transplantation, *vs.* blood stem cell, 447–456
Brain
  flt3, 26
  flt3 ligand, 26
Breast cancer, 280
  filgrastim, stem cell factor and, 37
  high-dose therapy for, 517–536
  MRD, 285–286
  purging cells from autografts, 296
Bronchiolitis obliterans, stem cell transplantation, 423
Burkitt tumor, 467
Burnet, Macfarlane, contribution of, 171
Burst-forming unit-erythroid, CD34⁺ cells, 324
Busulfan, 173, 419

c-*mpl*, in stem cell biology, 6
c-*mpl* genes, *tpo*, elimination in mice, 5
C57BL/6Sz-scid/scid, 201
Canine models, transplantation, gene therapy, 171–194
Carbonplatin, megakaryocyte growth and development factor, cyclophosphamide, 14
Carrel, Alexis, contribution of, 171
Cataract formation, 417, *418*
Cataracts, 414
CD8⁺ subset depletion, 440–441
CD18 deficiency, 307
CD34⁺ cell, 130, 141, 142–144, *143*
  allografts with, 245–247
  augmentation, 256–262
  culture, 303–320
  culture conditions, 326–330, *327, 328, 329*
  engraftment with, 242–245
  enrichment, isolex300, 297
  expansion, differentiation, 321–332
  intramedullar injection, 245
  from leukapheresis products, 296–297
  levels, stem cell factor, 38
  pediatric experience, 239–250
  posthaw viability, 236
  selection, immunomagnetic beads, 223
  surface marker, stem cell factor, 40
CD38⁻ cell, 141, 142–144, *143*
Cell motion, division, visualization of, 73–74
Cell signaling, by adhesion receptors, 125–136
Chediak-Higashi disease, 197, 538
Chemotherapy, 173
  with doxorubicin, ifosfamide, 15
  MPL ligand after, 14–15
  MRD response to, 280
Child, low birth weight, 419
Chills, 394
Chronic graft-*versus*-host disease, 414
Chronic granulomatous disease, 88, 101, 307, 538
Chronic myelogenous leukemia, 131–132, 254
Circulatory distress, 394
Clone size, 113
Cloning, of thrombopoietin, 2–4, *3*
CML. *See* Chronic myelogenous leukemia
Collection, autologous peripheral blood stem cell, engraftment, 457–478

Combined immune deficiency, 307
Conjunctivitis, stem cell transplantation, 423
Cord blood transplantation, 365
Costimulatory signal blockade, 440
Cyclophosphamide, 173
  megakaryocyte growth and development factor, 14
Cyclosporine A
  duration of engraftment, 258–259, *260*
  duration of early posttransplant morbidity, 261–262
  duration of GVHD, 259–261, *261*
Cytokine antagonists, 436–437
Cytokines
  development of megakaryocytic lineage, 2
  manipulation of, 436–439
  to megakaryocyte formation, serum-free murine marrow culture system, 4
  postnatal injection with, 209
Cytomegalovirus infection, 421
Cytoreductive therapies, hematological recovery following, 7

Delayed add back, donor cells, 437–439
Delivery, preterm, 419
Dendritic cells, 304
  from CD34 cells, 313–314
  flt3 ligand, effects on, 27
Dental caries, with stem cell transplantation, 423
Dermal manifestations, with stem cell transplantation, 423
Desquamative esophagitis, stem cell transplantation, 424
Diabetes mellitus, type I, 88
Differentiation, hematopoietic stem cells, 74–75
Diffuse large cell, 467
Diphtheria, immunization, 420
Dog, transplantation, gene therapy, 171–194
Donor eligibility, 334
Donor leukocyte infusion, after transplant, 246–247
Donor lymphocyte infusion, to induce graft-*versus*-malignancy, 367–369, 368t
Doxorubicin, chemotherapy, ifosfamide, 15
Dyspigmentation, with stem cell transplantation, 423
Dyspnea, 394

Elutriation, for primary graft modification, 253–256
Emotional distress, stem cell transplantation, 427
Endocrine abnormalities, 417–419
Endocrine conditions, 414
Engraftment
  autologous peripheral blood stem cell, 457–478
  failure of, 91
  requirements for, 91–93
Enzyme deficiencies, 88, 101
Eosinophils, 141
Epithelial cell, derived tumor cells, 141
Epo, principal bioactivity, 51
Epstein-Barr virus-associated, lymphoproliferative disorders, 427
Epstein-Barr virus (EBV), 546
Erythema, with stem cell transplantation, 423
Erythrocyte-lysing procedures, 138
Erythrocytes, 141
Erythroid, burst-forming unit, CD34$^+$ cells, 324
Erythropoiesis, 6
Esophageal complications, stem cell transplantation, 424
Estrogen levels, 419
Expansion, defined, 111
Expression of flt3 ligand transcripts and protein, widespread nature of, 25
Extrinsic regulation, stem cell maintenance, 117–121
Extrinsic stem cell support, mechanisms of, 119–120
Eyes, stem cell transplantation affecting, 421, 423

F-actin, integrins, 129
F-CSF, mobilization by, 240–241, *241*
Facilitating cells, color flow cytometric analysis for, 95
Fanconi's anemia, 88, 307, 538
  complementation group C MDR1, methyl transferase, 307
Fasciitis, stem cell transplantation, 423
Fertility, 419
Fetal liver, flt3, 26
Fetal liver cells, 155–159, *156, 157,* 157t, *158, 159*
Fibronectin, 126–127, *127*
  progenitors, integrin-mediated interactions, 127–129, *128*

Filgrastim, stem cell factor and, effect on tumor, 37
Flow cytometry, 137–152
    MRD, 276, 277–278
flt3
    cloning of, 24–25, 26t
    with granulocyte colony-stimulating factor, 27
    with granulocyte-macrophage colony-stimulating factor, 27
flt3 ligand, 23–30
    biological effects of, 25–27
    clinical utility of, 27
    effects on dendritic cells, 27
    expression of, 26
    fibroblasts, 26
    principal bioactivity, 50
Fludarabine, 569–573
Follicular center, 467
Fractures, 425

G-CSF. See Granulocyte colony-stimulating factor
G-CSF-mobilized peripheral blood progenitors, 322
Gastroesophageal reflux, stem cell transplantation, 424
Gastrointestinal manifestations, with stem cell transplantation, 424
Gastrointestinal tract, stem cell transplantation affecting, 421, 423
Gaucher's disease, 88, 101, 307, 538
Gene therapy, hematopoietic stem cells, 537–552
Germ cell tumor, CD34 cells, 243
Glucocerebrosidase deficiency, 307
Glycogenosis, 88
GM-CSF. See Granulocyte-macrophage colony-stimulating factor
    neutrophils, monocytes, effects of, 8
GM-stem cell factor, principal bioactivity, 51
Gonadal conditions, 414
Gonadal dysfunction, 419
Gonadotropins, menopausal symptoms, 419
Graft engineering, 361–382
Graft versus acute myeloid leukemia, 403–406, 404t
Graft-versus-host disease, 89–91, 176–178, 177, 254, 368
    acute, 395
    chronic, 396, 396t, 422–425
    lymphocyte add back, 435–446

Graft-versus-host reactivity, 389, 390, 391
Graft-versus-leukemia, graft-versus-host disease, distinguished, 368
Graft-versus-leukemia effect, 365, 389–391
Graft-versus-malignancy, effector cells of, 367
Graft-versus-malignancy, target antigens of, 366–367
Granulocyte colony-stimulating factor, 60
    effects on neutrophils, monocytes, 8
    and flt3, 27
    principal bioactivity, 51
Granulocyte-macrophage colony-stimulating factor, 60
    and flt3, 27
Granulomatous disease, chronic, 88, 101, 538
Graves' disease, 418
Growth abnormalities, 417–419
Growth and development, 414
Growth hormone deficiency, 418, 419
GVHD. See Graft-versus-host disease
Gynecological care, 419

H-ferritin, 59
    principal bioactivity, 51
Haemophilus influenzae conjugate, immunization, 420
Hair loss, with stem cell transplantation, 423
Headache, 394
Heart, flt3 ligand, 26
Hematological recovery
    following cytoreductive therapies, 7
    thrombopoietin, following marrow, stem cell transplantation, 8
Hematopoiesis
    defined, 125
    role of adhesive interactions in, 126–130
Hematopoietic assays, megakaryocytic cytokine characterization, 4
Hematopoietic blood stem cell. See also Blood stem cell
Hematopoietic chimeras, 153–170
Hematopoietic reconstitution, after PBSCT, 469–471, 470
Hematopoietic stem cell, identification of, 47–49, 48t
Hematopoietic stem cell candidates, characteristics of, 72–73
Hematopoietic stem cell commitment
    to blood cell lineages, 1
    stochastic nature of, to blood cell lineages, 1

Hematopoietic stem cell phenotype
  biological activity, 52–53
  CD34⁺ cells, 54
  cobblestone area-forming cell assay, 48
  colony-forming unit-spleen assay, 48
  cytokine modulation, 47–68
  cytokines
    biology of, 49–53, 50–51t
    predominant action, 50
  effects of cytokines, 50–51t, 53–60, 54t,
    55t, 56t
  flt3 ligand, 54–57
  inhibitors, 59–60
  long-term culture-initiating cell assay, 48
  production, 49–52
  proliferation, 49
  receptors, 52
  stem cell factor, 57–58
  Tpo, 58–59
Hemoglobinopathies, 538
Hemolytic anemias, 538
Heparan sulfate, 126–127, *127*
Hepatic manifestations, with stem cell trans-
    plantation, 423
Hepatitis B, immunization, 420
Hereditary immunodeficiency syndromes,
    101
Hereditary immunodeficiency syndromes se-
    vere combined immunodeficiency, 88
Histiocytosis, 88
Histocompatibility antigen, 245, 254
HIV, 545
  gene therapy, 553–568
  gene therapy against, target cells for, 556
  genome, 554
  life cycle of, *554*, 554–556
HIV-1 infection, 538
HIV competitors, ribozyme, and inhibitors
    (TAT decoy genes, antisense), 307
HLA. *See* Histocompatibility antigen
HLA-mismatched related pairs, transplants
    in, 245–246, 246t
Hodgkin's disease, 298, 571
  stem cell transplantation for, 479–498
Homing, hematopoietic stem cells, 69–86
Hormones, development of megakaryocytic
    lineage, 2
Hot flushes, 394
Human immunodeficiency virus. *See* HIV
Hunter's disease, 88, 307
Hurler's disease, 88, 101, 307
Hyperthermia, 394
Hypocalcemia, 394

Hypothyroidism, 417, 418
Hysteria, during apheresis procedure, 394

Identification, hematopoietic stem cell candi-
    dates, 70–72
Iduronato-s-sulfatase, 307
Ifosfamide, chemotherapy, 15
IL-1, principal bioactivity, 50
IL-2, principal bioactivity, 50
IL-3
  cultures containing, megakaryocyte forma-
    tion, 5
  granulocyte-macrophage-colony-
    stimulating factor, 130
  principal bioactivity, 50
IL-4, principal bioactivity, 50
IL-5, principal bioactivity, 50
IL-6, principal bioactivity, 50
IL-7, principal bioactivity, 50
IL-8, principal bioactivity, 50
IL-9, principal bioactivity, 50
IL-10, principal bioactivity, 50
IL-11, principal bioactivity, 50
IL-12, principal bioactivity, 50
IL-13, principal bioactivity, 50
IL-14, principal bioactivity, 51
IL-15, principal bioactivity, 51
IL-16, principal bioactivity, 51
IL-17, principal bioactivity, 51
IL-18, principal bioactivity, 51
Immunizations, after hematopoietic trans-
    plantation, 420
Immunodeficiency, 414, 419–420, 420t
Immunomagnetic beads
  CD34 selection, 223
  tumor cell contamination, stem cell isola-
    tion, 291–302
Immunospecific ferrofluid-coated cells, mag-
    netic properties, 146
Increased metabolic needs, stem cell trans-
    plantation, 424
Infection, 414
Inflammatory bowel disease, 88
Influenza, immunization, 420
Inhibin, principal bioactivity, 51
Integrin-mediated interactions, progenitors,
    fibronectin, 127–129, *128*
Interferon, alpha-beta, principal bioactivity,
    51
Interleukin. *See* IL
Intestine, flt3 ligand, 26
Intramedullar injection, CD34⁺ cells,
    245

In utero transplantation
  human, 197
  technique, *205, 206, 206*
Irradiation, total body, 172–173
Isolex300, allogeneic cell purification data,
  246
Isolex300, CD34$^+$ cell enrichment, 297

Kaposi's sarcoma, 553
Karnofsky Performance Scale, 416
Keratoconjunctivitis sicca, with stem cell
  transplantation, 423
Kidney, flt3 ligand, 26
Kidneys, transplantation of, experimental,
  171
Kinetics, initial mitosis of candidate hemato-
  poietic stem cells, *76, 76–79, 79*
Krabbe's disease, 88

Lansky Play-Performance Scale, 416
Large-volume leukapheresis, 342
Lentiviral vectors, 558
Lentiviruses, 545
Leukemia inhibitory factor, principal bioactiv-
  ity, 51
Leukocyte adherence deficiency, 307
Leukocyte adhesion defect, 538
Leukocyte defects, 538
Leukodystrophy, 88, 101
Leukoencephalopathy, 417
Lichen planus, with stem cell transplantation,
  423
LIF. *See* Leukemia inhibitory factor
Lifesaving procedure for variety of malig-
  nant and hereditary diseases, over-
  view, 69
Limbs, transplantation of, kidneys, experi-
  mental, 171
Liver, flt3 ligand, 26
Liver cells, fetal, 155–159, *156, 157,* 157t,
  158, 159
Liver function abnormalities, with stem cell
  transplantation, 423
Long-term survival, allogeneic graft engi-
  neering, 251–274
Loss of appetite, stem cell transplantation,
  424
Low birth weight children, 419
Lung, flt3 ligand, 26
Lungs, stem cell transplantation affecting,
  421, 423

Lymphoblastic leukemia, acute, CD34 cells,
  243
Lymphocyte add back, graft-*versus*-host dis-
  ease, 435–446
Lymphocyte infusion, post-bone marrow
  transplantation, 365
Lymphocyte-modified grafts, 253–256, *254,*
  254t, *255*
Lymphocytes, 141
  flt3 ligand, 26
Lymphoid development, flt3 ligand, 26
Lymphoma, filgrastim, stem cell factor and, 37
Lymphoproliferative disorders, Epstein-Barr
  virus-associated, 427
Lysosomal storage diseases, 88, 101, 538

Macrophage inflammatory protein-1 alpha,
  59
Maintenance, defined, 111
Malabsorption, stem cell transplantation, 424
Mantle cell, 467
Marrow progenitors, generation of platelets
  from, overview, 1
Mature platelet function, thrombopoietin and,
  8–9
  principal bioactivity, 51
Measles, immunization, 420
Medawar, Peter, contribution of, 171
Megakaryocyte development, physiology of,
  1–2
Megakaryocyte formation
  cultures containing IL-3, 5
  serum-free murine marrow culture system,
    4
  thrombopoietin and, 4–5
Megakaryocyte growth, development factor,
  9
  dose-response platelet effects of, 10
Megakaryocyte growth and development
  factor
  chemotherapy, with carbonplatin, cyclo-
    phosphamide, 14
  lineage specific, effect on blood, 10
  new platelet production, in patients receiv-
    ing, 11
  platelets generated in response to, 12
Megakaryocyte progenitors, 304
Megakaryocytic cytokine characterization, hematopoietic assays, 4
Megakaryocytic lineage, development of, 2
Megakaryopoietic activities, thrombopoietin,
  4

Menopausal symptoms, gonadotropins, 419

MGDF. *See* Megakaryocyte growth and development factor

Mineral density, in bone, decrease, 425

Minimal residual disease, 275–290, 292–293, *293*
   autologous stem cell transplantation, 280

MIP-1alpha. *See* Macrophage inflammatory protein-1 alpha

MK. *See* Megakaryocyte

MoMuLV-based vectors, with alternative envelopes, 544–545

Monoclonal antibodies, 173

Monocytes, 141
   flt3 ligand, 26
   GM-CSF, G-CSF, effects of, 8

Mouth, stem cell transplantation affecting, 421, 423

Mpl ligand
   clinical studies with, 9
   truncated pegylated, 9

MPS VII gene therapy murine model, 202–203

MRD. *See* Minimal residual disease
   in ASCT grafts, 282t, 282–284
   in stem cell-mobilization procedures, 281, 281t
   tumor purging, 284t, 284–285

Mucopolysaccharide deficiency, 307

Mucopolysaccharidoses, 538

Mucopolysaccharidosis murine model, in utero transplantation, 202–203

Multidrug resistance, in stem cell transplantation, 307

Multiple myeloma, stem cell transplantation for, 499–516

Multiple sclerosis, 88

Mumps-rubella, immunization, 420

Murine leukemia virus, 576

Murine model, in utero transplantation, 195–222

Murine retroviral vectors, 557

Muscle cramping, stem cell transplantation, 423

Muscles, stem cell transplantation affecting, 421, 423

Muscularskeletal pain, 394

Myelodysplastic syndrome, 88

Myelogenous leukemia, chronic, 131–132, 254

Myeloid leukemia, allogeneic transplantation, 403–412

Myeloma cancer, filgrastim, stem cell factor and, 37

Myesthenia gravis, 424

N-acetyl-Ser-Asp-Lys-Pro, principal bioactivity, 51

NADH oxidase deficiency, 307

Natural killer cells, flt3 ligand, 26

Neomycin phosphotransferase, 307

Neuroblastoma, 280, 307
   CD34 cells, 243
   MRD, 286

Neurological complications, 417

Neurological conditions, 414

Neutrophil progenitors, 304
   derived from CD34$^+$ cells, 309–312, *311*

Neutrophils, 141
   flt3 ligand, 26
   GM-CSF, G-CSF, effects of, 8

NK cells. *See* Natural killer cells

NOD/SCID, 201

Non-Hodgkin's disease, 298

Non-Hodgkin's lymphoma, CD34 cells, 243

Nondefective mice model, in utero transplantation, 203–215

Nonmalignant hematological disorders, 88, 100–101

Nonmyeloablative preparation regimens, 361–382

Nucleated erythrocytes, 141

Obstetrical care, 419

Obstetrical complications, 419

Obstructive lung defects, stem cell transplantation, 423

Ocular manifestations, stem cell transplantation, 423

Oral manifestations, with stem cell transplantation, 423

Oral sicca syndrome, with stem cell transplantation, 423

Osteoporosis, 425

Otitis media, 421

Ovarian cancer, filgrastim, stem cell factor and, 37

Ovary, flt3 ligand, 26

PBPC. *See* Peripheral blood progenitor cell

PBSC. *See* Peripheral blood stem cell

PBSCs, *vs.* factors influencing choice of allogeneic marrow, 349–350

Pediatric experience, CD34$^+$ cells, 239–250

Peptide Glu-Glu-Asp-Asp-Lys, principal bio-
    activity, 51
Periorbital exanthema, 394
Peripheral blood cells, 141
Peripheral blood progenitor cell, stem cell
    factor, after chemoradiotherapy, 35
Peripheral blood progenitor cells, composi-
    tion of collection products, 384–386,
    385t
Peripheral blood stem cell transplantation,
    392–397
    for allogeneic transplantation, 383–402
    for autologous transplantation, 457–478
    from normal donors, 333–360
Peripheral neuroectodermal tumor, CD34
    cells, 243
Peripheral neuropathy, 424
Pertussis-tetanus, immunization, 420
PF4, principal bioactivity, 51
Philadelphia chromosome, 131
Phosphotransferase, neomycin, 307
Photophobia, stem cell transplantation,
    423
PKH26 fluorescence, functional integrity of
    quiescent cells with, 79
Plasma glycocalicin levels, monitoring of,
    11
Platelet factor 4, 59
Platelet production, turnover, function,
    assays of, 11–13, 12
Platelet surface markers, variety expression,
    11
Platelets, 141
    generation of, from marrow progenitors,
        overview, 1
Pluripotent hematopoietic stem cell, 131
Pluripotent hematopoietic stem cells, re-
    quirements for engraftment of, 92–
    93
Poikiloderma, with stem cell transplantation,
    423
Poliovirus
    sabin, 420
    Salk, immunization, 420
Polymerase chain reaction, MRD, 276
Posthaw viability, CD34⁺ cells, 236
Preterm delivery, 419
Primitiveness, defined, 111
Progenitor growth, regulation of, 127–
    129
Progenitors, integrin-mediated interactions,
    fibronectin, 127–129, 128
Proliferation, defined, 111

Prostaglandin E1 and E2, principal bioactiv-
    ity, 51
Psoriasis, 88, 100
Psychosocial aspects, stem cell transplanta-
    tion, 427
Pulmonary infection, 421
    after discharge, 421
Pulmonary manifestations, with stem cell
    transplantation, 423
Purified adult human hematopoietic stem
    cells, 162–163

Radiotherapy, poor mobilization, 39
Recurrent leukemia, 426, 427
Regimen-related toxicities, 414, 417–419
Relapse of malignancy, 414
Requirements for hematopoietic stem cell
    engraftment, 87–110
Resistance, multidrug, in stem cell trans-
    plantation, 307
Reticulocytes, 141
Retinoblastoma, CD34 cells, 243
Retroviral vectors, targeting hematopoietic
    stem cells, 575–594
Retrovirus-mediated gene transfer, alpha-
    L-iduronidase-deficient dogs, 184–
    185
Retrovirus-mediated transduction
    canine marrow-derived stem cells, 181–
        183, 182
    peripheral blood-derived stem cells, 183–
        184
Rhabdomyosarcoma, CD34 cells, 243
Rheumatoid arthritis, 88, 100
    stem cell transplantation, 423
Ribozyme, HIV competitors, 307
Ribozymes, 559–562, 560, 561
Rubella, immunization, 420

Sabin poliovirus, 420
Salk poliovirus, immunization, 420
SCID, 197. See Severe combined immune de-
    ficiency
SCID mouse model, 201
Scleroderma, 88
Sclerosis, with stem cell transplantation, 423
Secondary malignancies, 180, 414, 425
Secondary sexual characteristics, develop-
    ment of, 419
Self-renewal, 112
    hematopoietic stem cells, 69–86
Serous surfaces, stem cell transplantation af-
    fecting, 421, 423

Serum-free murine marrow culture system, megakaryocyte formation, 4
Severe combined immunodeficiency disease, 196
Severe combined immunodeficient syndrome, 101
Sheep hematopoietic chimeras, 153–170
Sickle cell anemia, 88, 100–101, 307, 413, 538
Sinopulmonary infection, stem cell transplantation, 423
Sinuses, stem cell transplantation affecting, 421, 423
Sjogren's syndrome, 423
Skeletal muscle, flt3 ligand, 26
Skin, chronic GVHD affecting, 421, 423
Skin ulcers, with stem cell transplantation, 423
Spingolipidosis, 88
Spleen
    flt3, 26
    flt3 ligand, 26
Stem cell, functional properties of, 112–114
Stem cell factor, 31–46, 37t, 38, 130
    applications, related to CD34+, 42–43
    biology, 32–33
    blood CD34+ cell levels, 38
    CD34+ cell surface marker, 40
    engraftment, 40–42
    filgrastim, 36–40, 37t, 38
        hematopoietic reconstitution, 34
        on peripheral blood leukocytes, 36
    on hematopoiesis, 33
    mobilizing effects, plus filgrastim, 33–35
    mutations, 31
    peripheral blood progenitor cell, after chemoradiotherapy, 35
    phenotypic abnormalities, 32
    plus filgrastim
        mobilizing effects, 40
        in peripheral blood progenitor cell mobilization, 37
    preclinical studies, 33–35
    principal bioactivity, 50
    prior chemotherapy, 39
    studies, in humans, 36
    synergistic activity of, with filgrastim, 34
    systemic allergic-like reactions, 42
Stem cell transplantation, thrombopoietin in, 8
Stochastic nature, hematopoietic stem cell commitment, to blood cell lineages, 1
Stromal cells, 117–119
    flt3 ligand, 26

Symmetry, initial mitosis of candidate hematopoietic stem cells, 76, 76–79, 79
Syngeneic transplants, increased risk of relapse after, 365
Synovial effusions, stem cell transplantation, 423
Systemic lupus erythematosus, 88

T-cell, 467
T-cell clones, malignant cells, 365
T-cell-depleted bone marrow, graft rejection in patients receiving, 91–92
T-cell-depleted transplants, 364t, 364–365
    increased risk of relapse after, 365
T-cell depletion, 254, 391–392, 396–397, 397t
T-cell, manipulating, 439–440
T-malignant cells from autografts, immunomagnetic purging of, 293–296, 295
Talin, vinculin, and F-actin in focal contacts, integrins, 129
Tandem transplants, CD34-selected cells, 243–245, 245t
TAT decoy genes, 307
TCD. See T-cell depletion
Tendonitis, stem cell transplantation, 421, 423
Testis, flt3 ligand, 26
Tetanus, immunization, 420
Th2-type donor cells, 437
Thalassemia, 88, 100–101, 538
    and autoimmune disorders, 413
Thoracic pain, 394
Thrombocytopenia, 394
Thrombopoietin, 6–7, 7
    biology, 1–22
    clinical effects, 1–22
    cloning, 2–4, 3
    defined, 2
    effect on hematological recovery, following marrow, stem cell transplantation, 8
    hematological recovery following cytoreductive therapies, 7
    lineage specificity, 6
    mature platelet function, 8–9
    megakaryopoietic activities, 4
    other hematopoietic lineages, 7–8
    purification of, to homogeneity, 2
    in stem cell transplantation, 8
Thrombospondin, and fibronectin, 126–127, 127
Thymidine kinase suicide gene, 440

Thymus
    flt3, 26
    flt3 ligand, 26
Thyroid deficiency, 417–418
Thyroid gland, irradiation of, 417
Thyroid neoplasms, 417
Thyroiditis, 417
    autoimmune, 100
TNF, principal bioactivity, 51
Tolerance, transplantation, bone marrow chimerism and, 97–100, *99*
Total body irradiation, 172–173
Toxicities, regimen-related, 417–419
Tpo, principal bioactivity, 50
Tpo, c-mpl genes, elimination in mice, 5
Transcription factors, intrinsic regulation of stem cell behavior by, 116–117
Turnover, and function, platelet, assays of, 11–13, *12*
Tyrosine kinase family, role in hematopoietic system, 23
Tyrosine kinase receptor, flt3, 23–24

Ulcerative colitis, 100
Ursodeoxycholic acid, bile displacement therapy, 423
Uveitis, stem cell transplantation, 423

Vagina, stem cell transplantation affecting, 421, 423

Vaginal stenosis, with stem cell transplantation, 424
Varicella-zoster infection, 421
Vascular anastomosis, 171
Vinculin, and F-actin in focal contacts, integrins, 129
Violaceous papules, with stem cell transplantation, 423
Viral resistance or inactivation genes, 307

W^{41} mouse model, 200
Walter and Eliza Hall Institute of Medical Research, Melbourne, 5
Web formation, gastroesophageal reflux, stem cell transplantation, 424
Weight loss, stem cell transplantation, 424
Wilms' tumor, CD34 cells, 243
Wiskott-Aldrich syndrome, 88, 101, 538
W^{v} mouse model, 199

X-linked agammaglobulinemia, 538
X-linked SCID, 197
Xenogeneic mouse model, 201–202
Xenograft model, human, sheep, 155
Xerophthalmia, 423
Xerostomia, with stem cell transplantation, 423

Printed and bound by CPI Group (UK) Ltd, Croydon, CR0 4YY

23/10/2024

01778259-0006